The DIETETIC TECHNICIAN

Effective Nutrition Counseling
Second Edition

VIRGINIA ARONSON R.D., M.S.

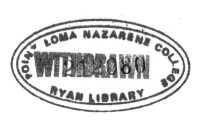

VNR VAN NOSTRAND REINHOLD
New York

Printed in the United States of America

Van Nostrand Reinhold
115 Fifth Avenue
New York, New York 10003

Chapman & Hall
2-6 Boundary Row
London SE1 8HN, England

Thomas Nelson Australia
102 Dodds Street
South Melbourne, Victoria 3205, Australia

Nelson Canada
1120 Birchmount Road
Scarborough, Ontario M1K 5G4, Canada

16 15 14 13 12 11 10 9 8 7 6 5 4 3 2 1

Library of Congress Cataloging-in-Publication Data

Aronson, Virginia.
    The dietetic technician : effective nutrition counseling /
Virginia Aronson. — 2nd ed.
        p.   cm.
    Bibliography: p.
    Includes index.
    ISBN 0-442-23343-4
    1. Diet therapy. 2. Nutrition. I. Title.
    [DNLM: 1. Allied Health Personnel. 2. Counseling. 3. Diet
Therapy. 4. Nutrition. WB 400 A763d]
RM216.A757 1989
615.8′54—dc19   88-36819
                                                              CIP

To my sister,
for skillfully typing the first edition of this text and for lending
support during the second edition

Contents

Contents continued

Contents continued

Preface

According to The American Dietetic Association (ADA), one of the primary goals of the programs that train dietetic technicians in the delivery of nutrition care is the development of competent dietetic personnel. Upon completion of the associate degree program, the dietetic technician is expected to be able to perform effectively in today's health care delivery system. Working directly under the supervision of a registered dietitian, today's practicing dietetic technician is responsible for assisting in the provision of effective nutrition care programs.

The curriculum for every dietetic technician program is based on the ADA's specific philosophies, goals, and behavioral objectives, as outlined by the program director. A combination of didactic lessonry and supervised field experience provides students with the various proficiencies required for the achievement of essential competencies. Throughout the program, students are guided in the development of the strong communication and teaching skills required for the provision of effectual nutrition care.

The first year's curriculum offers students an introduction to nutrition, nutrition care, and the health care field. Students begin to understand how they will be able to utilize their nutrition knowledge in individualized health care situations, and they learn what their roles will be as future members of the health care team. It is essential for students to examine who they are, how and why they eat what they do, and exactly what it is they are eating, so that they can transform self-understanding into effective counseling techniques. Basic nutrition (fact versus fallacy) and nutrition during the life cycle are taught, so that students can provide individualized diet counseling for healthy people of all ages. Role-play activities, as well as the opportunity for hands-on experience, are essential educational tools for the development of competent counseling skills.

The second year's curriculum focuses on nutrition care and diet therapy in disease. Emphasis is on patient care, individualized diet planning, and nutrition education, so that counseling can elicit the desired diet and behavioral changes for improved health. With supervised field experiences, students are able to apply the nutrition theory they receive in the classroom to the various individual situations they encounter in the health care setting. They can also polish and tone their skills as functioning members of the health care team.

The Dietetic Technician supplies both the background nutrition information and the counseling strategies needed by dietetic technician students throughout their educational program. The book can also be utilized by practicing dietetic technicians in a variety of nutrition care settings because it supplies much of the hands-on materials required for the provision of effective nutrition care programs. The information and activities supplied by this comprehensive text will assist today's dietetic technicians—students, educators, and practitioners—in this new and essential field of dietetics.

Acknowledgments: The author owes special thanks to those individuals who reviewed and criticized the manuscript prior to publication: Ruth Horgan, R.D., M.Ed.; Joyce Neely, R.D., M.S.; Joyce Nettleton, Sc.D., R.D.; and Mary Shea, R.D., M.S.

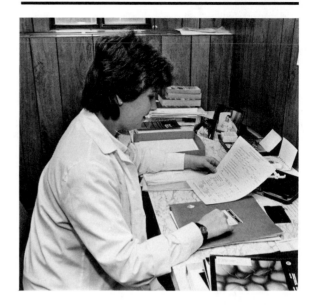

Who Are You?

As a first year student in an **ADA**-approved **dietetic technician** program, you are beginning an educational journey to specific career skills. Your chosen field is currently in great demand. As a relatively new avenue for allied health practitioners, the important role of the dietetic technician is being recognized by other members of the **health care team.** In fact, by the time you graduate from this program, a variety of satisfying and challenging employment opportunities should await you.

As a trained dietetic technician, it is important that you be able to satisfy the expectations of your employers, fellow health team members, and peers. As a dietetic technician in nutrition care, your ability to function successfully in the clinical setting is imperative. Thus, a workable knowledge of **nutrition** and **diet therapy** is essential, and the self-confidence which accompanies a well-practiced skill is crucial. A brief look at Fig. 0.1 can help you to see why *The Dietetic Technician* combines the nutrition theory with the use of practical skills.

ADA: The American Dietetic Association (founded in 1917), a national governing organization for the field of dietetics. All members are nutrition professionals.

dietetic technician: A technically skilled individual who has successfully completed an ADA-approved associate degree program with an emphasis either in Food Service Management or Nutrition Care. The "diet tech" assists dietitians and/or foodservice directors in the foodservice or clinical care setting.

health care team: A group of health care professionals—including physicians, nurses, pharmacists, nutritionists, social workers, occupational therapists, and physical therapists—who work together to provide coordinated services in order to enhance the health status of patients with various ailments.

nutrition: The science of food, the nutrients and other substances therein, their action, interaction, and balance in relation to health and disease, and the processes by which the organism ingests, absorbs, transports, utilizes, and excretes food substances. In addition, nutrition must be concerned with social, economic, cultural, and psychologic implications of food and eating (definition of the Council on Foods and Nutrition, American Medical Association).

diet therapy: The treatment of certain ailments using specific dietary modifications as prescribed by physicians and dietitians responsible for patient care. Modified diets are based on normal intake with those changes required to meet specific disease or metabolic demands.

We tend to remember:

10% of what we *read*

20% of what we *hear*

30% of what we *see*

50% of what we *see* and *hear*

80% of what we *say*

90% of what we *say* and *do*

Fig. 0.1 What is remembered.

Part I explains the particulars of your role as a dietetic technician; then, by closely examining your own diet and by reviewing the nutrition basics, you will be able to use this information in optimizing the diets of others. Once you know who *you* are, you can successfully administer dietary assistance to those in need of your expertise.

Chapter One

Your Role as a Dietetic Technician

CHAPTER BLUEPRINT

Step 1: Take the Pre-test on Your Role to begin reflecting on your responsibilities as a dietetic technician in nutrition care.

Step 2: Review the Summary of Competencies and follow the accompanying instructions.

Step 3: Read the ADA Definition of Your Role and complete the assignment.

Step 4: Examine the Position Descriptions and follow the accompanying instructions.

Step 5: Read the Role Delineation Study and follow the accompanying instructions.

Step 6: Read Using Medical Charts and complete the exercises on using SOAP.

Step 7: Review the Medical Professions from A to Z and complete the assignment.

Step 8: Read the material on Health Care Systems and complete the assignment.

Step 9: Participate in chosen Career Field Trips and write up the assigned reports.

Step 10: Complete the Self-Confidence Checklist.

Step 11: Take the Post-test on Your Role to evaluate the impact of this chapter on your understanding of the role of a dietetic technician.

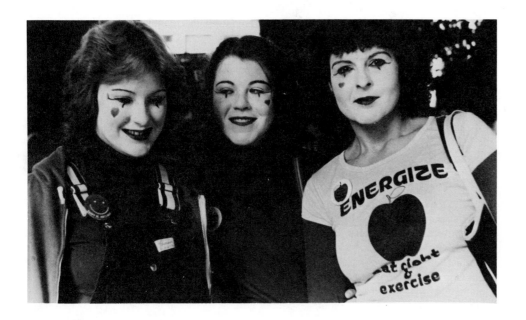

STEP 1: PRE-TEST ON YOUR ROLE

Answer the questions below as honestly and as concisely as possible. After completing this chapter, reread your answers and make any modifications you deem necessary. Discuss your answers with classmates or co-workers. Do you think that you will want to make additional revisions as your experience as a practicing dietetic technician expands?

1. What is your personal philosophy about the role of the dietetic technician as a health *professional?*

2. What is your personal philosophy about the role of the dietetic technician as an *assistant* to the dietitian(s)?

3. What is your personal philosophy about the role of the dietetic technician as a member of the *health care team?*

4. Why is *communication* important for you as a dietetic technician, and with whom must you effectively communicate?

5. What are some of the *skills* you employ as a dietetic technician (e.g., psychology in counseling and creativity in menu design)?

6. What are some of the *duties* you perform as a dietetic technician (e.g., nutritional assessment and menu planning)?

7. Why are you, as a dietetic technician, a more reliable source of nutrition information than a self-proclaimed "nutritionist"?

8. What are some of the positions in our *health care system* that you can obtain as a dietetic technician in nutrition care (e.g., assistant to out-patient dietitian, technician in nursing home facility, and in-patient clinical dietetic technician)?

9. How can you utilize some of the available *community nutrition resources* in your position as a dietetic technician in nutrition care?

10. How are *self-knowledge* and *self-confidence* important in your ability to function effectively as a dietetic technician? Do you know your own limitations?

STEP 2: SUMMARY OF COMPETENCIES

competencies: Skills or abilities that indicate legal qualifications.

As a dietetic technician in nutrition care, you will be expected to think, look, and act in a professional manner. Therefore, it is your responsibility to develop the specific **competencies** listed here. In order to carefully monitor your progress, consider each of these competencies and indicate ⟨✓⟩ those which you have already mastered. Then refer to this list later on in your training to check off the additional skills you have successfully adopted. Occasional rereading of the list of competencies (Table 1.1) required for the dietetic technician will assist you—as a student and as a practitioner—in maintaining the level of technical expertise others expect of you.

Table 1.1 Competencies of the Dietetic Technician

Competencies[a]—Successfully mastered ⊘	Date

A. Professional code of ethics
- ○ Respects the lifestyles, opinions, beliefs, and values of co-workers and patients.
- ○ Develops standards of behavior consistent with effective nutrition care.
- ○ Is aware of own limitations and is willing to seek assistance.
- ○ Understands the need for a team effort in the health care setting.
- ○ Seeks appropriate avenues for continuing self-development and education.
- ○ Maintains a healthy lifestyle which co-workers and patients can emulate and respect.

B. Communication skills
- ○ Assists **registered dietitian**(s) and other members of the health care team in planning, implementing, and evaluating the nutrition care provided in the health care facility.
- ○ Uses communication effectively in shared information and cooperative planning with peers and other personnel.
- ○ Develops rapport with all personnel to improve communications and morale within the department.
- ○ Participates in staff meetings at department or agency level.
- ○ Recognizes and uses intra- and inter-departmental communication patterns.
- ○ Participates in interview and selection of dietetic personnel.
- ○ Conducts programs for dietetic personnel to improve job performance and impart new knowledge.
- ○ Establishes and uses good interpersonal relationships with patients.
- ○ Teaches sound nutrition principles to patients and families.
- ○ Identifies and uses people and agencies with specialized services to help those with a problem or special need.

C. Professional skills
- ○ Understands the principles of normal nutrition and can apply these principles or their modification to assist in planning nutrition care programs.
- ○ Secures pertinent information for **diet histories** by interviewing patients and/or significant others, reviewing data recorded in the charts, and participating in health care team conferences.
- ○ Assists in **nutritional assessments.**
- ○ Develops and implements **nutrition care plans.**
- ○ Assists patients in selecting appropriate foods for their specific needs.
- ○ Assists dietitian(s) in referring clients requiring special diets.
- ○ Assists in the evaluation of nutrition care plans.
- ○ Calculates caloric and specific nutrient values as required in restricted modified diets.
- ○ Understands the principles of education and can apply educational techniques to both patient and employee teaching.
- ○ Assists dietitian(s) in teaching patients about meeting specific nutritional needs.
- ○ Assists dietitian(s) in developing and using teaching materials for in-service education.
- ○ Develops an understanding of the importance and interdependence of allied health disciplines.
- ○ Utilizes computer and other technology in the area of responsibility.

[a]Adapted from Horgan 1988.

registered dietitian (R.D.): A professionally trained nutritionist with a bachelor's degree in dietetics who has completed an ADA-approved training program, passed the registration board examination, and meets continuing education requirements. A clinical R.D. may work in a hospital, medical office, or health agency, whereas the administrative R.D. manages a foodservice and/or dietary department.

diet history: An organized diet sheet describing patient's dietary habits including meal patterns, food likes and dislikes, food preparation techniques and facilities, food intolerances, dietary restrictions, use of nutritional supplements, and social/financial/ethnic/religious lifestyle influences.

nutritional assessment: Comprehensive evaluation of physical status with particular attention to nutritional deficiencies and diet-related clinical conditions. Height, weight, triceps skinfold measurement, creatinine height index, serum albumin/transferrin, and total lymphocyte count reflect body protein/fat status to indicate need for diet therapy.

nutrition care plan: Specific individualized program of dietary treatment including subjective and objective observations, nutritional assessment, and plan of action.

STEP 3: ADA DEFINITION OF YOUR ROLE

The March 1982 issue of the *Journal of The American Dietetic Association* (ADA 1982) published the following report.

Role of the Dietetic Technician in Clinical Dietetics[1]

The American Dietetic Association is committed to the utilization of qualified support personnel in the delivery of nutrition care services. The Association supports the use of the title *dietetic technician* only for those who have satisfactorily completed an ADA-approved associate degree technician program. The Association further recommends that only those technicians who have an academic emphasis in nutrition care be employed for positions in **clinical dietetics** and that only qualified individuals be given the title of dietetic technician. Responsibilities appropriate to the dietetic technician in nutrition care practice are classified in the role delineation study into four conceptual levels analogous to those described for the registered dietitian.

At the *client* level the clinical dietetic technician assists the registered dietitian in clinical practice to provide direct nutrition service to patients or clients. The technician is responsible for

○ Using predetermined criteria in screening patients to identify those at **nutritional risk** and collecting specified data for use in assessment of dietary status.
○ Following guidelines established by the clinical dietitian to develop nutrition care plans for individual patients.
○ Providing technical services in the implementation of nutrition care plans.
○ Monitoring the effect of nutrition intervention and assessing patient food acceptance.
○ Utilizing opportunities for nutrition education and providing diet counseling for individuals not at nutritional risk.

Within the second level, *intra-professional* relationships, the dietetic technician cooperates with the clinical dietitian in promoting standards of quality practice and using current knowledge to solve nutrition problems of individual patients.

At the third or *inter-professional* level, the technician coordinates assigned nutrition care activities and is responsible for

○ Coordinating nutrition care of assigned patients/clients with other health services.
○ Coordinating designated nutrition care services with institutional food service activities.

At the *intra-organizational* level the dietetic technician utilizes established standards and procedures to implement the system of patient nutrition care. This responsibility includes

○ Utilizing established procedures for making available designated special food products and **dietary supplements.**
○ Supervising **diet clerks** and other patient food service personnel.
○ Developing and implementing a program of orientation, training, and in-service education for patient food service personnel.

clinical dietetics: The area of nutrition that focuses on diet therapy, incorporating normal/modified diet prescription, planning, and instruction while encouraging individualized dietary compliance.

nutritional risk: Any physical and/or emotional condition that jeopardizes nutritional status (e.g., pregnancy, diabetes, and post-surgery).

dietary supplement: Liquid or powder nourishment used to increase the nutritional or caloric content of the diet (e.g., protein powders and high-calorie pudding mixes); not to be used as sole dietary support.

diet clerk: A dietetic assistant not considered as part of the health care team. This clinical position entails such tasks as menu tallies, heading menus, distribution and collection of menus, transcription of meal patterns onto appropriate forms, answering the phone, and taking orders for new diets.

---

[1]From: *Position Paper on Clinical Dietetics.* Copyright The American Dietetic Association. Reprinted by permission from JOURNAL OF THE AMERICAN DIETETIC ASSOCIATION, Vol. 80:256, 1982.

For more information on being a dietetic technician, see Fig. 1.1.

Exercises on Dietetic Technician Role

As a dietetic technician,[1] you will assist the dietitian(s) at the client, intra-professional, inter-professional, and intra-organizational levels. From the following list, identify at which level you would be assisting the dietitian in performing the specified tasks. (Answers appear in Answer Key on p. 431.)

[1]As of 1985 the American Dietetic Association (ADA 1985) began enforcing their "Standards of Professional Responsibility of the American Dietetic Association," with which all practicing dietetic technicians should familiarize themselves.

Who is a <u>dietetic technician?</u>

An individual who has completed an ADA-approved Dietetic Technician program and earned an associate degree

What are areas of dietetic practice for the technician?

● *Foodservice management,* assisting in foodservice management under the supervision of an administrative dietitian or a consultant dietitian
● *Nutrition Care,* assisting in providing nutrition care services to individuals or groups under the supervision of a clinical or community dietitian

How many dietetic technicians are there in the United States?

There are more than 3,000 graduates of approved Dietetic Technician programs.

What are the employment opportunities for dietetic technicians?

Technicians are employed in hospitals, public health nutrition programs, long-term care facilities, child feeding programs, and foodservice management firms.

How can a technician become a member of The American Dietetic Association?

● A graduate from an ADA-approved Dietetic Technician program with an earned associate degree is eligible for membership in The American Dietetic Association.
● Technician members vote and hold appointed positions at national, state, and local levels.

What are the benefits for ADA members?

● Automatic membership in a state dietetic association
● Technical information exchange with other professionals in dietetic practice groups
● Reduced fees for ADA's annual meeting and other continuing education programs
● Discounted professional publications and merchandise
● Savings on health and malpractice insurance
● Scientific information in the Journal of The American Dietetic Association
● Opportunity for involvement in ADA's legislative network
● Public relations efforts
● Role delineations for technical and professional levels

Is there a credential for dietetic technicians?

Yes. Technicians who successfully write the Registration Examination for Dietetic Technicians are entitled to use the initials, "DTR", to signify professional competence. DTRs must earn 50 hours of continuing education every five years to maintain the credential.

For further information about the Registration Examination for Dietetic Technicians, write the Commission on Dietetic Registration, 216 West Jackson Boulevard, Chicago, IL 60606.

For further information about membership in The American Dietetic Association, careers in dietetics, or the knowledge and performance requirements for dietetic technicians and entry-level dietitians, contact ADA's Membership Development Department at 216 West Jackson Boulevard, Chicago, IL 60606 or call 1-800-621-6469 (in Illinois, call 312-899-0040).

Prepared September 1984 by the Committee on Association Membership, House of Delegates; updated September 1988.

Fig. 1.1   Dietetic Technician Fact Sheet.
Courtesy The American Dietetic Association

---

a. Client
b. Intra-professional
c. Inter-professional
d. Intra-organizational

_____ 1. Discuss appropriate weight for diabetic patient with dietitian.
_____ 2. Suggest patient referral to mental health department for assistance with alcohol problem.
_____ 3. Develop and present nutrition workshop for pregnant teens.
_____ 4. Take detailed diet history.
_____ 5. Read up on a special modified diet and report to dietitian.
_____ 6. Plan low-calorie Thanksgiving menu with foodservice department.
_____ 7. Teach a class on sanitation to foodservice personnel.
_____ 8. Attend and participate in medical rounds.
_____ 9. Request new high-protein supplement.
_____ 10. Develop individualized low-sodium diet plan.
_____ 11. Instruct diet clerks on proper meal tallies.
_____ 12. Record meal acceptance in patient chart.

After filling in the letters above, indicate (√) which tasks you feel able to accomplish. Tally the checks: _____. Do you think the number of responsibilities you can successfully undertake will increase? Tally again later on in your training to evaluate progress.

STEP 4: POSITION DESCRIPTIONS

It is a common error to expect that most people will understand what your role as a dietetic technician entails and that graduation from an approved training program will provide you with a working knowledge of your own duties. Unfortunately, many people—including experienced health professionals—have only a vague idea at best of the various responsibilities that a well-trained dietetic technician can handle. Therefore, it is up to you to familiarize yourself with your professional functions and to impart this information to fellow nutrition personnel, as well as to other health care team members, patients, and the community at large.

In 1981, The American Dietetic Association published their role delineation study for entry-level dietetics. This 15-month study was conducted in order to meet the ADA's increased demands for competent clinical dietetic practitioners, as well as to clarify the skill and knowledge requirements at the various levels of preparation and experience. "Role Delineation for Entry Level Clinical Dietetics 1980" (see References at end of chapter) has the official endorsement of the ADA, and serves to define just what dietetic personnel in nutrition care need to know and to practice in order to fulfill their expected obligations.

The following list summarizes the clinical dietetics hierarchy:

○   The director of the dietary department, in which the clinical dietetics section is situated, is a registered dietitian (R.D.). For departments headed by a nondietitian, the major and specific responsibilities still apply, but the manner of execution may vary, as required by the facility's needs. Nevertheless, the essence of each statement relates to departments headed by nondietitians, as well as registered dietitians.

○   The clinicial dietetic technician works under the supervision of a clinical dietitian (R.D.).

○   The role delineation for the clinical dietitian (R.D.) level subsumes responsibilities delineated for the clinical dietetic technician level.

○   The clinical dietitian (R.D.) will delegate the responsibilities delineated for the clinical dietetic technician when such technician is available.

○   Although diet clerk is not delineated as a level within the role of clinical dietetics, the functions of such a position are required to support a clinical dietetics section. (The diet clerk position should not be considered part of the clinical dietetic personnel hierarchy because responsibilities delineated for this clerical position do not require formal educational preparation in dietetics.)

To further clarify each of these specialized roles, the ADA has devised the following lists, called Position Descriptions.

Position Description: Clinical Dietitian—Entry Level

General Area of Performance

○   Assesses the nutrition status of individual clients/patients in health and disease throughout the life cycle.
○   Constructs and coordinates all aspects of nutrition care plan, including identification of short- and long-term goals, delineation of treatment modalities and education plans, establishment of procedures for implementation of the nutrition care plan, ongoing information gathering, and evaluation.
○   Communicates and monitors implementation of nutrition care plan; documents all aspects of nutrition care; verifies implementation of care plan.
○   Evaluates effects of intervention on individual client/patient nutrition status.
○   Plans, organizes, implements, and evaluates nutrition education for clients/patients; arranges for individual client/patient follow-up as needed.
○   Participates in applied research and related dietetic professional activities; uses research findings and current knowledge in nutrition care.
○   Communicates pertinent information to other health care professionals; discusses individual client/patient nutrition care needs with health team members; educates health team on nutrition-related topics.
○   Plans, reviews, provides consultation for the implementation of nutrition care on the systems level.

○ Develops short- and long-range plans for delivering quality nutrition care services while containing costs; maintains personnel and training functions for clinical dietetics section.
○ Identifies political, fiscal, and social factors influencing nutrition care and integrates these factors into system for delivering nutrition care.

Supervisory Controls

○ Responsible to the chief clinical dietitian or designate.

Limitations

○ Required to have basic understanding of, but not expertise in, subspecialty areas.

Position Description: Clinical Dietetic Technician—Entry Level

General Area of Performance

○ Assists in screening for individual clients/patients at nutrition risk; collects required data, performs calculations; assists in evaluating data.
○ Develops nutrition care plan, with consultation, for those not at nutrition risk; writes menus and substitutions under supervision for those at nutrition risk.
○ Performs delegated aspects of nutrition care plan to meet short- and long-term objectives and communicates relevant aspects orally and in writing.
○ Determines effects of intervention on individual client's/patient's nutrition status and revises plan for those not at nutrition risk.
○ Provides nutrition education and follow-up care for predetermined subpopulations of clients/patients.
○ Acquires current knowledge; maintains standards of technical dietetic practice.
○ Communicates with health team members; coordinates technical clinical dietetic activities with administrative dietetic activities.
○ Acquires special nutrition-related products.
○ Supports personnel functions; assists in ongoing quality assurance functions.
○ Orients co-workers and clients/patients to information networks and public agencies related to nutrition care.

Supervisory Controls

○ Responsible to a registered dietitian.

Limitations

○ Requires continuous supervision when performing delegated functions related to high risk patients.

Position Description: Diet Clerk

General Area of Performance—in Support of Clinical Dietetic Personnel

○ Tallies client/patient diet census by diet category.
○ Tallies number of food items selected for client/patient meals.
○ Reassembles/collates selective menu forms for regular and modified diet menus.
○ Writes name, date, and location of patient on individual patient menus and **supplemental feeding** forms.
○ Distributes and collects selective menu forms from individual clients/patients.
○ Transcribes prescribed meal patterns onto individual client/patient menu forms.
○ Transcribes prescribed **tube feeding** recipes onto individual client/patient supplemental forms.
○ Delivers and retrieves food preference/acceptance survey forms.
○ Answers telephone and records messages on phone log.
○ Notes written orders, telephone orders, verbal requests for new diets and diet changes.

supplemental feeding: Chemically defined and elemental diets that require minimal digestion but can be taken orally as source of extra protein/calories.

tube feeding: Method of ensuring proper nutrition by passing pliable tube through nasal cavity into stomach. Tube feeding may be indicated after dental or gastrointestinal surgery, with severe burns, paralysis, and cancer of the mouth or esophagus, or during coma or severe malnutrition.

Dietetic Technician Role Playing

role play: Educational activity in which participants act out assigned characters or functions to practice a skill or depict solutions to problem situations.

After careful examination of the preceding position descriptions, write a brief summary to describe each of the three levels of practice. Do you think that you are (or will be) well suited for the midlevel role of a dietetic technician? Are you willing to accept the added responsibilities of this position that differentiate it from the role of the diet clerk? Discuss the position descriptions and your own summaries with classmates or co-workers, and **role play** several situations in which the dietetic technician must make his/her level of expertise known to members of (1) the dietetics department, (2) the health care team, and (3) the community. Then write a brief summary of your thoughts on the three role-playing situations.

Summary of dietetics positions: _____

_____

Summary of your thoughts on the role-playing situations: _____

_____

STEP 5: ROLE DELINEATION STUDY

The ADA's "Role Delineation for Entry Level Clinical Dietetics 1980" (ADA 1981) defines your role as a dietetic technician in two separate ways: (1) the *actual* (i.e., currently accepted) entry role responsibilities; (2) the *appropriate* (i.e., what should be) entry role responsibilities and position description. (See Step 4 for the latter.)

A program of *appropriate* responsibilities for you as a practicing dietetic technician is outlined in Table 1.2 (ADA 1981). It incorporates the four practice levels (see Step 3) as the major areas of responsibility.

As a dietetic technician, it is your role to be able to actualize the *appropriate* responsibilities. In order to carefully monitor your progress, consider each of the responsibilities in Table 1.3 and indicate ⊘ those which you think you have already adopted. Discuss your list with a teacher/R.D. Then refer to this list later on in your training to check off the additional responsibilities you have assumed. Rereading the list of responsibilities every so often will assist you—as a student and as a practitioner—in fulfilling your role as a dietetic technician in nutrition care.

Table 1.2   Appropriate Responsibilities of Dietetic Technician

Nutrition Care Process: Client/Patient Level
    1.0   Nutrition Assessment
    2.0   Nutrition Care Planning
    3.0   Nutrition Care Implementation
    4.0   Nutrition Care Evaluation
    5.0   Nutrition Education and Referral
Nutrition Care Process: Intra-professional Level
    6.0   Professional/Educational Activity and Development
Nutrition Care Process: Inter-professional Level
    7.0   Health Team Functions
Nutrition Care Process: Intra-organizational Level
    8.0   Food Procurement, Productions, and Service
    9.0   Foodservice Systems Maintenance
         (in *actual* role only; deleted from *appropriate* role)
   10.0   Strategic Direction and Personnel Management
Plus
Nutrition Care Process: Inter-organizational Level
   11.0   Identification and Management of Extraneous Influences upon Nutrition Care

Table 1.3   Breakdown of Appropriate Responsibilities of Dietetic Technician[a]

Dietetic Technician's Responsibilities—Adopted ⊘	Date

Client level

○ **1.0**   *Nutrition assessment:*   Assists in screening for individual clients/patients at nutrition risk; collects required data, performs calculations; assists in evaluating data.

    ○ 1.1   Identifies individuals with special nutrition needs from total client/patient population using predetermined criteria.

    ○ 1.2   Assists in collecting nutritionally relevant data (e.g., laboratory data and **24-hour recall**) for individual clients/patients not at nutrition risk.

    ○ 1.3   Assists in collecting nutritionally relevant data from **medical history** of those clients/patients not at nutrition risk.

    ○ 1.4   Assists in collecting nutritionally relevant demographic (personal background) data (e.g., age and income) from individual clients/patients.

    ○ 1.5   Assists in collecting nutritionally relevant anthropometric (body measurement) data from individual clients/patients.

    ○ 1.6   Calculates nutrient and energy intake values and assists in evaluating data.

○ **2.0**   *Nutrition care planning:*   Develops nutrition care plan, with consultation, for those not at nutrition risk; writes menus and substitutions under supervision for those at nutrition risk.

    ○ 2.1   Selects appropriate source(s) of specific nutrients (e.g., food and food products) and develops/adjusts a diet pattern for individual clients/patients not at nutrition risk.

    ○ 2.2   Develops nutrition care plan, in consultation with a dietitian, for individual clients/patients not at nutrition risk, specifying diet, counseling, etc.; and documents in the **medical record.**

    ○ 2.3   Writes menu in accordance with diet pattern written by dietitian for individual clients/patients at nutrition risk; and makes appropriate substitutions in accordance with pattern.

○ **3.0**   *Nutrition care implementation:*   Performs delegated aspects of nutrition care plan to meet short- and long-term objectives and communicates relevant aspects orally and in writing.

    ○ 3.1   Communicates plan for nutrition care to individual client/patient and/or to individual client's/patient's family; and documents in the medical record.

    ○ 3.2   Communicates plan for individual client's/patient's nutrition care to health team members, and documents in the medical record.

    ○ 3.3   Communicates to appropriate personnel (e.g., foodservice, pharmacy, or central supply) the specific actions to implement client's/patient's nutrition care plan; and documents in the medical record.

    ○ 3.4   Implements diet orders in institutional settings.

    ○ 3.5   Maintains client/patient **Kardex** from diet order sheets.

    ○ 3.6   Verifies implementation of nutrition prescription for individual clients/patients (e.g., checking menus, diet orders, trays, and nourishments).

○ **4.0**   *Nutrition care evaluation:*   Determines effects of intervention on individual client's/patient's nutrition status and revises plan for those not at nutrition risk.

    ○ 4.1   Monitors and documents individual client's/patient's adherence to/tolerance of nutrition care (e.g., low-calorie diet).

    ○ 4.2   Evaluates individual client/patient acceptance of food.

    ○ 4.3   Monitors the outcomes of nutrition care for individual clients/patients, and documents in the medical record.

    ○ 4.4   Revises nutrition care plan for individual clients/patients not at nutrition risk, and documents in the medical record.

24-hour recall: A form on which a nutritionist records oral intake of patient during previous 24 hours to be used as educational and evaluative tool.

medical history: A form on which to record information on patient's health background and current physical status, including height and weight, clinical disorders, and medications.

medical record: Chart maintained by health care team to delineate information on patient's status and progress; daily entries are made by those in contact with patient using specified format.

Kardex: Organized file system with patient identification cards depicting information required by dietary personnel (e.g., name of patient, room number, diet prescription, and food likes and dislikes).

(continued)

Table 1.3   (Continued)

Dietetic Technician's Responsibilities—Adopted ⊘	Date

Client level (continued)

○ 5.0   *Nutrition education and referral:*   Provides nutrition education and follow-up care for predetermined sub-populations of clients/patients.

  ○ 5.1   Recommends nutrition education for clients/patients not at nutrition risk.
  ○ 5.2   Identifies all appropriate opportunities and settings for learning.
  ○ 5.3   Selects nutrition education materials/exhibits for clients/patients not at nutrition risk.
  ○ 5.4   Provides technical support for implementing and maintaining nutrition education processes (e.g., maintains files of materials for dissemination).
  ○ 5.5   Counsels individual clients/patients not at nutrition risk concerning nutrition concepts and desired changes in eating habits.
  ○ 5.6   Gives classes and lectures in basic nutrition to small groups of clients/patients.
  ○ 5.7   Evaluates effectiveness of nutrition education events for clients/patients not at nutrition risk and/or their significant others.
  ○ 5.8   Documents individual client's/patient's response to nutrition education.
  ○ 5.9   Arranges for follow-up or terminates nutrition care of individual clients/patients, in consultation with a dietitian.

Intra-professional level:

○ 6.0   *Professional/educational activity and development:*   Acquires current knowledge; maintains standards of technical dietetic practice.
  ○ 6.1   Uses current knowledge to solve client's/patient's nutrition problems.

Inter-professional level

○ 7.0   *Health team functions:*   Communicates with health team members; coordinates technical clinical dietetic activities with administrative dietetic activities.
  ○ 7.1   Contributes the nutrition-related expertise to the health team (e.g., physicians, nurses, pharmacists, and social workers) discussions of client's/patient's health status.
  ○ 7.2   Meets with health team members to integrate nutrition care of clients/patients.
  ○ 7.3   Coordinates clinical dietetic activities with administrative dietetic activities.

Intra-organizational level

○ 8.0   *Food procurement, production, and service:*   Acquires special nutrition-related products.
  ○ 8.1   Utilizes established standards and procedures for purchasing food for modified diets.
○ 9.0   *Foodservice systems maintenance:*   Traditionally, clinical dietetic personnel have assumed responsibilities in this area, but the expanding responsibilities of these personnel in client/patient-centered services require stationing clinical dietetic personnel in client/patient care areas, leaving kitchen-based duties to foodservice personnel.
○ 10.0   *Strategic direction and personnel management:*   Supports personnel functions; assists in ongoing quality assurance functions.
  ○ 10.1   Assists in an ongoing program of quality assurance for patient care and delivery of services to clients/patients.
  ○ 10.2   Implements orientation and training program for clinical dietetic personnel.
  ○ 10.3   Supervises and evaluates clerical personnel assigned to clinical dietetic functions (e.g., for productivity, quality, and integrity).
  ○ 10.4   Develops clinical dietetic personnel in nutrition care area.

Inter-organizational level

○ 11.0   *Identification and management of extraneous influences upon nutrition care:*   Orients co-workers and clients/patients to informational networks and public agencies related to nutrition care.
  ○ 11.1   Identifies programs and/or sources of outside funding related to the provision of nutrition care for individual clients/patients, in consultation with a dietitian.
  ○ 11.2   Informs health care team, in consultation with a dietitian, about laws, regulations, and professional guidelines related to nutrition care.

[a]The 1985 revised "Essentials" and "Guidelines" for Dietetic Technician programs and a Dietetic Technician Fact Sheet, which highlights employment roles and ADA functions, are available from ADA. Registration Maintenance Guidelines: Continuing Education Requirements for the Registered Dietetic Technician is available from ADA's Commission on Dietetic Registration. © American Dietetic Association. Used by permission.

STEP 6: USING MEDICAL CHARTS
(AHA AND ADA ON SOAP)

For the dietetic technician in nutrition care, the clinical setting requires a working knowledge of the proper use of medical records. Prior to visiting patients, attending medical rounds, or planning individual diets, it is essential for all members of the health care team to examine the pertinent medical charts. Upon completion of each nutritional assessment, patient visitation, diet history or 24-hour recall, diet instruction, and diet modification, it is essential for the attending dietetic technician to enter the appropriate information in the patient's chart. Proper organization of the pertinent data ensures maximal patient benefit as well as easy retrievability by interested medical professionals.

The American Hospital Association (AHA) has approved the use of the *problem oriented medical record* (**POMR**) with the so-called SOAP (Subjective data, Objective data, Assessment, Plan) method for making progress notes. As a practicing dietetic technician, you should find that the SOAP approach eases both your own charting responsibilities and the usability of your entries for others. Yet, this method is not excessively time consuming since abbreviations are used; sentences can be incomplete if comprehensible; and brevity is encouraged. Use the first set of guidelines to assist you in preparing for nutritional assessment and counseling (Before), and the final set to help you with recording the information in medical charts (After).

POMR: Problem oriented medical record. Medical charting technique in which notes are coded and entered based on a list of health care problems and needs, with the focus on intended plans of action.

Before Patient Visitation

1. Examine the **problem list** for diet-related information (e.g., overweight, weight loss/gain, diabetes, loss of appetite, food intolerance).
2. Examine the **progress notes** of other health care team members for any diet-related comments (e.g., patient refuses to eat, patient complained of heartburn after dinner).
3. Examine the diagnosis and meds (medications) list, and briefly review the rest of the chart to determine those factors that may influence the diet or necessitate diet modification.
4. Make all pertinent entries on your own record forms (see Parts III and IV of this book for sample forms).

problem list: A numbered, titled index in patient's medical chart of all health care related problems including symptoms, abnormal laboratory test results and physical findings, and diagnosis. List is modified as patient status changes.

progress notes: Follow-up notes in patient's medical chart using the problem list information and the SOAP format.

During Patient Visitation

See Parts III and IV of this book for guidelines.

After Patient Visitation

1. Enter pertinent information onto your own record forms (see Parts III and IV).
2. Record progress notes in patient's medical chart using SOAP format.

   S: Subjective data—how patient feels, the dietary problem from his/her point of view (or from information provided by significant others, nursing staff, or other referrals if necessary)
   O: Objective data—measurements of physical, physiological, and laboratory parameters relative to diet/nutritional status (may include diet order and/or specific nutrient needs)
   A: Assessment. For example, is the patient's dietary progress inacceptable? How so (e.g., diet not tolerated, patient unfamiliar with diet, diet not meeting specific nutrient/emotional/physical needs)?
   P: Plan—diet prescription/modifications and required nutrition education/ counseling sessions

3. Be sure to date and sign all chart entries; most health care facilities and individual departments have their own specific regulations for charting as well.

Suggested Readings on Using SOAP

AMERICAN HOSPITAL ASSOCIATION. 1976. Recording Nutrition Information in Medical Records, Technical Advisory Bulletin No. T0153M-2/81-7410. Chicago: AHA.
CHAPPELLE, M., and SCHOLL, R. 1973. Adapting the problem-oriented medical record to the psychiatric hospital. J. Am. Dietet. Assoc. *63*, Dec., 643.
OMETER, J. 1980. Documentation of nutritional care. J. Am. Dietet. Assoc. *76*, Jan., 35.
VOYTOVICH, A. 1973. The dietitian/nutritionist and the problem-oriented medical record, I: A physician's viewpoint. J. Am. Dietet. Assoc. *63*, Dec., 639.
WALTERS, F., and DEMARCO, M. 1973. The dietitian/nutritionist and the problem-oriented record, II: The role of the dietitian. J. Am. Dietet. Assoc. *63*, Dec., 641.
WILLS, B. 1985. Documentation: The missing link in evaluation. J. Am. Dietet. Assoc. *85*, Feb., 225.

Exercises on Using SOAP

Practice enhances the speed and ease with which you can make well-organized chart entries. The SOAP notes of the skilled dietetic technician help to ensure proper nutrition care for patients, as well as aid in smooth communication with other members of the health care team. Reading articles from the preceding Suggested Readings will help you answer the following questions and complete the Charting with SOAP case studies.

1. What are some typical examples of *subjective data* that you might be expected to record?

2. What are some typical examples of *objective data* that you might be expected to record?

3. What are some typical examples of *assessments* that you might be expected to devise and record?

4. What are some typical examples of *plans* that you might be expected to devise and record?

5. As a dietetic technician in nutrition care, to whom might you refer for assistance in the making and/or approval of your *plans*?

Charting with SOAP

Examine each of the following examples of simplified diet problem case studies. Note the given short-answer assessments (As) and plans (Ps), which can help you to fill in the blanks with appropriate As and Ps. Discuss your answers with classmates or co-workers. Also, try to keep in mind the fact that it does take time, experience, and education in nutritional assessment and diet therapy in order to become skilled at charting using the SOAP procedure.

hypertension: High blood pressure; excessive straining of blood against the walls of the arteries. The reading 140/90 is usually considered to be the upper limit of normal.

dehydration: Condition resulting from loss of essential body water, which may lead to fatal shock. Causes include prolonged fever, diarrhea, vomiting, severe injury, surgery, or certain medications.

hypokalemia: Deficient level of potassium in the blood.

Case A

Problem list
1. Overweight
2. **Hypertension**

Progress notes—2 (item 2 on problem list)
S: Feels uncomfortably full, bloated
O: Ht: 5′3″   Wt: 203
   Diet Plan: 1000 calories
A: May require sodium restriction
P: _____

Case B

Problem list
1. Diarrhea, chronic
2. **Dehydration**
3. **Hypokalemia**
4. Weight loss

Progress notes—3 (item 3 on problem list)
S: Weak, light-headed, dizzy
O: Ht: 5′3″   Wt: 110
   Diet Plan: House
A: _____
P: Discuss use of potassium supplements with dietitian/health care team

Case C

Problem list
1. **Anorexia nervosa**
2. Malnutrition
3. Underweight

Progress notes—1
S: Complains that meals are too large, unappealing
O: Ht: 5'3"   Wt: 72
    Diet plan: 2000 calories
A: Needs tasty high-calorie supplements/snacks, nutrition counseling
P: _____

Case D

Problem list
1. **Obesity**
2. **Chronic gallbladder disease**

Progress notes—2
S: Indigestion after meals
O: Ht: 5'3"   Wt: 203
    Diet plan: 1000 calories
A: _____
P: Suggest low-fat diet with smaller, more frequent meals to dietitian/health care team

anorexia nervosa: Loss of appetite due to emotional factors in which victim may self-starve into a state of emaciation, malnutrition, even death.

obesity: Excessive accumulation of fat tissue so that body weight is 20% or more above the range considered to be desirable for one's age, sex, height and frame.

chronic gallbladder disease: Repeated inflammation of the bile-storing saclike organ located below the liver, causing pain and indigestion, especially following heavy/fatty meals; may respond to diet/medication or require surgical removal of the gallbladder, especially if gallstones are present.

STEP 7: MEDICAL PROFESSIONS FROM A TO Z

Not only is it important for members of the health care team to be aware of your responsibilities as a dietetic technician, but it is essential for you to be familiar with their individual roles as well. In order to function as an effective team, health professionals must maintain an interactive and open relationship based on mutual respect and shared responsibilities. Communication and understanding are the keys to success in team efforts.

Using a medical dictionary and the references in Appendix V, (A) match the brief job descriptions for the listed medical professions with the appropriate job title; answers are given in the Answer Key at the end of the book. Then (B) define briefly each of the physician subspecialties. Which of these health professionals have you interacted with as a student or practicing dietetic technician? Can you visualize how each of these professionals is essential to the overall optimization of health care delivery?

A. Job Descriptions

a. Physician
b. Nurse
c. Pharmacologist
d. Speech pathologist
e. Physical therapist
f. Occupational therapist
g. Recreational therapist
h. Respiratory therapist
i. Medical technologist
j. Social worker
k. Psychologist
l. Medical records technician

_____ 1. Provides clinical services to patients with problems or disorders of communication, speech, language, or hearing. Certification requires bachelors and masters degrees in the field, supervised clinical practice, and passing a national board examination.

_____ 2. Performs the laboratory procedures to determine disease states and possible treatment measures. Certification requires bachelors degree, 1-year clinical training, and passing a national board examination.

_____ 3. Practices the healing arts after graduation from a college of medicine and licensure by the appropriate specialty board. The term doctor may also refer to the advanced medical student, medical intern, and medical resident.

_____ 4. Organizes and directs activity programs including athletics, music, dancing, drama, field trips, and games in order to aid mental rehabilitation through therapeutically beneficial play. Associates degree required.

_____ 5. Uses therapeutic techniques and equipment to assist/control patient breathing. Certification includes 1–2-year training program and passing a national board examination.

_____ 6. Evaluates levels of self-care (physical, mental, financial, familial, etc.) to plan and investigate appropriate avenues for placement during rehabilitation. Masters degree in social work usually required.

_____ 7. Evaluates the physically disabled, prepares therapeutic program in consultation with the physician, and instructs patient and others on function restoration and pain alleviation using exercise, massage, heat, cold, and other treatment modalities. Requires bachelors and/or masters degree and passing a state examination in order to be registered to practice.

_____ 8. Provides hands-on services required to aid physician in all aspects of health restoration and maintenance. Registration requires bachelors and/or masters degree, clinical competence, and passing a state board examination.

_____ 9. Evaluates patient's level of functioning in order to plan appropriate therapeutic activity program which includes music, crafts, industrial arts, daily living activities, and/or recreation. Registration requires bachelors and/or masters degree, 6 months clinical experience, and passing a national board examination.

_____ 10. Trained in maintaining, storing, and retrieving all medical documents which are kept for each patient treated at the medical care facility.

_____ 11. Specializes in the study of drug actions and interactions, therapeutic uses, and potential side effects. Licensure requires 5-year bachelors study or 6-year doctoral degree, clinical internship, and passing a state board examination.

_____ 12. Specializes in patient mental health evaluation, counseling, and rehabilitation therapy. Requires bachelors and masters degrees plus clinical experience in the area of specialization (e.g., clinical, child, or experimental).

B. Define Physician Subspecialties

m. Bariatrician _____

n. Cardiologist _____

o. Dermatologist _____

p. Internist _____

q. Neurologist _____

r. Obstetrician/Gynecologist _____

s. Ophthamologist _____

t. Orthopedic surgeon _____

u. Otolaryngologist _____

v. Pathologist _____

w. Podiatrist _____

x. Psychiatrist _____

y. Radiologist _____

z. Urologist _____

STEP 8: HEALTH CARE SYSTEMS

As a health care technician, your goal is to contribute to the control of disease through the application of scientific and medical knowledge. As a dietetic technician, you need to translate nutrition theory into diet therapy. Your ultimate concern is the preservation of health and the promotion of longevity by providing needed nutrition care and information. You are one cog in an important machine: the health care system.

Today's health care system offers a variety of medical facilities and services including hospitals, nursing homes, health maintenance organizations (HMOs) and clinics, hospices, home health care, and outreach programs. As a dietetic technician in nutrition care, each of these components of the overall health care system can be enhanced by the addition of your technical skills. Thus, it is important for you to understand the basic functions of these medical options, and to be able to visualize your own potential role within each operation.

Examine the following material so that you can complete the Evaluating a Health Care System questionnaire which follows.

The Components of a Health Care System

Hospital: Institute for the treatment of the physically and/or mentally ill.

Nursing Home: "Convalescent home" or "home for the aged" which provides room and board. Personal and/or nursing care may also be available.

HMO: Health Maintenance Organization which may vary in form but each includes comprehensive health care services provided by a group of medical professionals to pre-paid subscribers and their families. All medical care, except for extreme emergencies, must be provided by the HMO—including routine physical examinations and other preventive health care services.

Clinic: Free, sliding scale, or full payment out-patient medical service catering to the needs of a particular community.

Hospice: Institution designed to provide the terminally ill with a homelike environment and much psychological support.

Hospitals can be either **general** or **specialty** hospitals and be funded as **community, private,** or **public** institutions. The organizational relationships are illustrated in Fig. 1.2.

general hospital: Provides medical and/or surgical treatment for various conditions.

specialty hospital: Provides treatment for specific conditions such as diabetes, cancer, tuberculosis, or pregnancy/maternity.

community hospital: "Voluntary" hospital supported by patient and insurance payments plus private gifts; directed by board of trustees, religious order, or other nongovernmental group.

private hospital: "Proprietary" hospital owned by individual or corporation; operated for profit.

public hospital: "Government" hospital owned by a city, county, state, or federal agency.

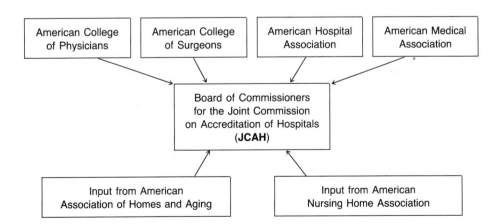

JCAH: Joint Commission on Accreditation of Hospitals; board of commissioners which establishes specific standards as minimum essentials for quality care in hospitals and other medical facilities.

Fig. 1.2 Hospital organizational relationships.

You may want to review "JCAH Standards of Quality Care for Hospitals" (AHA 1971) and the requirements for JCAH registration for hospitals, and discuss them with a teacher or R.D.

Some Characteristics of a Good Hospital

The characteristics that identify a good hospital according to Cornacchia and Barrett (1985) include the following:

1. Accredited by JCAH
2. Safe
3. Clean
4. Infection control and prevention
5. Complete medical records for all patients
6. Specific rules and regulations for medical staff
7. Specific hiring procedures and requirements for medical staff
8. Defined as a *teaching hospital* with medical school affiliation and various research programs
9. Defined as a *voluntary* hospital and operated on a nonprofit basis
10. Offering a wide range of diagnostic and treatment services and board certified specialists
11. Maintenance of standards with peer reviews and continuing education programs
12. Establishment of surgical evaluation committee (*tissue committee*)
13. Establishment of medical care evaluation committees
14. Required regular staff meetings
15. Employment of a patient services representative
16. Rapport with consumer representative(s) and involvement in community health improvement ventures

Checklist for a Good Hospital

Howard Berman, the vice-president of The Blue Cross Association's health care services department, suggests the following questions (Conniff 1973) as a checklist to determine if a hospital is a good one:

1. Is there a bathroom in, or located close to, every room?
2. What is the ratio of registered nurses to patients?
3. What is the quality of the food?
4. Is the range of services fully departmentalized? (Do they have their own laboratories, physical therapists, etc.?)
5. What is the range of specialists who have privileges to practice there, and are they board certified?
6. Does the hospital offer fully equipped and fully staffed emergency room service?
7. Does the hospital have an outpatient department?
8. Does it offer psychiatric service?
9. Does it have affiliation with a medical school?
10. Is there an intensive-care unit?
11. Does the hospital have accreditation from JCAH?
12. Does it meet all state and local fire and safety codes?
13. What is the type of ownership (physicians, private, nonprofit, or community)?
14. Does it have utilization review committees?
15. Does the hospital have medical audit committees?
16. Does the hospital have a (pathology) tissue committee?
17. Does it abide by the new AHA's Patient's Bill of Rights (see below)?
18. Is the average length of stay about the same as, or longer or shorter than, in other hospitals?
19. How do the basic daily room charge and laboratory charges compare with those in hospitals of similar size? (One good indicator of comparative costs is to examine maternity charges and those prevailing in similar-type hospitals.)
20. Does it require a deposit?

AHA's Patient's Bill of Rights

A good hospital abides by the AHA's Patient's Bill of Rights (Conniff 1973), which states that a patient has the right to the following:

1. Considerate and respectful care
2. Complete current information from his/her doctor about diagnosis, treatment, and prognosis in terms he/she (or an appropriate person in his/her behalf) can understand, and the name of the doctor handling the case
3. Information from the doctor that enables him/her to give informed consent before any procedure or treatment starts, and the name of the person administering it
4. Refusal of treatment to the extent the law allows, and knowledge of the medical consequences of doing so
5. Privacy in the medical care program that includes discreet conduct of examination and treatment, confidentiality in discussion of the case, and his/her permission for anyone not directly involved in his/her care to be present at case discussion, consultation, examination, and treatment
6. Assurance that communications and records concerning his/her case be kept confidential
7. Reasonable response to request for services, within the hospital's capacity, as indicated by the urgency of the case, and complete information as to the reasons for transfer to another institution if necessary (including the alternatives to such a transfer)
8. Information about any relationship between the hospital and other health care or educational institutions, as far as it concerns his/her case, and about any professional relationships among individuals (by name) who are treating him/her
9. Knowledge of the hospital's proposals to conduct human experimentation affecting his/her case or treatment, and to refuse to participate in such research projects
10. Reasonable continuity of care (including knowledge of what appointment times and doctors are available, and where), and having the hospital inform him/her of what the health care requirements will be after discharge
11. Examination and explanation of the bill regardless of who is responsible for payment
12. Knowledge of what hospital rules and regulations apply to his/her conduct as a patient

Nursing Homes

The characteristics of a nursing home are as follows:

Residential care: Provision for room and board plus certain other services such as laundry, housekeeping, recreation

Personal care: Residential care plus aid with daily living activities such as dressing, bathing, and feeding

Nursing care: Residential care and personal care plus medical care by licensed medical personnel including the administration of medications for patients recovering from acute illness or suffering from chronic conditions

The above can be provided by either of the following:

Skilled nursing facility: Provision for medical and/or long-term care for the elderly

Intermediate care facility: Provision for long-term care for elderly not in need of extensive nursing/medical care

To identify a "good" nursing home, use Table 1.4 (U.S. Dept. Health and Human Services, 1973; Bay Area Comprehensive Health Planning Council, 1974; AMA, 1971).

Table 1.4 Guidelines for Nursing Home Evaluation

Administration

- ○ Has current license from state
- ○ Is certified eligible for participation in government and other financial programs
- ○ Publishes admission and discharge policies and lists charges for care, extra charges, and others
- ○ Administrator has current state license, is well qualified, and is courteous and helpful
- ○ Administrator is on call 24 hours a day for problems or emergencies
- ○ Administrator spends much time at the facility. Attitude toward staff and patients is warm, friendly, and considerate
- ○ Is accredited by JCAH

Physical considerations

Location:

- ○ Acceptable to patient
- ○ Convenient for physician
- ○ Convenient for visiting
- ○ Proximity to a hospital

Accident prevention and fire safety:

- ○ Well-lighted, sturdy stairs, free of hazards
- ○ Handrails in hallways and grab-bars in bathrooms
- ○ Meets federal and/or state fire codes
- ○ Exits clearly marked, unobstructed, doors unlocked on inside

Rooms, halls, lobby, grounds, kitchen:

- ○ Pleasant, colorful, homelike
- ○ Clean, accessible drinking fountains, fresh drinking water at beds
- ○ Comfortable chairs and other furniture
- ○ Outdoor sitting and walking areas available and used
- ○ Adequate space in bedrooms, reading lights, room for wheelchair to maneuver
- ○ Books, magazines, tables on which to write

Activity and special-purpose rooms:

- ○ Rooms available
- ○ Space for physical examination or therapy

Services

Medical:

- ○ Physician available in emergency
- ○ Private physician allowed
- ○ Maintenance of medical records
- ○ Thorough physical examination before or on admission
- ○ Freedom to purchase medicines outside the home
- ○ Arrangement with nearby hospital for transfer when necessary
- ○ Quality medical staff; medical attention and facilities for medical care available

Health Maintenance Organizations

○ Prepaid Group Practice.   Group of physicians provide services for a fixed per capita payment to a specific enrolled population.

Examples: Kaiser-Permanente Medical Care Program (California); Group Health Association of Washington, DC; Group Health Association of St. Paul; Group Health Association of Puget Sound; Harvard Community Health Plan; Georgetown University Community Health Plan; Ross-Loos (southern California)

○ *Fee-for-Service* Individual Practice.   Physician in private office offers combination package of fee-for-service/fixed monthly payment.

Examples: San Joaquin Foundation for Medical Care (California); Physicians Association of Clackamas County (Oregon); Comprecare (Colorado); Physicians Health Plan (Minnesota)

Table 1.4 *(Continued)*

Nursing:

- RN responsible for nursing staff in skilled nursing home
- Nurse(s) on duty day and night in skilled nursing home
- Trained nurses' aides and orderlies on duty in homes providing some nursing care
- Director of nurses or nurse in charge warm, friendly, informative, and helpful
- Friendly, considerate, responsible, efficient nurses and aides
- Nursing stations in good viewing positions, call lights remain unanswered only for brief periods of time

Rehabilitation:

- Specialists in physical therapy available when needed

Food:

- Menus for patients on special diets and for regular patients planned by dietitians
- Variety of appetizing and attractively served meals
- Meals served at normal times
- Served promptly and hot
- Attractive dining room; used by most patients able to do so
- Meals delivered to patients' rooms when necessary
- Help with eating when needed
- Availability of snacks
- Kitchen, cooking area, and foodservice staff neat and clean

Costs

- All services covered in basic daily charges; if not, list of specific services not covered available
- Advance payments returned if patient dies or leaves

Psychological and social considerations

- Attempt made to achieve compatibility of roommates
- Well-lighted; pleasant, cheerful attitudes and atmosphere
- Staff members courteous, respectful, show interest in patients
- Staff members respond quickly to calls for assistance
- Patients appear alert, active (unless ill), ambulatory, out of bed, communicating freely
- Activities director or someone responsible for planning patient activities to meet needs of patients
- Variety of recreational, cultural, crafts, and other activities for individuals and groups, with posted calendar
- Visiting hours set for convenience of residents and visitors
- Arrangements made for religious services; religious observance a matter of choice
- Active use of community volunteers
- Barbers and beauticians available
- Patients look well-groomed and generally show care received
- Adheres to nursing home Patient's Bill of Rights

○ **Primary Care Network.** All medical care is from or through referral of participating primary care (generalist) physician.

Examples: Wisconsin Physicians Service Health Maintenance Program; SAFECO of Seattle; Blue Shield's Comprehensive Health Care Program (Pennsylvania); Group Health Plan of Northeast Ohio

Note: As a dietetic technician in nutrition care, employment with an HMO or work in an institution which offers an alternative health care delivery system may be unavailable. As a practitioner and an employee, however, it is important that you familiarize yourself with the various health care plans currently available.

Clinics, Home Health Care, and Outreach Programs

- ○ Diet therapy
- ○ Nutrition support
- ○ Dietary supplements
- ○ Nutrition education

Examples: Planned parenthood clinic; neighborhood clinic; youth shelter; dental clinic; weight loss clinic; family counseling clinic; visiting nurses association; home health care agency; **elderly site feedings; meals-on-wheels;** mobile medical/dental service

elderly site feeding and **meals-on-wheels:** Nutrition outreach programs with fees on sliding scale provide nutritionally balanced and special diets planned by R.D.s as (1) congregate meals in group setting for socially isolated/financially deprived who are mobile and (2) home-delivered meals for the homebound/physically incapacitated.

Hospices

The estimated 75–105 hospice services now operating in this country—in the at-home, in-patient, or hospital/nursing home setting—should include the following considerations [from Cornacchia and Barrett (1985)]:

1. Care of the dying patient should be accomplished at home if possible and should include pain management, instruction of family in basic nursing care, diet, medicine, exercise, and emotional support until death and through bereavement. Inpatient care in a special facility should be arranged if home care is impractical.

2. The services available should be provided 24 hours daily, 7 days a week, under the supervision of a licensed physician in cooperation with a family member designated to be in charge. Hospice teams should include nurses, mental health specialists, therapists, social workers, chaplains, and volunteers.

3. Emphasis should be placed on preserving the quality of life until the end without the use of heroic efforts to maintain life artificially. This does not rule out surgery, chemical treatment, or x-ray treatment if the goal is mainly to relieve pain. The use of certain painkilling drugs sometimes withheld in hospitals because of institutional policy may be encouraged.

Note: Reimbursement for home health aides, physical therapists, nurses, and certain other services may be available under certain insurance coverage plans.

Evaluating a Health Care System

After examining the preceding materials, complete the questionnaire which follows. Discuss your answers with classmates or co-workers. Do you find that your own values and goals differ somewhat from those of your peers?

1. What are some of the ingredients you consider to be essential to the effectiveness of any health care system?

2. What are some of the characteristics of a "good" hospital, one where you would choose to work (or to be a patient)?

3. What are some of the characteristics of a "good" nursing home, one where you would choose to work (or to be a resident)?

4. As a dietetic technician, what do you think your responsibilities, if any, would be as an employee in an HMO? an out-patient clinic? a hospice? a home health care program? an outreach program?

5. Where would you prefer to work and why?

6. How do you think our changing health care system will alter your future as a dietetic technician? as a potential patient/client/resident?

STEP 9: CAREER FIELD TRIPS

As a dietetic technician, you can apply your skills to a variety of opportunities for providing effective nutrition care. Depending on your physical location and the specific jobs available in your area, the various job options will have different pros and cons to be considered. Therefore, it is a wise idea to explore as many potential career paths as possible in order to determine your own individual preference and needs.

You would benefit from reading some of the pamphlets listed under Suggested Readings on a Dietetic Career and then selecting from the various field experiences available in your area (see lists that follow) and arranging to visit several of them. You should go with classmates or co-workers, schedule an appointment with dietetics staff member(s) at each site, and prepare a list of pertinent questions to ask during your visit. It is important for you to realize that a brief visit to a possible employment site cannot show you the full scope of an actual position as a dietetic technician there. Yet, it is usually both inspiring and enlightening to tour potential job sites in order that you may better visualize your future as a dietetic technician in nutrition care.

Clinical Care Field Experiences

Try to visit the dietetics department at one or more of the following sites:

○ Specialty research hospital (e.g., cancer center, diabetes center, metabolic research center)
○ Small community hospital
○ Veterans Administration hospital
○ Mental health institution
○ Pediatrics hospital
○ Long-term care facility (e.g., nursing home, extended care facility, prison)
○ Short-term facility (e.g., drug or alcohol detoxification center, hospice, detention center)

Make a list of questions to ask dietetics personnel.

1. _____

2. _____

3. _____

4. _____

5. _____

6. _____

7. _____

8. _____

9. _____

10. _____

Note: It is beneficial to arrange to meet with the foodservice director(s) to discuss diet aide/tray line duties and requirements. Also, try to meet with the director of nursing to discuss the duties of specialty teams within the institution (e.g., **TPN, ICU,** and **CCU**).

TPN: Total parenteral nutrition, or provision of total caloric and nutrient needs by intravenous route in those patients unable to take food orally.

ICU: Intensive care unit, used for continuous monitoring of patients with acute illnesses.

CCU: Coronary care unit, used for continuous monitoring of patients with acute cardiac disease.

Community Care Field Experiences

Try to visit one or more of the following sites:

○ Out-patient nutrition clinic (associated with HMO, hospital, doctors' office, public health agency, etc.)
○ Child nutrition program (**WIC,** day care, school foodservice, etc.)
○ Consumer health agency (**extension service** or **voluntary health agency** such as local chapters of the American Heart Association or American Diabetes Association)
○ Outreach nutrition program (for migrant agricultural workers, Indians, rural health education, etc.)

Make a list of questions to ask dietetics personnel.

1. _____

2. _____

3. _____

4. _____

5. _____

WIC (Women, Infants, Children): A federally supported funding program to provide nutrition services and supplemental food supplies to needy infants, children, pregnant women, and nursing mothers.

extension service: Nonprofit service agency associated with a department of agriculture (at federal, state, local, or university level) which provides consumer education and aid in various areas of concern.

voluntary health agency: Nonprofit organization which provides free information and aid in general or specific areas of health/ illness.

Alternative Field Experiences

Try to visit any of the following sites which may interest you:

○ **Metabolic unit** of a research center
○ Foodservice department of a school or college
○ Food research laboratory
○ Food industry which offers nutrition information for consumers
○ Nutrition-oriented public relations firm or private nutrition consulting company

Make a list of questions to ask dietetics personnel.

1. _____

2. _____

3. _____

4. _____

5. _____

metabolic unit: Specialized laboratory where metabolic balance studies are conducted by properly trained personnel on foods, diets, and nutritional/clinical relationships.

After visiting each of the job sites you have selected, prepare a brief report of your observations, the responses to your questions, and your overall reflections. Retain this for later referral during all fieldwork training, job searches, and placements in the field.

Suggested Readings on a Dietetic Career

AMERICAN DIETETIC ASSOCIATION (216 West Jackson Boulevard, Chicago, IL 60606) pamphlets available:

1977a. Essentials for coordinated undergraduate programs in dietetics.
1977b. Essentials of a dietetic assistant program.
1977c. Essentials of a dietetic technician program.
1980a. Be a dietitian.
1980b. Careers in dietetics.

1980c. Code of professional practice.
1980d. Dietetic internship post-baccalaureate essentials.
1980e. The dietitian.
1980f. Dietitians: The professionals in nutrition care.
1988. Dietetic technician: A dietetic professional

AMERICAN DIETETIC ASSOCIATION. 1981. Definitions: Dietetic technician and dietetic assistant. ADA Courier 20, Jul./Aug., 9.

AMERICAN DIETETIC ASSOCIATION COUNCIL ON PRACTICE CONTINUING EDUCATION COMMITTEE. 1988. Continuing education: Keeping pace with the changing scene. J. Am. Dietet. Assoc. 88, Oct., 1224.

BOBENG, B. 1986. Results of the 1985 dietetic needs assessment survey. J. Am. Dietet. Assoc. 86, May, 672.

HAUPTSCHEIN-RAPHAEL, M., et al. 1988. On-the-job training of clinical nutrition personnel to promote career mobility in the department. J. Am. Dietet. Assoc. 88, Sept., 1098.

KANE, J. 1987. Exploring Careers in Dietetics and Nutrition. New York: Rosen Publishing Group.

KLINE, A., and DOWLING, W. 1972. Delegation of duties to hospital dietary supportive personnel. J. Am. Dietet. Assoc. 60, Mar., 201.

LANZ, S. 1983. Introduction to the Profession of Dietetics. Philadelphia: Lea & Febiger.

LUMSDEN, J., et al. 1976. Delegation of functions by dietitians to dietetic technicians. J. Am. Dietet. Assoc. 69, Aug., 143.

SAYERS, S. 1986. Creating images of the future: A simulation game for dietetics students. J. Am. Dietet. Assoc. 86, Aug., 1052.

SIMONIS, P., SPEARS, M., and VADEN, A. 1983. Dietetic technicians' performance. J. Am. Dietet. Assoc. 82, Mar., 271.

WILLIAMS, C. 1977. Dietetic assistant/technician education, I: Historical background. J. Am. Dietet. Assoc. 70, Jan., 621.

STEP 10: SELF-CONFIDENCE CHECKLIST

In order to function as a contributing member of the health care team, it is important for you to be able to communicate effectively. Allied health professionals need to share their expertise with physicians and nurses. This leads to a cooperative effort which can prove beneficial to the patients' overall health care. It is essential for you to be able to participate freely in the patient care process and to be confident regarding your competence as a dietetic technician.

Table 1.5   Dietetic Technician Self-Confidence Checklist[a]

I am confident in my own ability to:	Often	Sometimes	Never
1. identify those at nutritional risk.	○	○	○
2. collect and calculate the data required for nutritional assessment.	○	○	○
3. help to develop nutrition care plans.	○	○	○
4. help to implement nutrition care plans.	○	○	○
5. monitor and evaluate the effect of nutrition intervention.	○	○	○
6. assess patient food acceptance.	○	○	○
7. provide effective nutrition education/diet counseling.	○	○	○
8. assist dietitian(s) to provide direct nutrition services to patients.	○	○	○
9. assist dietitian(s) to solve nutrition problems of individual patients.	○	○	○
10. coordinate patient nutrition care with other health services.	○	○	○
11. coordinate patient nutrition care with institutional foodservice activities.	○	○	○
12. acquire and utilize available special food products.	○	○	○
13. acquire and utilize available dietary supplements.	○	○	○
14. supervise diet clerks.	○	○	○
15. supervise other foodservice personnel.	○	○	○
16. develop and implement in-service education.	○	○	○
17. direct co-workers/patients to reliable sources of nutrition information/aid.	○	○	○
18. accept direct supervision from registered dietitian(s).	○	○	○
19. continue to update nutrition knowledge.	○	○	○
20. maintain the standards of technical dietetic practice.	○	○	○

[a]Based on ADA (1981) competencies for entry level dietetic technicians in clinical nutrition.

Self-confidence is built on knowledge and self-respect. Once you have a good working knowledge of your area of expertise (nutrition care) and are practiced in the art of disseminating required information (nutrition education and diet counseling), you should develop an overriding sense of trust in your own job capabilities. Of course, there will arise occasional periods of apprehension and/or personality conflicts inevitable within any working situation, but self-reliance and the ability to share with other health professionals should work to overshadow such temporary incidents. In fact, your self-confidence should be built in part upon your own belief that you will be able to properly handle the incidental and challenging circumstances which confront you as a practicing dietetic technician. It is also essential for you to be able to recognize your own limitations, and to handle these effectively as well.

Rate your current level of self-confidence by using the checklist. (Table 1.5). Later on, as you acquire more experience, fill out the checklist again in order to determine whether your self-confidence has grown. You should discover that practice, experience, and education will contribute to your ever-expanding equanimity as a skilled and competent dietetic technician.

STEP 11: POST-TEST ON YOUR ROLE

Select the best answer for each of the multiple-choice questions to evaluate your understanding of the information and learning experiences provided in Chapter 1. Answers are provided in the Answer Key at the end of the book. Have you developed a clearer conception of your role as a dietetic technician?

_____ 1. As a dietetic technician, it would be incompetent behavior for you to
(a) discontinue nutrition self-education upon completion of the dietetic technician training program. (b) smoke cigarettes in patient's view (or at all). (c) allow personal feelings to disrupt communication with another member of the health care team. (d) all of these.

_____ 2. At the inter-professional level, the dietetic technician is responsible for
(a) meeting with other members of the health care team. (b) supervising diet clerks. (c) developing an in-service program for diet clerks. (d) all of these.

_____ 3. The diet clerk is responsible for
(a) tally of patient diet census. (b) distribution and collection of menu forms to patients. (c) notation of orders for diet changes. (d) all of these.

_____ 4. The dietetic technician requires the supervision of a dietitian in planning the diets of high risk patients.
(a) True. (b) False.

_____ 5. It is an appropriate responsibility of the dietetic technician in nutrition care to
(a) know the performance standards for clinical dietetic personnel. (b) contact legislative personnel regarding nutrition-related issues. (c) know the goals of the health care facility where employed. (d) all of these.

_____ 6. As a dietetic technician in nutrition care, you might be responsible for community nutrition projects that could include helping dietitian(s) to
(a) develop a poster display on well-balanced dining. (b) conduct a workshop on weight control. (c) contact a local WIC (Women, Infants, Children) program regarding a pregnant client. (d) all of these.

_____ 7. "Patient is in need of an increase in the total amount of daily calories allowed on the prescribed weight reduction diet plan" is an example of
(a) a subjective notation you might make in the chart. (b) an objective notation you might make in the chart. (c) an assessment you might note in the chart. (d) a plan you might note in the chart.

_____ 8. "Patient has lost 5 lbs since the start of a weight reduction plan on 1/3/9X" is an example of
(a) a subjective notation you might make in the chart. (b) an objective notation you might make in the chart. (c) an assessment you might note in the chart. (d) a plan you might note in the chart.

_____ 9. "The patient complained of continued hunger following her luncheon meal" is an example of
(a) a subjective notation you might make in the chart. (b) an objective notation you might make in the chart. (c) an assessment you might note in the chart. (d) a plan you might note in the chart.
_____ 10. "Suggest to dietitian and/or patient's physician that caloric allowance be altered to 1200 calories per day" is an example of
(a) a subjective notation you might make in the chart. (b) an objective notation you might make in the chart. (c) an assessment you might note in the chart. (d) a plan you might note in the chart.
_____ 11. A psychologist and a psychiatrist have the same educational requirements.
(a) True. (b) False.
_____ 12. A physician who specializes in treatment of the obese is a(n)
(a) obstetrician. (b) nutritionist. (c) bariatrician. (d) dietitian.
_____ 13. A general hospital can
(a) be owned by an individual or organization. (b) provide medical diagnosis and treatment. (c) provide surgical treatment. (d) all of these.
_____ 14. The HMO is the commission responsible for the accreditation of hospitals and other health care facilities.
(a) True. (b) False.
_____ 15. As a dietetic technician in a weight loss clinic, your responsibilities would include
(a) prescribing vitamin/mineral supplements. (b) distributing printed diet sheets for a 350-calorie weight loss plan. (c) assisting the dietitian to plan menus and counsel clients. (d) all of these.

REFERENCES

AMERICAN DIETETIC ASSOCIATION. 1981. Role Delineation for Entry Level Clinical Dietetics 1980. Chicago: ADA.
AMERICAN DIETETIC ASSOCIATION. 1982. Role of the dietetic technician in clinical dietetics. J. Am. Dietet. Assoc. _80_, Mar., 259.
AMERICAN DIETETIC ASSOCIATION. 1985. Standards of Professional Responsibility of the American Dietetic Association. Chicago: ADA.
AMERICAN HOSPITAL ASSOCIATION. 1971. JCAH Standards of Quality Care for Hospitals. Chicago: AHA.
AMERICAN HOSPITAL ASSOCIATION. 1976. Recording Nutrition Information in Medical Records, Technical Advisory Bulletin No. T0153M-2/81-7410. Chicago: AHA.
AMERICAN MEDICAL ASSOCIATION. 1971. What to Look for in a Nursing Home. Chicago: AMA.
BAY AREA COMPREHENSIVE HEALTH PLANNING COUNCIL. 1974. Shoppers Guide to Nursing Homes in the San Francisco Bay Area. San Francisco: The BAHP Council.
CHAPPELLE, M., and SCHOLL, R. 1973. Adapting the problem-oriented medical record to the psychiatric hospital. J. Am. Dietet. Assoc. _63_, Dec., 643.
CONNIFF, J. 1973. How to tell a good hospital from a bad one. Today's Health, Nov., 71.
CORNACCHIA, H., and BARRETT, S. 1985. Consumer Health, 3rd Edition. St. Louis, MO: C. V. Mosby Co.
HORGAN, R. 1988. Summary of Dietetic Competencies of the Graduates of Labouré. Dorchester, MA: Labouré College.
U.S. DEPARTMENT OF HEALTH AND HUMAN SERVICES. 1973. Nursing Home Care. Washington, D.C.: Government Printing Office.
VOYTOVICH, A. 1973. The dietitian/nutritionist and the problem-oriented medical record, I: A physician's viewpoint. J. Am. Dietet. Assoc. _63_, Dec., 639.
WALTERS, F., and DEMARCO, M. 1973. The dietitian/nutritionist and the problem-oriented medical record, II: The role of the dietitian. J. Am. Dietet. Assoc. _63_, Dec., 641.

Chapter Two

You Are What You Eat

CHAPTER BLUEPRINT

Step 1: Take the Pre-test on Your Eating Habits to begin reflecting on your own food habits and beliefs.

Step 2: Complete the brief Medical History Assessment for a classmate or co-worker and identify any nutrition-related medical problems.

Step 3: Give a 24-Hour Recall to a classmate or co-worker and discuss your individual dietary intakes.

Step 4: Maintain a Food Diary for a week and answer the questionnaire about your food habits.

Step 5: Complete the Food Dislikes List and participate in the assigned group activity.

Step 6: Complete the Food Likes List and participate in the assigned group activity.

Step 7: Complete the Eating Behaviors Questionnaire and use the accompanying chart to determine your Reasonable Weight.

Step 8: Complete the Lifestyle Questionnaire, Foods from Different Cultures checklist, and the accompanying assignment.

Step 9: Begin to uncover your current nutrition knowledge by completing the questionnaire about your nutrition education background and the rest of the Post-test on Nutrition IQ.

Step 10: Compare the desired answers for the Pre-test (a Retake) on Your Eating Habits to your own, and participate in the assigned group discussion.

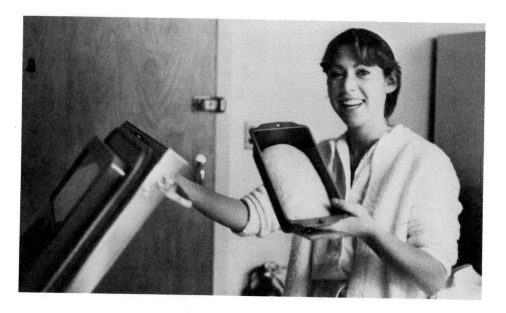

STEP 1: PRE-TEST ON YOUR EATING HABITS

In order to educate others effectively about balancing their diets and obtaining the 50 or so nutrients essential to good health, it is important for you to be able to optimize your own nutritional intake. It is also essential (as mentioned in Chapter 1, Step 2: Summary of Competencies) that your lifestyle reflects that which you recommend: healthy dietetic technicians tend to have a better chance at optimizing the lifestyle patterns of their patients than do their less health-conscious peers. After all, you would probably be more apt to respect the counsel of a nonsmoking physician who jogs regularly, a dentist with sparkling white teeth, and a financially successful tax advisor than the advice of professionals who appear not to practice what they preach.

How would you rate the nutritional status of *your* current diet? Is it varied and well balanced, or repetitive and nutritionally inadequate? There are approximately 10,000–20,000 different items offered in today's typical supermarket. With so many food products to choose from, it is relatively easy to build a varied, well-balanced diet for yourself—and to teach others how to do the same.

Diet History

In each statement below, insert the number which most closely approximates your typical dietary habits.

1. I usually include ____ servings of whole grain or enriched cereal, bread, pasta, rice, or other grains every *day*.
2. I usually include ____ servings of oranges, grapefruit, tomatoes, or their juices every *day*.
3. I usually include ____ servings of dark green leafy vegetables (collard greens, kale, mustard greens, spinach, Swiss chard, etc.) or bright yellow fruits or vegetables (carrots, pumpkin, squash, apricots, etc.) each *week*.
4. I usually include ____ servings of other fruits and vegetables every *day*.
5. I usually drink ____ cups of milk (include milk on breakfast cereals) every *day*; I eat ____ servings of cheese *daily*; I eat ____ cups of yogurt each *day*.
6. I usually include ____ servings of meat, poultry, or fish every *day*; I eat ____ eggs each *week*; I eat ____ cups of dried beans or peas (blackeye peas, cowpeas, lentils, navy beans, pea beans, etc.) each *week*.
7. I usually include ____ servings of one or more of the following each *week:* cake, candy, cookies, donuts, jam or jelly, gum, pastries, pies, soft drinks, sugar, syrups.
8. I usually include ____ servings of one or more of the following each *week:* chips, crackers, dips, dried or smoked meats, salted nuts, pickles, pretzels.
9. I usually drink ____ glasses of beer and ____ glasses of wine each *week*.
____ 10. I consider my own diet to be
(a) well balanced and varied. (b) unbalanced. (c) repetitive. (d) generally poor.

For each of the following statements, indicate whether in your case it is usually true (T) or false (F):

____ 11. I tend to avoid certain foods because they look or smell unappealing.
____ 12. I rarely attempt to try new foods.
____ 13. I rarely skip meals.
____ 14. I often attempt the latest "crash" weight loss diet.
____ 15. My lifestyle (school, socializing, homelife, etc.) has a negative effect on my diet.
____ 16. My culture, religion, and/or ethnic background has a negative effect on my diet.
____ 17. Food advertisements (e.g., magazines, newspapers, billboards, television, radio, store displays) greatly influence my food selections.
____ 18. Many food advertisements seem nutritionally misleading to me.
____ 19. Nutrition should be an integral component of educational programs beginning at the pre-school level.
____ 20. Eating should provide pleasure as well as nutrition.

STEP 2: MEDICAL HISTORY ASSESSMENT

As a practicing dietetic technician, obtaining a patient's medical history is an important aspect of your role. There are some specific medical questions you will need to have answered—either by the information provided in the patients' medical charts or by the patients themselves—in order to make a complete nutritional assessment and prepare the appropriate diet plan.

Modified diets are based on the physical, clinical, laboratory, and historical data which influence nutritional status and needs. Parts III and IV provide the medical history assessment forms for those requiring some of the most common modified diets. Even those following "normal" diet plans may require dietary alterations in order to optimize their nutritional status and overall health. As the technician with nutrition expertise, you may identify individuals with medical disorders requiring dietary care. It is important to develop your technical skills in acquiring informative medical assessments and reporting them to the health care team.

Select a partner (classmate or co-worker) to provide you with the information required to complete the following Medical History Form. Your partner may then use the same form to record your medical history. Are there any medical abnormalities that may require nutrition intervention? Report your findings to your peers as you would report the pertinent medical history information to the appropriate member(s) of your health care team.

Medical History Form

A.　Personal information:

Date _____　Reason for consult _____
Name _____
Address _____
Phone no. _____　Occupation _____
Education _____　Religion _____
Date of birth _____　Birthplace _____
Sex _____　Marital status _____
Physician _____
Address _____
Phone no. _____　Date of last check-up _____

B.　Medical background[a]

1.　Indicate ⊘ if patient has or has recently experienced any of the following on a frequent basis:

- ○ Nausea and/or vomiting
- ○ Loss of appetite
- ○ Pain or distress after eating
- ○ Unexplained weight loss (of 10 lb or more during the past month)
- ○ Need to urinate during the night
- ○ Excessive thirst
- ○ Excessive hunger
- ○ Periods of dizziness, weakness, and lightheadedness

- ○ Chronic fatigue
- ○ Constipation
- ○ Diarrhea
- ○ Alternating constipation and diarrhea
- ○ Black or bloody **stools**
- ○ Swelling in extremities
- ○ Painful, swollen joints
- ○ Undesirable weight gain

stool: Feces; body wastes discharged from the intestines.

[a]Note: If any of the answers to Part B are checked, you should inform patient's physician immediately; in the classroom/peer situation, if there is a ⊘, your partner should discuss the problem with his/her physician if he/she has not already done so.

2. Indicate ⊘ if patient has ever had any of the following disorders diagnosed by a physician:
   ○ Gastric, duodenal, or peptic **ulcer**
   ○ Gallbladder disorder
   ○ **Cancer** of the stomach, small intestine, colon, or breast
   ○ Sugar in the urine
   ○ High blood sugar
   ○ Diabetes
   ○ Anorexia nervosa
   ○ **Anemia**
   ○ **Lactose intolerance**
   ○ **Spastic colon** ("colitis," ulcerative colitis, Crohn's disease) or **diverticulitis**
   ○ High blood pressure
   ○ Decreased kidney function
   ○ Elevated blood **cholesterol** level
   ○ Elevated blood level of **triglycerides**
   ○ Arthritis
   ○ Obesity
   ○ **Thyroid** dysfunction

3. Indicate ⊘ if anyone in patient's immediate family now or in the past has been diagnosed as suffering from any of the following disorders:
   ○ Cancer
   ○ Diabetes
   ○ Lactose intolerance
   ○ Hypertension (high blood pressure)
   ○ Elevated blood level of cholesterol and/or triglycerides
   ○ Thyroid dysfunction
   ○ Obesity

C. Pertinent clinical data (Describe any visible abnormalities.):

Skin _____ Mouth _____
Hair _____ Eyes _____
Teeth _____ Other: _____

D. Other pertinent information:

Medications _____
Vitamin/mineral supplements _____
Height ____ Weight ____ Frame ____ Triceps skinfold thickness ____
Reasonable weight (See Reasonable Weight Chart, Table 2.1 in Step 7.) ____
Lab test results _____
Recent hospitalization(s) _____

STEP 3: 24-HOUR RECALL

In order to obtain a general picture of each patient's typical dietary intake, the dietetic technician can employ an evaluative tool called the 24-hour recall. By examining the dietary intake and associated behaviors for one 24-hour period, you can pinpoint some of the individual areas requiring dietary change. You can also help your patients to identify some of their personal dietary strengths and weaknesses, and show them how to maintain their own diet diaries.

To practice the technique of collecting diet-related information from others, select a classmate or co-worker to act as your patient. Ask your "patient" to recall everything consumed (solid or liquid) over the past 24 hours, starting with the last item entering the mouth. (For example, if the last item eaten was a midmorning snack, have your "patient" complete the recall for everything consumed during the time period from this most recent intake to the previous day at midmorning.) Also record the estimated amounts (if the "patient" cannot guesstimate in ounces or cups, try to determine the approximate amount in handfuls, bowlfuls, or by using food models), the date and time of consumption, and information to describe where, with whom, and associated activities. Your "patient" may then

---

ulcer: A localized defect on the lining of the mucosal surface; *peptic* ulcer, a term commonly used, refers to an ulcer of the inner wall of the stomach lining (gastric) or of the upper portion of the small intestine (duodenal) caused by acidic gastric juices.

cancer: Disease characterized by abnormal unregulated cell growth due to various and unknown factors.

anemia: A deficiency in blood quality and/or quantity which occurs as a symptom of various diseases.

lactose intolerance: Disorder characterized by the lack of an enzyme which breaks down lactose (milk sugar), resulting in cramps and diarrhea upon intake of lactose-containing foodstuffs.

spastic colon ("colitis," ulcerative colitis, Crohn's disease): Inflammation of the lower section of the large intestine characterized by cramps, constipation, or diarrhea, often caused by stress. Crohn's disease extends through the entire intestinal wall and may require surgical intervention.

diverticulitis: Inflammation of small pouches formed along the wall and lining of the colon, causing painful abdominal cramps.

cholesterol: A waxy fatlike substance manufactured by the liver and present in all foods of animal origin. Amount in diet may affect level in blood and lead to a buildup of fatty deposits in the arteries.

triglycerides: Most common form of fat in the diet and the usual storage form of fats in the body; excessive blood levels have been implicated in heart disease.

thyroid: Endocrine gland located in the neck which stores iodine and produces hormones required for growth and metabolism. Enlargement is called a goiter.

assume the dietetic technician role to obtain a 24-hour recall from you. Discuss your individual dietary intakes and associated behaviors with your peers. Do you consider your recall data to be typical of your own particular eating habits? Do you see any areas requiring dietary change? Could you now maintain a similar record for a period of a week?

24-Hour Recall Form

Date and time (over 24-hr period)	Food and amount	Where eaten[a]	Eaten with whom[b]	Associated activity[c]

[a]For example, at the kitchen table, at home—sitting at a desk, in a car, or at a restaurant.
[b]For example, with parents, friend(s), or a date.
[c]For example, while studying, driving, talking, or watching TV.

STEP 4: FOOD DIARY

Do you really know your own typical daily eating habits, meal patterns, and diet-related emotions? In order for you to be able to evaluate effectively the dietary behaviors of others, it is important for you first to examine your own. Perhaps *your* diet will need some alterations.

Before Record-Keeping

Before you begin your record-keeping, reflect on the questions below and answer each as honestly as possible. Discuss with your classmates or co-workers all of the individual influences on your dietary habits and eating patterns. Determine those influences which have undesirable results, and discuss possible methods for change.

Dietary Habits Questionnaire

1. Do you normally eat "health" foods? ____ "dietetic" foods? ____ convenience foods? ____ If so, list some examples: _____
2. Do you take vitamin/mineral supplements? _____ If so, indicate types, amounts, and reasons: _____
3. List any cultural/religious dietary practices: _____
4. Do you eat at regular meal times? ____ How many meals are eaten per day? ____ Do you snack regularly? ____ How many snacks are eaten per day? ____
5. Have you recently changed your usual food intake or intake pattern? ____ If so, indicate how and why: _____
6. Do you have any problems with food preparation or storage? ____ If so, explain (i.e., inadequate refrigerator or freezer space, lack of functioning range or oven): _____
7. Who is responsible for food purchase? _____ Preparation? _____ Menu planning? _____
8. For how long do you normally store fresh fruits/vegetables? _____
9. Do you normally boil vegetables? ____ In how much water? _____ For how long? _____
10. Do you include fried foods (e.g., fried seafood, meats, vegetables, or potatoes) in your diet? ____ How often? _____

11. How many meals per week do you eat away from home? _____
    Where? _____
12. List any physical activities routinely engaged in: _____
    Indicate type(s) and frequency: _____
13. List any hobbies/recreational activities: _____

Although it is generally understood that food records are not the most accurate reflections of nutritional intake, they can provide some insight into general eating habits and dietary patterns. Accuracy can be improved by recording each item consumed immediately after intake; trying to recall everything eaten and the approximate quantities at the end of the day or the next morning often results in major omissions and errors. And as you may have already learned from Step 3, it can be rather difficult to recall accurately a detailed food intake for a previous 24-hour period. Patients maintaining a food diary should therefore be encouraged to carry it with them at all times.

Not only can carefully maintained food diaries provide you and your patients with an overview of their diets, but the act of maintaining such records usually alerts patients to their food intake behaviors *as they occur.* In keeping the Food Diary for the next 7 days, you may notice how conscious you become of every morsel you put into your mouth. You may even find that you cut back your food intake, or select more of the nutrient-rich foods. Try not to alter your usual eating behaviors for the next week, but you will find it difficult to ignore the eating self-consciousness which accompanies food record-keeping.

In order to provide the space you need to maintain an accurate Food Diary for the next 7 days, copy the form onto seven or more sheets of notebook paper. Be sure to leave yourself plenty of room for comments. Recall the date and time of every meal and snack, all foods eaten and approximate amounts, plus the eating location, presence of others, and associated emotions; you may find that you are a fast eater, or that you often eat for emotional reasons rather than physical hunger. Be honest in recording your food intake and associated reflections. Insight is essential to improvement—for your own diet and for those of your patients.

After maintaining your Food Diary for seven consecutive days, you can take the Pretest on What You Eat in Chapter 3 to evaluate your own dietary habits. You may be surprised at the insight you will be able to gain into your own individual food-related behaviors. Do you think you will be able to assist others in gaining such insight?

Food Diary

Date and time (over 7-day period)	Duration of meal/snack (min)	Food and amount	Where eaten[a]	With whom[b]	Associated activity[c]	Associated emotions and comments[d]

[a]For example, at the kitchen table, at home—sitting at a desk, in a car, or at a restaurant.
[b]For example, with parents, friend(s), or a date.
[c]For example, while studying, driving, talking, or watching TV.
[d]For example, bored, tired, angry, frustrated, not hungry but food looked good, or ravenous.

STEP 5: FOOD DISLIKES LIST

Many of your patients will require assistance in the menu selection process. Ill patients may be suffering from appetite loss, yet still need special attention to their nutritional status, and possibly even a significantly increased intake of certain nutrients. Thus, it is especially important that you learn either to overcome or disguise your own food biases.

Do you avoid certain foods because they look unappealing? Do you often refuse to eat something if you have never tasted it before? In the Food Dislikes Chart, list ten of your *least* favorite foods. Indicate ⊘ whether each item is something that you (1) dislike intensely and rarely eat, if ever, or (2) simply avoid, for various reasons.

If possible, explain your reasons for disliking or avoiding these foods. A few samples have been illustrated for you in the Sample Food Dislikes Chart. You may have difficulty listing as many as ten foods which you dislike—some of us like everything as long as it is edible.

Sample Food Dislikes Chart

| Food Dislikes | Degree of Dislike √ | | Reasons/Comments |
	Dislike	Avoid	
1. Liver		√	Looks unappetizing
2. Fish		√	Smells unpleasant
3. Mexican food	√		Too spicy and hot
4. Lima beans	√		Texture is gross
5. Milk		√	Causes gastric distress

Food Dislikes Chart

| Food Dislikes | Degree of Dislike √ | | Reasons/Comments |
	Dislike	Avoid	
1.			
2.			
3.			
4.			
5.			
6.			
7.			
8.			
9.			
10.			

Have you ever tried any of the items you listed under Avoid? How long has it been since you sampled any of the items you listed under Dislike?

Compare your own list to those of your classmates or co-workers. Are there some food complaints that a number of you have in common? Prepare a meal based around several of those items that a majority of your peers tend to avoid. Include products that some of you have never tasted before. Assign one item for each dietetic technician to prepare and/or bring in, and provide the moral support needed by your peers so that everyone samples everything. Hopefully, your peers will provide the support *you* need to sample some of your own personal food dislikes.

Every individual has different tastes in life, including tastes for food. In making food choices and planning diets, it is important to consider individual tastes and distastes. With the wide variety of foods available to us, why miss out on potential favorites, new tastes, and flavor experiences? Keep an open mind, and open your mouth to new food experiences. Your openness will be transferred to your patients—as long as you encourage them to experiment for their own taste enjoyment instead of forcing them to eat what is supposed to be "good" for them. After all, do *you* enjoy eating only what is supposed to be "good" for you?

STEP 6: FOOD LIKES LIST

In order to compare your *food dislikes list* with the foods you really like to eat, complete the Food Likes Chart. List ten of your favorite foods and indicate approximately how often you eat each item (e.g., daily, weekly, 2–3 times per month, once a year). A few samples have been supplied for you in the Sample Food Likes Chart.

Sample Food Likes Chart

Food likes	Frequency of consumption
1. Ice cream	Weekly (in the summer)
2. McDonald's burgers	Weekly
3. Pizza	2 times per week
4. Beer	Weekends
5. Lobster	2–3 times a year (in the summer)

Food Likes Chart

Food likes	Frequency of consumption
1.	
2.	
3.	
4.	
5.	
6.	
7.	
8.	
9.	
10.	

Discuss your list with classmates or co-workers. Are there a number of food favorites which many of you share? Prepare a meal based around several of the more popular fare. Assign one item for each dietetic technician to prepare and bring in. Remember, alcoholic beverages may be considered the favorite "foods" for some, but their consumption may not be allowed in your classroom or workplace.

STEP 7: EATING BEHAVIORS AND REASONABLE WEIGHT

In assessing the dietary patterns of others, it will be common for you to encounter specific eating behaviors which lead to faulty dietary habits. It is currently estimated that over one-third of the American population is overweight—and this "figure" is growing "fatter" every year. The majority of persons with weight problems can attribute their excess poundage to faulty dietary behaviors. This particular dietary disorder will be discussed in detail in Chapter 10.

A significant aspect of your role as a practicing dietetic technician in nutrition care is to provide diet counseling. Since a sizable percentage of your patients suffer from weight problems, you need to be able to counsel them effectively in the area of eating behavior modification. It is therefore essential that you first familiarize yourself with your own eating behaviors, particularly those which may be undesirable and/or contributory to a weight problem. If you *are* overweight, you might want to begin immediately on a reputable weight reduction program. Maintenance of a **reasonable weight** (see Table 2.1) can contribute to your credibility as a dietetic technician while improving your overall health and self-esteem. (See Chapter 10 for further direction and references.)

reasonable weight: That weight at which most people will live the longest, as determined by insurance actuarial data.

Table 2.1 Reasonable Weight Chart[a]

Height (without shoes)	Weight (without clothing)		Height (without shoes)	Weight (without clothing)	
	Normal range	Obesity level		Normal range	Obesity level
Men			Women		
5 ft 3 in.	118–141	169	5 ft 0 in.	100–118	142
5 ft 4 in.	122–145	174	5 ft 1 in.	104–121	145
5 ft 5 in.	126–149	179	5 ft 2 in.	107–125	150
5 ft 6 in.	130–155	187	5 ft 3 in.	110–128	154
5 ft 7 in.	134–161	193	5 ft 4 in.	113–132	158
5 ft 8 in.	139–166	199	5 ft 5 in.	116–135	162
5 ft 9 in.	143–170	204	5 ft 6 in.	120–139	167
5 ft 10 in.	147–174	209	5 ft 7 in.	123–142	170
5 ft 11 in.	150–178	214	5 ft 8 in.	126–146	175
6 ft 0 in.	154–183	220	5 ft 9 in.	130–151	181
6 ft 1 in.	158–188	226	5 ft 10 in.	133–156	187
6 ft 2 in.	162–192	230	5 ft 11 in.	137–161	193
6 ft 3 in.	165–195	234	6 ft 0 in.	141–166	199

[a]For persons 20 years and older, as adapted from USDA (1960).

Answer the questions in the following chart as honestly as you can, and utilize the weight tables to determine your current body weight status. If several of your classmates or co-workers are overweight, you may want to form a weight loss support group or join a local reputable weight loss program together. Even if you find that your current weight is within the acceptable range, you may identify certain eating behaviors which need to be altered. As a dietetic technician, you are certainly not expected to have "perfect" dietary habits, merely eating behaviors deserving of respect. In the following Eating Behaviors Questionnaire, indicate ⊘ the answer for each of the following questions which is most applicable to your own behaviors. (You may want to examine your charts from Steps 3 and 4 in this chapter to assist you in answering these questions as accurately as possible.)

Eating Behaviors Questionnaire

calorie: A unit of measurement of heat [1 calorie = the amount of heat required to raise 1 kg (kilogram) of water 1°C (centigrade)] used to express the energy value of food.

fats: Solid or liquid compounds abundant in meats and dairy products which yield 9 calories per gram and act as a storage form of energy in the body.

Always	Usually	Rarely		Do you tend to
○	○	○	1.	Moderate your intake of foods high in **calories**?
○	○	○	2.	Moderate your intake of foods high in calories but with little nutrient value?
○	○	○	3.	Moderate your intake of foods high in **fat**?
○	○	○	4.	Moderate your intake of alcoholic beverages (not more than one or two drinks per day)?
○	○	○	5.	Eat moderate portion sizes of food?
○	○	○	6.	Avoid taking seconds or thirds or more helpings of food?
○	○	○	7.	Know those foods or beverages which tempt you to overindulge?
○	○	○	8.	Avoid overindulgences on holidays and when dining out?
○	○	○	9.	Avoid all-you-can-eat restaurants and other situations which encourage overindulging?
○	○	○	10.	Buy and prepare only the quantity of food required, in order to avoid leftovers?
○	○	○	11.	Plan meal contents ahead of time and adhere to a shopping list?
○	○	○	12.	Read labels carefully when food shopping?
○	○	○	13.	Avoid buying sweets and tempting high-fat snack-foods?
○	○	○	14.	Avoid eating when not physically hungry (i.e., you do not eat according to the clock)?
○	○	○	15.	Avoid unconscious nibbling (e.g., after meals, during meal preparation, or while watching TV)?
○	○	○	16.	Avoid indulging in activities other than eating during food consumption?
○	○	○	17.	Avoid substituting food for less desirable activities (e.g., homework, housework, or errands)?
○	○	○	18.	Deal with boredom in ways other than food consumption?
○	○	○	19.	Deal with anger in ways other than food consumption?
○	○	○	20.	Deal with anxiety or stress in ways other than food consumption?
○	○	○	21.	Deal with fatigue in ways other than food consumption?
○	○	○	22.	Socialize without making food the focus of your attention?
○	○	○	23.	Refuse to eat out of guilt (due to the influence of parents, host(ess), family, or friends)?
○	○	○	24.	Relax during mealtime, taking time out from eating to chat or rest?
○	○	○	25.	Take your time eating (i.e., eating a meal lasts at least 20 minutes)?
○	○	○	26.	Avoid going for long periods of time without eating?
○	○	○	27.	Avoid significant swings in weight (gain and/or loss)?
○	○	○	28.	Exercise at least several times a week for 20 minutes or more?
○	○	○	29.	Maintain your weight within the Reasonable Weight Chart range for your age, sex, and height (Table 2.1)?
○	○	○	30.	Consider yourself someone with a weight or eating problem?

STEP 8: LIFESTYLES

In addition to particular food likes or dislikes and individual eating behaviors, dietary patterns are also influenced by lifestyles. For some people, the way they live detracts from their nutritional status (e.g., the busy executive who skips lunch and indulges in several martinis every evening, the weight conscious young female who skips breakfast and has "dietetic" candy bars for dinner). Some people have lifestyles which regularly result in overindulgences, often leading to overweight (see the Eating Behaviors Questionnaire in Step 7). Those who live alone may exist almost exclusively on **convenience foods,** while the fast pace of today's society leads others to rely on **fast food** for daily sustenance. Some people attempt to derive a diet from "**natural**" foods grown "**organically.**" **Vegetarian, Kosher, macrobiotic,** and other cultural practices set limitations on the dietary intake of many Americans. As a practicing dietetic technician, it is your responsibility to help build individualized diets around specific lifestyles and to provide nutrition education for people with all kinds of backgrounds and living patterns.

Prior to counseling others, it is important for you first to examine the influence of your own lifestyle on your dietary habits. Do you have any special beliefs or practices which affect your food intake? Complete the questionnaire below in order to gain a general idea of those lifestyle factors which help to form your own individual dietary patterns. You may want to refer to your charts from Steps 3 and 4. Discuss your answers with classmates or co-workers prior to undertaking the assignments which follow.

Lifestyle Questionnaire

1. How does your school/job influence your dietary patterns?
   - ○ How many meals and snacks do you eat at school/work each day? _____
   - ○ Do you eat these meals/snacks at the school/office, in a restaurant, in a cafeteria, or do you go home? _____
   - ○ Do you eat breakfast before going to school/work, at school/work, or not at all on school/work days? _____
   - ○ How many coffee breaks do you take each day? ____ What do you usually eat and/or drink at this time? _____
   - ○ Do you keep food at your desk? ____ Do you snack while working? _____
   - ○ Do you ever utilize the food vending machines at your school/office? _____
   - ○ What vending machine items do you buy? _____
2. How does your home life influence your dietary patterns?
   - ○ How many meals and snacks do you eat at home each day? _____
   - ○ Do you eat at regular times each day? _____
   - ○ Do you prepare your own meals? ____ Your family's meals? _____
   - ○ Do you find yourself eating during meal preparation/clean-up? _____
   - ○ Do you eat alone? ____ Do you eat any meals/snacks with others? _____
     For approximately how many minutes do your meals last?
     Breakfast ____ Lunch ____ Dinner ____ Others: _____
   - ○ Approximately how many hours of television do you watch each day? _____
     And, do you usually eat while watching television? _____
3. Do you have any religious and/or cultural beliefs which influence your dietary patterns?
   - ○ Do you follow any of the following dietary practices:
     - ____ Kosher
     - ____ Vegetarian
     - ____ Macrobiotic
     - ____ **Seventh Day Adventist**
     - ____ "Natural," "organic" foods diet
     - ____ Others: _____
   - ○ Due to your cultural background, do you follow a diet based on any of the following types of foods:
     - ____ Chinese/Japanese   ____ Indian
     - ____ Italian   ____ Soul
     - ____ Spanish-Mexican   ____ Other: _____
     - ____ Puerto Rican

"dietetic": Product adapted for use in modified diets; may indicate reduction in sodium, calories, and/or sugar.

convenience food: Food partially prepared and packaged so that it requires minimal at-home effort before cooking and serving.

fast food: Food prepared and served quickly at take-out restaurants (e.g., hamburgers, pizza, tacos, fried chicken).

"natural": Existing or produced by nature; term used to describe foods supposedly produced and packaged without chemical additives.

"organic": Of, relating to, or containing carbon; of, relating to, or derived from living organisms. Term used to describe foods supposedly grown and packaged without chemical additives.

vegetarian: Nonmeat eating practice, based on certain beliefs about health, ethics, economics, religion, and/or ecology. Lacto-ovo vegetarian includes milk products and eggs, lacto includes milk products.

Kosher: Sanctioned by Jewish law. Food ritually fit according to Jewish law.

macrobiotic: "Large as life." Vegetarian diet (and lifestyle philosophy) based on grains and some vegetables which restricts use of dairy products and certain other foods.

Seventh Day Adventist: Follower of a Christian religious philosophy which observes the Saturday Sabbath day and restricts the intake of animal foods to lacto-ovo vegetarianism.

4. Are there other lifestyle patterns and personal beliefs which influence your dietary habits?
    ○   Do you eat convenience foods? ____ List any which you eat regularly: _____
    _____
    ○   Do you grow any of your own foods? ____ List any which you are currently growing: ____
    ○   Do you eat so-called dietetic foods? ____ List any which you eat regularly: ____
    _____
    ○   Do you eat at fast food restaurants? ____ How often? _____
    ○   Do you eat at other types of restaurants? ____ List any kinds which you attend regularly (e.g., seafood, steak house, salad bar, pancake house, ethnic) and indicate approximately how often you visit each: _____
    _____

5. Do you have any financial constraints that influence your diet?
    ○   Do you adhere to a food budget? ____ If so, describe: _____
    _____
    ○   Do you utilize any of the following food shopping aids?
        ____ Unit pricing ____ Advertised sales ____ Generic products
        ____ Discount coupons ____ Store-brand products ____ Food cooperatives/bulk food buys ____ Other: _____

6. Do you have unhealthy lifestyle habits?
    ○   Describe any lifestyle habits you now have which might be considered as unhealthy: _____
    ○   Do you plan on changing these habits? ____ If so, describe your future plans for improving your lifestyle: _____

Like lifestyle, culture (the characteristics of a particular group of people) is an important factor in determining what one eats. This is influenced by the physical environment, which determines the foods prevalent in the diet. What is eaten customarily by one generation is often passed down as tradition to the succeeding generations. When there is a mixture of peoples of different origins in one area, there are usually many different varieties of foods consumed. Migration of ethnic groups to various parts of the world has led to the disappearance of the strong identification of some foods with particular cultures; there are often many different versions of such foods, the origins hard to trace, some even assigned to the wrong group. Increased travel opportunities provide a range of eating experiences, often causing ethnic foods to be adopted and absorbed into different cultures.

Patterns of eating and the uses of certain foods are still generally associated with particular cultures. The kinds of foods, ways they are prepared, their grouping in meals, and the manner of serving and eating constitute the food customs characteristic of a country or region. Although these vary widely, they can meet nutritional needs equally as well. Specific foods, the methods of preparation and serving, and the times at which foods are eaten acquire symbolic meanings associated with religious beliefs and ceremonies, social usages, status, ethnic and family traditions, maturity levels, and masculine and feminine roles.

Whatever a culture defines as "good food" comes to the individual at birth and throughout a lifetime in the form of a particular set of eating habits. People may feel very strongly about what foods are "good" or not good ("bad"). It is not up to the dietetic technician to change a person's cultural beliefs.

What is *your* attitude regarding foods that are from different cultures, different areas of this country, or just plain different? Take an honest look at your food attitudes. In the following chart, check ⊘ the columns you feel are appropriate. An awareness of the exact meanings of cultural food terminology can help to improve your counseling techniques with individuals from other walks of life.

Foods from Different Cultures—Likes and Dislikes

Food	Have eaten	or Would eat	Acceptable food item	Unacceptable food item	Food	Have eaten	or Would eat	Acceptable food item	Unacceptable food item
Squirrel	○	○	○	○					
Snails	○	○	○	○	Pinto beans	○	○	○	○
Bagels	○	○	○	○	Watermelon	○	○	○	○
Grits	○	○	○	○	Eggplant	○	○	○	○
Venison	○	○	○	○	Mango	○	○	○	○
Pigs feet	○	○	○	○	Papaya	○	○	○	○
Turnip greens	○	○	○	○	Coconut	○	○	○	○
Head cheese	○	○	○	○	Café au lait	○	○	○	○
Hominy	○	○	○	○	Flan	○	○	○	○
Tamales	○	○	○	○	Spinach pie	○	○	○	○
Grape leaves	○	○	○	○	Tongue	○	○	○	○
Lard	○	○	○	○	Locusts	○	○	○	○
Refried beans	○	○	○	○	Avocado	○	○	○	○
Buckwheat	○	○	○	○	Challah	○	○	○	○
Zucchini	○	○	○	○	Knockwurst	○	○	○	○
Polenta	○	○	○	○	Bratwurst	○	○	○	○
Goats' milk	○	○	○	○	Sauerkraut	○	○	○	○
Buttermilk	○	○	○	○	Water chestnuts	○	○	○	○
Raw fish	○	○	○	○	Mint julep	○	○	○	○
Litchi nuts	○	○	○	○	Petits fours	○	○	○	○
Yogurt	○	○	○	○	Beer	○	○	○	○
Olive oil	○	○	○	○	Pheasant	○	○	○	○
Catfish	○	○	○	○	Caviar	○	○	○	○
Figs	○	○	○	○	Gefilte fish	○	○	○	○
Plantain	○	○	○	○	Mutton	○	○	○	○
Blackeye peas	○	○	○	○	Prosciutto	○	○	○	○
Octopus	○	○	○	○	Tempura	○	○	○	○
Ham hocks	○	○	○	○	Potato latkes	○	○	○	○
Lox	○	○	○	○	Strudel	○	○	○	○
Dandelions	○	○	○	○	Chitterlings	○	○	○	○
Borscht	○	○	○	○	Pigs intestine	○	○	○	○
Miso sauce	○	○	○	○	Taco	○	○	○	○
Soy sauce	○	○	○	○	Dried codfish	○	○	○	○
Squid	○	○	○	○	Mussels	○	○	○	○
Brains	○	○	○	○	Cornmeal	○	○	○	○
Pork jowl	○	○	○	○	Sardines	○	○	○	○
Tortillas	○	○	○	○	Liver	○	○	○	○
Matzoth	○	○	○	○	Paté de foie gras	○	○	○	○
Bamboo shoots	○	○	○	○	Dumplings	○	○	○	○
Kasha	○	○	○	○	Baked beans	○	○	○	○
Knish	○	○	○	○	Heart	○	○	○	○
Blintz	○	○	○	○	Oppossum	○	○	○	○
Chili peppers	○	○	○	○	Sweet potatoes	○	○	○	○
Leeks	○	○	○	○	Baklava	○	○	○	○
Okra	○	○	○	○	Flapjacks	○	○	○	○
Syrian bread	○	○	○	○	Curry	○	○	○	○

Ethnic Foods

Examine the terms below to familiarize yourself with some of the food terms you may hear as a practicing dietetic technician.

Chinese

Bok choy. Cabbage
Carambola. Starfruit
Chayote. Pear squash
Congee. Thin rice gruel
Daikon. Radish
Dim sum. Stuffed, steamed dumplings
Loquat. Smooth fruit
Lotus root. Tuber from water lilies
Lychee (litchee). Small juicy fruit
Ramaki. Chicken livers wrapped in bacon
Taro. Rough brown tuber

Tofu. Soybean curd
Wonton. Pork stuffed dumpling

Cantonese. Cooking style in Southern China; rice and rice flour used extensively
Mandarin. Cooking style in Northern China; uses mostly wheat products, including noodles and millet, and highly seasoned foods
Shanghai. Cooking style in Central China; rice predominates
Szechuan. Cooking style of southwestern province; dishes are spicy, oily, very peppery

Italian

Cacciatore. Browned in oil, simmered in wine, tomato sauce
Cannelloni. Hollow pasta filled with cheese, tomato sauce
Cannoli. Cream-filled pastry
Farfalleti dolci. Dough fried in fat
Manicotti. Large hollow pasta filled with cheese, meat, tomato sauce
Minestrone. Thick soup with vegetables, chick peas, pasta

Mortadella. Bologna
Parmigiana. Baked with parmesan cheese, usually breaded and served in tomato sauce
Pasta e fagioli. Soup with noodles and beans
Polenta. Thick cornmeal mush served plain or in casserole with sausage, cheese, tomato sauce
Prosciutto. Cured ham
Torta. Cake
Zabaglione. Soft custard

Japanese

Miso. Fermented soybeans used as paste or sauce
Nori. Seaweed

Tamari. Thick soy sauce made from miso
Tempura. Batter coated and deep-fat fried

Jewish

Bagel. Doughnut-shaped hard yeast roll
Blintz. Thin rolled pancake filled with cheese or fruit mixture
Borscht. Beet soup
Bulke. Light yeast roll
Challah. Light egg bread, usually braided
Farfel. Matzo pieces
Gefilte fish. Chopped highly seasoned white fish
Kasha. Buckwheat groats served as cooked cereal or pasta substitute
Knish. Pastry filled with ground meat
Kreplach. Dumplings filled with ground meat
Kugel. Noodles, often served as a cold pudding or casserole
Latkes. Thin potato pancakes

Leckach. Honey cake
Lox. Smoked salmon
Lukshen. Noodles
Matzo. Unleavened bread
Schav. Soup with spinach and sorrell leaves
Schmaltz. Chicken fat
Teiglach. Small pieces of dough cooked in honey

Conservative. Sect which normally observes laws but makes distinctions within and outside the home
Orthodox. Sect which places great value on tradition and ceremonial rituals and always observes dietary laws
Reform. Sect which minimizes significance of dietary laws

Puerto Rican/Cuban/Spanish

Annato. Yellow coloring used with rice
Arroz con pollo. Chicken with rice
Bacalao. Dried codfish
Café con leche. Strong coffee with milk
Calabaza. Yellow squash
Cuchifritos. Fried pigs' intestines

Gazpacho. Cold vegetable soup
Granos. Legumes
Salcocho. Pigs' intestines stewed with vegetables
Sofrito or refrito. Sauce made with green pepper, tomato, garlic, and lard
Viandas. Starchy vegetables including plantain

Southern United States _____

Chitterlings.   Intestines
Hoecakes.   Cornbread, originally baked on a hoe

Hominy grits.   Grain from hulled corn
  with germ removed

Spanish American/Mexican _____

Atole.   Cornmeal gruel
Burrito.   Soft flour tortilla filled with beans or meat,
  rolled, fried or baked with various sauces
Chilies.   Chili peppers
Chorizo.   Seasoned sausage
Enchilada.   Corn tortilla, rolled, filled with beef
  or cheese and baked with various sauces
Frijoles.   Refried beans, mashed and seasoned
Guacamole.   Avocado dip with chilies
Jicama.   Starchy, crisp vegetable
Mangoes.   Green peppers (different from the fruit)
Masa.   Dried corn, soaked in lime water
  (which adds appreciable amounts of calcium),
  ground into dough
Nopalitos (Nopales).   Prickly pear cactus leaves
  sliced in strips and cooked with spices.

Quesadilla.   Flour tortilla filled with cheese and
  baked or fried
Salsa.   Chili sauce
Sapote.   Mexican custard apple
Taco.   Crisp, fried corn tortilla folded in half,
  filled with ground beef, cheese,
  chopped tomatoes and lettuce
Tamale.   Corn masa wrapped around beef-chili filling
  and served with various sauces
Tortilla.   Masa which is flat and baked
Tostada.   Fried tortilla topped with various layers
  of meat, poultry, beans, chili, cheese,
  chopped tomatoes and lettuce

Near East _____

Arab bread or Syrian bread.   Flat, unleavened bread
  which can be filled with meat, cheese,
  and/or vegetables
Baklava.   Pastry with nuts and honey
Dourglour.   Cracked whole wheat

Filo.   Thin, crisp dough layered in main dish pies
  and desserts
Shashlik.   Mutton or lamb marinated
  in garlic, oil and vinegar, roasted on skewers

Exercise on Lifestyle Effects on Diet

As a dietetic technician in nutrition care, you may encounter peoples of different cultures whose dietary patterns detract from their nutritional status. Select an area/culture, perhaps of special interest to you, and prepare a brief presentation in order to explain the dietary habits of this particular population group to your classmates or co-workers. You may want to use the following reference list. Discuss the foods popular with your particular group, and note any nutritional problems and special dietary customs. Bring in a sample food native to your area or culture, explain its cultural and nutritional significance, and share it with your peers. You might just discover a new item to add to your Food Likes List—or to your Food Dislikes List (see Steps 5 and 6).

Selected References on Ethnic Food Composition[1]

AMBEGAOKAR, S. D., SESHADRI, S., SHAH, H. C., SHINDE, V. P., ADHIKARI, H. R., PATEL, S. M., and RADHAKRISHNA RAO, M. V. 1964. Studies in nutritive value of Indian foodstuffs. I. Proximate principles, minerals and vitamins. J. Nutr. Dietet. *1*, 269.

ASENJO, C. F., DE HERNANDEZ, E. R., RODRIGUEZ, L. D., and DE ANDINO, M. G. 1968. Vitamins in canned Puerto Rican fruit juices and nectars. J. Agric. Univ. Puerto Rico *52*, 64.

ASENJO, C. F., DE HERNANDEZ, E. R., RODRIGUEZ, L. D., and DE ANDINO, M. G. 1970. Proximate analysis and vitamin content of canned Puerto Rican native dishes. J. Agric. Univ. Puerto Rico *54*, 305.

BURROUGHS, A. L., and CHAN, J. J. 1972. Iron content of some Mexican-American foods. J. Am. Dietet. A. *60*, 123.

CAMPBELL, J. A., SABRY, Z. I., COWAN, J. W., and SHADAREVIAN, S. 1963. Food composition tables for use in the Middle East, Publ. No. 20. Division of Food Technol. and Nutr., American Univ., Beirut, Lebanon.

FARMER, F. A., and NEILSON, H. R. 1970. The nutritive value of canned meat and fish from northern Canada. J. Can. Dietet. A. *31*, 102.

FOOD AND AGRICULTURE ORGANIZATION OF THE UNITED NATIONS. 1975. Food composition tables: updated and annotated bibliography, p. 181. Nutrition Policy and Program Service, Food Policy and Nutrition Division, Rome.

[1]From USDA (1974).

GOPLAN, C., RAMA SASTRI, B. V., and BALASUBRAMANIAN, S. C. 1971. Nutritive Value of Indian Foods. Natl. Inst. of Nutr., Indian Council of Med. Res., Hyderabad, India.

HO, M. L., FARMER, F. A., and NEILSON, H. R. 1972. Sodium, potassium and magnesium content of birds, fish and mammals of northern Canada. J. Can. Dietet. A. *33,* 164.

HOPPNER, K., LAMPI, B., and PERRIN, D. E. 1972. The free and total folate activity in foods available on the Canadian market. J. Inst. Can. Sci. Technol. Aliment. *5,* 60.

I.C.N.N.D. 1959. Chemical Composition of Alaskan Foods. An Appraisal of the Health and Nutritional Status of the Eskimo, p. 83. Interdepartmental Commission on Nutr. for Natl. Defense, Natl. Inst. of Health, Bethesda, MD.

INTENGAN, C. L., ABDON, I. C., ALEJO, L. G., and PALAD, J. G. 1964. Food Composition Table: Recommended for Use in the Philippines. Natl. Inst. Sci. Techn., Natl. Sci. Development Board, Manila, Philippines.

JOSEPH, S., GOLDBERG, A., and GUGGENHEIM, K. 1962. Composition of Israeli mixed dishes. J. Am. Dietet. A. *40,* 125.

KIGHT, M. A., REID, B. L., FORCIER, J. I., DONISI, C. M., and COOPER, M. 1969. Nutritional influences of Mexican-American foods in Arizona. J. Am. Dietet. A. *55,* 557.

KOREA FAO and NUTR. ASSOCS. 1970. Korean Food Composition Table. Applied Nutrition Project, Korea FAO Association and Korea Nutrition Association.

LANTZ, E. M., GOUGH, H. W., and JOHNSON, M. M. 1953. Nutritive Values of Some New Mexico Foods. New Mexico Exp. Stn. Bull. No. 379.

LEUNG, W.-T. W. 1968. Food Composition Table for Use in Africa. Health Services and Mental Health Administration, U.S. Dept. Health and Human Services, Bethesda, MD.

LEUNG, W.-T. W., BUTRUM, R. R., and CHANG, F. H. 1972. Food Composition Table for Use in East Asia. Health Services and Mental Health Administration, U.S. Dept. Health and Human Services, Bethesda, MD.

LEUNG, W.-T., and FLORES, M. 1961. Food Composition Tables for Use in Latin America. Interdepartmental Commission on Nutr. for Natl. Defense, Natl. Inst. of Health, Bethesda, MD.

LOPEZ, H., NAVIA, J. M., CLEMENT, D., and HARRIS, R. S. 1963. Nutrient composition of Cuban foods, III. Foods of vegetable origin. J. Food Sci. *28,* 600.

MILLER, C. D., and BRANTHOOVER, B. 1957. Nutritive Values of Some Hawaii Foods. Hawaii Agric. Exp. Stn., Circ. No. 52. Univ. of Hawaii, Honolulu.

MILLER, C. D., BRANTHOOVER, B., SEKIGUCHI, N., DENNING, H., and BAUER, A. 1956. Vitamin Values of Foods Used in Hawaii. Hawaii Agric. Exp. Stn., Univ. of Hawaii, Honolulu.

NAVIA, J. M., LOPEZ, H., CIMADEVILLA, M., FERNANDES, E., VALIENTE, A., CLEMENT, I. D., and HARRIS, R. S. 1955. Nutrient composition of Cuban foods, I. Foods of Vegetable Origin. Food Res. *20,* 97.

NAVIA, J. M., LOPEZ, H., CIMADEVILLA, M., FERNANDEZ, E., VALIENTE, A., CLEMENT, I. D., and HARRIS, R. S. 1957. Nutrient composition of Cuban foods, II. Foods of vegetable origin. Food Res. *22,* 131.

ONATE, L. U., ARAGO, L. L., GARCIA, P. C., and ABDON, I. C. 1970. Nutrient composition of some raw and cooked Philippine vegetables. Philippine J. Nutr. *23,* 33.

WENKAM, N. S., and MILLER, C. D. 1965. Composition of Hawaii Fruits. Hawaii Agric. Exp. Stn. Bull. No. 135. Univ. of Hawaii, Honolulu.

YU, J. Y., YUN, S. R., KIM, K. K., KWON, H. H., KIM, I. P., and AHN, K. O. 1973. Studies on the nutritive value of Korean foods. Korean J. Nutr. *6,* 11.

Note: A helpful reference for nutrition counseling is "Asian Foods Guide for Teachers" (Dairy Council of California 1981). The University of Minnesota Cooperative Extension offers materials for use in counseling Vietnamese individuals. Highly recommended as a self-study aid is The Cultural Teaching Kit #2, 1982, available from the state of California Health and Welfare Agency, WIC, 714/774 P Street, Sacramento, CA 95814. Also recommended is Cross-Cultural Counseling: A Guide for Nutrition and Health Counselors (1986), available from the National Maternal and Child Health Clearinghouse, 38th and R Streets NW, Washington, D.C. 20057.

World food problems and national food issues are important topics with which to become acquainted. For more information concerning hunger and food policy, write to (1) World Hunger Year, 350 Broadway, Room 209, New York, NY 10013 and (2) Bread for the World, 32 Union Square E., New York, NY 10003.

The excellent although somewhat dated film entitled "Hunger in America" can be ordered from AV Center, Indiana University, Bloomington, IN 47401.

The following references are worth reading for an in-depth study: (1) Lappé, F.M., 1977, Food First: Beyond the Myth of Scarcity (Boston: Houghton Mifflin); (2) Mayer, J. (Editor), 1978, World Nutrition: A U.S. View (Washington, D.C.: Voice of America Forum); (3) Mayer, J., and Dwyer, J. (Editors), 1979, Food and Nutrition Policy in a Changing World (New York: Oxford University Press); (4) American Dietetic Association, 1986, Timely Statement: Hunger—A Worldwide Problem, J. Am. Dietet. Assoc. *86,* Oct., 1414; (5) Brown, J. L., 1986, Physician Task Force on Hunger in America (Boston: Harvard University School of Public Health).

A new reference of interest is K. Sucher's Food and Culture in America: A Nutrition Handbook (New York: Van Nostrand Reinhold, 1989).

STEP 9: POST-TEST ON NUTRITION IQ

Perhaps even more than individual characteristics—such as food likes or dislikes, lifestyles, or beliefs—knowledge about nutrition has a profound influence on diet and nutritional status. Use the check sheet which leads off the post-test (questions 1 and 2) to depict your own background in nutrition education. As a dietetic technician in nutrition care, you may want to use similar questions for your prospective patients in order to discover their general levels of knowledge and interest in nutrition. Then complete the rest of the post-test in order to evaluate your understanding of the information and learning experiences provided in Chapter 2. Answers are provided in the Answer Key at the back of the book. Do you agree with the chapter title? If so, do *you* want to be what you eat?

1. I have
    ○ little or no nutrition education.
    ○ received some nutrition education in high school (e.g., in home economics, science, health class).
    ○ been in nutrition workshop(s).
    ○ taken college level course(s) in nutrition.
    ○ a college degree in nutrition: __ A.S. __ B.S. __ M.S. __ other
2. In all honesty, I
    Often   Rarely   Never
    ○   ○   ○   read magazine and/or newspaper articles about nutrition.
    ○   ○   ○   read books about nutrition.
    ○   ○   ○   discuss nutrition with others.
    ○   ○   ○   think about my own diet, the changes I can make, and the overall effect of nutrition on my health.

Select the best answer for each of the statements below.

____ 3. A complete medical history assessment should include
    (a) date of last medical check-up. (b) pertinent clinical data, such as observable skin abnormalities. (c) vitamin/mineral supplements being taken. (d) all of these.
____ 4. The 24-hour recall gives an accurate representation of a patient's typical dietary habits.
    (a) True. (b) Not always; it gives more of a general picture of typical intake.
____ 5. In maintaining an accurate food diary, it is important to write down the entire day's food intake at the end of each day.
    (a) True. (b) False.
____ 6. Dedicated dietetic technicians attempt to
    (a) avoid eating any foods they think they might not like. (b) eat only those foods they like. (c) include a wide variety of foods in their diets.
____ 7. Reasonable weights are based on
    (a) age. (b) sex. (c) height. (d) all of these.

STEP 10: PRE-TEST (A RETAKE) ON YOUR EATING HABITS

Compare the ideal answers given here with your own for the Step 1: Pre-test on Your Eating Habits, p. 30. Then participate in a classroom or peer group discussion to compare your own answers with those of fellow dietetic technicians. Discuss each question and the reasons for your individual response, then speculate on whether you believe your answers will change as your experience in the field of nutrition expands.

Ideal answers to Diet History Test (p. 30):

1. 4 or more; day
2. 1 or more; day
3. 3 or more; week
4. 3 or more; day
5. *x; x; x* (*x* + *x* + *x* = total = 3 for adults, 4 for teens; day.)
6. 2, day; 3 or less, week; 1 or more, week
7. The lower the numbers, the better; week
8. The lower the number, the better; week
9. The lower the number, the better; the lower the number the better; week
10. a. 11. F. 12. F. 13. T. 14. F. 15. F. 16. F. 17. F. 18. T. 19. T. 20. T.

REFERENCES

AMERICAN DIETETIC ASSOCIATION. 1986. Timely Statement: Hunger—A Worldwide Problem. J. Am. Dietet. Assoc. *86,* Oct., 1414.

BROWN, J. L. 1986. Physician Task Force on Hunger in America. Boston: Harvard University School of Public Health.

DAIRY COUNCIL OF CALIFORNIA. 1981. Asian Foods Guide for Teachers. Los Angeles: Dairy Council of California.

LAPPÉ, F. M. 1977. Food First: Beyond the Myth of Scarcity. Boston: Houghton Mifflin.

MAYER, J. (editor). 1978. World Nutrition: A U.S. View. Washington, D.C.: Voice of America Forum.

MAYER, J., and DWYER, J. (Editors). 1979. Food and Nutrition Policy in a Changing World. New York: Oxford University Press.

SUCHER, K. 1989. Food and Culture in America: A Nutrition Handbook. New York: Van Nostrand Reinhold.

U.S. DEPARTMENT OF AGRICULTURE. 1960. Heights and Weights of Adults in the United States. USDA Home and Garden Bulletin No. 74. Washington, D.C.: Government Printing Office.

U.S. DEPARTMENT OF AGRICULTURE. 1974. Composition of Foods Used by Ethnic Groups, Selected References to Sources of Data. Washington, D.C.: Agriculture Research Service, USDA.

Chapter Three

What Is in What You Eat?

CHAPTER BLUEPRINT

Step 1: Read the Pre-test on What You Eat and take the test to reevaluate your food intake patterns as illustrated by your week-long Food Diary.

Step 2: Read the Nutrients and Calories materials and complete the accompanying chart.

Step 3: Become familiar with the Basic Food Groups by examining the materials and completing the assignments.

Step 4: Examine the Carbohydrate Comparison Chart and participate in the assigned activities.

Step 5: Examine the Protein vs. Fat Chart and participate in the assigned activities.

Step 6: Examine the Fat Sources Chart and participate in the assigned activities.

Step 7: Memorize the High in Vitamins Chart.

Step 8: Memorize the High in Minerals Chart.

Step 9: Examine the Water-Weight Contents table and complete the accompanying assignment.

Step 10: Take the Post-test on What You Eat to determine the degree to which this chapter has helped to elevate your nutrition IQ.

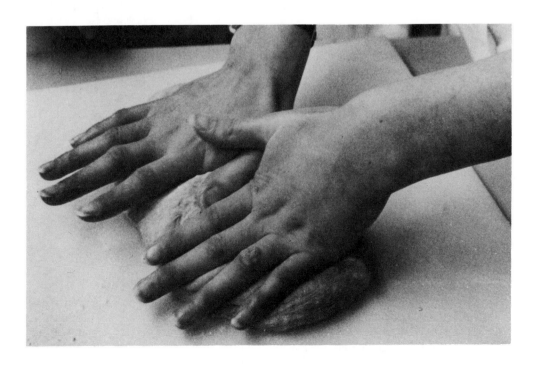

STEP 1: PRE-TEST ON WHAT YOU EAT

As a dietetic technician, it is essential for you to be able to balance your own diet, as well as to become adept at assisting others in optimizing their individual nutrient intakes.

After maintaining an accurate and honest Food Diary for one week, you can evaluate your current dietary pattern by comparing your actual intake to the suggested food intake as outlined in the Pre-test (a Retake) on Your Eating Habits from Chapter 2 (see p. 46). Simply fill in the following chart for each of the seven Food Diary days, complete the computations, and examine the results. Was this particular week's food intake varied and well balanced? Compare your results to your answers in the Chapter 2 Pre-test: Were you able to accurately summarize your typical food intake prior to maintaining a Food Diary?

Also examine your typical eating rate(s) (*duration of meal/snack*), dining location(s), eating companions (if any), and associated activities for the week. Can you now pinpoint any specific eating habits that might be contributing to a less-than-desirable diet?

Pre-test—Food Diary Evaluation

A.   According to my food diary, I

On day:

	1	2	3	4	5	6	7
1. included (give number for each day throughout the week) __ servings of whole grain or enriched cereal, bread, pasta, rice, or other grains.							
2. included __ servings of oranges, grapefruit, tomatoes, or their juices.							
3. included __ servings of dark green leafy vegetables or bright yellow fruits/vegetables.							
4. included __ servings of other fruits and vegetables.							
5. drank __ cups of milk and/or ate __ servings of cheese and/or __ cups of yogurt (total no: __).							
6. included __ servings of meat, poultry, fish or eggs and/or __ cups of dried beans or peas (total no: __).							
7. included __ servings of one or more of the following: cake, candy, cookies, donuts, jam or jelly, gum, pastries, pies, soft drinks, sugar, syrups.							
8. included __ servings of one or more of the following: chips, crackers, dips, dried or smoked meats, salted nuts, pickles, pretzels.							
9. drank __ glasses of beer, wine, or other alcoholic beverage.							

B.   To compute your week's intake, complete the following equations:

○ Total columns for Day 1–7 for part A items 3, 7, 8, and 9; put answers in chart that follows.

○ Total columns for Day 1–7 and divide by 7 for part A items 1, 2, and 4–6; put answers in chart that follows.

	Your Answer	Desired Answer (from Chapter 2)
1.	_____	4 or more
2.	_____	1 or more
3.	_____	3 or more
4.	_____	3 or more
5.	_____	Total = 3 or more (4 for teenagers)
6.	_____	Total = 2 or more
7.	_____	The lower the total, the better.
8.	_____	The lower the total, the better.
9.	_____	The lower the total, the better.

After maintaining your Food Diary for 7 consecutive days, you should now be able to evaluate your own dietary habits. Did the overall contents of your diet for those 7 days come as a surprise to you? Was your diet as well balanced and varied as you had expected? Might *you* need to revamp your diet before attempting to assist others with theirs? Summarize your thoughts regarding your Food Diary: _____

_____

_____

STEP 2: NUTRIENTS AND CALORIES

As a dietetic technician in nutrition care, you will need to have a basic understanding of the 50 or so nutrients essential for good health. It is also important for you to be able to evaluate both the nutritive and the caloric contents of foods. As a brief overview, read the Nutrition Summary provided here, and use the nutrient values charts in Appendix V [see e.g., USDA (1977)] in order to complete the Calorie and Nutrient Values Chart on page 54.

Note that nutrient and caloric values are merely estimates and that foods may vary due to the influences of climate, soil, harvesting, processing, and storage. Also note that careful use of nutrient values charts is an essential aspect of your role as a practicing dietetic technician.

Nutrition Summary

There are approximately 10,000 to 20,000 different items offered by today's average supermarket. With so many products to choose from, it may prove difficult for some people to select foods wisely in order to eat a well-balanced diet. Yet, a well-balanced diet can be obtained with a bit of knowledge about the basics of nutrition.

Nutrition is the science of food and the role of nutrients in health, and deals with how the body uses food. Nutrients are the chemical substances the body obtains from food during digestion which are essential for

○ energy for the body.
○ the growth, upkeep, and repair of all body tissues.
○ the regulation of body processes.

No single food contains all of the 40 some nutrients the body requires in amounts adequate for proper growth and health. However, all of the nutrients needed by the body can be obtained by eating a wide variety of foods. A well-balanced diet contains the proper array of nutrients: since foods vary in the kinds and amounts of nutrients they provide, such a diet always includes a variety of foods each day.

Nutrients are separated according to their chemical compositions into six categories:

Protein	Vitamins
Carbohydrate	Minerals
Fat	Water

carbohydrates: Chemical compounds comprising starches and sugars which yield 4 calories per gram and act as a ready source of energy for the body.

Protein, carbohydrate, and fat all provide energy (calories), while vitamins, minerals, and water are noncaloric. Protein provides approximately 4 calories/gram (or 115 calories/ounce), as does carbohydrate. Fat, however, provides more than twice this amount: 9 calories/gram, or 250 calories/ounce. Obviously, foods that are high in fat content provide more calories than the lower fat items.

Alcohol, while generally not considered a food, does provide calories, about 7 calories/gram (more than protein and carbohydrate, less than fat), or about 200 calories/ounce.

Protein

Protein is required for life itself, and is found in the cells of all plants and animals. Next to water, protein is the most abundant substance present in the healthy, nonobese body, contributing around 20% of total body weight. Protein helps to form muscles, skin, bones, hair, and nails. Protein is essential for the proper function of oxygen transport in the blood, blood clotting, the regulation of blood sugar and fats, and protection against infection. Protein also forms enzymes which speed up body processes, and hormones which regulate body processes. Plants make their own special protein while animals, in most cases, must rely on food for protein. To most Americans, protein means meat, but high quality protein is also provided by poultry, fish, eggs, cheese, milk, yogurt, and specific plant combinations.

Carbohydrate

The major function of *carbohydrate* is the provision of energy, but carbohydrate foods also serve as carriers of other important nutrients and fiber. Carbohydrates exist as sugars and starches: the former are simple in chemical structure and the latter are complex chains of simple sugars. The world's major carbohydrate sources are as follows:

Cereal grains   Cassava (tapioca)
Potatoes   Sugar cane
Fruits and vegetables   Sugar beet
Dried beans and peas

Many processed foods are also rich in carbohydrates, including such products as the following:

Breads and other baked goods   Molasses, honey, syrups, table sugar
Pastas   Desserts
Jams and jellies   Dried fruits

Fat

Fat is an integral dietary component, an essential nutrient that provides the following:

○ Calories for body energy
○ Fatty acids essential for growth
○ Transport of certain vitamins, cholesterol, and other substances in the bloodstream
○ Palatability to enhance the flavor of food
○ Satiety value (to enhance the feeling of "fullness")

Fats are both visible (e.g., butter, margarine, shortening, lard, salad dressing, mayonnaise, vegetable oil, bacon and other fatty meats, and greasy fried foods) and hidden in foods such as meat and poultry, eggs, whole milk and cheeses, ice cream, nuts and peanut butter, avocado, chocolate, olives, nondairy creamers, and many processed foods.

Vitamins and Minerals

Vitamins and *minerals* help to regulate numerous body processes. The vitamins now known to be required by humans include the fat-soluble vitamins A, D, E, K; and water-soluble vitamin C and the Bs (thiamin, riboflavin, niacin, B_6, folacin, B_{12}, biotin, and pantothenic acid).

Those minerals currently recognized as essential nutrients include the macro-minerals (needed in relatively large amounts) calcium, phosphorus, magnesium, potassium, sulfur, sodium, and chloride, and the micro-nutrients or trace elements (needed in tiny amounts), iron, zinc, selenium, manganese, molybdenum, copper, cobalt, iodine, chromium, and fluoride. Note: The element boron is believed to play a role in body function, but has not been established as a required nutrient (Nielson, 1988).

Water

Perhaps because it is not thought of as "food" per se, *water* is the nutrient category which is most often overlooked. Actually, the body contains more water than anything else; water accounts for about 60% of total body weight. Water is present inside all body cells (*intracellular*) and bathes the outside of body cells (*extracellular*). Water performs all of the following essential body functions:

○ Acts as the body's transportation system
○ Helps to absorb shocks to the body
○ Lubricates joints
○ Carries digestive juices
○ Cools body down and helps regulate body temperature
○ Removes body wastes

People can survive for weeks without food, but not without water. On a hot, dry day, most people would probably be unable to survive for longer than several hours without water.

All the nutrients work together to provide the body with energy, growth, and health itself. Deficiency in any one nutrient can affect the function of other nutrients. Obviously, it is important to obtain an adequate amount of *all* required nutrients. What about calories?

Calories and Energy

Most Americans are concerned about gaining undesirable poundage, and many are constantly trying to shed pounds by using a wide variety of methods. The majority of weight loss efforts are not permanently successful, usually because dieters hold false concepts of how and why the body gains and loses fat. There is really no need to undertake costly, dangerous, and rarely successful fad diets, "crash" programs, or quick weight loss schemes. Instead, weight can be kept under control, successfully and permanently, using nutrition knowledge and a basic understanding of how food provides energy and how the body uses this energy.

In terms of body energy, the unit for measurement is the *calorie.* Foods do not contain calories the way they contain nutrients. Rather, foods provide energy which is measured in calories.[1]

If a food has few calories, then it provides little energy. A food high in caloric content, however, serves as a good source of energy. Vitamins do not provide calories. Adequate vitamin intake assists in the maintenance of health and, although good health can make people feel more energetic, true body energy is only provided by calorie-containing foodstuffs.

---

[1]The term calorie is used to describe the energy potential of foods. However, energy is actually measured in thousands of calories, so the more accurate term is kilocalorie. But since calories are actually too small to use conveniently (e.g., an apple would have 60,000 calories vs. 60 kilocalories), and the term kilocalorie is too long to use conveniently, we measure in kilocalories yet talk in calories.

The basic formulas for determination of weight gain and loss are as follows:

Energy Intake > Energy expenditure → Weight gain

Energy intake < Energy expenditure → Weight loss

Energy intake = Energy expenditure → Weight maintenance

Energy is never "lost," but is used up by or stored in the body. If more energy is taken in than is used up, the extra is stored as body fat. To get rid of the energy stores, an energy deficit must be created; when energy intake is appropriately low, the body then turns to its fat stores for energy.

In terms of calories, the formulas for weight gain and weight loss are the same:

Calories provided (by food) > Calories used (by bodily function and physical activity)

→ Weight gain

Calories provided < Calories used up → Weight loss

Calories provided = Calories used up → Weight maintenance

Thus, it is important to be wary of diet claims which promise weight loss along with unrestricted caloric intake. Such diets usually only result in loss of body fluids, not body fat. To dispose of body fat stores, more calories must be used up than are provided by the diet.

In numerical terms, the key number is 3500: approximately 3500 calories of energy are furnished by 1 pound of body fat. It takes an excess of 3500 calories to create a pound of body fat, and a deficit of 3500 calories to lose a pound of body fat.

The body is constantly at work performing such involuntary activities as digestion, thought, heartbeat, and respiration. Individual bodies work at different rates, depending on age, sex, body size, physical activity, and personal and genetic factors. Body rates decrease with age after infancy. Males usually have faster body rates than females. Lean people tend to have quicker body rates than their fatter counterparts, and physically and/or nervously active persons have body rates which are more rapid than the sedentary and/or relaxed types. Chronic dieters typically have sluggish metabolic rates because the body adapts to a low energy supply by slowing down. Energy is required to support the body's work. Unless involved in strenuous physical work or athletic activity, the body rate accounts for most of the energy (calories) used.

The need for calories gradually declines after the first birthday and, after growth, drops around 5% with each decade. Dieters with chronically restricted caloric intakes have a significantly decreased need for calories, but the decline is reversible with proper nutrition and exercise. Muscle uses more energy than fat, so most males require more calories than females, and those who are physically "in shape" need a greater amount of calories than their fatter counterparts. There are also some strong hereditary influences on caloric needs, including the body's facility for fat storage and body composition; individuals with greater fat storage capacities tend to be overweight, as do those with the *endomorph* body composition. Table 3.1 summarizes *somatotypes*, or body composition categories. Most people are a combination of types.

Table 3.1   Body Composition Categories

| Somatotype | Physical description | | | |
	Body frame	Body characteristics	Appetite	Activity level
Endomorph	Rounded, pear-shaped figure	Pudgy hands and feet, bulky abdomen and hips, great fat storage capacity	No distinct appetite cutoff	Inactive, slow, tendency to rest for long intervals
Ectomorph	Slight, thin	Long thin hands and feet with narrow fingers, wiry muscles, little fat storage capacity	Distinct appetite cutoff	Active, fidgety
Mesomorph	Broad shoulders, heavy bones	Blunt hands and fingers, sturdy legs, well-formed muscles, fat storage capacity greater than ectomorph and less than endomorph but evenly distributed	No distinct appetite cutoff	Tendency for bursts of activity

Body weight is more easily controlled and metabolism is kept boosted when a program of regular physical activity is undertaken. Yet, the physical activity level of most Americans is *sedentary* or *light*. The typical American lifestyle does not incorporate much daily exercise; people drive or take public transportation to work and on errands, opt for elevators instead of stairs, utilize numerous household gadgets to save time (and energy), and spend far more time in front of the television than out walking or bicycling.

Do you consider *your* general lifestyle to be *sedentary/light* in activity; *moderately* active; or physically *strenuous*? Use Table 3.2 as a general guideline for determining activity levels.

Individuals also vary in the intensities with which they indulge in activities as shown in Table 3.3.

Table 3.2 Activity Level Guidelines

Activity level	Typical activities
Sedentary/light:	Sitting, standing, watching television, eating, driving, sewing, ironing, cooking, dusting, washing, shopping, painting, typing, lab work, garage work, golfing, sailing, walking 2–3 mph
Moderate:	Walking 3–4 mph, gardening, heavy housework, dancing, tennis, bowling
Strenuous:	Pick and shovel work, logging, ball games, swimming, climbing, bicycling, skiing, running

Table 3.3 Intensity of Activity

Activity	Method of participation
Tennis	Play doubles, let partner do most of the retrieval or
	Play singles, constantly in motion
Golf	Ride in golf cart or
	Caddy own clubs on foot
Walking	Saunter casually, never hurriedly or
	Step briskly at a quick pace (3–4 mph)
Cycling	Ride slowly, coasting often or
	Pedal constantly at a quick pace (12–15 mph)
Dancing	Fox trot, waltz, etc., or
	Square dance, disco, jitterbug, etc.
Skiing	After one run spend day in lounge or
	Many brisk runs
Swimming	Slow, relaxing float or
	Many brisk laps
Sailing	Let others sail and relax with a beer or
	Constantly in motion, at tiller and sails

Height–weight charts do not account for the wide degree of variation between individuals, but merely depict body weights without consideration of body fat. Try the following methods for more accurate estimation of body fat levels:

Pinch test. There are certain areas of the body where the thickness of the fat deposits under the skin reflect rather accurately the total amount of fat stored in the body; pinch the skin midway between shoulder and elbow—can you pinch an inch? More?

Mirror test. This is the most revealing way to determine the need for weight loss; individuals should examine themselves unclothed in a full-length mirror to check for obvious body fat deposits.

The simplest mathematical method for determining weight goals is to use one of the following formulas:

Males: 106 lb for the first 5 ft of height + 6 lb for each additional inch.
Females: 100 lb for the first 5 ft of height + 5 lb for each additional inch.
If body frame is large boned, add an additional 10%.

Some individuals prefer to set their own goals, using specific weights at which they once felt comfortable (e.g., weight at age 18, weight at high school graduation, weight on marriage day). It is important to set a realistic weight goal that is practical and can provide physical benefits when reached and maintained, and it is necessary to avoid a goal that will ultimately result in discouragement and feelings of failure.

For each of the items in the Calorie and Nutrient Values Chart, use a nutrient values chart selected from the references in Appendix V [e.g., USDA (1977)] to determine the caloric and nutrient contents for the indicated portion sizes. You may have to use a bit of math (and/or a calculator) since some of the portions differ from those given in the various charts. Compare your answers to those of classmates or co-workers and recheck any answers that are not the same as those determined by your peers.

Calorie and Nutrient Values Chart

Food and amount	Calo-ries (kcal)	Pro-tein (g)	Fat (g)	Carbo-hydrate (g)	Calci-um (mg)	Phos-phorus (mg)	Iron (mg)	Potas-sium (mg)	Vita-min A (IU)	Thia-min (mg)	Ribo-flavin (mg)	Niacin (mg)	Ascorbic acid (mg)
Pizza, ⅛ of 12-in. pie													
Bagel, wheat													
Muffin, bran													
Brownie, commercial, 3½-in. square													
American cheese, 1½ oz													
Cottage cheese, creamed, large curd, ½ cup													
Cottage cheese, low-fat (2%), ½ cup													
Cream cheese, 1 oz													
Sirloin steak, lean, 6 oz													
Chicken, broiled, 6 oz													
Bacon, crisp, 2 slices													
Butter, 1 Tbsp													
Margarine, 1 Tbsp													
Mayonnaise, 1 tsp													
Italian dressing, 2 tsp													
Orange juice, frozen, 6 oz													
Watermelon, 2 × 4 in. wedge													
Cashews, roasted, ½ cup													
Popcorn, plain, 3 cups													
Potato chips, 15													
Fruit-flavored yogurt, 8 oz													
Jello, 1 cup													
Vanilla shake, 11 oz													
Root beer float (½-cup vanilla ice cream, 12-oz root beer)													

STEP 3: BASIC FOOD GROUPS

The easiest method for you to plan out well-balanced diets—including your own—and to educate others on doing so, is by using the Basic Food Groups. Since there are some 40 nutrients known to be required by the body, and so many different foods to choose from, nutritionists have eased the burden of diet planning by incorporating both the bodily needs of individuals and the nutrient values of foods into the Basic Food Groups. These groups separate foods according to the similarities in their nutrient compositions. Thus, you can ensure an adequate intake of the nutrients required by healthy individuals by basing a diet around the recommended number of servings of a variety of foods chosen from the following Basic Food Groups:

Fruits and vegetables   Milk and cheeses
Breads and cereals   Meats and alternates

Some foodstuffs are composed of a combination of several groups (e.g., pizza, taco, cheese omelet), while certain other foods do not fit into any of the groups. The former products can make substantial nutritional contributions to the diet, whereas the latter are usually more caloric than nutritive in value. After obtaining total daily nutrient needs with the recommended servings from the Basic Food Groups, additional caloric requirements can be met with the other, less nutritious foodstuffs (i.e., fats, sweets, and alcoholic beverages). There is no need to eliminate such foods from the diet (unless so prescribed by a physician). Such foodstuffs can be considered as "extras," or fun foods to enjoy on occasion, once nutrient needs have been met.

Examine the following excerpt from the illustrated brochure prepared by the U.S. Department of Agriculture's Food and Nutrition Service: "Building a Better Diet" (USDA 1979) explains the Basic Food Groups in lay terms. It is an excellent example of the kind of literature you should have available as handouts for your patients interested in simple guidelines for balancing their diets.

Fruits and Vegetables

Fruits and vegetables are good sources of vitamin A, vitamin C, and fiber.

Vitamin A helps keep the skin healthy. It protects against night blindness and helps you see well. Vitamin A also helps the body grow.

Vitamin C builds the material which connects the body's cells. The body needs it for healthy gums and to resist infection.

Fiber some experts say may help prevent constipation and some diseases of the large intestine. It may also help control your weight.

Different fruits and vegetables will give different amounts of these and other nutrients, so it is a good idea to vary the ones you eat.

Dark green and deep yellow vegetables like squash, carrots, broccoli, and greens give vitamin A. Most dark green vegetables also supply vitamin C, but only if they are not overcooked. Citrus fruits like oranges and grapefruit give lots of vitamin C.

Some greens—collards, kale, mustard, turnip, and dandelion—give calcium and iron, as well as vitamins.

Nearly all fruits and vegetables are low in fat, and none has cholesterol unless animal fat is added in cooking.

Breads and Cereals

Enriched breads and cereals, especially whole grain products, are important sources of the B vitamins, iron, and fiber. They also supply some protein—a good thing to remember if you are cutting down on meat or do not eat it.

The *B vitamins* help our bodies grow at a normal rate.

Most breakfast cereals have nutrients added at levels higher than those which are there naturally. Some vitamins like vitamins A, B_{12}, C, and D are added which are not naturally found in cereals. You can find out which nutrients are in which cereals by reading the nutrition label on the box.

Foods included in the group are whole grain and enriched breads, biscuits, muffins, waffles, pancakes, cooked and ready-to-eat cereals, cornmeal, flour, grits, macaroni and spaghetti, noodles, rice, rolled oats, barley, bulgur, and corn and flour tortillas.

Milk and Cheeses

Milk and milk products supply most of the calcium in the average American diet. Milk and its products also give vitamin A and protein. Most milk you buy has vitamin D added to it.

Calcium is the mineral which builds strong teeth and bones.

Vitamin D helps your body absorb the calcium you need.

Low-fat or skim milk products are better choices than whole milk products. With vitamins A and D added they have the same nutrients as whole milk products, but fewer calories and less fat.

You can buy milk in many forms: whole, skim, low-fat, evaporated, buttermilk, and nonfat dry milk. Milk products also include yogurt, ice cream, ice milk, and cheeses, including cottage cheese.

If you or members of your family prefer the taste of whole milk but not the calories it gives, try mixing it half and half, with skim milk or nonfat dry milk and water, made according to the package directions.

Meats and Alternates

These foods are important sources of protein, iron, and other minerals and vitamins.

Protein is vital to all living cells and helps build and repair all body tissues like skin, bone, hair, blood, and muscle.

Iron helps build healthy blood.

Because each food offers different combinations of nutrients, along with protein, try to eat a variety of the foods in this group. Lean, red meats not only give protein, they supply iron and several of the B vitamins. Liver and egg yolks are valuable sources of vitamin A. Dried peas and beans, soybeans, and nuts supply magnesium, which helps your body change food into energy. Fish and poultry are excellent choices because they are relatively low in calories and fat, and high in vitamins and minerals.

Foods in this group include beef, veal, lamb, pork, poultry, fish, shellfish, organ meats (such as liver and kidneys), dried beans and peas, soybeans, lentils, eggs, seeds, nuts, peanuts, and peanut butter.

All meat contains cholesterol. Fish and shellfish, except shrimp, are relatively low in cholesterol. Egg yolks and organ meats have the most cholesterol.

Examine the Serving Size Chart in Table 3.4 for a simplified illustration of the appropriate serving sizes for each of the Basic Food Groups. Does this clarify your Pre-test—Food Diary evaluation results? Can the Serving Size Chart (Table 3.4) assist you in making more complete evaluations of the food intake patterns of your patients—and in more careful analysis of your own diet? Examine your Pre-test answers once again to ensure that each of the "servings" you recorded approximates those serving sizes given in the Serving Size Chart.

Basic Food Group Match Game

Complete the following match game to illustrate your understanding of the Basic Food Groups. For each item from the left column, select the appropriate food group(s) from the column on the right. Note that some foodstuffs are composed of a combination of several groups, while other items do not fit into any of the four groups. In each such case, indicate all of the groups which make up the product, or select the "Others" group (fats, sweets, alcoholic beverages) choice. Discuss your answers with classmates or co-workers, and try to derive several other tricky foodstuffs to classify.

Note: Highly suggested as a study aid for Basic Food Groups is "Colorado's Self-Teaching Module—No. 1," available from Nutrition Services, Office of Health Care Services, Colorado Department of Health, 4210 East 11th Avenue, Denver, CO 80220.

Table 3.4   Serving Size Chart

Basic food group	No. servings per day	Serving size	Food sources
Fruits and vegetables	4–6	$\frac{1}{2}$ cup cooked $\frac{1}{2}$ cup juice 1 cup raw $\frac{1}{3}$–$\frac{1}{2}$ cup	Citrus fruit or juice daily Dark green leafy vegetables or bright yellow fruit/vegetables 3–4 times weekly Starchy vegetables—corn, lima beans, peas, potato, pumpkin, winter squash
Breads and cereals	4–6	1 slice $\frac{1}{2}$–$\frac{3}{4}$ cup $\frac{1}{2}$ cup	Bread—whole grain or enriched Cereal—cooked, dry, flours, grains Pasta—macaroni, noodles, spaghetti
Milk and cheeses	3–4 (Adult) 3 (Child) 4 (Teen)	1 cup 1$\frac{1}{2}$ oz 1 cup	Milk—buttermilk, skim, whole Cheese (calcium contents are higher in harder varieties) Yogurt
Meats and alternates	2	2 oz cooked 2 1$\frac{1}{2}$ oz 1 cup 4 tbsp. 1 cup	Meat, poultry, fish Eggs Cheese Cottage cheese Peanut butter, nuts Dried beans or peas
Others	—	Fats Sweets Alcoholic beverages	Butter, margarine, oils, salad dressings, shortening, bacon, cream, olives, avocado Candy, cake, cookies, donuts, jam, jelly, pastries, pies, soft drinks, sugars, syrups Beer, wine, liquor, liqueurs, cordials

Basic Food Group Match Game

__ a. **Chayote**
__ b. **Millet**
__ c. Avocado
__ d. Pineapple yogurt
__ e. Coffee
__ f. **Tofu**
__ g. Orange-flavored Jello
__ h. Bean **burrito**
__ i. **Fettucini alfredo**
__ j. Spaghetti and meatballs
__ k. Cornbread
__ l. Gin and tonic
__ m. Chef's salad (ham, turkey, cheese, croutons on greens)
__ n. Shrimp
__ o. Sour cream
__ p. Spanish omelet

1. Fruits and vegetables group
2. Breads and cereals group
3. Milk and cheeses groups
4. Meats and alternates group
5. "Others" group

chayote: A tropical American squashlike vegetable.

millet: A grasslike staple grain popular in Africa, India, and China.

tofu: Soybean curd; good source of protein and calcium.

burrito: Soft tortilla wrapped around beans/cheese/meat/other fillings; popular food item in Mexican populations.

fettucini alfredo: Italian noodle dish with white sauce, butter, and slivers of ham.

More examples: Select several food choices which include ingredients from two or more of the five groups.

__ q. _____
__ r. _____
__ s. _____
__ t. _____
__ u. _____

__ v. _____
__ w. _____
__ x. _____
__ y. _____
__ z. _____

STEP 4: CARBOHYDRATE COMPARISON CHART

As a dietetic technician practitioner, it is important for you to be able to assist others in optimizing both nutritional status and overall health. The current consensus of the nutrition community is that nutrition is a new and ever-changing science; thus, dietary guidelines cannot be concrete. As a technician in this rapidly developing field, it is your responsibility to keep up with the latest developments and the most recent research results.

Examine Table 3.5 to obtain a broad view of the various dietary sources of carbohydrate and their caloric/nutrient values. Then read the information provided on carbohydrates and participate in the indicated activities. Once you have a thorough understanding of dietary carbohydrate, you will be better equipped to educate others on the subject.

Although most of the world's population obtains around 70% of their total caloric intake as carbohydrate, Americans only consume around 45% of total calorie intake in this form. We tend to include less carbohydrate in our diets because we

○ mistakenly consider all carbohydrate foods to be high in calories and low in nutritional value.
○ consume large amounts of protein, often more than twice the required quantity.
○ regard carbohydrate foods as unnecessary expenses, even though they are economical to produce in abundance.

Thus, carbohydrates can actually prove to be a nutritional, psychological, and economical boon to the diet.

monosaccharide: A carbohydrate ("simple" sugar) which cannot be broken down into simpler substances.

disaccharide: A carbohydrate ("simple" sugar) which can be broken down into two monosaccharide units.

polysaccharide: A "complex" carbohydrate (starch) which can be broken down into ten or more monosaccharide units.

fiber: Complex carbohydrates which cannot be completely broken down during digestion; found in varying amounts with different properties in various plant foods.

Carbohydrates in the diet are in the form of sugars and starches. The simple sugars (**monosaccharides**) are the building blocks for most common carbohydrates. They double up to form double sugars (**disaccharides**) and connect in chains of three or more to form the more complex starches (**polysaccharides**). In order to be able to be used by the body, carbohydrates are broken down during digestion into simple sugars. The carbohydrate material which the human body is unable to completely break down is known as **fiber.** Fiber does not provide energy or nutrients, but is an important dietary constituent, essential for the proper function of the gastrointestinal system. Fiber assists in digestion and elimination, and may play a role in the prevention and/or control of certain diseases.

In order to identify carbohydrates, some familiarity with the following terms is helpful:

Simple sugars (monosaccharides):	Glucose ("blood sugar") Fructose ("fruit sugar") Galactose
Double sugars (disaccharides):	Glucose + Fructose = Sucrose (table sugar, brown sugar, honey, syrups) Glucose + Galactose = Lactose (milk sugar) Glucose + Glucose = Maltose (malt products)
Starches (polysaccharides):	Digestible (starch, dextrins) Partially digestible Indigestible (fiber, cellulose, hemicellulose, pectin)

Refined table sugar (sucrose) is derived from sugar cane and/or beet, and is basically pure carbohydrate. Table sugar provides calories without any accompanying nutrients. Brown sugar, "raw" sugar (which is actually refined by law), and honey provide, in addition to carbohydrate, trace amounts of a few nutrients. Molasses contains an appreciable amount of iron.

Table 3.5 Carbohydrate Comparison Chart

Food	Fiber source	Calories	Notable nutrients
Cereals, 1 cup (uncooked)			
Barley	Good	696	Potassium, B vitamins
Buckwheat	Good	340	Potassium
Corn	Good	137	Potassium, vitamin A
Millet	Good	760	Potassium, B vitamins
Oats	Good	312	Potassium, B vitamins
Rice (brown)	Good	666	Potassium, B vitamins
Rye	Good	364	B vitamins
Wheat	Good	400	Potassium, B vitamins
Legumes, 1 cup			
Dried beans	Good	224	Iron, potassium, B vitamins
Dried peas	Good	230	Iron, potassium, B vitamins
Lentils	Good	212	Iron, potassium, B vitamins
Soybeans	Good	234	Iron, potassium, B vitamins
Starchy vegetables, 1 cup			
Lima beans	Good	189	Calcium, iron, potassium, vitamin A, B vitamins
Parsnips	Good	139	Potassium, B vitamins
Peas	Good	114	Potassium, vitamin A, B vitamins
Potato	Good	145	Iron, potassium, vitamin C
Sweet potato	Good	161	Potassium, vitamin A
Breakfast cereals, 1 cup			
Bran with raisins	Good	105	Iron, potassium, B vitamins
Corn flakes	Fair	95	Usually fortified
Shredded wheat	Fair	90	B vitamins
Presweetened varieties	Poor	115–155	Usually fortified
Breakfast sweets			
Danish, 1 avg	Poor	275	—
Doughnut, raised, 1	Poor	205	—
Muffin, bran, $2\frac{3}{8}$-in. diam.	Good	105	Iron, potassium, B vitamins
Toaster pastry, avg size	Poor	200	Usually fortified
Candy, 1 oz			
Milk chocolate	Poor	145	—
Fudge, chocolate	Poor	115	—
Hard candy	Poor	110	—
Desserts			
Angel food cake, avg slice	Poor	135	—
Apple pie, avg slice	Fair	345	Potassium, B vitamins
Brownie, $1\frac{3}{4} \times 1\frac{3}{4}$ in.	Poor	85	—
Chocolate chip cookie, $2\frac{1}{4}$-in. diam.	Poor	50	—
Chocolate sandwich cookie, $1\frac{3}{4}$-in. diam.	Poor	50	—
Fig bar, $1\frac{5}{8}$-in. sq.	Fair	50	Iron
Oatmeal-raisin cookie, $2\frac{5}{8}$-in. diam.	Fair	50	Iron
Pound cake, avg slice	Poor	160	—
Sugars, 1 Tbsp			
Jelly	Poor	50	—
Honey	Poor	65	—
Corn syrup	Poor	60	—
Brown sugar	Poor	45	—
Granulated sugar	Poor	45	—

Try to guess the nutrient equivalency for the following food: In order to obtain the amount of calcium provided by one cup of skim milk, you would have to consume _____ tablespoons of honey.

(a) 2–3   (b) 10   (c) 296

The answer is (c). Since 1 cup of skim milk provides less than 90 calories, whereas 296 Tbsp of honey is equivalent to nearly 19,000 calories, it is indeed difficult to obtain much of your nutrient needs from honey—or other refined sugars.

Sweet foods have not been shown to directly cause obesity, but sweet foods *can* be high in calories. Compare the caloric contents of some carbohydrate foods which are low in sugar with the calories in some of our popular sweets:

Wheat bread, 1 slice	70 calories
Donut, plain	150 calories
Danish pastry	270 calories
Pancake, 3-in. diam.	80 calories
Pancake with syrup, 3 Tbsp	230 calories
Pumpkin, mashed	80 calories
Pumpkin pie, $\frac{1}{8}$ of 9-in. pie	240 calories
Pumpkin pie with whipped cream, 3 Tbsp	315 calories

Note that some of the more caloric items above contain a considerable amount of fat, which also contributes to total calories (see Step 6 that follows).

STEP 5: PROTEIN VS. FAT CHART

As a dietetic technician practitioner, it is important for you to be able to assist others in optimizing both nutritional status and overall health. The current consensus of the nutrition community is that nutrition is a new and ever-changing science; thus, dietary guidelines cannot be concrete. As a technician in this rapidly developing field, it is your responsibility to keep up with the latest developments and the most recent research results.

Examine Table 3.6 to compare the fat contents of some typical "protein foods" to the actual protein contents. Then read the information provided and participate in the indicated activities. Once you have a thorough understanding of dietary protein, you will be better equipped to educate others on the subject.

Protein Quiz

Try the following quiz in order to determine what you already know about protein by indicating whether the following statements are true (T) or false (F).

_____ 1. There are five essential amino acids that must be obtained through diet.
_____ 2. High quality protein contains adequate amounts of all of the essential amino acids.
_____ 3. Meat is the only valid source of high quality protein.
_____ 4. Plant proteins do not contain adequate amino acids, so cannot serve as a valid protein source.
_____ 5. Protein undernutrition is fairly common in America today.
_____ 6. Athletes need much larger quantities of dietary protein than normally required by the body.

Protein is composed of 22 building blocks known as *amino acids* linked together in various combinations. The number of possible combinations is almost infinite, and tens of thousands of the same amino acids may be repeated in a single protein. Thus, amino acids can form a wide variety of patterns.

During digestion, the amino acid chains in protein foods are broken, and later rearranged to form body proteins. In order to build body protein efficiently, a well-balanced mixture of amino acids must be present. If the amino acids available are not properly balanced [i.e., certain amino acid(s) are low or missing], protein cannot be built and the amino acids are wasted.

Table 3.6 Protein vs. Fat

Food, amount	Total calories	Fat calories
Almonds, 10	60	50
Peanut butter, 1 tbsp	90	70
Peanuts, 10	110	80
Bologna, 1 oz	80	60
Bacon, 2 slices	90	70
Frankfurter, 1 small	130	100
Sausage, 1 link	170	140
Steak, flank, 6 oz	330	110
Steak, sirloin, 6 oz	660	490
Steak, T-bone, 10.4 oz	1400	1150
Tuna, in water, 3 oz	120	8
Tuna, in oil, 3 oz	150	60
Chicken, thigh, 3 oz	120	50
Egg, 1 medium	80	50
Cheese, cottage, $\frac{1}{2}$ cup	110	40
Cheese, cheddar, 1 oz	110	80
Cheese, cream, 1 oz	120	100
Milk, skim, 1 cup	90	2
Milk, whole, 1 cup	160	80
Ice cream, 1 cup	260	180

Certain of the 22 necessary amino acids can be manufactured by our bodies, but eight to ten cannot be synthesized at a rate sufficient to meet our needs. These *essential* amino acids must be provided by foods, while the other *nonessential* amino acids can be manufactured within the body from ingested dietary protein.

A high quality protein provides all of the essential amino acids in those proportions required by the body. Because the composition of the animal body is similar to that of the human body, the amino acid balance of animal foods (meat, poultry, fish, eggs, cheese, milk, yogurt) is of higher quality than that of plant foods. Plant proteins do *not* contain the proper assortment of amino acids in the amounts sufficient to support bodily growth. Therefore, plant foods should be combined with animal foods in order to improve the quality of the available protein.

However, *complementary* plant foods can contribute high quality protein to the diet. For example, combine (1) corn with beans, peanuts, or soy; (2) rice with beans or peanuts; (3) wheat with all legumes; (4) oats with peanuts; (5) rye with soy; and (6) sesame with garbanzos or soy to get high quality protein. Also, whenever any of these plant foods are combined with animal foods, the resulting protein is of high quality.

Protein undernutrition is rare in America today. Most people consume two to three times as much protein as they really require. Although a continual supply of dietary protein is desirable since the body has little protein reserve, if more protein is consumed than is needed, the excess will be used for energy if necessary, or stored as body fat.

The need for protein is heightened only when the body is building new tissue at a rapid rate (e.g., during infancy and pregnancy), and following tissue destruction (e.g., after hemorrhage, burns, or surgery). Contrary to popular belief, athletes require little extra protein in their diets. From the standpoint of energy production, only 5–15% of total energy in the well-nourished individual is from protein breakdown. Thus, the protein used for muscle power is actually quite small so that, except for the small amount of protein required by developing muscles during conditioning, protein requirements are not increased significantly for the athlete. And since most Americans obtain more protein than they actually need anyway, it is unlikely that the well-nourished athlete will require extra or supplemental protein.

Use Table 3.7 to assist you in determining the approximate number of grams of protein required each day in order to meet individual needs. In order to convert body weight in pounds into kilograms (kg), simply divide by 2.2. The recommended amounts were determined by the National Research Council's Food and Nutrition Board (1980).

Table 3.7   Daily Protein Needs

Individual status	Recommended daily intake of protein in grams
Infancy–6 months[a]	2.4–2.0/kg body weight
6 months–1 year	2.0/kg body weight
Childhood–Adolescence[a]	2.0–0.8/kg body weight
Adulthood	0.8/kg body weight
Pregnancy	0.8/kg body weight + 10 g
Lactation	0.8/kg body weight + 20 g

[a]Note that protein requirements decline gradually with age.

STEP 6: FAT SOURCES CHART

As a dietetic technician practitioner, it is important for you to be able to assist others in optimizing both nutritional status and overall health. The current consensus of the nutrition community is that nutrition is a new and ever-changing science; thus, dietary guidelines are not concrete. As a technician in this rapidly developing field, it is your responsibility to keep up with the latest developments and the most recent research results.

Examine Table 3.8 to obtain a broad view of the various sources of fat. Then read the information provided on fat and participate in the indicated activities. Once you have a thorough understanding of the sources, kinds, and amounts of fats in your diet, you will be better equipped to educate others on the subject.

Table 3.8   Fat Sources

High in polyunsaturated fats	Moderately high in polyunsaturated fats	High in monounsaturated fats
Safflower oil	Cottonseed oil	Peanut oil
Corn oil	Soft, non-corn oil margarines	Peanuts
Soft corn oil margarine	Commercial salad dressings	Peanut butter, old fashioned[a]
Walnuts	Mayonnaise	Olive oil
Soybeans		Olives
Sunflower seeds		Almonds
Sesame seeds		Pecans
Soybean oil		Cashews
Sunflower oil		Brazil nuts
Sesame oil		Avocados

hydrogenation: Chemical process used to convert fats from liquid to semisolid form in order to enhance shelf life.

[a]Made from ground peanuts without the addition of **hydrogenated** shortening.

omega-3 fatty acids: Polyunsaturated fatty acids abundant in cold water fish and fish oils.

Note: Fish oils are rich in polyunsaturated fats called **omega-3 fatty acids** with possible roles in disease prevention (more in Chapter 12).

The average American diet contains around 15% of the total calories as protein, and approximately 40% as fat. It has been recommended, however, that the amount of fat be reduced—the amount of **saturated fat** in particular—to comprise no more than 30% of the total calories (Table 3.9). This would leave 55% of total caloric intake to be supplied by carbohydrate.

saturated fat: Usually hard at room temperature and found primarily in animal products or in solid and hydrogenated vegetable fats.

Unsaturated fats contribute the same amount of calories as saturated fats per serving, but are preferable fat sources because intake does not elevate blood fats and cholesterol. However, a diet high in total fat content—saturated and/or unsaturated—is not healthful and can lead to weight gain.

unsaturated fat: Usually liquid at room temperature and found primarily in plant seed oils, fish and fish oils.

Table 3.9 Sources of Saturated Fat

Food	Approximate % saturated fat	Comments
Red meat		
Prime grade	50–60	
Choice grade	35–40	
Good grade	25–35	
Young beef	Least of all grades	
Ground meat		
Regular	30–35	
Lean	20–25	
Extra lean	15–20	
Prepared meats		
Sausage	35–40	Some special brands (made from soybeans) do
Precooked sausage	10–15	not contain any saturated fat or cholesterol.
Cured meat	35–40	
Luncheon meat	35–40	
Poultry		
Chicken	30–35	Remove skin (rich in fat).
Turkey	30–35	Remove skin (rich in fat).
Fish	20–30	
Milk		
Whole	3.5	
Low-fat	2	
Skim	0	
Cheese		
Hard	45–50	Alternatives now available with low/no saturated
Part-skim	30	fat/cholesterol contents include: skim-milk
Processed food, spread	20–30	cheeses, Dorman's Lo-Chol, Lite 'n Lively, Life-
Cream	50–60	time, Weight Watchers, Lite Line, and others.
Ice cream	10–20	
Ice milk	10	
Cream	50–60	
Butter	55	
Palm oil		
Coconut oil	50–90	Many food labels indicate only "vegetable oil," which includes these highly saturated products.
Cocoa butter		
Shortening		Common ingredients in processed foods—more
Hydrogenated oils	50	stable than unsaturated fats.
Nuts	Varying, 5–50	Dry roasted and raw nuts do not contain cholesterol, and have less total fat than those roasted in oils.
Fried foods	Varying, 25–50	Unless otherwise labeled, most commercially fried foods are prepared in hydrogenated oils.

It is important to keep in mind the following concepts:

○ Heart disease is the number one killer in America today, accounting for more deaths than all other diseases combined.

○ Every known culture which follows a diet rich in saturated fat and cholesterol demonstrates a high rate of **atherosclerosis.**

○ A high-fat, high-cholesterol diet produces atherosclerosis in many species of laboratory animals.

○ Recent studies indicate a possible relationship between a high-fat diet and cancer of the colon and breast.

atherosclerosis: Disease in which fatty deposits build on artery walls to cause narrowing, possibly resulting in heart attack or stroke.

Most sources of saturated fat are of animal origin and are usually solid at room temperature. Because they spoil less rapidly than most liquid fats, saturated fats are often included in processed foods. By being able to identify the presence of saturated fats in foods, it is possible to control the amount included in the daily diet.

"Sneaky" Sources of Saturated Fats

Check food labels carefully for

Coconut oil	Partially hydrogenated oil
Palm oil	Shortening
Vegetable oil (type unidentified)	Lard
Hydrogenated oil	Chicken fat (and other meat fats)

Table 3.10   Vitamin Food Sources

Vitamin	Major function(s) in the body	Best food sources
A	Increases resistance to infection; maintains normal skin; promotes healthy eyes and eye adaptation in dim light; aids growth.	Fish-liver oils, liver, margarine, butter, whole and fortified milk, cheese, cream, egg yolk, dark green leafy vegetables, bright yellow fruits and vegetables
D	Promotes bone development.	Fish-liver oils, fortified milk
E	**Antioxidant:** protects cell structure.	Vegetable oils, margarine, nuts, dried beans and peas, wheat germ
K	Promotes proper blood clotting.	Dark green leafy vegetables, cauliflower, cereals
Thiamin (B_1)	Aids in energy use; promotes healthy skin, eyes, nerves, appetite, and digestion.	Lean pork, organ meats, whole grains, wheat germ, dried beans and peas, milk, peanuts
Riboflavin (B_2)	Aids release of energy from food; promotes healthy eyes, skin.	Milk, organ meats, lean meats, eggs, dark green leafy vegetables
Niacin (B_3)	Aids release of energy from food; promotes healthy skin, nerves, digestion.	Lean meat, poultry, fish, organ meats, whole grains, dark green leafy vegetables, peanuts, milk
Pyridoxine (B_6)	Involved in protein synthesis.	Wheat germ, lean meat, organ meats, milk, whole grains, legumes, corn
Folic acid	Forms red blood cells; prevents anemia.	Organ meats, dark green leafy vegetables, legumes
B_{12}	Involved in blood formation; promotes growth; aids health of nervous system.	All foods of animal origin (meat, milk, dairy products), specially prepared fermented yeasts and soy products
C	Strengthens blood vessels; speeds wound healing; increases resistance to infection; aids in iron use.	Citrus fruits, tomatoes, strawberries, cantaloupe, cabbage, broccoli, potatoes, green peppers

antioxidant: A substance which can inhibit the oxidation (breakdown) of other compounds.

STEP 7: HIGH IN VITAMINS CHART (TABLE 3.10)

Americans spend millions of dollars every year on self-prescribed vitamin supplements. Yet for the majority of individuals, supplementation is unnecessary. Due to popular misconceptions, many consumers now purchase unneeded vitamins—all sorts of brands and forms—in quantities and at costs which can boggle the mind of the dietetic technician. The myths and facts about vitamin supplementation will be discussed in detail in Part II.

In order to acquaint yourself with the functions and the best food sources of some of the essential vitamins, memorize Table 3.10. It is probably unnecessary for you to memorize vitamin quantities per serving of food sources, but you may find that during nutrition counseling and/or education sessions, it is helpful to be able to rapidly recall the information provided in this chart.

STEP 8: HIGH IN MINERALS CHART

Although vitamins are the more common dietary supplement, American consumers have become convinced of the need to take mineral supplements as well. Like vitamins, minerals occur in tiny, yet sufficient quantities in our foods. A balanced, varied diet can fulfill the daily needs of most individuals for those minerals essential for good health. The myths and facts about minerals will be discussed in detail in Part II.

The 17 minerals now known to be essential to humans perform two basic functions: (1) Minerals help to build the skeleton and all soft tissues. (2) Minerals regulate body systems (e.g., heartbeat, blood clotting, oxygen transport, and nerve conduction).

However, the 17 minerals are separated into two categories not by function but by the quantities needed in human nutrition.

Macrominerals

Minerals needed by the body each day in amounts greater than 100 milligrams (mg) are known as *macrominerals.* The seven macrominerals are

Calcium	Sodium	Potassium	Sulfur
Phosphorus	Chloride	Magnesium	

Microminerals

Those minerals needed by the body in daily amounts no greater than a few milligrams are called *microminerals,* or *trace elements.* The ten trace elements are

Iron	Copper	Zinc	Chromium	Selenium
Manganese	Iodine	Cobalt	Fluoride	Molybdenum

The body also contains minute quantities of minerals not known to be essential for growth and health in humans. Some of these "nonessential" minerals include

Aluminum	Tin	Barium	Mercury
Silver	Lead	Gold	Boron

In order to acquaint yourself with the functions and the best food sources of some of the various minerals, memorize Table 3.11. It is probably unnecessary for you to memorize mineral quantities per serving of food sources, but you may find that during nutrition counseling and/or education sessions, it is helpful to be able to rapidly recall the information provided in this chart.

Table 3.11   Mineral Food Sources

Mineral	Major function(s) in the body	Best food sources
Calcium	Provides structure to teeth and bones; vital to proper function of nerves and muscles	Milk and milk products; sardines, green leafy vegetables (except spinach and chard)
Phosphorus	Present with calcium in bones and teeth; important for body energy	Meat, poultry, fish, eggs, whole grains
Sodium	Helps to maintain body fluid balance	Table salt, most processed foods, meat, poultry, fish, milk, eggs
Chloride	Present in gastric juice; important in digestion	Table salt, most processed foods
Potassium	Helps to maintain body fluid balance; certain **diuretics** cause depletion	Bananas, citrus fruits, melon, strawberries, tomatoes, potatoes, lean meats, bran, oatmeal
Magnesium	Essential to nerves and muscles	Dried beans and peas, nuts, green leafy vegetables, whole grains
Sulfur	Important for protein utilization; essential component in certain vitamins	Eggs, meat, milk, cheese, nuts, dried beans and peas
Iron	Important in oxygen transport; deficiency can result in anemia	Liver, meats, dried beans and peas, clams, oysters, dried fruits
Manganese	Necessary for tendon and bone structure	Bran, coffee, tea, nuts, dried beans and peas
Copper	Important in red blood cell formation	Organ meats, shellfish, nuts, dried beans and peas
Iodine	Essential to thyroid gland; deficiency results in **goiter**	Iodized table salt, seafood
Zinc	Important in transport of carbon dioxide; deficiency results in loss of taste sensation and poor wound healing	Meat, poultry, fish, egg yolk, milk
Cobalt	Essential component of vitamin B_{12}	Meat, eggs, dairy products
Chromium	Important in blood sugar regulation	Liver, whole grains
Fluoride	Contributes to formation of strong teeth and bones; can reduce incidence of tooth decay, possibly **osteoporosis**	Fish, tea, fluoridated water
Selenium	Works with vitamin E; may play preventive role in cancer; excessive intake can be toxic	Foods grown in selenium-rich soils, seafood, whole grains
Molybdenum	Important in protein metabolism; deficiency in humans unknown	Meat, whole grains, dried beans and peas

diuretic: A substance which stimulates the flow of urine and rids excess body fluid accumulations; coffee, tea, and "water pill" medications impart diuretic action.

goiter: Enlargement of the thyroid gland, primarily due to a lack of dietary iodine.

osteoporosis: Bone disease common with aging which causes thinning of the skeleton; due to a lack of physical activity, hormonal influences, and a low-calcium diet.

STEP 9: WATER IN FOODS

The American Medical Association advises us to consume a minimum of 1–2 quarts of liquid every day. Fortunately, this does not mean that we must force down eight glasses of tap water day after day. In fact, it is relatively simple to obtain a large percentage of the water needed each day from the foods we eat. Thus, even if you—or your patients—do not care for the taste of plain water, the typical diet can provide the fluids required for good health.

Avoiding Dehydration

Advise your patients to avoid dehydration by adhering to the rules listed here . . . and remember to follow the suggestions yourself:

○ Thirst is usually the best indication of the body's need for fluids; when the amount of water in the body is low, we feel thirsty, and when the amount of water in the body is too high, the kidneys work to rid the body of the excess. This ability is often reduced in the aged.

○ Drink more fluids during fever and illness. Fresh fruit and vegetable juices are a nutritious alternative to colas and ginger ale.

○ Do not restrict fluid intake when taking diuretic medications. A glass of grapefruit or orange juice will help to replace any accompanying potassium losses. Use of diuretic drugs for weight loss purposes is inadvisable, as results are due to temporary fluid loss.

○ During hot weather or physical activity, be sure to replenish lost body fluids. Do not be afraid to drink water while exercising; studies show that athletes actually perform better and have more endurance if they continuously replace fluid losses during performance. (With exercise, thirst is not always a reliable indicator for dehydration.)

○ Increase fluid intake when eating high-protein or salty foodstuffs. Cheese and crackers, nuts, and chips really do need to be washed down with a beverage. Moderation in protein and salt intake is a wise idea anyway, for a number of reasons related to overall health.

○ Keep in mind the fact that alcoholic beverages can lead to dehydration. Athletic performance can be hindered when beer or other alcohol is the beverage chosen to quench thirst during activity.

Assessing Fluid Intake

Examine Table 3.12, which depicts the water-weight content for various foodstuffs. It is often surprising to see the percentage of total food-weight provided by water, especially in those foods we consider as solids.

Table 3.12   Water-Weight Contents

Food	Approximate percentage water
Bread	35
Cheese	35–50
Meat	45–55
Eggs	65–75
Fish	65–75
Potatoes	80
Fruit	85
Vegetables	75–90
Milk	90
Fruit juices	90

As a practicing dietetic technician, it is important for you to be able to assess the fluid intake of your patients. In order to do so effectively, practice by recording your own fluid intake for a 24-hour period using the following Fluid Intake Chart. Include water, milk, juices, coffee, tea, soft drinks, alcohol, and any other beverages consumed during the course of one day. Did you obtain the recommended daily fluid intake? What types of fluids did you tend to consume? Did you include fluid-rich foodstuffs as well? Discuss your own chart results with those of your classmates or co-workers. Would you be able to assist patients in determining their own fluid intakes?

Fluid Intake Chart

Date/time	Beverage type	Amounts in ounces

Total = ____ ounces

Total ÷ 8 = ____ cups

STEP 10: POST-TEST ON WHAT YOU EAT

Select the best answer for each of the multiple-choice questions below in order to evaluate your understanding of the material provided by the information, charts, and learning experiences in Chapter 3. Answers are given in the Answer Key at the back of the book. Have you developed a better understanding of the basics of nutrition so that you can effectively educate others about the Basic Food Groups, the caloric and nutrient values of foodstuffs, and the components of a well-balanced diet?

____ 1.   There are approximately ____ different items available in the typical supermarket.
(a) 1000–2000. (b) 5000–8000. (c) 10,000–20,000. (d) 100,000–120,000.

____ 2.   There are ____ categories of nutrients, ____ of which provide calories.
(a) 5, 3. (b) 3, 3. (c) 6, 6. (d) 6, 3.

____ 3.   Alcohol furnishes ____ calories per gram, which is more than that provided by ____ but less than that of ____.
(a) 4; protein; fat. (b) 7; protein; carbohydrate and fat. (c) 9; carbohydrate; fat. (d) 7; protein and carbohydrate; fat.

____ 4.   Some foods are high in energy content yet low in calories.
(a) True (T). (b) False (F).

____ 5.   Approximately ____ calories of energy are required to create or lose a pound of body fat.
(a) 350. (b) 1000. (c) 3500. (d) 10,000.

____ 6.   Individual body rates vary, depending on
(a) age. (b) sex. (c) body size. (d) physical activity. (e) personal/genetic factors. (f) all of these.

_____ 7. Several examples of "strenuous" exercise include
(a) dancing and tennis. (b) eating and watching television. (c) swimming and running. (d) dancing and swimming.

_____ 8. According to available nutrient values charts, there are _____ calories in $\frac{3}{4}$ cup cottage cheese than in 1 average slice of pizza.
(a) more. (b) less.

_____ 9. Two examples of choices from the Fruits and Vegetables Group are
(a) sweet potato pie and whipped cream. (b) chayote and collards. (c) figs and peanuts. (d) carrot cake and avocado.

_____ 10. Two examples of choices from the Breads and Cereals Group are
(a) peanut butter and wheat bread. (b) bran flakes and milk. (c) millet and kasha. (d) tortilla chips and onion dip.

_____ 11. Two examples of choices from the Milk and Cheeses Group are
(a) kefir and part-skim mozzarella cheese. (b) poached egg and sliced American cheese. (c) egg salad and skim milk. (d) buttermilk and tofu.

_____ 12. Two examples of choices from the Meats and Alternates Group are
(a) fried eggs and bacon. (b) tofu and oysters. (c) hamburger and french fries. (d) fish and chips.

_____ 13. Two examples of foodstuffs which contribute more calories than nutrients are
(a) pizza and "light" beer. (b) popcorn and "diet" cola. (c) hamburger and milkshake. (d) Danish and coffee with cream and sugar.

_____ 14. The more nutritious carbohydrate-rich food choice is
(a) jelly. (b) toaster pastry. (c) cornbread. (d) pound cake.

_____ 15. Foods high in protein are usually negligible in fat content.
(a) True (T). (b) False (F).

_____ 16. Vegetable oil cannot be a source of saturated fat.
(a) True (T). (b) False (F).

_____ 17. Thirst is always the best indicator of the body's need for water.
(a) True (T). (b) False (F).

_____ 18. The American Medical Association recommends a daily water intake of around
(a) 1–2 cups. (b) 3–5 cups. (c) 4–8 cups. (d) 4 quarts or more.

_____ 19. Complete the matching exercise below by indicating the best food sources on the right for each of the vitamins listed on the left. If you have memorized the chart (Table 3.10) in Step 7, this exercise should be relatively easy.

Vitamin	Best Food Sources
_____ A	a. Fish-liver oils, fortified milk
_____ D	b. Lean pork, organ meats, whole grains
_____ E	c. Citrus fruits
_____ K	d. All foods of animal origin
_____ Thiamin	e. Fish-liver oils, liver, margarine, bright yellow fruits and
_____ Riboflavin	vegetables
_____ Niacin	f. Wheat germ, legumes, corn
_____ Pyridoxine	g. Lean meat, poultry, fish, organ meats, peanuts
_____ Folic acid	h. Dark green leafy vegetables, cauliflower
_____ B$_{12}$	i. Organ meats, dark green leafy vegetables, legumes
_____ C	j. Milk
	k. Vegetable oils

_____ 20. Complete the matching exercise that follows by indicating the major functions from the list on the right for each of the minerals listed on the left. If you have memorized the chart (Table 3.11) in Step 8, this exercise should be relatively easy.

Mineral	Major Function(s) in the Body
____ Calcium	a. Helps to maintain body fluid balance
____ Phosphorus	b. Certain diuretics cause depletion
____ Sodium	c. Deficiency results in loss of taste sensation and poor wound healing
____ Chloride	
____ Potassium	d. Important in blood sugar regulation
____ Magnesium	e. Present in gastric juice
____ Sulfur	f. Important in red blood cell formation
____ Iron	g. Essential compound of vitamin B_{12}
____ Manganese	h. Deficiency results in goiter
____ Copper	i. Essential to nerves and muscles
____ Iodine	j. Provides structure to teeth and bones
____ Zinc	k. Deficiency can result in anemia
____ Cobalt	l. Necessary for tendon and bone structure
____ Chromium	m. Essential component in certain vitamins
	n. Present with calcium in teeth and bones

REFERENCES

COLORADO DEPARTMENT OF HEALTH. 1981. Colorado's Self-Teaching Modules, No. 1. Denver: Nutrition Services, Office of Health Care Services, CDH.

NATIONAL RESEARCH COUNCIL/FOOD AND NUTRITION BOARD. 1980. Recommended Dietary Allowances, 9th Edition. Washington, D.C.: National Academy of Sciences.

NIELSON, F. 1988. Boron: An overlooked element of potential nutritional importance. Nutrition Today 23, Jan./Feb., 4.

U.S. DEPARTMENT OF AGRICULTURE. 1977. Nutritive Values of American Foods. Home and Garden Bulletin No. 456. Washington, D.C.: Government Printing Office.

U.S. DEPARTMENT OF AGRICULTURE. 1979. Building a Better Diet, Program Aid No. 1241. Washington, D.C.: Food and Nutrition Service, USDA.

Part II

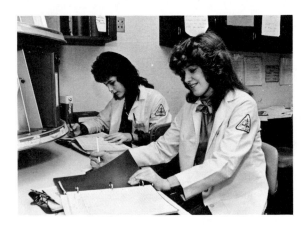

What Can *You* Say to *That?*

What you fail to understand about nutrition sense and nonsense can have a significant impact on your life—as well as on the overall health of your nutritionally naive patients. As a dietetic technician in nutrition care, you will often be asked to elaborate on many of the common nutrition concerns currently plaguing the health-conscious public. Thus, it is your responsibility to be able to separate nutrition myth from scientific fact, in order to protect your patients and yourself from the potential dangers of health **quackery.**

quackery: Claims or actions of an untrained or fraudulent practitioner of medicine.

Due to the increased use and capabilities of mass communication, nutrition "information" has become widespread. Unfortunately, much media attention is focused on invalid nutrition theories and false diet remedies which are based on testimonial "evidence" rather than scientific research. Marketed to the public as "guaranteed to work," many of the proposed diet "cures" are derived for sales purposes, not to improve public health status.

Although you may already have a strong grasp on the basics of nutrition, it is sometimes difficult to differentiate between valid science and pseudoscience. For example, reflect for a minute on your own thoughts regarding the following "hot potatoes":

○ "Organic" foods are nutritionally superior to their supermarket counterparts.
○ Some examples of "junk" foods include cookies, pizza, and fast foods.
○ Sugar is fattening and the main cause of **diabetes**.
○ Vegetarian diets are low in certain essential nutrients.
○ **Laetrile** has been proven to cure cancer.
○ The best dietary advice for arthritis sufferers is to lose weight if overweight, and avoid all food fads.

diabetes (mellitus): Metabolic disorder characterized by elevated levels of glucose in blood and urine due to inadequate production or use of insulin (see Chapter 11).

laetrile: Amygdalin, derived from apricot pits; contains cyanide, fatal in large doses; also known as "vitamin" B_{17}.

Except for the last statement (which is true), each of these nutrition myths is often considered to be factual. Adherents to such false beliefs can waste their money, unbalance their diets, and damage their overall health—even to a fatal extent. Yet, dietary mythology continues to flourish, with economic gains for proponents but without any demonstrable benefit to the public.

The decisions you make concerning your own health, and the nutrition guidance you supply to your patients, should be based on the most recent findings supported by the established medical, scientific, and nutrition communities. As a practicing dietetic technician, you need to first build up a working knowledge of substantiated nutrition concepts, and then adopt the most practical methods for the effective nutrition education of others. Part II can assist you in learning to separate nutrition fact from fancy, so that you are able to enlighten others on topics such as those listed above.

Chapter Four

Are There 'Good' Foods and 'Bad' Foods?

CHAPTER BLUEPRINT

Step 1: Take the Pre-test on Nutrition Sense to begin reflecting on your political stance as a technician in the field of nutrition.

Step 2: Complete the Food Fallacies Checklist and consider your answers while reading the accompanying reprint.

Step 3: Examine the Health Foods Chart and participate in the assigned group discussion.

Step 4: Read the material on Junk Foods and complete the accompanying quiz.

Step 5: Read the Supplementary Information and complete the accompanying quiz.

Step 6: Read the material on Food Additives and prepare a brief oral report for your peers.

Step 7: Read the material on sugar and participate in the Hidden Sugar activity.

Step 8: Read the material on sodium and participate in the Hidden Salt activity.

Step 9: Read the material on Liquid Libations and complete the accompanying assignment.

Step 10: Take the Post-test on Nutrition Sense in order to evaluate what you have learned from Chapter Four.

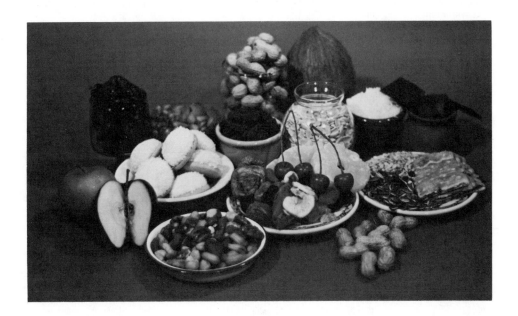

STEP 1: PRE-TEST ON NUTRITION SENSE

In order to effectively educate others on the facts about nutrition, it is essential for you to be able to distinguish between nutrition sense and nonsense. The first goal, therefore, is to equip yourself with a working knowledge of the fundamentals of nutrition and dietetics (as you should have accomplished in Part I). The next task is to prepare yourself for the multitude of "hot" nutrition controversies currently bubbling full force in our society.

Where would you place yourself on this scale regarding your nutrition beliefs?

○——Radical——Liberal——Middle-of-the-road——Moderate——Conservative——○

Although you may consider yourself to be of a certain "political" stance, others may view you differently, and eventually you may reevaluate your political position in the field. To examine some of the political positions of others in the field, read several of the Suggested Readings that portray differing viewpoints; discuss your reactions with classmates or co-workers.

Suggested Readings on Political Positions on Nutrition

AMERICAN DIETETIC ASSOCIATION. 1980. Nutrition Policy—A Position Paper. Chicago: ADA.

DWYER, J., and MAYER, J. 1975. Beyond economics and nutrition: The complex basis of food policy. Science, May 9, 566.

EGAN, M. 1986. Nutrition public policy: The process and the challenge. J. Nutr. Ed. *18*, Dec., 246.

GUSSOW, J., and CLANCY, K. 1986. Dietary guidelines for sustainability. J. Nutr. Ed. *18*, Feb., 1.

HEATH, E. 1985. The politics of food. Nutrition Today *20*, Sept./Oct., 21.

MANOFF, R. 1980. Communications perspectives for the 1990s: The new politics of nutrition education. J. Nutr. Ed. *12*, Supp.-1, 112.

MILLER, S., and STEPHENSON, M. 1987. The 1990 National Nutrition Objectives: Lessons for the future. J. Am. Dietet. Assoc. *87*, Dec., 1665.

NATIONAL ACADEMY OF SCIENCES. 1980. Toward Healthful Diets. Washington, D.C.: NAS.

SHORTER, E. 1987. The Healthy Century. New York: Doubleday & Co.

SORENSON, A., KAVET, J., and STEPHENSON, M. 1987. Health objectives for the nation: Moving toward the 1990s. J. Am. Dietet. Assoc. *87*, Jul., 920.

TRUSWELL, A. 1987. Evolution of dietary recommendations, goals, and guidelines. Amer. J. Clin. Nutr. *45*, Supp.-5, 1060.

TUDGE, C. 1980. Future Food: Politics, Philosophy, and Recipes for the 21st Century. New York: Harmony Books.

U.S. DEPARTMENT OF AGRICULTURE. 1985. Nutrition and Your Health: Dietary Guidelines for Americans, Home and Garden Bulletin No. 232. Washington, D.C.: Government Printing Office.

U.S. DEPARTMENT OF AGRICULTURE and U.S. DEPARTMENT OF HEALTH AND HUMAN SERVICES. 1986. Nutrition Monitoring in the United States: A Progress Report. Washington, D.C.: Government Printing Office.

U.S. DEPARTMENT OF HEALTH AND HUMAN SERVICES. 1979. Healthy People: The Surgeon General's Report on Health Promotion and Disease Prevention, PHS Publication No. 79-55071. Washington, D.C.: Government Printing Office.

U.S. DEPARTMENT OF HEALTH AND HUMAN SERVICES. 1988. The Surgeon General's Report on Nutrition and Health. Washington, D.C.: Government Printing Office.

U.S. SENATE SELECT COMMITTEE ON NUTRITION AND HUMAN NEEDS. 1977. Dietary Goals for the United States, 2nd Edition. Washington, D.C.: Government Printing Office.

WHITE, P. 1986. Setting new diet and health directions. Nutrition Today *21*, Jul./Aug., 4.

Nutrition Beliefs Questionnaire

After reading several of the Suggested Readings and discussing your reactions with classmates or co-workers, complete the following brief questionnaire. Do your answers, like your political self-image, differ from those of your peers? Who and what may influence your viewpoint—now and in the future—in your practice as a dietetic technician in nutrition care?

1. Briefly describe the "conservative" viewpoint on contemporary nutrition policy:

2. Briefly describe the "liberal" viewpoint on future nutrition policies:

3. Compare the overall conclusions provided by the Dietary Goals (U.S. Senate Select Committee on Nutrition and Human Needs 1977), Healthy People (DHHS 1979), Toward Healthful Diets (NAS 1980), Dietary Guidelines (USDA 1985) and The Surgeon General's Report (DHHS 1988). Do you agree or disagree with these conclusions?

4. Draw up your own list of general dietary advice for Americans in the 1990s:

5. Compose a brief essay entitled "Foods and Nutrition, 2000":

STEP 2: FOOD FALLACIES

Where have *you* obtained most of your nutrition knowledge so far? Complete the checklist below to indicate the most important sources of nutrition information on which/whom you have relied in the past, and to begin to re-evaluate the scientific validity of your beliefs. Then read the reprint entitled "The Truth about Nutrition and Health Rip-Offs" (Herbert and Barrett 1982a). Have you been harboring long-held nutrition myths? Have you fallen for any "new" diet claims? As a dietetic technician in nutrition care, it is one of your overall responsibilities to be well informed on the facts about diet and health so that you can assist others to identify nutrition nonsense—and successfully avoid falling prey to potentially dangerous health claims yourself. (More guidelines for evaluating nutrition information are provided in Chapter 6.)

Food Fallacies Checklist

Indicate ⊘ the resources from the following list from which you have often obtained nutrition information (more than one resource may be checked), and provide examples whenever possible.

○ 1.   Magazines or journals.   List any you read which regularly offer diet advice:

○ 2.   Newspaper articles.   List any regular diet/nutrition columns you read:

○ 3.   Television and/or radio programs.   List examples:

○ 4.   Books/brochures from "health" food stores.   List any favorite titles or authors:

○ 5.   "Nutritionists" without traditional training (e.g., "health" food store personnel, **clinical ecologists,** supplement salespersons).   List:

○ 6.   Nonprofessional associates (e.g., relatives, friends, neighbors).   List:

○ 7.   Health professionals (e.g., physicians, dietitians, professors).   List:

○ 8.   Books from bookstores or libraries.   List any favorite titles/authors:

○ 9.   Seminars or workshops.   Identify sponsors:

○10.   Classes.   List course titles and intended audiences:

Separate nutrition facts from fakes by indicating whether you think each of the following statements is true (T) or false (F). Most of the answers should already be obvious to you from the information provided in Part I.

_____ 11.   "Health" foods are safer, more nutritious alternatives to supermarket fare.
_____ 12.   Refined sugar has been shown to cause chronic **hypoglycemia** and diabetes.
_____ 13.   Athletes need to purchase nutrition supplements, particularly because they require a significantly increased intake of protein and other nutrients.

clinical ecologist: Practitioner of unrecognized medical specialty based on the theory that many physical and psychological disorders are due to "allergies" to food, pollutants, and other environmental factors.

hypoglycemia: Condition in which the blood glucose level is abnormally low due to malfunction in insulin regulation and/or environmental factors such as fasting, alcoholic beverages, or exercise.

cellulite: Term used to describe the dimpled fat primarily found on hips, thighs, and buttocks of overweight females (which is actually ordinary fat); can be eliminated via sound reducing diet and exercise.

RNA: Ribonucleic acid; controls cell synthesis.

holistic: Pertaining to the theory that organisms function as units and cannot be treated in separate parts.

chelation: Process of causing a binding of chemicals, usually involving metal.

_____ 14. "Health" food stores can supply the youth-promoting products that elderly people need to purchase.

_____ 15. Herbs have magical curative properties.

_____ 16. Specific dietary manipulations can eliminate unwanted **cellulite.**

_____ 17. Bee pollen is a rich source of unusual dietary factors.

_____ 18. Naturally fertilized soil produces more nutritious produce than that grown in synthetically cultivated soil.

_____ 19. Organically grown foods are pesticide-free.

_____ 20. Older persons should purchase **RNA** tablets for enhanced youthfulness.

_____ 21. **Holistic** medicine is untainted by myths and frauds.

_____ 22. Arthritis can be cured by special diets.

_____ 23. Arthritis can be cured with **chelation** therapy.

_____ 24. Enzyme supplements aid in digestion and are especially helpful to the older population.

_____ 25. Laetrile has been proven as a safe, effective cure for cancer.

_____ 26. Two essential B vitamins for which we require supplementation include "B_{15}" and "B_{17}."

_____ 27. An effective method for identifying a vitamin deficiency is hair analysis.

_____ 28. False claims for specific foods, diets, and health practices are easy to identify and avoid.

_____ 29. "Health" foods, "organic" produce, and "natural" items are "good" foods and should form the basis of one's diet.

_____ 30. Fast foods, snacks, sweets, and "junk" foods are "bad" foods and should never be included in one's diet.

Each of the preceding food fallacies is an example of the many possible nutrition misconceptions held by certain patients you may need to counsel. Use the nutrition facts that follow and the rest of the information provided in Part II in order to strengthen your own understanding of some popular nutrition "rip-offs" and evaluate your own sources of health advice. Begin an on-going review of the nutrition/diet information currently available to the public via newspapers, magazines, television, radio, etc. It is interesting and edifying to keep an active file on misleading nutrition/diet information promoted by the media.

The Truth about Nutrition and Health Rip-offs[1]

Victor Herbert, M.D., J.D., is both a doctor and a lawyer. Chief of the Hematology and Nutrition Laboratory, Bronx VA Medical Center, he is a member of the Food and Nutrition Board of The National Academy of Sciences. Stephen Barrett, M.D., a psychiatrist, is board chairman of the Lehigh Valley Committee Against Health Fraud, Inc., a member organization of the Consumer Federation of America. Here, excerpts from their book, "Vitamins and 'Health' Foods: The Great American Hustle."

1. Some herbal teas sold in health food stores can cause hallucinations and other severe reactions.

Two teas with diuretic action should be avoided because of their toxic effects. _Juniper_ berries can irritate the gastrointestinal tract and _Shave grass_ or _horsetail_ plants contain nicotine and thiaminase; in horses and other grazing animals these plants have caused excitement, loss of appetite and muscular control, diarrhea, labored breathing, convulsions, coma, and death.

Herbal teas containing _buckthorn_ bark and _senna_ leaves, flowers, and bark have caused severe diarrhea. Dock roots and _aloe_ leaves are also powerful laxatives available as teas. Aloe is a particularly strong laxative widely used in veterinary medicine.

Ingestion of half a cup of _burdock root_ tea purchased in a "health" food store has resulted in typical anticholinergic symptoms of blurred vision with enlarged pupils, dry mouth, inability to urinate, and bizarre behavior and speech, including hallucinations.

2. Hypoglycemia (low blood sugar) is extremely rare and most likely not the cause of your fatigue or depression.

[1]From Herbert and Barrett (1982a). Reprinted with permission of the George F. Stickley Company, Publishers.

Today, hypoglycemia is fashionable as a socially acceptable diagnosis to explain away certain symptoms of neurotic nervousness or fatigue. This condition, which is extremely rare, should be diagnosed only after careful interpretation of a blood-sugar test. A diagnosis of functional hypoglycemia should not be considered unless a person gets symptoms two to four hours after eating, and low blood sugar and symptoms occur together.

3. Extra protein cannot increase your vigor or improve athletic performance.

The "health" food industry would have us believe that protein plays a special role in the nutrition of athletes or active people. The scientific facts are otherwise: Proteins are broken down, by digestion, to amino acids, which are needed to build or maintain muscles. But muscle-building is not *caused* by eating extra protein. It is stimulated by increased muscular work.

4. Gerovital H3 (GH3) is not the fountain of youth. Its main ingredient can cause convulsions.

Although GH3 is promoted as an anti-aging substance, controlled use of it has failed to demonstrate any improvement in elderly patients. Additional claims have been made that GH3 can prevent or relieve disorders including arthritis, depression, and impotence but none of these claims has been verified.

The main ingredient is procaine, a local anesthetic that can cause convulsions and other serious side effects when rapidly absorbed.

5. Some of the components of ginseng, claimed to be a sexual enhancer, act like steroid drugs.

Take heed. Ginseng contains a variety of potentially toxic chemicals. Among its toxic effects are diarrhea, skin eruptions, insomnia, nervousness, and severe mental confusion. Ginseng also contains small amounts of **estrogens** and has been reported to cause swollen, painful breasts.

estrogen: Female sex hormone.

6. There is no such thing as "cellulite," and treatments for it are a rip-off.

The term "cellulite" is sometimes used to describe the dimpled fat found in the hips and thighs of many women. Cellulite is promoted as a special type of fat that is resistant to diet and exercise. The simple truth about it is that it doesn't exist—it is ordinary fat that can only be lost as part of an overall reducing program.

7. Bee-pollen tablets and wheat germ oil do not improve athletic performance.

Neither contains any nutrients that cannot be supplied less expensively in a balanced diet.

8. Natural fertilizers cannot produce more nourishing foods.

The only "extra" you may get from animal fertilizers is a good case of **salmonella** diarrhea or intestinal parasites. Moreover, "natural" foods are more likely to have molds growing on them that produce potent carcinogens.

salmonella: Bacteria which can induce gastritis and lead to potentially fatal food poisoning.

9. Organically grown foods are not free of **pesticides.**

Organic promoters imply that the use of pesticides is bad and dangerous, and that foods grown under "organic" conditions will contain no pesticides. But they do. Over the years, many laboratories have found little difference in the level of pesticide residues between foods that are labeled "organic" and those that are not.

pesticide: Chemical used to kill pests.

10. It is simply not true that RNA (ribonucleic acid) can increase your energy or make you look younger.

RNA, a compound we produce in our bodies, is part of the reproductive apparatus of all cells. When taken by mouth, as a food supplement, it is broken down by a pancreatic enzyme and doesn't even get into the cells of the body, but one of the products of the breakdown can produce a dangerous elevation of the **blood uric acid** level.

blood uric acid: Found in plasma; factor indicative/causative for gout.

11. There is no cure for arthritis or any special diet that *totally* relieves the symptoms.

There is hardly a food item that has not been promoted at one time or another as a cure for arthritis. Medical research has found only one form of arthritis (gout) for which symptoms are partially related to the type of food eaten. Diets based on raw foods, foods without chemical additives, and other supposedly "natural" nutrition items are being hustled by the "health" food industry. "Natural" faddists overlook the fact that prehistoric man, who certainly ate no additives, also suffered from arthritis.

12. "Chelation therapy" can destroy the kidneys—and kill you.

"Chelation therapy"—injection of disodium EDTA into the bloodstream where it supposedly cleans out unwanted mineral deposits from various parts of the body before exiting via the kidneys—can, in fact, cause death from kidney destruction. A course of treatment consisting of 20–50 injections can cost thousands of dollars. According to its promoters, it may be helpful in kidney and heart disease, arthritis, Parkinson's disease, emphysema, **multiple sclerosis, gangrene, psoriasis. . . .**

multiple sclerosis: Chronic, progressive disease of the nervous system, the cause as yet unknown.

gangrene: Tissue death due to deficient blood supply.

psoriasis: Chronic, reoccurring skin infection characterized by dry red scales.

Note: Chelation therapy (except for heavy-metal poisoning) and treatment with GH3 (see number 4) do not have FDA approval, and physicians who use these treatments may be operating on the fringes of the law. Steer clear of anyone who even recommends these methods.

13.   "Enzyme tablets," sold as digestion aids, have no beneficial effect, unless you have pancreatic disease.

Enzymes taken by mouth are broken down into their component amino acids by digestion in the stomach and intestines and therefore do not even function as enzymes within the body.

14.   Laetrile heads the all-time list of quack cancer remedies.

cyanide: Deadly poison found in the seeds of certain fruits including apricots and apples.

It is a trade name for the chemical amygdalin, a substance abundant in the kernels of plants—including apricots, peaches, bitter almonds, and apple seeds. The seeds are dangerous to eat because amygdalin is six percent **cyanide** by weight and releases cyanide when broken down within the stomach and intestine.

Although amygdalin has been used against cancer for over 100 years, there is no evidence that it is effective. The fundamental problem with laetrile chemotherapy is not that laetrile can't kill cancer cells but that the dose needed to kill cancer will also kill the patient.

15.   "B_{15}" (pangamate) and "B_{17}" (laetrile) sound like vitamins but are not—they are dangerous and should be avoided.

Laetrile contains cyanide and has poisoned people (see above). Pangamate is not even a single substance but is merely a label applied to differing product mixtures marketed by various manufacturers. Recent experiments have shown that ingredients in some of the most widely sold "pangamates" can cause mutations in bacteria—which means they may cause cancer in humans.

16.   Hair analysis is a waste of money when it is used for diagnosing vitamin or mineral deficiencies.

The state of the body's health may be completely unrelated to the chemical composition of the hair. Hair analysis may have some limited usefulness in the diagnosis of lead, cadmium, arsenic, or mercury poisoning, but using it as a routine test is a waste of money.

There are no vitamins in hair except at the root (below the surface of the skin). The mineral composition of hair can be affected by a person's age, natural hair color, and rate of hair growth, as well as by the use of hair dyes, bleaches, and shampoos.

STEP 3: HEALTH FOODS CHART

"There is no human society that deals rationally with food in its environment, that eats according to the availability, edibility, and nutritional value alone," stated Dr. Hilde Bruch (1973), an expert on food-related behaviors, in her prominent book "Eating Disorders." With the affluence and the wide availability of foods in America today, her statement helps to explain the national attraction to nutrition nonsense. Many consumers appear to be somewhat irrational concerning diet and health. Nutrition nonsense and health rip-offs abound, and many individuals who should be well informed about nutrition abandon common sense in favor of health fads. Why?

Nutrition is a relatively new science. In earlier years, medical researchers experimented with "food cures" and—if they lived to tell about it—they made amazing dietary claims. Since scientists and the medical community were still nutritionally naive, the medical quacks of earlier times were often left undisputed—and the equally naive public suffered, often fatally.

Today, however, there is little reason to fall for nutrition nonsense. Science and medicine have advanced at a rapid pace during the past few decades, and the facts of nutrition are gradually being uncovered. In recent years, nutrition education has begun to be promoted in school systems, universities, medical schools, and—to a limited and questionable extent—the media. Yet, we are spending more money than ever before on fad diets, unnecessary nutrition supplements, and costly "health" foods.

As a nutrition educator, it is important for you to recognize that food philosophies often have an emotional basis. Thus, many individuals hold strong personal beliefs about diet and nutrition. When it comes to health, some people tend to shove scientific, logical thought aside and believe whatever they *want* to believe.

Common-sense nutrition is the best defense against food faddism. "Health" food stores offer an array of nutritious products, along with costly items of questionable health value. In order to obtain a better understanding of some of the popular "health" food hustles, examine the Health Foods Chart (Table 4.1) to again compare nutrition fact with fallacy. Discuss the use of "health" foods with classmates or co-workers: Are there some you would recommend to specific patients, and are there any you would counsel patients to be wary of?

Table 4.1 Health Foods Chart

"Health" food	Claim(s)	Scientific fact(s)
Acerola cherry	Excellent source of vitamin C	Citrus fruits more readily available
Acidophilus	Helps restore normal intestinal flora	Intestinal flora function well in normal healthy people
Alfalfa	Has minerals lacking in shallow-root plants	Subsoils have fewer nutrients than topsoils
Bee pollen	Rich in nourishing factors and enzymes	No special nutrients; mostly fruit sugar
Biotin	Prevents baldness and restores hair	No known deficiency in humans; no proven effects on hair growth
Blackstrap molasses	Enriches blood, provides energy	High in iron and sugar
Bone meal	Halts muscle pain, menstrual cramps, nervous problems	Source of calcium, but may contain toxic metals
Bran	Prevents appendicitis and cancer of the colon	Increases bulk, aids digestion and elimination; excessive intake can cause nutrient losses, possibly intestinal blockage
Brewer's yeast	Lifts depression, restores genes	High in protein, B-complex vitamins
Brown rice	Adequate alone to maintain life	More nutrients than white rice but protein incomplete
Carob	Unrefined, nutritious chocolate substitute	Dried powder of seed pod (contains no caffeine); often added to high-fat, high-sugar foods
Choline	Enhances memory	No known deficiency in man; body makes own supply
Cider vinegar	Balances body's acid-ash content; cures kidney disease and overweight	Contains potassium which is widely distributed in foods
"Coaches' formula"	Rebuilds muscle tissue; easily digested	Contains skim milk powder, sugar, enzymes; amino acid content may be unbalanced
Dessicated liver	Helps body to make vitamin B_{12}	May conceal anemia; contains only some of the nutrients in liver
Dolomite	Cures nerve and muscle disorders	Source of calcium, but may contain toxic metals
Enzymes	Aid digestion, decrease gas	Broken down during digestion; body makes own supply
Fertilized eggs	Better amino acid content	Equal nutritionally to unfertilized eggs

(continued)

Table 4.1 *(Continued)*

"Health" food	Claim(s)	Scientific fact(s)
Garlic	Cures hypertension, cancer, skin disease; halts aging	Odor is absorbed into blood, breathed out through lungs; health benefits with large intakes only
Ginseng	Increases energy; enhances sexual potency and immunities	Noncaloric herb; may elevate blood pressure
Glutamic acid	Inhibits gene breakdown, aids memory	Broken down during digestion; body makes own supply
Goats' milk	Highly nutritious and disease-free	No more nutritious than cows' milk; dangerous if unpasteurized
Granola	High in nutrients and fiber	High in calories, sugar, and fat
Honey	Cures arthritis, high in nutrients, useful for diabetics	Nutritionally similar to table sugar
Inositol	Clears blood of fat and cholesterol	No known deficiency in man; widely distributed in food
Kelp	Natural source of iodine, other minerals	High in sodium
Lecithin	Dissolves cholesterol and clears blood of fat	Phospholipid in all cells; body makes own suppy
Minerals	Cure variety of health problems and diseases	Widely distributed in food; can build up in body to toxic levels
"Organic" food	More nutritious than supermarket foods	Usually more expensive
Pantothenic acid	Calms anxiety, speeds healing, combats cancer	Deficiency unknown in man; widely distributed in food
Papain	Aids digestion, decreases gas	Broken down during digestion and deactified
Protein powders	Build muscle tissue	Nutritionally similar to skim milk powder; amino acid content may be unbalanced

STEP 4: JUNK FOODS

In talking to friends, reading the popular press, or counseling patients, you may encounter the term "junk" food as often as you hear or see the term "health" food. Both terms are equally meaningless. The dictionary defines "junk" as "useless stuff, trash, rubbish" (and describes "food" as "any substance taken into the body to maintain life and enable growth"), so "junk" food could actually be defined as the rubbish we take in to keep ourselves going—hardly a sensible term. Actually, *all* foods are "health" foods, if they are eaten as part of a balanced diet; and *all* foods can become "junk" if eaten in excess, crowding out of the diet other foods necessary for a balanced diet. If you only ate candy to the point that your diet failed to include a variety of foods from the Basic Food Groups, your nutritional balance would be upset. Yet, if you only drank milk to the extent that you excluded other foodstuffs, then your diet would also be unbalanced, deficient in important

Table 4.1 (*Continued*)

"Health" food	Claim(s)	Scientific fact(s)
Raw cheese	More nutritious than pasteurized cheese	Dangerous if aged less than 60 days
Raw egg	More nutrients, easily digested	Nutritionally equivalent to cooked eggs; chance of food poisoning from bacterial contamination
Raw meat	More nutritious than cooked meat	Nutritionally equivalent to cooked; danger of parasites and illness
Raw milk	More nutritious than pasteurized milk	Nutritionally equivalent to pasteurized; danger of tuberculosis and other diseases
Raw nuts	More nutritious than roasted nuts	Nutritionally equivalent to cooked; often contaminated with molds
Raw sugar	Unrefined, with high nutrient content	Refined, with trace amounts of molasses on crystals
Rutin	Aids in complete utilization of vitamin C	Accompanies vitamin C in food sources
RNA/DNA	Inhibits gene breakdown, halts aging	Broken down during digestion; body makes own supply
Sea salt	Unrefined; source of iodine, other minerals	Refined; high in sodium
Seeds	Excellent source of protein and energy	Incomplete protein; high in fat, calories
"Tiger's milk"	High in protein, vitamins, energy	Contains skim milk powder, sugar, calories
Vitamins	Inadequate in food supply, prevent and cure a variety of ills	Sufficiently available in food supply; excesses can cause side effects, sometimes toxic
Wheat germ	Nutritious, low-calorie, high-energy supplement	Good source of protein, vitamins; available in whole grain products

nutrients. Thus, *any* food can be considered a "junk" food if it restricts dietary balance and limits the variety of foods eaten.

Foods commonly thought of as "junk" foods include fast foods like hamburgers, shakes, and pizza, snack foods like chips and soft drinks, and sweets such as cookies or cake. Although many of these foods can serve as significant sources of fat and calories, the concept that these calories are "empty" or totally nutrient free is an exaggeration.

Read through the following commonly asked questions and the answers which most nutritionists would provide, after completing the brief quiz that follows. Do you and your peers agree with the current scientific viewpoint on "junk" foods? Do you enjoy an occasional slice of pizza, a few cookies, or a burger? It is essential that, as a dietetic technician in nutrition care, you are able to convey to others the following concept: Food is meant to provide pleasure, as well as nutrients.

Preliminary Quiz

Indicate whether you consider each of the following statements to be true (T) or false (F). Answers can be found throughout the remainder of Step 4 and are listed in the Answer Key at the end of the book.

_____ 1. Foods like cake and pizza do not provide any nutrients.
_____ 2. Eating a "junk" food will jeopardize nutritional balance.
_____ 3. Fast foods do not contribute nutrients to the diet.
_____ 4. Submarine sandwiches can be nutritionally adequate food choices.
_____ 5. It is better to skip breakfast than to eat at a fast food outlet in the morning.
_____ 6. Schools offering fast foods usually increase lunch program participation significantly.
_____ 7. Fast foods are to be avoided by those watching their weight.

Junk Food Questions Answered by a Nutritionist

Q. Should all candy, soft drinks, and other "junk" foods be excluded from children's diets?

A. Eating is not merely a biological event, it is also one of life's many pleasures. Thus, it is acceptable to eat certain foods simply to enjoy them. Moderation is the key—that is, inclusion of a variety of different foods in moderate amounts. This means eating foods from all of the Basic Food Groups, including sweets and "junk" foods.

Absence of choice does not teach moderation. Banning foods from children's diets will not stop them from obtaining their favorite goodies elsewhere. Rather than resulting in the ability to enjoy all different sorts of foods in moderation, food bans can lead to eating disorders, food obsessions, diet myths, and lack of pleasure in eating.

Just as there should be rules about bedtime and hours allotted for television viewing, so should there be rules about what, when, and how much is eaten. Children should not be allowed to eat whatever they choose whenever they happen to think of it—in unlimited amounts. As long as snacks do not interfere with consumption of well-balanced meals and as long as sweets are used as occasional after-meal treats, healthy children need not eliminate all "junk" foods. With overweight children, however, these treats are the first foods to limit. There is still no need to prohibit them completely; children should be encouraged to increase their activity levels rather than restrict their diets.

Q. Do "junk" foods provide any nutrients, or do they merely threaten health?

A. Some "junk" foods are relatively high in nutrient value (e.g., milkshakes, hamburgers, and pizza), and few are totally nutrient free. In addition to calories, many of these products provide carbohydrate, some contribute protein, and several offer vitamins and/or minerals as well. Upon careful evaluation, "junk" foods may be seen to be composed of nutritious ingredients. Consider the following examples:

- ○ Pie—wheat flour, fruit, nuts, or custard (milk)
- ○ Cake—whole wheat, milk, eggs, sometimes fruit or nuts
- ○ Hamburger—lean beef (bun has wheat flour)
- ○ Cookies—wheat flour, milk, eggs, sometimes oats, nuts, or fruit
- ○ Potato chips—potatoes, vegetable oil
- ○ Popcorn—corn
- ○ Pizza—wheat flour, cheese, tomatoes, sometimes other vegetables

Q. Do "junk" foods interfere with proper nutrition?

A. "Junk" foods do not have to interfere with good nutrition, but can be enjoyed in addition to other foods as part of a well-balanced diet. Only if "junk" food favorites crowd out the variety of foods necessary for a well-balanced diet will health be threatened. Moderate amounts of sweets, alcoholic beverages, and fast foods are nutritionally acceptable and, in today's society, practically unavoidable.

Q. What are fast foods, and do they offer any nutritional value?

A. "Fast food" can be defined as relatively low-cost food, eaten out of hand, and sold at outlets featuring over-the-counter, quick, convenient service—without any frills. Such foods are not devoid of nutritional value and, if eaten as *part* of a well-balanced diet, provide some nutrients as well as eating pleasure. If one eats a wide variety of other foods in addition to fast food fare, it is most likely that the diet is nutritionally adequate.

Q. How can a nutritious meal be selected at a fast food restaurant?

A. Most fast food restaurants offer a limited variety of foods, but many are now expanding their menus to include salads, vegetables, fruit, whole grain products, and vegetarian fare. Thus, a well-balanced meal can be selected from most any fast food menu, if the following concepts are kept in mind:

1. Choose a variety of different items; avoid getting trapped in the hamburger-and-soft-drink habit.
2. Limit intake of greasy, fried foods such as french fries, fried chicken, fried fish, sausage, and pepper steaks.
3. The dessert choices often contain considerable amounts of calories and sugar with little accompanying nutrient value.
4. Avoid salting fast food items since most already contain a significant amount of sodium.
5. Select fruit juice or milk (preferably skim or low-fat), especially if watching caloric intake.
6. Ask for lettuce, tomato, onion, green pepper, mushrooms, and other vegetables on sandwiches or pizza; order coleslaw, or try out the salad bar where available.
7. Look for vegetarian fast food restaurants, "light" fast food franchises with low-fat menus, and innovative fast food outlets offering whole grain buns and other nutritious options.
8. Be sure that fast foods are only *part* of a well-balanced diet, rather than forming the basis of the overall diet.

Q. Is it nutritionally unwise to lunch on submarine sandwiches?

A. An occasional submarine sandwich (sub, hoagie, grinder, wedge, hero, bomber, etc.) can serve as a nutritious luncheon choice. As long as the fillings are varied from day to day, one need not worry about a lack of variety. However, the typical sandwich of this size may pose a few problems worth considering:

○ Caloric content can be high.
○ Fat, cholesterol, and sodium (salt) content can be high.
○ Fiber content can be low.

Sub sandwiches can still be included in the diet, however, if selected wisely. The following tips are helpful when pondering over submarine sandwich menus:

○ Syrian bread is a lower-calorie alternative to sub rolls, and half-size subs are often available.
○ Turkey, lean roast beef, tuna, and chicken are all low-calorie, low-fat, low-cholesterol choices—but only if made with limited amounts of mayonnaise.
○ Vegetarian sandwiches offer much fiber for little caloric cost.
○ Raw vegetables (e.g., low-calorie items such as lettuce, tomato, peppers, mushrooms, and onions) can be added to subs to increase both fiber and nutrient content.
○ Milk can enhance a sub meal, and is sometimes available in the skim or low-fat forms.

Q. Is it better to skip breakfast than to have a fast food meal on work days?

A. A good day begins with a good breakfast. Morning fatigue and lack of energy are more apt to afflict breakfast skippers, and it is more likely that they will end the day with an insufficient total nutrient intake. Yet, today's typically fast-paced lifestyles have led to a large-scale shift away from the sit-down, family-style, bacon-and-eggs morning meal. More and more consumers are opting for quick, solitary breakfasts consisting of ready-to-eat breakfast cereals, toast and coffee, and a glass of juice. When one is unable to find the time to eat breakfast at home, a quick stop at a fast food outlet can provide a nutritious meal, as long as care is taken to make wise food choices.

Many fast food breakfast selections are undesirably high in calories, fat, cholesterol, salt, and/or sugar. It is best to minimize intake of fried foods, pastries, and fatty meats by limiting consumption of hash browns, pancakes, waffles, Danish pastries, donuts, sausages, bacon, and fried and scrambled eggs. Some of the preferable fast food breakfast choices include:

○ Muffins (corn, bran, or fruit)—although sometimes higher in fat than the home-made kinds, these donut shop choices are relatively low in calories and high in nutrient value.

○ English muffins—without added butter, since the fast food variety tends to come drenched with it.

○ Dry cereals—including bran varieties, served with skim or low-fat milk.

Depending on geographical location, some restaurants offer yogurt, scones, bagels, or biscuits. Thus, as long as lunch and supper meals are well balanced, a fast food breakfast can certainly contribute to an overall healthy diet.

Q.   Is it unwise (nutritionally) for school cafeterias to offer fast foods?

A.   Since the early 1970s, a number of school districts around the country have incorporated fast food menus into their foodservice. In an attempt to increase food acceptance and decrease food waste, school foodservice directors have capitalized on the popularity of fast foods among students. Reports have shown that the school use of fast foods has increased participation in lunch programs and decreased both food waste and cost per student. When included as *part* of a nutritionally balanced daily intake, fast foods can provide nutrients, energy, and fun. After all, a lunch eaten is far more helpful and healthful than one wasted due to disinterest.

Q.   Should dieters eliminate fast foods?

A.   Fast foods do tend to be higher in calories (and fat) than a lot of other meal and snack items, but they can certainly be included as *part* of a well-balanced diet. Calorie counters can use Table 4.2 to select the lower calorie versions of favorite fast foods, or get a copy of "How to Stay Slim and Healthy on The Fast Food Diet" by Judith Stern (1980), which lists the caloric contents for some of the various items offered by many fast food restaurants. Waist watchers can order small portions, choose the regular burgers over the giant-size specials, and request that items be prepared plain, unbuttered, and unsauced.

Table 4.2   Caloric Contents of Select Fast Foods

Fast food	Approximate no. of calories	Fast food	Approximate no. of calories
Arby's junior roast beef sandwich	220	McDonald's English muffin (unbuttered)	140
Burger King hamburger	295	McDonald's hamburger	255
Dairy Queen cone, small	110	McDonald's french fries (small)	210
Dunkin' Donuts cake donut, plain	240	Pizza Hut Thin 'n Crispy cheese, 2 slices	340
Dunkin' Donuts Munchkin, raised and glazed	35	Pizza Hut Thick 'n Chewy cheese, 2 slices	390
Friendly's Junior Fribble, vanilla	450	Taco Bell taco	160
Jack in the Box taco	190	Taco Bell tostada	205
Kentucky Fried Chicken drumstick	115	Taco Charley tortilla chips (1.27 oz)	170
Kentucky Fried Chicken thigh	260	Wendy's chili	230
Long John Silver's scallops (6 pieces)	260	Wendy's hamburger, single	470
Long John Silver's shrimp (6 pieces)	270	Wendy's hamburger, triple with cheese	1035!

STEP 5: SUPPLEMENTARY INFORMATION

During this century, a great deal of progress has been made in treating and preventing infectious diseases. Several great medical mysteries, such as the cause of **tuberculosis** and the prevention of **polio,** have been solved by sudden decisive advances in medical technology, that is, the identification of a disease agent or the discovery of a vaccine.

Today, we find that our chronic physical and mental diseases generally have more than one cause, which makes health research much more complex, and the long wait for definitive answers becomes even longer. Americans are extremely anxious to receive news of cures and preventions and, therefore, are ready and eager to accept any solutions that find their way into the headlines of the popular press. Unfortunately, too many individuals are able to publish partial evidence—or in some cases, mere hunches—and the public perceives this as fact.

One of the most popular (and costly) myths into which Americans are putting their trust (and earnings) are nutrition supplements. Hoping for a short-cut to health, or even a miracle cure for illness, consumers purchase billions of dollars worth of unnecessary vitamin and mineral pills, protein powders, herbal concoctions, and other dietary supplements. Unless prescribed by a physician for a clinically diagnosed deficiency, such supplementation is unnecessary—and may prove harmful.

As a dietetic technician in nutrition care, you will encounter patients with diagnosed nutritional deficiencies. In such cases, nutrition supplements will be prescribed. (See more on diet modifications in Parts III and IV.) However, you will also encounter many ill patients, as well as healthy individuals, who have questions regarding the need for and use of nutrition supplements. It is important to prepare yourself by obtaining a working knowledge of the scientific facts regarding nutrition supplementation. Therefore, after you complete the brief quiz that follows, read through the accompanying commonly asked questions and the answers that most nutritionists would provide. Do you and your peers agree with the scientific viewpoints on nutrition supplements? Do *you* take supplements? If so, were they prescribed by your physician? Discuss your personal supplementation practices with your classmates or co-workers; will the information provided in Step 5 influence your current supplementation practices?

tuberculosis: Infectious disease typically affecting respiratory system which is acquired due to contact with a carrier or by consumption of contaminated (raw) milk.

polio: Poliomyelitis, an infectious inflammation in the spinal cord, often causing paralysis.

Preliminary Quiz

Indicate whether you consider each of the following statements to be true (T) or false (F). Answers are provided throughout the remainder of Step 5, and are given in the Answer Key at the end of the book.

_____ 1. Megavitamins have been proven effective in the treatment of a number of diseases and disorders.
_____ 2. Everyone should take vitamin supplements to ensure good health.
_____ 3. Vitamin C has never been proven as a cure for the common cold.
_____ 4. Vitamin E has not been shown to be the "sex vitamin" that advertisements claim.
_____ 5. Mineral supplements are expensive, unnecessary, and potentially harmful in large doses.
_____ 6. Women should routinely take an iron supplement.
_____ 7. "Health" food supplements—such as wheat germ, brewer's yeast, bee pollen, and royal jelly—can be expensive sources of the nutrients amply provided by a well-balanced diet.
_____ 8. Excessive intakes of any nutrient will simply be excreted, not stored in the body.

Supplementation Questions Answered by a Nutritionist

Q. Do large doses of vitamins help to protect against illness and disease?

A. If a little bit of a vitamin is good, then must a great deal of it be even better? Such is the philosophy of vitamin salespersons who advocate large doses of specific vitamins for an endless list of ailments. They appear to be quite successful in their efforts: according to a recent national survey, three-fourths of adult Americans believe that vitamins promote extra "pep" and energy, and can generally lead to improved health.

Vitamin salespeople convince the public that everyone could benefit from routine dietary supplementation. The truth is that most everyone can obtain all of the required nutrients simply by eating a moderate amount of a wide variety of foods.

Q. Is it possible to take an excessive amount of vitamins?

A. Definitely! An excess could be defined as anything exceeding the Recommended Dietary Allowances of the National Research Council. Symptoms of excessive vitamin intakes are varied and sometimes vague. The known hazards of vitamin A overdose include loss of appetite, flaking of the skin, increased brain pressure (imitating a brain tumor), and abnormal bone growth. Vitamin C in megadoses is especially dangerous for pregnant women, causes gastrointestinal disturbances, and can lead to scurvy-like symptoms upon discontinued use. Overdoses of vitamin D can lead to hypercalcemia (excess calcium in the blood) in infants. The B vitamins in large amounts can also cause a number of undesirable symptoms.

A number of deaths and cases of unnecessary surgery have been recorded as directly related to taking high potency preparations, combining too many different kinds of supplements, or taking more than the recommended dosage.

Q. Does the average healthy adult need to take vitamin supplements to ensure good health?

A. Despite claims to the contrary—usually made by vitamin salespersons—healthy people rarely need to take vitamin supplements. A varied diet usually provides adequate amounts—not only of vitamins, but of other required nutrients as well. Although vitamins and other types of nutrition supplements are useful in the treatment of certain diseases and occasionally in recovery from illness, most healthy individuals should simply eat a well-balanced diet. The necessary vitamins are available in today's food supply—far more pleasantly and much less expensively than in a pill bottle.

Q. Is vitamin C really helpful in treating the common cold?

A. Most of the researchers and physicians whose field of expertise includes the many viruses that can cause colds (or influenza) disagree with the concept that large doses of vitamin C are either preventative or curative with regards to colds or flu. There have been many well-controlled studies conducted on the subject which indicate that the benefits of vitamin C therapy are minimal at best.

The body requires only a very small amount of this vitamin in order to function properly and remain healthy. One glass of orange juice, a wedge of cantaloupe, a sliced tomato, or a serving of broccoli will provide the recommended daily requirement, along with various other nutrients.

Q. Do vitamin E supplements improve sexual function?

A. Illness in humans due to a lack of vitamin E in the diet is unheard of, and there are no known human illnesses caused by a lack of vitamin E, nor illnesses requiring treatment with vitamin E. Those who recommend—and usually sell at exhorbitant prices—vitamin E for increased sexual potency, prevention or treatment of heart disease, muscle cramps, or any other ailment, lack supportive evidence to back such claims.

Vitamin E is so plentiful in the foods currently available (e.g., vegetable oils, whole grains, leafy vegetables), that it is almost impossible to develop a deficiency, providing the diet is well balanced. Yet, because of the myriad undocumented claims of curative powers, vitamin E sales continue to expand. Health professionals, however, warn that vitamin E will not cure a nonexistent deficiency.

Q. Are mineral supplements necessary to replace the nutrients lost due to over-processing of modern foods?

A. There is no need for healthy consumers to take mineral supplements, as all of the minerals required can be obtained via a well-balanced and varied diet. It is safer to meet nutrient needs by eating a wide variety of foods; foodstuffs contain minerals in balanced proportions, while supplements can lead to unhealthy mineral imbalances. For example, a daily megadose of phosphorus can upset the body's calcium balance, and zinc supplementation can aggravate a copper deficiency.

In excessive doses, minerals can have toxic effects, especially the trace minerals required only in very small amounts. Selenium, a favorite among supplement salespersons, is toxic in amounts only slightly above the trace amounts needed. Large doses of zinc, another popular supplement, can cause nausea, vomiting, and intestinal bleeding.

Obviously, diet is a more favorable means of obtaining required minerals, and in the amounts the body needs. Although the less-processed foods—dairy products, meat, vegetables, whole grains—tend to be richer in mineral content, convenience foods, frozen vegetables, fast food fare, and other processed products also provide various minerals.

The only exceptions to the no-need-to-supplement rule is with the minerals iron and fluoride; iron is difficult to absorb, and both iron and fluoride can be scarce in the diet. Therefore, for those people requiring extra iron—pregnant women and women of childbearing ages—a supplement may be required. The need for iron supplementation should always be diagnosed by a physician. In locations where the fluoride content of the water supply is low, a supplement may be prescribed.

Q. Is there any truth to the claim that the use of bone meal supplements is dangerous?

A. Heavy metals such as lead are stored in bones. The amount stored depends on the lead content of the forage, other food, and water consumed by the animal; commercial bone meal is usually prepared from the bones of cattle or horses. Thus, there is a good chance that the lead—or other heavy metal—content of available supplements is dangerously high. Nutritionists now warn "health" food users of the potential for health damage with use of such supplements.

Q. Is there any value in using a high-potency protein supplement in daily milk shakes?

A. All of the protein the body requires can be obtained through a well-balanced dietary intake. Meat, poultry, fish, eggs, milk, and cheese (as well as certain plant food combinations) provide more than enough of the protein essential for good health. Protein supplements are an unnecessary expense, and some can unbalance nutritional status by providing incomplete amino acid supplies or excessive amounts of protein.

Q. Is wheat germ an essential food supplement?

A. Wheat germ is a source of some valuable nutrients: protein, B vitamins, vitamin E, several minerals, and fiber. But wheat germ is not a miracle cure-all food, nor is it a dietary essential. It is provided in whole wheat products, but can be relatively high in calories and fat if consumed as a supplement.

Q. Is brewer's yeast as healthful as many claim?

A. A good source of protein and of several of the B vitamins, yes; a miracle food, no.

Q. What about bee pollen and royal jelly—is it true that they have health-giving properties?

A. Only their manufacturers claim that such products are "health-giving." They also fail to express just what composes these overpriced items, and conveniently omit labeling of specific nutritional value. Bee pollen is good for bees, and royal jelly is the food of queen bees, but their use to humans is unknown. Such supplements are really not much more than a waste of money.

Food is meant to supply nutrients in the required amounts, and to provide pleasure and satisfaction. Food is not meant to be used as a drug. As a dietetic technician in nutrition care, you will manipulate diets to aid in overall health care. Other members of the health care team will prescribe nutrition supplementation based on diagnosed needs. In counseling healthy persons, however, it is your responsibility to steer them clear of worthless supplements and the potentially dangerous side effects. Immoderate intakes of supplementary vitamins and minerals can damage the body—as can excessive amounts of carbohydrate, protein, or fat, which may be stored as body fat. Despite the many claims to the contrary made by vitamin salespersons, "health" food promoters, and self-proclaimed "nutritionists," a well-balanced diet can provide all of the nutrients required to maintain good health.

STEP 6: FOOD ADDITIVES

The term *food additive,* as defined by the Federal Food, Drug, and Cosmetic Act, is applied to any substance which can be reasonably expected to result—directly or indirectly—in becoming a component of or otherwise affecting the characteristics of any food. This means that any natural or synthetic substance which is added intentionally or accidentally to any food is considered a food additive.

The Food Protection Committee of the Food and Nutrition Board of the National Research Council's National Academy of Sciences has defined food additive as "a substance or mixture of substances other than a basic foodstuff, which is present in food as a result of any aspect of production, processing, storage, or packaging." Food additives are manufactured in laboratories and from natural sources. Often, man-made additives are chemically identical to natural food constituents; examples would include vitamins and minerals. Other food additives are derived from natural sources, such as lecithin from corn and soybeans, and carotene from yellow fruits and vegetables.

Food additives, like anything else, are not completely risk free. Yet, due to the strict food safety laws required by our government, the level of risk associated with common usage is low. Food scientists have the moral responsibility to ensure that the risk is as low as possible. You have the responsibility to reassure the public of this fact and to keep up to date on the latest research in order to inform your patients about any undesirable food additives.

Additive Questions Answered by a Nutritionist

Q.   There are so many rumors about food that it has become difficult to be sure exactly which foods are safe and which foods are not. Are food additives harmful or not?

A.   Food additives make up only about 1% of the total amount of food consumed—excluding sugar and salt—and all have been tested for safety before being used in our foods (which is more than can be said for the "natural" foods we eat). Some individuals have sensitivities to some additives, and certain people are sensitive to some of the "staple" foods, but most Americans can enjoy safe, varied diets that include food additives.

Concerns about food are certainly nothing new. From Biblical times, people have complained about the food served to them. In the past, food panics have focused on the safety of milk, meat, fish, coffee, vegetables, fruit, and a number of other items common to our weekly shopping lists.

The prospects of contracting disease or facing death have always created enough fear-provoking connotations to ensure that any "recommended solution" will be examined carefully by some portion of a population. Fear interferes with any attempt to examine food scare statements in a rational manner.

If one is concerned about the safety of a particular food, information can be obtained from established professionals in the nutrition field, such as individuals working in universities, state health departments, hospitals, or for the Food and Drug Administration (FDA). Also, the historical aspects of food faddism should be noted when considering the current concern about additives. Today's "panic in the pantry" phenomenon may just be the latest chapter in the thick volume of unfounded food scares.

Q.   Could the American food supply exist as is, even without food additives?

A.   Without the use of food additives, America would be forced to the old concept of bakery freshness: good today, stale tomorrow.

Additives are used to enhance the color and flavor of foods. Food color is a dynamic entity—rapidly changing colors would not appeal to wary consumers who prefer recognizable foods. Thus, permanent color is often added to foods to retain the aesthetic appeal. A wide variety in food flavors is available, but natural flavors do not always exist in large enough quantities to meet public demand. Thus, many flavors are synthesized.

Additives also help to preserve food and enhance the nutritional value. Without preservatives, products made from wheat and rye, potatoes, and many other foods could cause serious health problems. Nutritional deficiency diseases have been virtually eliminated due to food enrichment and fortification—with nutrient additives.

It is not very sensible, in consideration of the facts, to eliminate use of all food additives.

Q. Why do so many people think that food additives are "bad" and that "natural" foods are safe?

A. Many people think that additives have not been tested and are simply dumped haphazardly into our foods—solely for the convenience and economic advantages of the food industry. In reality, however, more is known about additives than is known about the chemistry of food itself. This is because food additives, especially the newer ones, have survived rigid testing procedures not applied to many of the ingredients of "natural" products.

As far as "natural" foods are concerned, such a label is relatively meaningless, since "natural" may or may not ensure that additives and/or preservatives are not present.

Q. How are food additives approved?

A. Any substance newly proposed for addition to food must undergo strict testing. Information has to be presented to the FDA depicting the chemical composition of the new additive, the manufacturing process, and the methods to be used to detect and measure actual presence in the food supply at the levels of expected use. Data must establish that the proposed testing methods are sufficiently sensitive to ensure compliance with appropriate regulations.

There also must be data to establish that the additive in question will accomplish the intended effect in the food, and that the amount proposed for use is no higher than that required to accomplish this effect.

Finally, data must be provided to establish that the additive is safe for the intended use. This requires scientific evidence obtained from feeding studies and other tests, using the proposed additive at various levels in the diet of two or more species of animals.

Q. How is the "safe dose" of an additive determined?

A. For many centuries, the rule of **toxicology** has been *sola dosis facit venenum,* or "only the dose makes the poison." Arsenic is used in small quantities as a therapeutic agent; curare, a deadly poison used by certain South American Indians, is used as a muscle relaxant; and the heart stimulant digitalis has saved thousands more lives than it ever threatened as part of the poisonous foxglove plant.

Safe is a relative term. Pre-clearance testing procedures ensure the lowest effective level of the additive used, and extensive animal testing—along with years of use by humans—are evidence to indicate that a safe dose has been achieved.

Scientists cannot "prove" the ultimate safety of anything, but can only take a reasonable approach based on present knowledge of the advantages and disadvantages of a substance—its benefits versus any possible risks. The acceptable percentage of the substance in the human diet is set at one-hundredth of the no-adverse-effect level in animals, that is, a one hundredfold margin of safety.

toxicology: Science dealing with poisonous substances including their detection, antidotes, and the development of treatment/prevention.

Q. What is the GRAS list?

A. Certain substances, which have been added to food for many years and which qualified scientists "generally recognize as safe" under the conditions of intended use, are exempt from the expensive pre-marketing clearing requirements required by law for acceptable food additives. This includes chemicals used prior to January 1, 1958, without any evidence of health hazards. The FDA has published listings of the substances recognized as GRAS. Some familiar items are sugar, salt, vinegar, and some spices. In all, these chemicals number more than 600. And whenever new research on food chemicals is reported—by scientists both inside and outside the food industry—which indicates a possible health risk, the FDA may revoke the GRAS classification of the chemical and relabel it as an unapproved food additive. The FDA can then require that a series of experiments be conducted to "prove" that the chemical is "safe" for its intended use. If these tests support the earlier suspicions, FDA can then move to prohibit or restrict use of the chemical. Both cyclamate and saccharin were once listed as GRAS substances, yet were removed later from the list when tests failed to "prove" that they were "safe."

In reality, tests cannot ever "prove" something, but can only indicate that a concept is probably true. A chemical cannot be guaranteed as "safe," but it can be demonstrated that the substance is probably harmless in moderate quantities. Yet, there is "safety in numbers"; that is, the wider the variety of foods eaten, the greater the number of different chemical substances consumed, and possibly the less the chance that any one chemical will reach a hazardous level in the diet. It is for this reason that many scientists believe that neither cyclamate nor saccharin should be banned. (By banning cyclamate, for example, larger amounts of saccharin—then the only available artificial sweetener—were consumed.) The "safety in numbers" principle should be applied to all chemicals, including sweeteners. Now that aspartame has been marketed, allowance of all three sweeteners for public consumption could further increase the safety margin.

Q. Why are there so many chemicals in foods today?

A. There always have been and always will be chemicals in food, given that all foods are naturally made of chemicals. The simple potato, for example, is actually a complex chemical aggregate of at least 150 distinct chemical substances. All "natural" foods are similarly complex, as are our modern day processed products. Our diet is composed of over 99% naturally occurring food chemicals, with less than 1% as food additives.

Q. Are all "natural" foods safe?

A. If the FDA were to ban or severely restrict all foods which contain traces of poisons, toxins, or cancer-causing agents, consumers would be forced to starve to death. Natural foods, like man-made foods, are composed of chemicals. And most chemicals can pose health threats—depending, of course, on the dose ingested.

Who would want to eat something composed of the following ingredients: water, triglycerides of stearic, palmitic, oleic, and linoleic acids, myosin, actin, glycogen, collagen, lecithin, cholesterol, dipotassium phosphate, myoglobin, and urea?

Many people would, if they realized that these chemicals comprise steak. How about a beverage with a label listing the following components: acetone, methylacetate, furan, diacetyl, butanol, methylfuran, isoprene, methylbutanol, caffeine, essential oils, methanol, acetaldehyde, methylformate, ethanol, dimethyl sulfide, and propionaldehyde? This is only a partial list of the hundreds of natural chemicals which make up coffee.

Food is made up of chemicals, as are all living things including humans. Not all chemicals are "bad," whether natural or man-made. In fact, there are many very poisonous chemicals which are naturally present in our foods, while some of the chemicals most important for our health and safety are synthesized in the laboratory. The body is unable to distinguish between a natural and a synthetic chemical, but will simply derive the benefits and the detriments provided by both.

Q. Do food additives, especially artificial colorings and flavorings, cause **hyperactivity** in children?

A. In 1974, the late Dr. Benjamin Feingold, once Chief of the Allergy Department of the Kaiser-Permanente Medical Center in Oakland, California, wrote a book entitled, "Why Your Child Is Hyperactive." His treatise was that the major cause of hyperactivity in children is ingestion of food additives, mainly artificial flavorings and colorings, plus the chemical salicylate found in many medications and foods—including aspirin, apples, apricots, cherries, grapes, nectarines, oranges, peaches, plums, prunes, raisins, raspberries, strawberries, cucumbers, tomatoes, and tea. His proposed diet virtually eliminates all processed foods: most condiments must be avoided and convenience foods are generally restricted. Thus, eating in school cafeterias, restaurants, fast food outlets, and even in others' homes becomes nearly impossible. Homemade foods prepared from "scratch" become a requirement for all family meals, and Dr. Feingold even recommended that all family members follow the diet (so that the hyperactive child will not feel "different"). This is a lot of work for the homemaker, and quite a project for the family to take on, representing a major alteration in family dynamics.

The results of adherence to the Feingold diet have always been open to question. Large-scale studies failed to prove that salicylates or artificial colors and flavors have the dramatic impact on hyperactivity that Dr. Feingold claimed. If these chemicals do affect behavior, the relationship seems to be a minor one. The evidence indicates that a few hyperactive children, perhaps a fraction of 1%, may experience a mild adverse reaction to one or several artificial colors or flavors present in foods. However, the magnitude of any relationship that may exist is so small that changes in food processing and food labeling—in an effort to prevent or control hyperactivity—are probably unnecessary.

hyperactivity: Hyperkinesis, or excessive activity, typically in young children and symptomatic of a behavior disorder; usually lessens with age and disappears during adolescence.

Q. If a diet is not the cause of hyperactive behavior in children, then why do so many parents insist that the Feingold diet helps their children?

A. Hyperactivity is characterized by a variety of symptoms, not all of which are necessarily present in each case. A hyperactive child is very restless, excitable, easily distracted, and emotionally unstable. The child is often irritable, aggressive, disruptive, and uncoordinated. It is estimated that 5–10% of all school age children in America are hyperactive, but quite often such "problem" children are improperly diagnosed.

There are many theories on the causes of hyperactivity, but none have been proved. Treatments are varied, including counseling, drugs, and diet. The Feingold diet is particularly attractive to parents because it removes their own guilt for their childrens' behavior and attaches it to our impersonal industrial complex. Also, it offers a "natural" alternative to drug therapy.

In analyzing the use of diet therapy in hyperactivity, research scientists have discovered what most parents fail to recognize: adherence to the diet regimen causes significant changes in family social patterns and lifestyle which could affect the child's behavior. The alterations in family dynamics which occur when the Feingold diet is adopted can contribute to a reduction in hyperactivity. Plus, the child's own sense of self-responsibility—he or she must take charge of food choices at school, friends' houses, and social events—can reduce fidgity behavior.

The Feingold diet, because it excludes so many common foods, could prove to be harmful to health. Planning meals to fulfill the day's nutritional needs becomes difficult. The possible benefits resulting from psychological influences must be weighed against the potential harm of instilling in children the false belief that their behavior is controlled by what they eat. Fortunately, most children "grow out of" hyperactivity as they get older.

Q. If additives are not poisonous chemicals, are pesticides safe as well?

A. Pesticides are poisonous chemicals, and that is why they work. They are poisonous for the insects, worms, rats, weeds, and other living pests against which they have been designed to be directed. Strictly enforced regulations aim to minimize any hazard to man from pesticide residues on foods.

Table 4.3 Additives Chart

Maintain or improve quality

Nutrients	Preservatives	Anti-oxidants
Ascorbic acid (vitamin C)	Ascorbic acid (vitamin C)	Ascorbic acid (vitamin C)
Beta carotene (vitamin A)	Benzoic acid	BHA (butylated hydroxyanisole)[a]
Iodine	Butylparaben	BHT (butylated hydroxytoluene)[a]
Iron	Calcium lactate	Citric acid
Niacinamide	Calcium propionate	EDTA (ethylenediamine tetraacetic acid)[a]
Potassium iodide	Citric acid	Propyl gallate
Riboflavin	Heptylparaben	TBHQ (tertiary butylhydroquinone)
Thiamin	Lactic acid	Tocopherols (vitamin E)
Tocopherols (vitamin E)	Methyl paraben	
Vitamin D	Potassium propionate	
	Potassium sorbate	
	Propionic acid	
	Propylparaben	
	Sodium benzoate	
	Sodium diacetate	
	Sodium erythorbate	
	Sodium nitrate[a]	
	Sodium nitrite[a]	
	Sodium propionate	
	Sodium sorbate	
	Sorbic acid	

nutrients: Enrich (replace vitamins and/or minerals removed in processing) or fortify (add nutrients which may be low in typical diet).

preservatives: Prevent spoilage, extend shelf life, or protect natural odor and/or flavor.

anti-oxidants: Prevent or delay rancidity or enzyme-caused browning.

(continued)

Table 4.3   (*Continued*)

Affect food appeal

	Flavor enhancers	Flavors	Colors	Sweeteners

flavor enhancers: Change or increase original taste and/or aroma without donating own taste.	Disodium guanylate
	Disodium inosinate
	Hydrolyzed vegetable protein
	MSG (monosodium glutamate)
	Yeast—malt sprout extract
		Paprika
		Salt
		Spices
		Turmeric (oleo resin)
		Vanilla, vanillin
			Annotto extract
			Beta-apo-8′ carotenal
			Beta carotene
			Canthaxanthin
			Caramel
			Carrot oil
			Citrus red #2[a]
			Cochineal extract
			Corn endosperm
			Dehydrated beets
			Dried algae meal
			FD&C colors[a] (blue #1,
			  red #3, red #40,
			  yellow #5)
			Grape skin extract
			Iron oxide
			Paprika
			Riboflavin
			Saffron
			Tageles (Aztec Marigold)
			Titanium dioxide
			Toasted, partially de-
			  fatted, cooked cotton-
			  seed flour
			Turmeric (oleo resin)
			Ultramarine blue
				Aspartame[a]
				Corn syrup
				Dextrose
				Fructose
				Glucose
				Invert sugar
				Mannitol
				Saccharin[a]
				Sorbitol
				Sucrose

flavors: Increase or restore flavors.				
colors: Add desirable or characteristic color.				
sweeteners: Change or increase sweetness of taste and/or aroma.				

Aid in processing or preparation

	Emulsifiers	Stabilizers, texturizers, thickeners	Leavening agents	pH-control agents	Humectants

emulsifiers: Improve consistency, stability, texture.
 	
stabilizers, texturizers, thickeners: Give body, improve texture and consistency.
 	
leavening agents: Affect texture and volume.
 	
pH-control agents: Change or maintain acidity or alkalinity.
 	
humectants: Cause moisture retention.
 	
anti-caking agents: Prevent lumping of crystalline or powdered substances.
 	
maturing and bleaching agents, dough conditioners: Speed up aging and improve baking qualities.
	Carrageenan
	Diglycerides
	Dioctyl sodium
	  sulfosuccinate
	Lecithin
	Monoglycerides
	Polysorbates
	Sorbitan mono-
	  stearate
	
	Anti-caking agents
	
	Calcium silicate
	Iron–ammonium
	  citrate
	Mannitol
	Silicon dioxide
	Yellow prussiate
	  of soda
		Ammonium algi-
		  nate
		Arabinogalactan
		Calcium alginate
		Carrageenan
		Carob bean gum
		Cellulose
		Gelatin
		Guar gum
		Gum arabic
		Gum ghatti
		Karaya gum
		Larch gum
		Locust bean gum
		Mannitol
		Modified food
		  starch
		Pectin
		Potassium algi-
		  nate
		Propylene glycol
		Sodium alginate
		Sodium calcium
		  alginate
			Calcium phosphate
			Sodium aluminum
			  sulfate
			Sodium bicarbonate
			
			Maturing and bleaching agents, dough conditioners
			
			Acetone peroxide
			Azodicarbonamide
			Benzoyl peroxide
			Calcium bromate
			Hydrogen peroxide
			Potassium bromate
			Sodium stearyl
			  fumarate
				Acetic acid
				Adipic acid
				Citric acid
				Lactic acid
				Phosphates
				Phosphoric acid
				Propylene glycol
				Sodium acetate
				Sodium citrate
				Tartaric acid
					Glycerine
					Glycerol mono-
					  stearate
					Sorbitol

[a]Currently under research to ensure safety.

Exercise on Food Additives

Read through the preceding commonly asked questions and the answers which most nutritionists would provide. After examining the additive charts in Table 4.3, prepare a brief oral report on one additive. You can use the reference list in Appendix V at a local library—medical school, hospital, or university branches are best—to gather your facts. Explain the background, uses, food sources, advantages and possible disadvantages of the chosen additive. Discuss your additive with classmates or co-workers and, if possible, learn the facts from them on other food additives. Is there a need to rely on "health" foods and "natural" products claiming to be free of additives? Is there reason to advise your patients to base their diets on such products? Discuss your views with peers.

STEP 7: HIDDEN SUGAR

Sugar is not poisonous, nor is it a proven health hazard. However, refined sugar provides only nutrient-free calories. Devoid of nutritional value and yet a significant source of calories, many sugar-rich foods are palate pleasers which tempt overindulgence. A diet

Table 4.4   Hidden Sugar Chart

Meal	Food and amount	Sugar (tsp)	Subtotal (tsp)
Breakfast:	Instant breakfast drink, 4 oz	4	
	Granola, commercial, $\frac{3}{4}$ cup	1	
	Toast, 2 slices	Trace	
	with jelly, 1 Tbsp	3	
	Coffee with cream	1	
			9
Midmorning snack:	Glazed donut	6	
	Coffee with cream	1	
			7
Lunch:	Sandwich: bread, 2 slices	Trace	
	with peanut butter, 1 Tbsp	Trace	
	and jam, 1 Tbsp	3	
	Yogurt, fruit-flavored, 1 cup	5	
	Applesauce, 1 cup	9	
			17
Midafternoon snack:	Chewing gum, 2 sticks	1	
	Fudge, 1 oz	5	
			6
Cocktail hour:	Butter crackers, 10–12	1	
	Whiskey sour, 6 oz, 2	6	
			7
Dinner:	Hamburger, lean, 3 oz	0	
	with noodle mix, 1 cup,	9	
	and catsup, 2 Tbsp	1	
	Corn, canned, $\frac{1}{2}$ cup	1	
	Salad with French dressing	1	
	Fig bars, 2	10	
	Sherbet, $\frac{1}{2}$ cup	4	
			26
Bedtime snacks:	Fruit, canned in syrup, 1 cup	9	
	Chocolate cake, 1 avg slice	10	
	Cider, 1 cup	6	
			25
	Total sugar:		97

with an excess in calories from sugar—or from starch, protein, or fat—can lead to overweight. A diet high in refined sugar can also be detrimental to dental health, especially if the sweets which are eaten are sticky and remain in the mouth for considerable amounts of time.

Thus, sugar does pose dietary drawbacks. It has been recommended by various nutrition advisory panels that Americans reduce their intake of refined sugar (see Appendix III). Yet, sugar is the country's most popular additive: each of us consumes over 100 lb of sugar and corn sweeteners (which are also low in nutrient value) every year. Those who protest that they "never eat sweets" may not realize that around two-thirds of the ingested sugar is already hidden in our foodstuffs while only one-third is purposely added by consumers, because sugar is used not only to add flavor, but to preserve foods and improve appeal.

Exercise on Hidden Sugar

As a dietetic technician in nutrition care, you need to be aware of the scientific facts on sugar in order to evaluate diets properly and educate your patients.

Examine the Hidden Sugar Chart (Table 4.4). Are you surprised at the total quantity of sugar in the sample menu? Determine the caloric content of the *total* sugar, and remember that the sugar itself provides only energy. How could you advise an overweight person to curtail sugar intake? What would you advocate for the healthy, normal weight individual regarding refined sugar intake?

Using sugar packets or teaspoonfuls of sugar, demonstrate for friends or family the quantity of sugar contained in the menu from the Hidden Sugar Chart: teaspoon by teaspoon, pile up the total sugar hidden in this menu on a tray for your audience to view. Do you think such an intake is desirable? or necessary? or possible to alter? Discuss the answers to these questions and the audience's responses to your sugar demonstration with classmates or co-workers.

STEP 8: HIDDEN SALT

Sodium is an essential nutrient which comprises about 40% of the common compound table salt (sodium chloride). Because the mineral sodium is present in so many foodstuffs (including water), it is rare for a deficiency to occur in the normal, healthy individual. Dietary intakes vary from culture to culture, with some Oriental diets containing 30–40 grams (g) of salt per day, while the typical American diet may include 6–18 g. Since sodium is more abundant in animal foods than in plants, vegetarians usually consume less than do meat eaters.

Although the exact mechanism is still uncertain, sodium intake is thought to play a role in hypertension. For those with a tendency to develop high blood pressure and a sensitivity to salt, a diet excessively high in sodium may lead to hypertension; for those with elevated blood pressure, a high-sodium diet may exacerbate the problem. Loss of excess body weight can help to lower elevated blood pressure, as can a low-sodium diet and (possibly) an adequate intake of calcium with a desirably high potassium-to-sodium ratio. It is important to realize that one-fourth to one-half of the typical American's sodium intake comes from processed food, which means that a significant percentage of dietary sodium is hidden in our foods.

Exercise on Hidden Salt

As a dietetic technician in nutrition care, you need to be aware of the scientific facts on sodium in order to evaluate diets properly and educate your patients. (More on the regulation of dietary sodium appears in Chapter 12.) Examine the Hidden Salt Chart (Table 4.5)

Table 4.5   Hidden Salt Chart

Food and amount	Approximate amount of sodium (mg)
Tomato juice, canned, 1 cup	486
Egg, fried	155
Bacon, 2 slices	306
Cornflakes, 1 cup	251
Milk, skim, $\frac{1}{2}$ cup	64
Pumpernickel bread, 2 slices	364
Margarine, 2 tsp	92
Milk, skim, $\frac{1}{2}$ cup	64
Bouillon, 1 cup	960
Crackers, oyster, 20	166
Hot dog	627
Roll	202
Butter, 1 Tbsp	140
Catsup, 1 Tbsp	156
Mustard, 2 tsp	126
Relish, 1 Tbsp	107
Dill pickles, 3 spears	1276
Potato chips, 1-oz package	191
Cola, 12-oz can	54
Martini	Trace
Olives, 2	136
Crackers, butter type, 6	216
Cheese, processed American, 2 oz	922
Peanuts, $\frac{1}{2}$ cup	301
Big Mac	1510
Tossed salad	Trace
Italian dressing, 2 Tbsp	628
Chocolate pudding, 1 cup	335
Beer, "light," 2 cans (12 oz each)	112
Pretzels, thin, 10	504
Peanut butter 'n crax (Nab), 2-oz package	592
Total sodium:	11,043

and consider the following questions: Are you surprised at the total quantity of sodium in the chart? What would you advise a patient who may be prone to hypertension regarding sodium intake? What would you advocate for the healthy, nonhypertensive individual regarding dietary sodium?

Using quarter-teaspoonfuls of salt (1 tsp salt contains approximately 2000 mg sodium), demonstrate for friends or family the quantity of salt contained in the menu given as the Hidden Salt Chart (Table 4.5): gradually pile up the total salt hidden in this menu on a tray for your audience to view. Do you think such an intake is desirable? or necessary? or possible to alter? Discuss the answers to these questions and the audience's responses to your salt demonstration with classmates or co-workers.

Sodium is an essential nutrient required by the body for proper functioning (see Chapter 3). Since sodium is naturally present in most foods, the amount needed each day is easily obtained through a well-balanced diet. However, most Americans tend to consume far more sodium than required through excessive use of salt at the table and in cooking.

Table 4.6 High-Sodium Foods

Fruits and vegetables

Frozen lima beans, mixed vegetables, peas	Sauerkraut
Pickled beets	Seasoned vegetables (frozen)
Pickled salad mix	Tomato juice
	Vegetable juice cocktail

Breads and cereals

Breadsticks (unless unsalted)	Pretzels
Crackers (unless unsalted)	Rolls, salted top
Popcorn (commercial)	

Meats and alternates

Bologna	Anchovies
Chipped beef	Canned fish
Corned beef	Caviar
Dried meat	Dried fish
Frankfurters	Herring
Ham	Sardines
Kosher meats	Spread cheese
Luncheon meats	Nuts, salted
Pastrami	
Pickled meats	
Sausage	
Smoked meat or fish	
Smoked tongue	
Stew, canned	

And then there's

Bacon	Fast foods
Bouillon	Olives
Chips (corn, potato, cheese-flavored, etc.)	Soups (canned, frozen, dry package)
Dips	

Condiments: catsup, horseradish, mustard, pickles, relishes, salad dressings, and sauces (barbecue, chili, meat, soy, tartar, Worcestershire)

Seasonings: cooking wines, gravies, meat marinades, meat tenderizers, meat/vegetable extracts, monosodium glutamate, salts (celery salt, garlic salt, Kosher salt, onion salt, sea salt, seasoned salts)

Most processed foods also contain substantial amounts of sodium in the form of

○ Salt—Sodium chloride
○ MSG–monosodium glutamate
○ Additives–benzoate of soda, disodium phosphate, sodium benzoate, sodium bi-carbonate, sodium propionate, sodium saccharin, sodium silico aluminate, etc.

Does your diet actually contain more sodium than you think? The medical community currently advises a moderate daily salt intake of around 5 g, or 2 g of sodium. Examine the items listed in the High-Sodium Foods chart (Table 4.6) to determine some common sources of excess sodium.

Obviously, it is easy to consume a large amount of sodium without even shaking a salt shaker. Because so many processed foods contain added sodium and processed foods may make up a significant proportion of the diet, it would be impossible (and unnecessary) to avoid salt entirely. The key is to be aware of salt intake, and thereby consume only a moderate amount. Table 4.6 can serve as a helpful guide for identifying high-sodium foods.

STEP 9: LIQUID LIBATIONS

Food is not the only source of nutrients—and of oral satisfaction. Beverages, too, provide energy (calories), various nutrients, and liquid refreshment. They replace lost body fluids, quench thirst, and often play a central role in our overall social environment. After all, what's a coffee klatch without the coffee? Or a social tea without the tea? Or any party without the punch?

As with food, there are fallacies and confusion surrounding some of our common beverages. Coffee is sometimes condemned due to caffeine-phobia, tea is similarly slotted, and the topic of alcohol is surrounded by a multitude of health fears. Many consumers currently sip their favorite drinks—be it cola, coffee, tea, beer, or martini—with feelings akin to those their forebears held when entering the local speakeasy!

Coffee and tea both contain caffeine—as do several other products, including most cola beverages, chocolate, cocoa, and certain headache or cold remedies. Although many stories about the hazards of caffeine are exaggerated, caffeine does exert certain physical effects.

Alcohol too exerts druglike effects on the body. Heavy and regular alcohol abuse is accompanied by some very definite health risks. However, these risks must be viewed in perspective. In moderate amounts, alcohol may be compatible with good health. Again, moderation in intake seems to be the wisest choice.

As a dietetic technician in nutrition care, it is essential that you become aware of your patients' liquid—as well as solid—dietary intakes. The caloric, caffeine, and alcoholic contents of the diet can prove to be of relevance to overall health status (more on alcohol in Chapter 14). After you read the following commonly asked questions and the answers which most nutritionists would provide, you can complete the Beverage Nutrient/Caloric Value Chart in this section in order to compare several common beverages.

Beverage Questions Answered by a Nutritionist

Q. Why is coffee such a popular beverage?

A. Coffee can be low in calories (depending on the addition of cream, milk, or sugar), it has a taste which appeals to many people, and it may help some individuals to stay awake. In this country, the "coffee break" is the time period used to "perk up" and prepare for the work ahead. Although coffee has been America's most popular source of caffeine, sales have declined somewhat in recent years while sales of tea, soft drinks, and cocoa have increased. Yet, the major reason for the continued popularity of coffee is that it contains caffeine, a physically and psychologically addictive drug.

Q. How does caffeine affect the body?

A. Caffeine can function as a diuretic, a mild antidepressant, and a stimulant for the central nervous system, heart, and rate of body metabolism. Caffeine is not stored in body tissues, but is efficiently metabolized so that, in only a few seconds, the caffeine from coffee (or other source) can reach the brain and, in a few minutes, will appear in other body tissues (to be then excreted).

The metabolic effects of caffeine depend on the dosage, as well as individual tolerance and state of health. The average healthy adult is less sensitive to caffeine than are children and ill or elderly persons. There is also some question as to how caffeine may affect an unborn fetus since it will cross the **placenta** and accumulate in the fetus' brain tissue, taking 20–30 times longer than normal to be eliminated. Although there is no evidence as yet which shows that caffeine intake by pregnant humans causes birth defects, tests in laboratory rats show that large doses can cause fetal abnormalities.

placenta: Structure in the uterus through which the fetus is able to derive nutrients and oxygen and can dispose of wastes.

Q. Does coffee really provide "pep" and energy?

A. Coffee has essentially no calories (only around 2 calories per cup), but due to the stimulating effects of caffeine, coffee is used by many as a quick "pepper-upper." Moderate doses can increase work output and lengthen physical performance.

Table 4.7 Caffeine Contents of Foods and Drugs (mg)

Coffee (6 oz)		Tea (6 oz)		Cocoa	
Automatic drip	181	Iced tea	69	Chocolate candy (2 oz)	45
Automatic perk	125	Red Rose:	weak, 45	Baking chocolate (1 oz)	45
Instant	54		medium, 62	Milk chocolate candy (2 oz)	12
Decaffeinated	3		strong, 90	Cocoa powder (6 oz)	10
Soft drinks (12 oz)[a]		Tetley:	weak, 18	Drugs (tablet)	
Mountain Dew	54		medium, 48	Nodoz	100
Mellow Yellow	51		strong, 70	Anacin	32.5
Dr. Pepper	38	English Breakfast:	weak, 26	Midol	32.4
Pepsi Cola	38		medium, 78	Coricidin	30
Coca Cola	33		strong, 107		
Tab	32				
RC Cola	26				

[a]Unless labeled as caffeine free.

Q. Will drinking coffee at bedtime cause insomnia?

A. While some individuals claim that caffeine does not inhibit their ability to fall asleep, most people find that after-dinner or bedtime coffee consumption can keep them awake. Even those who do not notice major sleep disturbances may take longer to fall asleep and can experience a poorer quality of sleep whenever caffeine is consumed at bedtime.

Q. What are "coffee nerves"?

A. The problem of "coffee nerves" may occur in susceptible individuals who drink more than 4 or 5 cups of brewed coffee per day (or 10–12 cups of instant coffee, 10–12 cups of tea, or 12 cans of caffeinated soft drinks), while certain individuals may even react to only 1 or 2 cups. The symptoms include tremors, poor motor coordination, insomnia, visual disturbances, and a ringing in the ears. Thus, "coffee nerves" are sometimes confused with **anxiety neurosis.** Chronic coffee consumption may aggravate **psychoses** in the mentally ill.

anxiety neurosis: Mental disorder characterized by excessive and nonspecific anxiety.

psychosis: Mental disorder characterized by loss of contact with reality.

Q. Does caffeine irritate the gastrointestinal tract?

A. Certain individuals with gastrointestinal problems—including ulcers and colitis—should avoid caffeine because it stimulates gastric acid secretions to cause further irritation. Recent evidence indicates that decaffeinated beverages can also increase gastric secretions.

Q. Does coffee consumption cause cancer of the pancreas?

A. Despite some stories promoted by the media, caffeine intake has not been linked by scientific studies to degenerative diseases. A report which claimed an association between coffee and pancreatic cancer was based on only one study of hospitalized patients (MacMahon *et al.* 1981). The fact that unhealthy coffee drinkers were more apt to have cancer of the pancreas than unhealthy noncoffee drinkers is hardly evidence on which to base a claim against moderate coffee consumption by healthy individuals.

Q. Does tea contain caffeine?

A. Caffeine is a chemical which is present in coffee, tea, cocoa, chocolate, certain soft drinks, and some medications (see Table 4.7). Most teas contain less caffeine than coffee, and there are a number of noncaffeinated varieties of tea (and coffee) available. The longer the tea is steeped, the higher the caffeine content. Weak tea is often tolerated by those who need to avoid coffee.

Table 4.8   Caloric Contents for Common Alcoholic Beverages and Mixers

Alcoholic beverage	Proof	Amount (oz)	Approximate no. of calories	Mixer, 6 oz	Approximate no. of calories
Liquor, distilled	80	1½	95	Tonic	55
	86	1½	105	Collins	60
	90	1½	115	Ginger ale	60
	100	1½	125	Seven-up	75
				Cola	75
Beer, "light"	3%	12	95	Fruit punch	80
Beer, regular	4%	12	150	Bitter lemon	85
Ale	5%	12	165	Cream	385
Wine, table	12%	3½	90		
Wine, fortified (sherry, port)	19%	3½	140		

Q.   Of what nutritional value are alcoholic beverages?

A.   Alcoholic beverages were used in ancient and prehistoric times for nourishment, as well as for religious and social purposes. Unfortunately, such drinks are virtually devoid of nutrients and provide mostly calories. No longer used extensively for religious purposes, alcohol plays a major role in many social functions and is used for relaxation by millions of Americans. Therefore, it is important to be aware that there is no such thing as a noncaloric alcoholic beverage, and all have negligible nutritional value (unless nutritious mixers are used).

Q.   What does proof mean and can it indicate caloric values?

A.   The alcoholic content of distilled spirits—gin, rum, vodka, whiskey—is expressed in terms of proof. In this country, the *proof* represents twice the alcohol content by volume. Thus, 100 proof means 50% alcohol and 80 proof is 40% alcohol. White table wines usually contain about 12% alcohol, red wines about 14%, and fortified wines have 20–24% (due to the addition of alcohol as neutral spirits).

Liqueurs range from 40 to 55% alcohol content. Beer—including ale, lager, and stout—contains anywhere between 3 and 5% alcohol, with the "light" beers down toward the lower end of the spectrum.

The remainder of an alcoholic beverage which is not alcohol consists mainly of water and congeners, the substances which impart specific flavors to each beverage. A simple formula for determining the caloric content of an alcoholic beverage (without mixer) is as follows:

$$0.8 \times \text{proof} \times \text{ounces} = \text{calories}$$

The higher the proof, the more calories per ounce. Remember, however, that beer is usually consumed in 12-oz servings, wine is sipped in 4- or 5-oz glasses, and the typical hard drink contains about 1–1½ oz of alcohol.

Table 4.8 depicts the alcohol and caloric contents for common alcoholic beverages, and the caloric contributions made by 6 oz of a variety of popular mixers.

Q.   If alcohol is high in calories, why are so many alcoholics underweight?

A.   For reasons that are not yet clearly understood, alcohol does not provide caloric food value equivalent to that contributed by food. Although alcohol provides about 7 calories per gram and carbohydrate yields 4, laboratory studies have shown significantly less weight gain with alcohol diets compared to calorically equivalent carbohydrate diets. Substituting alcohol for carbohydrate for half of the total calories in an otherwise balanced diet resulted in weight loss. It appears that chronic alcohol intake diminishes the body's ability to utilize the calories from alcohol. Also, alcohol in sustained high amounts tends to suppress the appetite. Eventually, alcohol interferes with normal digestion and metabolism so that the body is unable to properly use those nutrients which are consumed.

Q. Is it wiser to drink beer or wine rather than hard drinks?

A. Some people believe that they are automatically consuming less alcohol if they drink wine or beer rather than distilled liquor. But alcohol is alcohol, be it in beer, wine, or martinis. And it is the quantity of alcohol consumed, not the type of beverage, which is important. Thus, moderation in the consumption of all alcoholic beverages is best.

Q. What health damages will alcoholic beverages cause?

A. Unlike foods, alcohol is not digested but is absorbed from the stomach directly into the bloodstream, the rate dependent on individual size and metabolism, amount and speed of alcohol consumption, and the presence of food in the stomach. If alcohol is imbibed faster than it can be metabolized, it accumulates in the blood and body tissues causing the symptoms of drunkenness. The long-term health effects of alcohol are many, but research indicates one general conclusion: There are definite risks which accompany regular heavy use of alcohol.

cirrhosis: Chronic liver disease primarily due to nutritional deficiencies and/or chronic alcoholism.

Since alcohol is oxidized by the liver, long-term heavy consumption may damage this organ, causing **cirrhosis** and interfering with normal functioning. About 10% of all heavy drinkers develop this condition.

There is no substantial evidence that alcohol alone causes cancer, but studies do indicate that alcohol may act as a co-carcinogen in conjunction with cigarette smoking: A heavy drinker who smokes has an increased risk of developing cancer of the esophagus or oral cavity. Preliminary studies also indicate a possible link between alcohol intake and breast cancer in women (Rosenberg et al. 1982; Schatzkin et al. 1987; Willet et al. 1987).

Q. Will alcohol intake during pregnancy have any effect on the baby?

A. Nutrition is extremely important during pregnancy, and if alcohol is part of the diet, it is a vital consideration. Alcohol, like nutrients, will pass through the placenta to enter the bloodstream of the fetus. Overindulgence means excessive fetal intake, with potentially dangerous consequences.

Fetal alcohol syndrome is the term used to describe the severe form of physical and mental birth defects which have been found in babies born to women who drink excessively during pregnancy. The affected babies are abnormally small at birth and, unlike other small newborns, they never catch up to achieve normal growth. Many show degrees of mental deficiency, and physically they appear jittery and poorly coordinated. Evidence shows that the IQs do not improve with age, almost half have heart defects which sometimes require surgery, and all have deformed facial features with narrowed eyes, low nasal bridges, and short upturned noses.

It is estimated that there are over one million alcoholic women of childbearing age in the United States today—and this number is increasing, particularly among adolescents. Fetal alcohol syndrome is a tragedy, but a preventable one. All women of childbearing age can prevent the birth defects caused by excessive use of alcohol.

Q. How much alcohol is too much for the average healthy male or nonpregnant female?

A. Alcohol can be part of a pleasant, relaxing atmosphere and may contribute to good health. Used in moderation, alcoholic beverages can enhance social occasions, reduce stress, and add pleasure to meals. On the other hand, if alcohol is abused, serious physical and social problems can result. The amount of alcohol each person should consume is an individual matter, depending on general health, both mental and physical.

For most individuals, a moderate daily intake of a favorite cocktail is not a threat to life. In fact, those who enjoy a drink or two tend to live longer than teetotalers. It is important to ensure that the calories in alcoholic beverages do not replace the foods necessary to build a well-balanced diet. Moderation in both food and drink is an essential factor for attaining and maintaining good health.

Exercise on Beverages

After reading the preceding questions and the answers which most nutritionists would provide, complete the Beverage Nutrient/Caloric Value Chart in order to compare several common beverages. Do you think that such a chart could be helpful for guiding patients in the selection of nutritious liquids for dietary inclusion? Prepare a bright poster based on the data from this chart for use in educating others (see Figs. 4.1–4.4).

Beverage Nutrient/Caloric Value Chart

Beverage and amount	Calories[a]	Notable nutrients[a]	Caffeine or alcohol (√)
1. Beer, light, 12 oz			
2. Beer, regular, 12 oz			
3. Wine, dry, 3½ oz			
4. Wine, sherry, 3½ oz			
5. Cola, 12 oz			
6. Sugar-free cola, 12 oz			
7. Milkshake, vanilla, 11 oz			
8. Hot chocolate, 8 oz			
9. Milk, chocolate, 8 oz			
10. Milk, skim, 8 oz			
11. Scotch, 1½ oz, and soda, 3 oz			
12. Tomato juice, 6 oz			

[a]Use caloric/nutrient values from reference(s) provided in Appendix V.

STEP 10: POST-TEST ON NUTRITION SENSE

There may arise a number of situations in which your expertise in nutrition will be called upon in order to answer certain questions or clear up specific misconceptions. Therefore, it is important for you to have a working knowledge of the scientific facts and an up-to-date understanding of the ubiquitous nutrition fallacies. Complete the following post-test for a general evaluation of your current level of understanding about nutrition sense versus nonsense. Answers are given in the Answer Key. Remember that nutrition is a relatively new and ever-changing science, so it is essential for practitioners to constantly monitor both the latest nutrition research and the newest dietary fads.

Indicate whether you think each of the following statements is true (T) or false (F).

_____ 1. Food is either good for you or bad for you.
_____ 2. It is essential to try to examine impartially all sides of any nutrition controversy.
_____ 3. According to Herbert and Barrett, the "health" food store is an inexpensive place to shop.
_____ 4. Ginseng, like certain other herbs, can cause ill side effects.
_____ 5. Pizza is a good example of a popularly maligned "junk" food which can actually be nutritious.
_____ 6. Vitamin and mineral supplements should not be self-prescribed.
_____ 7. Most food additives are injurious to health.
_____ 8. Sugar has been shown to be the direct cause of a number of degenerative diseases.

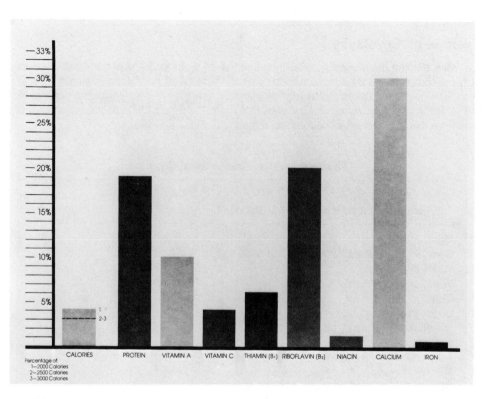

Fig. 4.1 Skim milk's contribution to U.S. Recommended Daily Allowances. One cup, 8 fl oz (244 g) fortified with Vitamins A and D; 86 calories.
Comparison Cards, courtesy of NATIONAL DAIRY COUNCIL ®

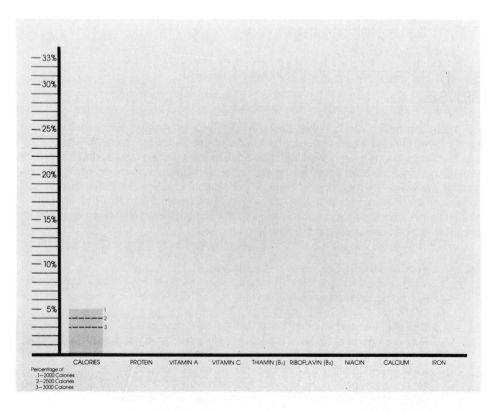

Fig. 4.2 Soft drink's contribution to U.S. Recommended Daily Allowances. One cup, 8 fl oz (246 g) cola; 96 calories.
Comparison Cards, courtesy of NATIONAL DAIRY COUNCIL ®

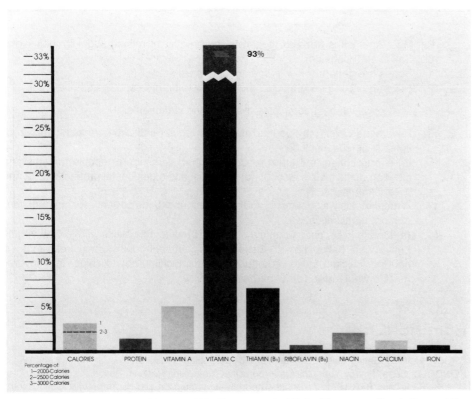

Fig. 4.3 Orange juice's contribution to U.S. Recommended Daily Allowances. One-half cup, 4 fl oz (125 g) frozen reconstituted; 56 calories.
Comparison Cards, courtesy of NATIONAL DAIRY COUNCIL ®

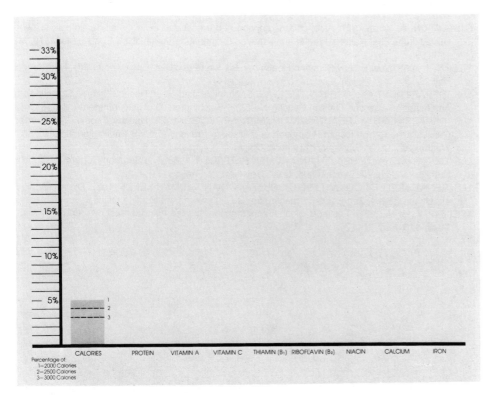

Fig. 4.4 Highball's contribution to U.S. Recommended Daily Allowances. Ten fluid ounces, 1½ oz (42 g) 80-proof whiskey with soda and ice cubes; 97 calories.
Comparison Cards, courtesy of NATIONAL DAIRY COUNCIL ®

_____ 9. Most Americans need to moderate the amount of refined sugar in their diets.

_____ 10. Salt is 100% sodium.

_____ 11. Soups are generally low in sodium content.

_____ 12. Beverages containing alcohol may pose health threats to pregnant women.

Select the answer which best completes the following statements:

_____ 13. Beverages which may be inadvisable for regular intake by pregnant women or some ill persons include

(a) strong coffee and other products high in caffeine. (b) double martinis and other products high in alcohol. (c) skim milk and other low-fat products. (d) a and b. (e) all of these.

_____ 14. A meal that is well balanced and best conforms to the current recommendations of most nutritionists is

(a) tomato juice, cheese omelet, coffee. (b) vegetable sticks with low-fat yogurt, broiled fish, baked potato, tossed salad, oatmeal cookies, and fresh fruit. (c) bouillon, chicken salad on lettuce bed, dill pickles, potato chips, fruit-flavored gelatin, whole milk. (d) all of these.

REFERENCES

BRUCH, H. 1973. Eating Disorders. New York: Basic Books.

FEINGOLD, B. 1974. Why Your Child is Hyperactive. New York: Random House.

HERBERT, V., and BARRETT, S. 1982a. The truth about nutrition and health rip-offs. Good Housekeeping, April.

HERBERT, V., and BARRETT, S. 1982b. Vitamins and "Health" Foods: The Great American Hustle. Philadelphia: George F. Stickley Co.

MACMAHON, B., et al. 1981. Coffee and cancer of the pancreas. New Engl. J. Med. *304*, Mar. 12, 630.

NATIONAL ACADEMY OF SCIENCES. 1980. Toward Healthful Diets. Washington, D.C.: NAS.

ROSENBERG, L., et al. 1982. Breast cancer and alcoholic beverage consumption. Lancet *1*, Jan. 30, 267.

SCHATZKIN, A., et al. 1987. Alcohol consumption and breast cancer in the epidemiologic follow-up survey of the First National Health and Nutrition Examination Survey. New Engl. J. Med. *316*, May 7, 1169.

STERN, J. 1980. How to Stay Slim and Healthy on the Fast Food Diet. Englewood Cliffs, NJ: Prentice-Hall.

U.S. DEPARTMENT OF AGRICULTURE. 1985. Nutrition and Your Health: Dietary Guidelines for Americans, Home and Garden Bulletin No. 232. Washington, D.C.: Government Printing Office.

U.S. DEPARTMENT OF HEALTH AND HUMAN SERVICES. 1979. Healthy People: The Surgeon General's Report on Health Promotion and Disease Prevention, PHS Publication No. 79-55071. Washington, D.C.: Government Printing Office.

U.S. DEPARTMENT OF HEALTH AND HUMAN SERVICES. 1988. The Surgeon General's Report on Nutrition and Health. Washington, D.C.: Government Printing Office.

U.S. SENATE SELECT COMMITTEE ON NUTRITION AND HUMAN NEEDS. 1977. Dietary Goals for the United States, 2nd Edition. Washington, D.C.: Government Printing Office.

WILLET, W., et al. 1987. Moderate alcohol consumption and the risk of breast cancer. New Engl. J. Medi. *316*, May 7, 1174.

Chapter Five

Can Vegetarianism Meet Your Needs?

CHAPTER BLUEPRINT

Step 1: Take the Pre-test on Vegetarianism to begin reflecting on your beliefs regarding meat-eating versus vegetarianism.

Step 2: Examine the Possible Pros and Cons to determine whether your own diet might be altered.

Step 3: Examine the Complementarity Charts for assistance in planning a well-balanced vegetarian diet.

Step 4: Read some of the current literature on macrobiotics, complete the accompanying questionnaire, and participate in the assigned group discussion.

Step 5: Examine the Vegetarian Guidelines and complete the accompanying questionnaire.

Step 6: Take the Post-test on Vegetarianism in order to evaluate what you have learned from Chapter 5.

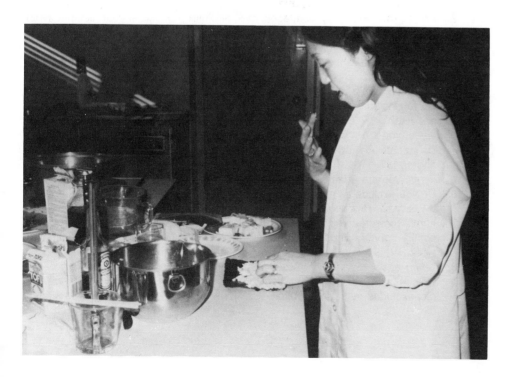

STEP 1: PRE-TEST ON VEGETARIANISM

Recent surveys of American eating habits have revealed the trend toward "lighter" foods, with a swing away from the traditional meat-and-potatoes fare. When dining out, Americans are often choosing vegetables, salads, fish, and crêpes over hamburgers and steak. Although meat consumption can still be a sign of affluence in this country, there has occurred a definite movement towards the vegetarian-type lifestyle. There are several reasons for this shift in food choice:

- ○ Ethics—some believe in the philosophy that meat-eating requires unnecessary killing.
- ○ Economics—meat is more costly than most other protein-rich alternatives.
- ○ Ecology—the process of converting land to meat is more wasteful than eating the plant foods grown there (e.g., 1 acre of land will, in one year, produce 77 days worth of the RDA for protein as beef, 236 days of protein as milk, 877 days of protein as whole wheat, and 2224 days of protein as soybeans).
- ○ Health—meat is higher in calories, fat, saturated fat, and cholesterol than most of the protein source alternatives; vegetarians tend to have a lower incidence of heart disease and certain other illnesses with possible dietary links.

If undertaken knowledgeably, vegetarianism can bypass faddism as a healthy alternative to the traditional American way. But if adopted without regard to nutrition facts, a meatless diet can prove to be a threat to overall health. Thus, as a dietetic technician in nutrition care, you should be adequately prepared for assisting vegetarian patients in balancing their diets. You should also be able to provide the nutrition information required for those seeking to make the decision whether to switch to a vegetarian way of life. Why not begin with yourself?

Examine your Food Diary from Chapter 2 before answering the questions below. As you complete the Pre-test, keep in mind the following question: Could you—realistically speaking—eliminate meat from your diet, and do you really want to do so? Discuss your feelings and your Pre-test answers with classmates or co-workers. Answer yes (Y) or no (N) where applicable, and fill in the remaining answers to the questions that follow.

_____ 1. Do you include meat, poultry, fish, eggs, milk, and milk products in your daily diet?
       If yes, you are a *nonvegetarian.*

_____ 2. Do you include poultry, fish, eggs, milk, and milk products in your diet, but avoid red meat?
       If yes, you are a *semivegetarian.*

_____ 3. Do you include fish, eggs, milk, and milk products in your diet, but avoid meat and poultry?
       If yes, you are a *piscivegetarian.*

_____ 4. Do you include eggs, milk, and milk products in your diet, but avoid meat, poultry, and fish?
       If yes, you are a *lacto-ovo vegetarian.*

_____ 5. Do you include milk and milk products in your diet, but avoid meat, poultry, fish, and eggs?
       If yes, you are a *lacto-vegetarian.*

_____ 6. Do you exclude all animal products from your diet?
       If yes, you are a *vegan,* a strict vegetarian.

      7. If you answered yes to question 1 or 2, approximately how much meat and/or poultry do you eat daily? _____ oz. How often do you eat poultry? _____ times a week. Would you find it difficult to eliminate these foods from your diet? _____

      8. If you answered yes to question 3, approximately how much fish do you eat weekly? _____ oz. How many eggs do you eat weekly? _____ How long has your diet excluded meat and poultry? _____ Explain briefly why you adhere to such a diet:

9. If you answered yes to question 4 or 5, approximately how much milk do you drink every day? ___ cups. How much cheese do you eat daily? ___ oz. How much yogurt do you eat? ___ cups per ___ day/week/month. List other milk products you include in your diet and estimate how often (e.g., milkshakes once a week, custard once a month):

    Explain briefly why you adhere to such a diet:

10. If you answered yes to question 6, briefly explain how you balance your diet (e.g., drink soy milk, eat "complementary" proteins):

    How long has your diet excluded all animal products?

    Explain briefly why you adhere to such a diet; if you are a member of a specific vegan group (e.g., **Zen macrobiotics**), please indicate:

In the following checklist indicate if you have ever eaten Ⓥ the listed products, and if so, how often you usually do so:

Vegetarian Foods Checklist

Food	Frequency[a]	Food	Frequency[a]
○ **Alfalfa**		○ Milk, soy	
○ Bran, unprocessed		○ Milk, special high-protein	
○ Bran cereal		○ Millet	
○ Bran muffins		○ **Miso**	
○ Bread, high-protein		○ Molasses, blackstrap	
○ **Brewer's yeast**		○ Nut butters	
○ Buckwheat		○ Pasta, soy or high-protein	
○ Bulgur (cracked wheat)		○ Seaweed	
○ Carob		○ Soybeans	
○ Cornbread		○ Sprouts	
○ **Hummous**		○ **Tahini**	
○ Kasha (buckwheat groats)		○ Tofu	
○ **Kefir**		○ **TVP**	
○ **Kelp**		○ Wheat germ	
○ Legumes		○ Yeast, fortified	
○ **Meat analogs**		○ Other:	

[a]Frequency of consumption (per day, week, month, or year).

Indicate in the chart below any nutrition supplements you take, the doses, and the frequencies. If possible, explain why you are taking each supplement.

Nutrition Supplement Chart

Nutrition supplement and brand	Dose (g or mg)	Frequency (per day, week, month)	Reason for taking

Zen macrobiotics: Specific sect of macrobiotics in which a ten-step diet plan is followed to gradually reduce food intake to 100% whole grains, supposedly to achieve spiritual enlightenment; long-term adherence can be fatal.

alfalfa: Deep-rooted plant grown for hay and forage.

brewer's yeast: Yeast used for brewing beer, dried and used as a source of B vitamins; does not rise like regular yeast.

hummous: Chickpea and sesame paste flavored with garlic.

kefir: Liquid yogurt, usually flavored.

kelp: Large brown seaweed, used as a source of iodine.

meat analogs: Fabricated foods which are composed of textured vegetable protein (TVP) but resemble meats in flavor and appearance.

miso: Fermented soybean paste or sauce.

tahini: Sesame seed paste.

TVP: Textured vegetable-protein; product prepared from soybeans and/or other plant proteins which offers high quality protein to be eaten alone (in casseroles, patties, etc.) or used as meat extenders.

STEP 2: POSSIBLE PROS AND CONS

In order to be adequately prepared for making lifestyle altering decisions, it is essential to consider all of the possible impacts on the future, both positive and negative. Complete the chart below, which lists some of the possible positive (*pros*) and negative (*cons*) factors associated with a vegetarian lifestyle. List any additional factors, both pro and con, that you can think of which may affect your decision. Discuss your answers with classmates or co-workers. Did they list any additional pros or cons which you might want to consider? Total your *possible pros* and your *possible cons* to determine whether your own decision should be a yes or a no.

Possible Pros and Cons Chart

Possible Pros ⃠ (for adoption of a well-balanced nonmeat diet)

○ I want to keep my blood cholesterol level low.
○ I want to keep my blood pressure low.
○ I want to lower my overall risks for developing heart disease.
○ I want to lower my risks for developing other diseases of high incidence in meat-eating countries (e.g., cancer of the colon).
○ I want to lose weight.
○ I want to lessen the incidence of constipation.
○ I want to decrease my food bills/my family's food bills.
○ Other: _____

Possible Cons ⃠ (for adoption of a well-balanced, nonmeat diet)

○ I may require supplementation (since I am an infant/child/pregnant woman).
○ I may develop nutritional deficiencies (since I am/will become a strict vegetarian).
○ I may develop caloric deficiencies (since I am an infant/child/pregnant woman/underweight person/athlete/problem eater).
○ I may encounter burdensome social difficulties (at restaurants, dinner parties, family meals, etc.).
○ I may encounter difficulties with increasing meal frequency (less dietary fat can cause more frequent hunger pangs).
○ I may dislike the need to frequent the bathroom more often (due to increased dietary fiber).
○ I may dislike the need for special care in food selection and preparation.
○ My family refuses to let me change my diet.
○ Other: _____

Total Pros: _____
Total Cons: _____

If the preceding chart indicated that you *do not* wish to adopt a vegetarian way of life, you may want to consider the following suggestions:

○ Diet plays an important role in determining your state of health and well-being.
○ Excessive calories, dietary fat, and cholesterol may have an effect on your health.
○ Meats and other animal products contain varying amounts of fat and cholesterol.
○ It is wise to be moderate in the consumption of animal foods, particularly those high in fat and/or cholesterol.

If the Possible Pros and Cons Chart indicated that you *do* want to switch to a non-meat-eating lifestyle, you may first want to consider the following suggestions:

○ Be sure to include a wide variety of foods in your diet and avoid food faddism (more in Step 4).
○ Do not purchase self-prescribed supplements.

○ Consider the benefits—nutritional and social—of opting for the semi- or lacto-ovo vegetarian diet in favor of the more restrictive lifestyles.

○ Be sure to obtain a sufficient amount of vitamin B$_{12}$ through intake of some animal foods, fortified products, or a physician-prescribed supplement.

○ Include sufficient dietary iron—especially important for women during child-bearing years, as well as for infants, children, and pregnant women—and note that phytates present in whole grain products can inhibit iron absorption; iron supplements should be prescribed by a physician.

STEP 3: COMPLEMENTARITY CHARTS

Since the elimination of an entire food group will diminish the overall variety present in the diet, reduce nutrient intake, and pose social problems (e.g., restaurant dining, visiting nonvegetarian friends, catered meals), the most convenient and least radical option is to moderate meat intake. By choosing meat selections wisely, minimizing intake of high-fat meats, and regularly substituting meatless alternatives, it is possible to follow a well-balanced and sensible diet. Whether you—and your patients—select this particular dietary option or choose instead to adopt a vegetarian lifestyle, the use of Complementarity Charts can assist in diet planning.

The charts below provide the following information:

○ High-fat meat choices (Table 5.1)
○ How to obtain complete protein from plant foods (Table 5.2)
○ How to complement proteins (Table 5.3)
○ Plant food definitions (Table 5.4)
○ An easy reference for complementing proteins (Table 5.5)
○ Ethnic examples of complementary proteins (Table 5.6)

Table 5.1 Complementarity Chart No. 1: Fatty Meats[a]

Top loin steak	Capon
Rib roast	Duck
Brisket	Goose
Short ribs	Bacon
Veal breast	Bologna
Pork roast	Corned beef
Lamb rib/blade chop	Frankfurter
Salami	Sausage

[a]*Note:* Trim all meats of all visible fat and remove skin from poultry, and prepare by baking, boiling, broiling, or roasting on a rack without any added fats; organ meats are high in cholesterol.

Table 5.2 Complementarity Chart No. 2: Complementary Plant Foods

Corn ⟷	Beans, peanuts, soy
Rice ⟷	Beans, peanuts
Wheat ⟷	All legumes
Oats ⟷	Peanuts
Rye ⟷	Soy
Sesame ⟷	Garbanzos, soy

Table 5.3 Complementarity Chart No. 3: Complementary Proteins

Any combination of			Specific plant food complements
Animal foods	and	Plant foods[a]	
Meats, lean		Grains	
		Legumes ⟶	Nuts and seeds/grains; wheat
Cheeses, skim and part-skim		Beans ⟶	Rice; corn
		Soybeans ⟶	Corn; rye; sesame
Milk, skim and low-fat		Garbanzos ⟶	Sesame
Yogurt, low-fat		Nuts	
		Peanuts ⟶	Corn; oats; rice
Eggs (3–4 per week)		Seeds	

[a]*Note*: Use the plant food definitions in Table 5.4 for further assistance.

Table 5.4 Complementarity Chart No. 4: Plant Food Definitions

Grains and cereals	Include barley, buckwheat, bulgur, corn, millet, oats, rice, rye, wheat, and their products.
Legumes	Include black beans, broad beans, chickpeas (garbanzos), cowpeas, kidney beans, lentils, lima beans, mung beans, navy beans, pea beans, soybeans, tofu, white beans.
Nuts	Any kind.
Seeds	Include pumpkin, sesame, squash, sunflower.

Table 5.5 Complementarity Chart No. 5: Complementary Proteins Easy-Reference Chart

Plant foods	+	Animal foods
Legumes	+	Grains
Legumes	+	Grains + nuts
Legumes	+	Nuts
Legumes	+	Nuts + seeds
Legumes: Soy, garbanzos	+	Seeds: Sesame

Table 5.6 Complementarity Chart No. 6: Ethnic Complements

Ethnic group	Popular dish(es)
Italian	Spaghetti with parmesan cheese, pizza, pasta e fagioli (wheat and kidney beans), fettucine (wheat and cheese)
Puerto Rican	Rice and beans
Cuban	Black beans and rice
Mexican	Bean burrito/**taco**/**tortilla**/**enchilada**
American Indian	Succotash (corn and lima beans), baked beans and cornbread
American	*GORP* (good old raisins and peanuts, plus seeds), cereal with milk, macaroni and cheese, baked beans and brown bread
African	**Couscous** with chickpeas
Middle Eastern	Hummous (sesame seeds with chickpeas)
Chinese	Bean curd and rice
Japanese	Miso sauce on rice

taco: Spanish/Mexican-style sandwich composed of crisp tortilla folded over filling, usually ground beef and/or beans, plus cheese, lettuce, tomatoes, and chili peppers.

tortilla: Round thin cake of cornmeal or flour, usually consumed with toppings or fillings containing ground meat, beans, cheese, and/or vegetables.

enchilada: Tortilla rolled around filling of meat, beans, and/or cheese with vegetables and chili peppers.

couscous: Finely ground hard wheat or semolina.

For centuries, people from all over the world have consumed the majority of their protein in the form of complementary protein foods. People eat this way naturally, without even realizing the scientific principles behind combining plant proteins. Table 5.6 gives some popular complementary protein dishes from various ethnic groups.

You may want to make copies of Tables 5.1–5.6 for use at home or in future diet counseling settings.

STEP 4: MACROBIOTICS

Vegetarianism, in and of itself, is not a fad diet. Yet, vegetarians—just like meat eaters—can become food faddists. A food faddist believes that certain foods offer special properties while other foodstuffs must be totally avoided; they believe that, despite the lack of scientific evidence to support such concepts, certain foods are "good" while other foods are "bad." Certain foods, some of which are listed in the Vegetarian Foods Checklist, are often mistakenly thought of as magically health promoting (e.g., alfalfa, brewer's yeast, carob, kelp, seaweed, wheat germ, and honey). Some individuals attribute all sorts of undocumented properties to nutrition supplements, and they may take excessively large doses. The potential dangers of food faddism, self-prescribed supplements, and health quackery were described in Chapter 4 and will be discussed further in Chapter 6. Faddism and the vegetarian diet are not synonymous, but when vegetarianism is carried to an extreme, it can become unbalanced and dangerous.

The vegan diet requires supplementation in order to provide all of the nutrients required for good health. Thus, this restrictive form of vegetarianism can pose nutritional drawbacks, while the other forms of vegetarianism are less apt to be nutritionally unbalanced. Vegans require careful diet counseling (see Step 5).

The most excessive form of the vegetarian diet is illustrated by Zen macrobiotics. The Zen macrobiotic diet is highly unbalanced, scientifically unsound, and potentially fatal. Another phase of the dangerous Zen macrobiotic diet is the (non-Zen) macrobiotic diet. Articles published in nutrition magazines and journals can provide you with a review of these vegetarian fads, Zen and non-Zen, and their nutritional implications.

Suggested Readings on Macrobiotics

AMERICAN ACADEMY OF PEDIATRICS. 1977. Nutritional aspects of vegetarianism, health foods, and fad diets. Pediatrics 59, Mar., 460.
COWMEADOW, O. 1987. Introduction to Macrobiotics. Northamptonshire, England: Thorsons Publishing Group.
KREY, S. 1982. Alternate dietary lifestyles. Primary Care 9, Sept., 595.
KUSHI, M. 1985. The Macrobiotic Way. Wayne, NJ: Avery Publishing Group.
SONNENBERG, L., ZOLBER, K., and REGISTER, U. Food for Us All—A Vegetarian Diet Study Kit. Chicago: American Dietetic Association. (Contains an extensive bibliography on macrobiotics and vegetarianism.)

Discuss the implications of the following letter from Stare and Aronson (1982). Do you agree that zealous, strict vegetarianism can mean faddism?

Dear Dr. Stare:

I have a 23-year-old daughter of excellent intelligence, formerly skeptical mind, and good education, up to the point where she got "into" the "counter-culture" and dropped out of college after one year. She now has two children, a little girl three years old and a baby eight months old. These children are being raised on the macrobiotic diet—or were; the parents appear to have relaxed a little.

The older child was fed only breast milk for about a year. After that she was fed exactly what her parents ate and was given no milk in any form—on the theory that we are unkind to our cows, breeding them only to take their calves away from them, and cow's milk is intended by nature only for little cows!

While being breastfed, the little girl seemed to be doing well enough, although she was small and somewhat slower in her development than other children. My daughter reassured me that children on this diet do develop at a slower rate than children on a "straight" diet, but that they come along better in the end. I tried to console myself with the fact that children do indeed develop at different rates.

For a few months after breast-feeding was stopped, the child continued more or less all right, then she began to slow up. She didn't seem to grow or gain weight, went back to crawling, and finally gave up on her efforts to walk altogether. She was fretful, with little appetite. At this point her parents became disturbed enough to take her to a doctor (**homeopathic**) who thought the trouble was with her nervous system. When the food supplement he prescribed didn't seem to work, they took her to a pediatrician who immediately put her in the hospital for tests. These revealed, among other things, soft and porous bones full of tiny fractures which the doctor attributed to deficiencies of vitamin D and calcium. With proper supplements, she is doing much better; she's sleeping better, has an enormously increased appetite, has grown four inches, gained six pounds, and is walking pretty well for the length of time she has been at it. I would say her mental development does not seem to have been affected. She has a very quick understanding, a good vocabulary, and talks as well as most children her age.

Following this experience, her parents have modified the diet, though they do not appear to have given up on it altogether. They have added cheese and many fruits and vegetables, especially citrus—but also tomatoes, avocados, and other such things that one does not encounter on a strict macrobiotic diet. They continue to give vitamin supplements to the little girl, but still no eggs or milk. While my daughter admits the child's trouble was attributed to elements missing from her diet, she seems

homeopath: Practitioner of alternative medicine which uses very small doses of specific drugs plus nutrition counseling.

to believe more firmly that the real cause lies elsewhere; that is, for some reason the little girl was unable to absorb and assimilate much of the missing elements available in her diet. She says she knows plenty of children raised on this diet who are as healthy as anyone could want.

My concern is, of course, to try to wean them away from this diet altogether, so that the little girl will continue to improve, the baby will not similarly suffer, and the parents' health will not be harmed. Any suggestions you can give me will be appreciated.

M.J.H.

You may want to read one or two of the preceding Suggested Readings before answering the following questions. Discuss your answers with classmates or co-workers.

Questionnaire on Strict Vegetarianism

1. How would you counsel a pregnant woman who refuses to alter her vegan diet?

2. How would you counsel a vegetarian woman who wants to have her infant adhere to her own macrobiotic regime?

3. How would you counsel a teenage girl who had been following the Zen macrobiotic diet for several weeks?

4. How would you counsel a male college student who was interested in adopting a vegetarian diet and was planning on moving into a macrobiotic household?

5. In each situation, would you call upon other members of the health care team for assistance? ____ Why or why not?

STEP 5: VEGETARIAN GUIDELINES

If you found it difficult to complete the questionnaire in Step 4, the information provided below should help to improve your confidence—and skills—regarding your counseling abilities. After examining the following Suggested Readings and Counseling Guidelines, try to answer the revised Vegetarianism Questionnaire at the end of this step.

This step includes suggested strategies to use in counseling vegetarians. The following references may prove helpful.

Suggested Readings on Vegetarianism

AMERICAN DIETETIC ASSOCIATION. 1981. Vegetarian diets. In Handbook of Clinical Dietetics, pp. A33–A50. New Haven, CT: Yale University Press.

AMERICAN DIETETIC ASSOCIATION. 1988. Position of The American Dietetic Association: Vegetarian Diets. J. Am. Dietet. Assoc. 88, Mar., 351.

AMERICAN SOCIETY FOR CLINICAL NUTRITION. 1988. First International Congress on Vegetarian Nutrition. Am. J. Clin. Nutr. 48, Sept. Supp., entire issue (pp. 707–927).

ANDERSON, J. (Editor). 1982. Nutrition and Vegetarians. Chapel Hill, NC: Health Sciences Consortium.

BALLANTINE, R. 1987. Transition to Vegetarianism. Honesdale, PA: Himalayan International Institute.

BODWELL, C., ADKINS, J., and HOPKINS, D. 1982. Protein Quality in Humans. Westport, CT: AVI Publishing Co.

DEBRUYNE, L., and ROLFES, S. 1986. Diet planning for the vegetarian. Nutrition Clin. 1, Oct., 1.

DWYER, J. 1980. Vegetarianism. New York J. Med. 80, Mar., 660.

DYER, J. 1982. Vegetarianism: An Annotated Bibliography. Metuchen, NJ: Scarecrow Press.

FREELAND-GRAVES, J., et al. 1986. Health practices, attitudes, and beliefs of vegetarians and nonvegetarians. J. Am. Dietet. Assoc. 86, Jul., 913.

HARTBARGER, J., and HARTBARGER, N. 1981. Eating for the Eighties: A Complete Guide to Vegetarian Nutrition. Philadelphia: W. B. Saunders Co.

KOWALSKI, R., et al. 1987. Congress investigates vegetarian nutrition. Nutrition Today 22, Aug., 30.

LABINE, P., BURRILL, G., and NOLFI, J. 1980. The Homegrown Vegetarian. Burlington, VT: Center for Studies in Food Self-Sufficiency.

LAPPÉ, F. M. 1982. Diet for a Small Planet, 10th Edition. New York: Ballantine.

NATIONAL RESEARCH COUNCIL/FOOD AND NUTRITION BOARD. 1982. Alternative Dietary Practices and Nutritional Abuses in Pregnancy: Summary Report. Washington, DC: National Academy of Sciences.

NELMAN, A., and DARNTON-HILL, I. 1987. Vitamin and iron status in new vegetarians. Amer. J. Clin. Nutr. *45,* Apr., 785.

ROBERTSON, L., FINDERS, C., and RUPPENTHAL, B. 1986. Laurel's Kitchen: A Handbook for Vegetarian Cookery and Nutrition, 2nd Edition. Berkeley, CA: Ten Speed Press.

SEVENTH-DAY ADVENTIST DIETETIC ASSOCIATION. 1982. Vegetarian Diet Manual, 6th Edition. Loma Linda, CA: SDADA.

SOCIETY FOR NUTRITION EDUCATION. 1982. Vegetarians and Vegetarian Diets. Oakland, CA: SNE.

TRUESDELL, D., and ACOSTA, P. 1985. Feeding the vegan infant and child. J. Am. Dietet. Assoc. *85,* Jul., 837.

TRUESDELL, D., WHITNEY, E., and ACOSTA, P. 1984. Nutrients in vegetarian foods. J. Am. Dietet. Assoc. *84,* Jan., 28.

VEGETARIAN TIMES EDITORS. 1984. The Vegetarian Times Cookbook. New York: Macmillan.

WHITNEY, E. 1987. Vegetarian Diet Planning. Tallahassee, FL: Nutrition and Health Association.

For further information:

General Conference of Seventh-Day Adventists, 6840 Eastern Avenue NW, Washington, DC 20012.
Seventh-Day Adventist Dietetic Association, Box 75, Loma Linda, CA 92354.
Worldwatch Institute, 1776 Massachusetts Avenue NW, Washington, DC 20036.

Counseling Guidelines—Vegetarians

Table 5.7 outlines the steps for diet counseling for vegetarians. The following material gives the details of each step.

Table 5.7 General Outline for Counseling Vegetarians

I. Initial Session
  A. General Guidelines
  B. Patient Records
    1. Medical History Form
    2. Weight Chart
    3. 24-Hour Recall Form
  C. Assignments
    1. Food Intake Record
    2. Diet History
  D. Technician's Notes
II. Follow-up Session(s)
  A. General Guidelines
  B. Handouts
    1. Personal Diet Plan
    2. Learning Assessment Quiz
  C. Technician's Notes

I. Initial Session

I. A. General Guidelines

1. Use Medical History Form to assess patient's nutritional status. Evaluate health and social histories affecting nutrient intake, digestion, or absorption. (Lab Data should be confirmed by client's physician).
2. Weigh patient and record on Weight Chart. The chart is a helpful tool for visualization of patient's weight status.
3. Assist patient in recording 24-hour recall of food intake using 24-Hour Recall Form. This will aid patient in keeping an accurate Food Intake Record.
4. Instruct patient to keep daily Food Intake Record until next session so that typical food intake patterns can be evaluated. Advise patient not to deviate from normal eating pattern. Stress the importance of recording food intake immediately after eating.
5. Instruct patient to complete Diet History. This provides for a basic evaluation of food intake patterns. (Use Pre-test in Step 1.)
6. Record assessment and recommendation(s) using the SOAP method (Chapter 1, Step 6) in Technician's Notes. This form can be kept in your files with a copy in the patient's medical records.

I. B. Patient Records

1. Medical History Form

Date _____ Referred by _____

Name _____ Date of birth _____

Address _____ Phone no. _____

Occupation _____ Hours per work week _____ Work phone no. _____

Educational background _____ Religious/ethnic background _____

Sex ____ Marital status _____

Household composition: Live alone _____ Spouse _____ Children/No. _____ Other: _____

General health status:

Physician _____ Address _____
Phone no. _____ Date of last visit _____
Ambulatory care required? _____ If so, describe: _____
Neuromuscular problems? _____ If so, how is eating affected? _____
Visual/auditory problems? _____ If so, describe: _____
Chewing difficulties? _____ If so, describe: _____
Appetite typically good? _____ Fair? _____ Poor? _____
Digestion/elimination difficulties? _____ If so, describe: _____
Food intolerances? _____ If so, describe: _____
Other: _____

Height ____ Weight ____ Frame ____
Triceps skinfold thickness _____ Mid-arm circumference _____
Mid-arm muscle circumference _____
Weight changes/problems? _____ If so, describe: _____

Clinical signs of nutritional status:

Skin _____ Mouth _____
Hair _____ Eyes _____
Teeth _____ Other: _____

Lab data:

Blood pressure _____
CBC _____
Serum albumin _____
Other: _____

Medications taken regularly: _____
Prescribed by: _____ Date(s) prescribed: _____
Nutrition supplements taken regularly: _____
Prescribed by: _____ Date(s) prescribed: _____
Special diet prescription: _____
Prescribed by: _____ Date of prescription: _____
How closely is diet followed? Always adhered to ___ Sometimes ___ Rarely ___ Never ___

Type of housing: Room ____ Apartment ____ Home ____ Institution ____
Prepare own meals? _____ Dine out? Often (more than once a day) _____ Rarely _____
Food shopping done independently? _____ If not, describe required assistance: _____
_____
Eligible for food stamps? _____ If so, are they currently being used? _____
Cigarette smoker? _____ If so, how much: _____
Exercise regularly? _____ If so, describe: _____
   No. times per week _____ No. minutes per session _____

Comments: _____

2. Weight Chart

Starting weight: ____ Desired weight: ____

Date	Weight	Comments

3. 24-Hour Recall Form

Date and time (over 24-hr period)	Food and amount	Where eaten[a]	Eaten with whom[b]	Associated activity[c]

[a]For example, at the kitchen table, at home—sitting at a desk, in a car, or at a restaurant.
[b]For example, with parents, friend(s), or a date.
[c]For example, while studying, driving, talking, or watching TV.

I. C. Assignments

1. Food Intake Record

Date and time	Duration of meal (min)	Food and amount	Where eaten[a]	With whom	Associated activity[b]	Associated emotions[c]

[a]Such as work, restaurant, kitchen, living room.
[b]For example, watching television, reading, socializing, driving, talking on the phone, cooking.
[c]Attitude: bored, anxious, frustrated, depressed, happy, angry, tense, etc.

2. Diet History

Use Pre-test on Vegetarianism on pp. 106–107.

I. D. Technician's Notes

Patient: _____   Date: _____

S   (Subjective data—how patient feels):
O   (Objective data—physical measurements including diet/nutritional status):
A   (Assessment—acceptability of dietary progress/nutritional status):
P   (Plan—diet prescription and instruction):
Comments:

II. Follow-up Session(s)

II. A. General Guidelines

1. Weigh patient and record on Weight Chart.
2. Review assignments and discuss.
3. Individualize Personal Diet Plan and instruct patient in its use. (Note that high sodium content of meat analogs may prohibit their inclusion in sodium restricted diets.)
4. Assign Learning Assessment Quiz to evaluate counseling process and to determine if additional counseling is needed.
5. Record assessment and recommendation(s) using the SOAP method in Technician's Notes. This form can be kept in your files with a copy in the patient's medical records.

II. B. Handouts

1.   Personal Diet Plan (See Table 5.8.)

Name _____

How to use diet plan:

1. Balance the diet by including a wide variety of foods in moderate amounts.
2. Include combinations of foods providing all the essential amino acids at each meal (called *complementary essential amino acids*). Some foods already contain all the essential amino acids (called *complete protein foods*), and may be eaten alone or in combination with any plant food.
3. Include foods which are good sources of iron.
4. Include foods which are good sources of calcium.
5. If no animal products are included, supplement the diet with B_{12} or include B_{12}-fortified foods.
6. If milk and milk products are excluded and exposure to sunlight is minimal, include foods which are good sources of vitamin D.

2.   Learning Assessment Quiz

Answer true (T) or false (F) to the following statements:

_____ 1. It is not possible for a vegetarian to follow a nutritionally sound diet.
_____ 2. The lacto-ovo vegetarian diet includes milk and eggs.
_____ 3. Essential amino acids are manufactured by the body as needed.
_____ 4. An adequate intake of calories guards against the utilization of protein for energy.
_____ 5. Foods of plant origin are usually complete in their essential amino acid contents.
_____ 6. Gelatin is an acceptable vegetarian food selection.
_____ 7. All foods sold in "health" food stores are nutritionally superior to comparable items sold in local supermarkets.
_____ 8. Eggs, milk, and cheese are complete protein foods.
_____ 9. Some meat analogs and soy milks do not contain complete protein.
_____ 10. Nuts are a good source of vitamin B_{12}.
_____ 11. The amino acid contents of dried peas/beans and grains are complementary.

Select the best answer to the following statements:

_____ 12. Foods high in iron include
(a) mustard greens. (b) baked beans. (c) apricot juice. (d) prunes. (e) sweet potato. (f) all of these.
_____ 13. Foods rich in calcium include
(a) yogurt. (b) cream cheese. (c) soybeans. (d) crabmeat. (e) tofu. (f) cheddar cheese. (g) a, c, e, f. (h) all of these.
_____ 14. Some good sources of vitamin D are
(a) sunshine. (b) cod liver oil. (c) fortified soy milk. (d) all of these.

Table 5.8 Vegetarian Diet Plan

Food combinations with complementary essential amino acids:
Legumes (dried beans and peas) *plus* Grains (barley, corn, oats, rice, rye, wheat)
Legumes *plus* nuts
Legumes *plus* seeds

Essential amino acids:

Isoleucine	Phenylalanine	Histidine[a]
Leucine	Threonine	Arginine[a]
Lysine	Tryptophan	
Methionine	Valine	

Complete protein foods:

Meat, poultry, fish	Soy products[b]
Eggs	Meat analogs[b]
Milk, cheese, yogurt	

Foods high in iron:

Meat, especially organ meats	Dried fruits and their juices
Oysters, clams	Dark green leafy vegetables
Legumes	Potato, sweet potato
Whole grain and enriched breads and cereals	Foods cooked in iron cookware

Foods high in calcium:

Milk	Dark green leafy vegetables
Hard cheeses	Almonds
Yogurt	Soybeans, fortified soybean milk products
Sardines, salmon (with bones)	

Foods high in vitamin D:

Fish oils	Liver
Salmon, sardines	Fortified milk products
Egg yolks	

[a]For children only.
[b]Containing all essential amino acids.

II. C. Technician's Notes

Patient: _____   Date: _____

S (Subjective data—how patient feels):
O (Objective data—physical measurements including diet/nutritional status):
A (Assessment—acceptability of dietary progress/nutritional status):
P (Plan—diet prescription and instruction):
Comments:

Vegetarianism Questionnaire

Keeping in mind the preceding Suggested Readings on Vegetarianism and Counseling Guidelines, try to answer this expanded version of the Questionnaire on Strict Vegetarianism from p. 112 (with several new counseling settings requiring guidance), and discuss with your classmates or co-workers. As a dietetic technician in nutrition care, do you consider yourself capable of conducting effective counseling sessions with patients following vegetarian diets or contemplating the adoption of a vegetarian lifestyle? Do your own dietary patterns reflect the nutrition advice you include in diet counseling sessions?

1. How would you counsel a pregnant woman who refuses to alter her vegan diet?

2. How would you counsel a vegetarian woman who wants to have her infant adhere to her own macrobiotic regime?

3. How would counsel a teenage girl who had been following the Zen macrobiotic diet for several weeks?

4. How would you counsel a male college student who was interested in adopting a vegetarian diet and was planning on moving into a macrobiotic household?

5. In each of the four preceding situations, would you call upon other members of the health care team for assistance? ____ Why or why not?

6. How would you counsel a healthy lacto-ovo vegetarian adult female?

7. How would you counsel a healthy lacto-vegetarian adult male?

8. How would you counsel a healthy teenage girl who was considering lacto-ovo vegetarianism?

9. How would you counsel a healthy older female who had been a vegetarian for several decades?

10. In each of the four situations above, would you call upon other members of the health care team for assistance? ____ Why or why not?

STEP 6: POST-TEST ON VEGETARIANISM

In order to evaluate your understanding of vegetarianism, complete the following Post-test: Section I is the Learning Assessment Quiz (pp. 116–117) for vegetarian patients. (If the diet counselor is unable to complete this test successfully, how can the patient be expected to?); Section II incorporates much of the material from this chapter. Answers are given in the Answer Key. Is the title of this chapter applicable to you and your vegetarian patients? Can vegetarianism meet your needs?

Section I: Complete the Learning Assessment Quiz. Check your answers with the Answer Key.

Section II: Indicate whether you think the following statements are true (T) or false (F). Check your answers with the Answer Key.

____ 1. A vegan diet can pose difficulties in achieving dietary balance.
____ 2. A vegetarian diet may result in a lowered risk of certain illnesses including heart disease.
____ 3. Vegans should consult their physicians for diagnosis of possible nutritional deficiencies and prescription of necessary supplements.
____ 4. Whole grains are a good source of readily absorbed iron.
____ 5. The macrobiotic diet is high in calcium.
____ 6. Long-term adherents to the Zen macrobiotic regime may require medical attention as well as nutrition counseling.

Select the answer which best completes the following statements and check your answers with the Answer Key.

____ 7. Many Americans are altering their diets and incorporating more nonmeat choices due to
(a) personal philosophies about life. (b) the current economic situation. (c) ecological considerations. (d) health factors. (e) all of these.
____ 8. Examples of complementary plant proteins are corn and
(a) navy beans. (b) peanuts. (c) soy beans. (d) tofu. (e) all of these.
____ 9. An example of an ethnic complementary protein meal is
(a) bean burrito. (b) couscous. (c) fettucine. (d) a and c. (e) all of these.
____ 10. Counseling an individual following a lacto-ovo vegetarian diet should include
(a) a discussion on how to balance the diet. (b) the completion of both a medical history and a diet history. (c) an explanation of complementary proteins. (d) a list of good food sources of iron. (e) a learning assessment quiz. (f) all of these.

REFERENCE

STARE, F. J., and ARONSON, V. 1982. Dear Dr. Stare: What Should I Eat? Philadelphia: George F. Stickley Co.

Chapter Six

Can Diet 'Cure' All Ills?

CHAPTER BLUEPRINT

Step 1: Take the Pre-test on Politics of Nutrition to continue reflecting on your political stance as a technician in the field of nutrition.

Step 2: Read the materials on Dietary "Cures" and participate in the assigned activity.

Step 3: Examine the Diploma Mill Exposé and complete the accompanying assignment.

Step 4: Read the information describing How to Spot Nutrition Fraud and prepare the assigned handout.

Step 5: Examine the outline on Whom to Trust and prepare the assigned handout.

Step 6: Take the Post-test on Nutrition Fraud in order to evaluate what you learned from the information and activities provided in Chapter 6.

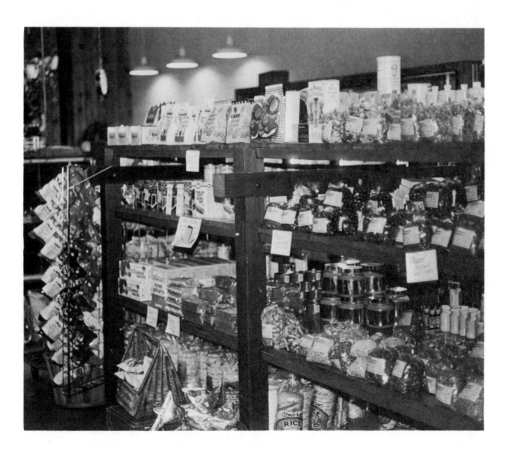

STEP 1: PRE-TEST ON POLITICS OF NUTRITION

For the Pre-test on Nutrition Sense in Chapter 4, you placed yourself on a scale to delineate your approximate position in the politics-of-nutrition scene. You may want to reexamine your position after reading and discussing with classmates some of the following Suggested Readings.

Suggested Readings on the Politics of Nutrition Fraud

AMERICAN ACADEMY OF PEDIATRICS. 1977. Nutritional aspects of vegetarianism, health foods, and fad diets. Pediatrics 59, Mar., 460.

AMERICAN COUNCIL ON SCIENCE AND HEALTH. 1988. The unhealthy alliance: Crusaders for "health for freedom." Nutrition Today 23, Jul./Aug., 26.

AMERICAN DIETETIC ASSOCIATION. 1984. ADA blasts nutrition quackery. ADA Courier 23, 1.

AMERICAN DIETETIC ASSOCIATION. 1985. Statement by the ADA on assuring credible nutrition information for the American public. J. Am. Dietet. Assoc. 85, Jan. 94.

AMERICAN DIETETIC ASSOCIATION. 1988. Position of The American Dietetic Association: Identifying food and nutrition misinformation. J. Am. Dietet. Assoc. 88, Dec., 1589.

BENDER, A. 1986. Health or Hoax? Buffalo, NY: Prometheus Books.

CAMPBELL, T.C., and O'CONNOR, T. 1988. Scientific evidence and explicit health claims in food advertisements. J. Nutr. Ed. 20, Mar./Apr., 87.

COOPER, R. 1986. Health claims on foods. Am. J. Clin. Nutr. 44, Oct., 560.

CORDARO, J. B., and DICKINSON, A. 1986. The nutrition supplement industry: Realities and opportunities. J. Nutr. Ed. 18, Jun., 128.

DARBY, W. 1986. Nutrition: Gastronomy, mythology, or science? Nutrition Today 21, Sept./Oct., 4.

GUSSOW, J., and THOMAS, P. 1986. The Nutrition Debate: Sorting out Some Answers. Palo Alto, CA: Bull Publishing Co.

GUTHRIE, H. 1986. Supplementation: A nutritionist's view. J. Nutr. Ed. 18, Jun., 130.

HARPER, A. 1988. Nutrition: From myth and magic to science. Nutrition Today 23, Jan./Feb., 8.

HERBERT, V. 1987. Health claims in food labeling and advertising: Literal truths but false messages. Nutrition Today 22, Jun., 25.

HURLEY, L. (Editor). 1987. Special Issues in Nutrition. Bethesda, MD: American Institute of Nutrition.

JARVIS, W. 1980. Coping with food faddism. Nutrition and the MD 6, Nov., 1.

KUROWSKI, K. 1981. Coping with Controversy: Professional Perspectives. Ithaca, NY: Cornell University Division of Nutrition Sciences.

LOWELL, J., KENNEY, J., and RASMUSSEN, A. 1987. Nutrition Assessment: Separating Fact, Fiction, and Fraud. Tucson, AZ: Nutrition Information Center.

MCGEE, G. (Editor). 1987. Nutrition Misinformation and Mythology. Van Nuys, CA: PM, Inc.

MCNUTT, K., and SLOAN, A. E. 1985. Of flies and honey and vinegar. J. Nutr. Ed. 17, Aug., 105.

NATIONAL DAIRY COUNCIL. 1981. Nutrition misinformation. Dairy Counc. Dig. 52, Apr., 19.

NATIONAL DAIRY COUNCIL. 1986. Nutrition labeling and health claims. Dairy Counc. Dig. 57, Nov./Dec., 31.

PASSMORE, R. 1988. Food propagandists: The new Puritans. Nutrition Today 21, Mar./Apr., 17.

SCHRODER, A. J. 1986. Health claims in advertising: An industry perspective. Am. J. Clin. Nutr. 44, Oct., 567.

SCHUFTAN, C. 1982. Ethics, ideology, and nutrition. Food Policy 7, 159.

SLOAN, A. E. 1987. Educating a nutrition-wise public. J. Nutr. Ed. 19, Nov./Dec., 803.

WATSON, D. 1985. Nutrition: Society's latest buzzword. J. Am. Dietet. Assoc. 85, Apr., 485.

WATSON, D., and SCHUCKMAN, R. 1985. Nutrition quackery. J. Am. Dietet. Assoc. 85, Jun., 721.

WHITE, P., and SELVEY, N. 1982. Nutrition and the new health awareness. J. Am. Med. Assoc. 247, Jun. 4, 2914.

Political Self-Image Pre-test

After reading about the politics of nutrition fraud from the preceding Suggested Readings, complete this questionnaire to rate your current political self-image as it compares to the political stance of others. Is your political position any different from your approximation of Chapter 4? Do you think that your experiences as a dietetic technician in the coming years will cause your politics regarding nutrition to undergo further change?

○——Radical——Liberal——Middle-of-the-Road——Moderate——Conservative——○

1. Why do you think nutrition is such a controversial field?
2. Why do you think consumers and professional nutritionists disagree on controversial issues?
3. Scan several recent newspapers and magazines; then briefly comment on the role the media currently plays in "the new health awareness." How could nutritionists influence this situation? and be effective as local political forces?
4. Prepare a statement which summarizes your own views on the best nutrition policy for protecting society from fraud. Perhaps you can use this statement with patients who are curious about the political viewpoint of a dietetic technician.

STEP 2: DIETARY "CURES"

Nutrition has always been a popular field for faddists and hucksters. The public has long served as a ready market for money-making diet claims. The current "health" industry is a billion dollar business which advertises a multitude of nutrition cures for every ill known to humans. Yet, because self-proclaimed "nutritionists" often present their claims under a guise of scientific truth, it is quite difficult to separate nutrition fact from fantasy. Only a small percentage of the many popular diet claims are based on the results of documented research, and few prove to be effective. After all, not all illnesses are diet related, nor can every disease be cured through diet.

Nutrition fraud can be a profitable endeavor for clever entrepreneurs who overlook scientific fact while successfully selling dietary fiction. Unfortunately, it is often the sick, the elderly, and the poor who become the victims of nutrition sales hype and the accompanying damages—to both budget and health.

Cancer and **arthritis** are two examples of diseases which all too often draw gullible sufferers into the ensnarement of health hucksters promising magical cures. **AIDS** (the acquired immune deficiency syndrome) also serves as fertile ground for the promotion of unproven medical therapies. Special dietary aids are often bought up en masse by the victims of serious illnesses searching for the means to miraculous recovery. Only the salespersons of false hopes find what they are looking for: sales profits from health gimmickry.

As a dietetic technician, your expertise in the area of diet in disease will encourage questions from associates, family, and friends, as well as patients, regarding various nutrition claims. Because of the popularity of diets promising to cure cancer, arthritis, and other degenerative diseases, you may often need to explain the scientific facts behind the fallacies. Therefore, it is essential that you maintain a working knowledge of the most current medically sound and scientifically supported diet therapies, while simultaneously remaining up to date on the facts behind the prevailing allegations for diet "cures."

arthritis: Painful inflammation of the joints.

AIDS: The acquired immune deficiency syndrome, a fatal infectious disease caused by the human immunodeficiency virus which attacks white blood cells required for resistance to infection; first identified in 1981, this devastating disease has increased dramatically in incidence and mortality rate.

Exercise on Dietary "Cures"

To gain some insight into several popular dietary "cures," read up on **"vitamins" B$_{15}$** and **B$_{17}$** and on diet therapies used with cancer and arthritis—some suggestions for references follow.

Then, if you can, visit several "health" food stores in your area to: (1) look through the supplement sections for these two "vitamins"; (2) search the book/magazine section for information on dietary "cures" for cancer, arthritis, and other ills; and (3) compare products and written claims with scientific studies on the role of diet in the prevention and treatment of cancer, arthritis, and other health problems.

Prepare a brief report of your discoveries and discuss it with classmates or co-workers.

"vitamin" B$_{15}$: Pangamic acid or calcium pangamate, this chemical compound contains a variety of substances, none of which are vitamins or nutrients.

"vitamin" B$_{17}$: Laetrile (which has never been established as a vitamin).

Suggested Readings on Dietary "Cures"

AMERICAN CANCER SOCIETY. 1984. Nutrition and Cancer: Cause and Prevention. New York: ACS.

AMERICAN CANCER SOCIETY. 1984. Nutrition, Common Sense, and Cancer. New York: ACS.

AMERICAN CANCER SOCIETY/FLORIDA DIVISION. 1987. The Good Book of Nutrition. Lakeland, FL: ACS/Publix Supermarkets, Inc.

AMERICAN CANCER SOCIETY/OREGON DIVISION. 1986. Simply Nutritious: Recipes and Recommendations to Reduce the Risk of Cancer. Portland, OR: ACS.

AMERICAN COUNCIL ON SCIENCE AND HEALTH. 1981. Vitamin B_{15}: Anatomy of a Health Fraud. New York: ACSH.

AMERICAN INSTITUTE FOR CANCER RESEARCH. 1984. Dietary Guidelines to Lower Cancer Risk. Chicago: American Dietetic Association.

ARJE, S., and SMITH, L. 1976. The Cruelest Killers. In The Health Robbers, Stephen Barrett (Editor), pp. 1–15. Philadelphia: George F. Stickley Co.

BRIGHT-SEE, E. 1987. Diet and the prevention of cancer. J. Canadian Dietet. Assoc. 48, Feb., 13.

CASSILETH, B. 1982. After laetrile, what? New Engl. J. Med. 307, Jun., 1482.

CREASEY, W. 1985. Diet and Cancer. Philadelphia: Lea & Febiger.

DER MARDEROSIAN, A., and LIBERTI, L. 1987. A Clinical Guide to Natural Products in Medicine. Philadelphia: George F. Stickley Co.

DWYER, J., et al. 1988. Unproven therapies for AIDS: What is the evidence? Nutrition Today 23, Mar./Apr., 25.

HERBERT, V. 1980. Nutrition Cultism, pp. 93–97. Philadelphia: George F. Stickley Co.

HERBERT, V., and BARRETT, S. 1981. Vitamins and "Health" Foods: The Great American Hustle, pp. 108–115. Philadelphia: George F. Stickley Co.

LINDSAY, A. 1988. The American Cancer Society Cookbook. New York: Hearst Books.

MOERTEL, C., FLEMING, T., and RUBIN, J. 1982. A clinical trial of amygdalin (laetrile) in the treatment of human cancer. New Engl. J. Med. 307, Jan., 201.

NATIONAL CANCER INSTITUTE. 1984. Diet, Nutrition, and Cancer Prevention: A Guide to Food Choices. Washington, DC: Government Printing Office.

NATIONAL CANCER INSTITUTE AND NATIONAL INSTITUTES OF HEALTH. 1986. Diet, Nutrition, and Cancer Prevention: The Good News. Washington, DC: Government Printing Office.

NATIONAL NUTRITION CONSORTIUM. 1987. Vitamin-Mineral Safety, Toxicity, and Misuse. Chicago: American Dietetic Association.

NEWELL, G. 1982. Nutrition and the etiology of cancer. Primary Care 9, Sept., 573.

MARSHALL, C. 1983. Non-Vitamins and Phony Vitamins. In Vitamins and Minerals: Help or Harm? pp. 32–39. Philadelphia: George F. Stickley Co.

PALMER, S., and BAKSHI, K. 1983. Diet, nutrition, and cancer: Interim dietary guidelines. J. Nat. Cancer Inst. 20, 1153.

PANUSCH, R. 1984. Controversial arthritis remedies. Bull. Rheumatic Dis. 34, 5, 1.

PARKE, A., and HUGHES, G. 1981. Rheumatoid arthritis and food. British Med. J. 282, Jun. 20, 2027.

RELMAN, A. 1982. Closing the books on laetrile. New Engl. J. Med. 306, Jan. 28, 236.

SEGAL, M. 1987. Defrauding the desperate: Quackery and AIDS. FDA Consumer 21, Aug., 17.

SHILS, M., and HERMANN, M. 1982. Unproven dietary claims in the treatment of patients with cancer. Bull. New York Acad. Med. 58, Apr., 323.

SOCIETY FOR NUTRITION EDUCATION. 1988. Book review: Authentic Arthritis Diet and the Problem of Alkalosis. J. Nutr. Ed. 20, Apr., 96.

TOUGER-DECKER, R. 1988. Nutritional considerations in rheumatoid arthritis. J. Am. Dietet. Assoc. 88, Mar., 327.

WOLMAN, P. 1987. Management of patients using unproven regimens for arthritis. J. Am. Dietet. Assoc. 87, Sept., 1211.

YETIV, J. 1986. Popular Nutritional Practices: A Scientific Appraisal, pp. 23–27, 43. Toledo, OH: Popular Medicine Press.

STEP 3: DIPLOMA MILL EXPOSÉ

Health quackery is flourishing in today's health-conscious society. And health hucksters will continue to prosper—at the expense of the gullible consumer—as long as the right to free speech exists in America. However, there are positive steps you can make as a dietetic technician involved in providing effective nutrition care and reliable diet information.

The following exposé by this author [see Aronson (1983)] is an example of the on-going professional pursuit to interrupt shady operations that foster the dissemination of nutrition misinformation.

Bernadean University: A Nutrition Diploma Mill

Upon reading a magazine article expounding the advice of a local megavitamin and "health" food salesman, I became curious about Bernadean University, the school that had awarded his nutrition "credentials." I decided to find out what courses were offered there and what type of "degrees" were being granted. Thus began my first nutrition espionage adventure, one I conducted undercover, posing as a "health" food enthusiast with limited nutrition education.

The U.S. Department of Education has defined a diploma mill as "an organization that awards degrees without requiring its students to meet educational standards for such degrees established and traditionally followed by reputable educational institutions." Bernadean University appears to fit this description. Originally housed in Nevada, it was never approved or accredited to offer any courses or degrees. After being closed down in 1976 by the Nevada Commission on Postsecondary Education, Bernadean reopened in California, a state where the only requirement for "authorization" of a school is the filing of an affidavit describing the school's program and stating that there are at least $50,000 in assets. Until recently, however, Bernadean did not even apply for authorization.

Using a local address to remain incognito, I sent for Bernadean's catalogue. In addition to nutrition, health services courses can be taken towards certificates in naturopathy, massage, **iridology, reflexology,** acupuncture, diabetes, cancer research, and even natural childbirth. Courses are also offered towards "bachelors' degrees" in psychology, history, literature, language, mathematics, economics, government, sociology, astronomy, botany, accounting, home economics, horticulture and "self-fulfillment." Training in law is also offered, and the "College of Theology" grants a 6-credit-hour "degree," with optional ordination as a minister. Holders of a bachelor's degree can obtain a master's degree if they "write a thesis or some short course for the school." According to the catalogue, any student who satisfactorily completes a course may apply for the designation as a "school mentor" who can tutor new students. Mentors are also referred to as "Adjunct Professors."

How many people so far have received "degrees" from Bernadean? When I wrote to ask, the "Office Administrator" responded as follows:

> Regarding you [sic] request as to the number of students we have, all I can tell you is that we have many, many students all over the country and world..The students start taking one course and then going [sic] into many others. It is really impossible to give you the breakdown.

The "Nutritionist" course, in which I enrolled, consisted of two lessons costing $41.00 apiece and based on the $12.50 "textbook" by [the late] Paavo Airola, author of "Stop Hair Loss," "Swedish Beauty Secrets," "How to Keep Slim, Healthy and Young with Juice Fasting," and "Are You Confused?" After reading his books, one may well be! Airola is a naturopath who, according to his book jacket, "studied ancient, herbal and alternative healing methods during his worldwide travels." Sample quotes from "How to Get Well" are given in Table [6.1].

Each lesson included an open-book exam to be sent back to the University for grading. For Lesson One, I answered the 35 true–false questions correctly in accordance with nutrition facts. Some of the questions are listed in Table [6.2]. Since nearly one-third of my answers contradicted information given in the school's lessons, I expected to get a grade of 70 or below. However, my test was returned with a grade of 90, with a letter from the "office administrator" stating: "You may use the book for answers as it is an open book course. I just seem to feel that you put the answers in the wrong column."

iridology: Study of alterations in the eye (iris) to determine disease states; method is often used to promote specific diets and/or nutrition supplements.

reflexology: Study of involuntary bodily stimulus response, often used to promote specific diets and/or nutrition supplements.

Table 6.1   How to Get Well—Dr. Airola's Handbook of Natural Healing[a]

Page no.	Quote
43	Raw goat's milk is excellent in fresh or soured form, up to a quart a day. I have known patients who cured themselves of arthritis by drinking one quart of goat's milk each day.
49	[for baldness] Raw egg yokes [sic] twice a week.
51	[for baldness] Mix 3 oz of cayenne pepper (red pepper powder) with one fifth of Romanoff Vodka or pure alcohol. Leave for two weeks, agitating the bottle each day. Strain through several layers of fine cheesecloth. Rub a small amount into the scalp twice a day. *Keep away from eyes!*
57	Total vitamin and mineral supplementation is advised but particularly the following anti-cancer vitamins: C and A in large doses; C, up to 5,000 mg; A, preventative dose 50,000 units. (If subjected to strong carcinogens—100,000 units. In a short therapeutic program—up to 2 months—250,000 units.)
60	[for colds] Barefoot walking on sand, gravel and/or wet grass is strengthening in chronic conditions.
77	Of course, the ideal way of eating is to eat only one food at a meal, whether it is cereal, salad, fruit or protein meal. Such eating will help even further in eliminating gas and other digestive disorders. . . . Never eat raw fruits and raw vegetables at the same meal—they require a different set of enzymes and will only "confuse" the digestive processes and cause indigestion.
87	[for **emphysema**] . . . move to a 100% smog-free environment.
90	[for **epilepsy**] . . . live outdoors all of the time, day and night.
101	Okra, the slippery vegetable containing the viscous mucilage, is beneficial in atherosclerosis in that it helps to reduce blood vessel friction. . . . Asparagus is beneficial for an enlarged heart.
103	[for heart disease] . . . periodic blood letting can be considered.

[a]From P. Airola. 1974. How to Get Well. Handbook of Natural Healing. Health Plus Publishers, Phoenix, AZ.

emphysema: Chronic pulmonary disease causing breathlessness; often caused by cigarette smoking.

epilepsy: Brain disorder characterized by sudden brief attacks, usually as convulsive seizures.

Table 6.2   Sample Test Questions[a]

No.	Test Question	Answer graded as correct by Bernadean
1	There are three basic foods in the Airola Diet.	True
7	The protein of potatoes is a complete protein of great value.	True
10	75% to 80% of the diet should consist of foods in natural form.	True
11	The body needs only $\frac{1}{2}$ of the usual recommended amount of protein in the daily diet if protein foods are eaten raw—not cooked.	True
15	Organically grown foods (without chemical fertilizers and without dangerous sprays during the growing period) have been found to have anti-malignancy factors.	True
16	It is safe to purchase and use food with additives or preservatives.	False
18	Goats' milk contains both anti-arthritic and anti-cancer factors not found in cows' milk.	True
26	Mental illness may be caused by much eating of meat.	True

[a]From Nutritionist Lesson #1, Bernadean Univ., Van Nuys, CA.

Lesson Two included a 5-page supplement based mainly on quotes by Rachel Carson and other crusaders against processed food. Some sample quotes are given in Table [6.3]. Since I answered all of the short-answer questions correctly, my grade—based on information given in the "text" and supplement—should have been a zero. To my surprise, I received a grade of 100% and an accompanying note congratulating me on the "excellent manner in which you have completed the Nutrition course." I then sent $10.00 for the "Nutritionist" certificate to hang on my office wall. . . . Although the certificate contains an attractive gold seal and indicates that I graduated "Cum Laude," my Harvard colleagues do not appear particularly impressed with it.

Table 6.3   Sample Quotations from Supplement[a]

Pesticides have been proved to damage the liver and to reduce the supply of B-vitamins, thus leading to an increase in the "endogenous" estrogens, or those produced by the body itself.

If non-organic food is used containing preservatives or grown with synthetic chemicals, tiny doses of poisons enter the body. The liver has to change these into **bile** and excrete or throw them off as best it can. In time, these poisons affect the cells of the liver and the liver actually starts to break down and to harden and undergo cellular changes that produce symptoms such as **gastritis,** indigestion, **acidosis,** and allied results.

bile: Secretion from the liver stored in the gallbladder and used during digestion of fats.

Meats: Meats should be broiled or barbecued. This eliminates frying, which is bad because the oil used is generally over-fried to the point where poisons are formed that become part of the meat and enter the body.

gastritis: Inflammation of the stomach characterized by pain, nausea, and vomiting; due to infection, alcohol abuse, or faulty diet.

Soups: Soups are best when they are eaten alone. Soups dilute stomach acids and ferment, and therefore reduce the likelihood of other food being fully mixed with the digestive enzymes.

acidosis: Excessive acidity of the body's fluids.

Potatoes: The heavy starchy potato should be reserved for the vegetable meals, such as plain salads or steamed vegetables.

[a]From Nutritionist Lesson #2, Bernadean Univ., Van Nuys, CA.

Bernadean's most prominent "graduate" is probably Richard Passwater, "Ph.D.," author of several books and director of research for the Solgar, Co., Inc., a food supplement manufacturer. In 1981, *People* magazine published an article on Passwater's views of the benefits of large doses of vitamins, selenium, and zinc. Victor Herbert, M.D., J.D., complained to the National News Council (a journalistic peer review organization) that the article misled the public by giving an undeserved appearance of reliability to Passwater and his "degree." After determining that Bernadean University was not legally authorized to grant degrees in the states in which it operated, the Council concluded that *People* had "failed to exercise elementary and necessary journalistic responsibility that would put the public on notice."

According to a consultant to California's Office of Postsecondary Education, the "University" is little more than a dilapidated old building and had been ordered to cease operations a few months prior to the time I enrolled as a student. But the combination of permissive laws, bureaucratic roadblocks, and legal delays enabled it to keep operating. Even the U.S. Postal Service, charged with public protection against mail fraud, had decided that Bernadean's activities "did not meet its investigative criteria."

Bernadean failed in an attempt to obtain authorization due to lack of ability to meet the legal requirements. Thus, the "University" should no longer be in operation. Too bad, as I had hoped to buy myself a Ph.D.

Exercise on Nutrition Fraud

After reading the preceding personal account of an attempt to expose one source of nutrition fraud, gather as much information as you can find on a similar health fraud currently available to the public. At a local "health" food store: (1) peruse health magazine advertisements for a health-related degree-by-mail, dietary cure-all, or super-supplement; (2) send for information on one of these items; and (3) write up a brief evaluation.

You might even investigate a local "health" claim by locating—from billboards at "health" food stores, supermarkets, or coffeeshops—and visiting a super-health spa or a workshop on macrobiotics.

Present your findings to classmates or co-workers, and discuss possible avenues for exposing health fraud.

Steps 4 and 5 provide you with suggestions for follow-up on any fraudulent health claims you may uncover. It is up to *you,* as a practicing technician in the field of nutrition, to take the active steps required to help the public to protect themselves from the dangers of health fraud.

STEP 4: HOW TO SPOT NUTRITION FRAUD

More often insidious than obvious, health quackery can be difficult to identify. In order to be able to assist others in separating nutrition sense from nonsense, it is essential for you to be able to spot health fraud.

List some of the common characteristics which could help you to decide whether a health claim is questionable. Then read the following questions, and the answers which would be provided by most nutritionists, in order to uncover a number of ways to spot nutrition fraud; redo your list as a handout for your patients. (See sample on page 130.)

How to Spot Nutrition Fraud

1.

2.

3.

4.

5.

6.

7.

8.

9.

10.

11.

12.

Q. Did nutrition fraud originate in America?

A. Nutrition fraud in this country dates back to the 1600s—and has made a significant amount of progress since that time—but was prevalent in other countries even before that. In 1630, a resident of the Massachusetts Bay Colony was fined for vending sea water as a cure for scurvy. Over 300 years later, in 1961, the Food and Drug Administration backed a six-state roundup of Atlantic Ocean water, bottled by the Florida Sea-Brine Laboratories and sold for $1.69 per pint.

Q. To what extent are medical doctors involved in health fraud?

A. Fortunately, the numbers are relatively few, but there do exist a number of M.D.s who seem to have abandoned scientific thought. Because these doctors hold licenses to practice medicine, the public has confidence in them. Unfortunately, such respect is abused in favor of fast money and unprofessional advice. It is up to consumers to be wary.

Q. How can an unreliable medical practitioner be identified?

A. The following tips may assist in discerning promoters of nutrition nonsense.

    1. He/she claims that all our foods are nutritionally poor, overprocessed, de-vitalized, and poisonous.

    2. He/she claims to have an unusual understanding of health and disease, and believes that most of our ills are due solely to poor diets.

    3. He/she often has a product to sell, such as vitamin supplements, protein powders, mineral pills, or "natural" foods.

    4. He/she promises quick results, offers "testimonials" from other "cured" patients as supportive evidence, and denounces the medical profession, the Food and Drug Administration, and often the scientific community in general.

Q. Why are "nutrition" promoters and purveyors of health nonsense so common these days?

A. Probably because they are so successful financially! Health promotion is a lucrative business and money can be made by everyone—"wellness" advisors, "health" food store employees, self-proclaimed "nutritionists," etc.—except for the victimized consumer. A clever individual can—despite a lack of education in the field of nutrition, and sometimes a complete lack of any education—convince a multitude of educated people that he/she is a nutrition expert offering dependable dietary advice. Because these seemingly professional and appealingly enthusiastic individuals are able to promise cures for every ill, many hopeful consumers want to believe in them, and so end up supporting them—both theoretically and financially. Convincing salespeople with overpriced products and unattainable guarantees, they use sensationalism and scare tactics to provide the fuel for their promotions. Yet, nutrition is science, not magic. And nutrition facts are neither sensational nor panaceas for all human ills.

Q. How can the work of a nutrition phony be distinguished from that of a reliable nutrition professional?

A. There are a number of methods for distinguishing nutrition science and identifying health nonsense. Fortunately, one need not obtain an advanced degree in nutrition in order to become adept at separating diet fact from fancy. By using some common sense and employing the guidelines of nutrition professionals, you can learn to spot nutrition fraud. The following guidelines may prove helpful.

Recognizing a Faddist Nutrition Publication

In Stephen Barrett's (1980) informative book entitled, "The Health Robbers," guidelines for characterizing faddist publications are given by Dr. H. W. Blackburn, Professor of Medicine at the University of Minnesota. According to Dr. Blackburn, the typical nutrition faddist sells written materials that can easily be identified by the following characteristics:

- ○ The book jacket is designed for popular, not scholarly appeal.
- ○ There is collaboration with a popular-style writer, though this is not always noted, or at least not prominently.
- ○ It appeals to a mass market—clear and simple enough to be grasped by the layman, and basic enough for anyone "interested in his own health and the health of his children."
- ○ Provision is made for self-diagnosis and self-treatment along with a cure-all.
- ○ There are undocumented claims of success using testimonial-type evidence.
- ○ A semblance of authority exists using promotional methods: "world's leading authority," a bogus degree, or a recognized degree in a professional discipline but without relevance to the field in which the book is written.
- ○ Research and practice are cited from institutions which may or may not be renowned in the field.
- ○ There exists respectability due to association with well-known institutions and individuals.
- ○ There are complaints of lack of recognition, and persecution is hinted at.
- ○ Controversy is fostered with unqualified theses.
- ○ Seemingly plausible scientific mechanisms are developed.
- ○ Assurances which spread false hope follow outright misinformation.
- ○ Devils are exorcised (big government, taxes, overworked soil, processed foods, white sugar, and white flour are favorites).
- ○ Missionary zeal is prominent.
- ○ Claims are made for the enhancement of sexual potency.
- ○ Recommendations are made for specific dosages, and available products are given by name.

Recognizing a Reliable Nutrition Professional

Victor Herbert, M.D., J.D., has identified two major ways to recognize a credible nutrition publication (Herbert 1980):

1. The author has real scientific credentials in nutrition, rather than phony nutrition credentials.

2.   Most everything on nutrition written by the author was forged in the fire of peer review by competent nutrition scientists, passed that review, and was published in scientific journals indexed in the National Library of Medicine's Medlars Search Computer.

The American Medical Association (AMA 1979) gives consumers some sensible suggestions for recognizing health frauds. They warn the public to beware of self-styled medical "experts" who do the following:

- ○   Use a special or secret formula they claim can cure disease
- ○   Guarantee a quick cure
- ○   Advertise or use case histories or testimonials to promote their cures
- ○   Clamor constantly for medical investigation and recognition
- ○   Claim that representatives of organized medicine are persecuting them or are afraid of their competition.

The Sample Handout lists tips for recognizing nutrition frauds.

Sample Handout

Tip List for Recognizing Nutrition Frauds[1]

1.   Advises that you go out and buy something which you would not otherwise have bought: *the sales pitch.*
2.   Is a fake specialist with imposing "front" titles: *the nutritionist hoax.*
3.   Says that most disease is due to a bad or faulty diet: *the diet-causes-all-ills myth.*
4.   Says that most people are poorly nourished: *the poor American diet pitch.*
5.   Tells you that soil depletion and the use of chemical fertilizers cause malnutrition: *the nutrient-poor soils myth.*
6.   Alleges that modern processing methods and storage remove all nutritive value from food: *the nutrient-poor foods myth.*
7.   Tells you that under stress, and in certain diseases, your need for nutrients is increased: *the sales pitch.*
8.   Says that you are in danger of being poisoned by food additives and preservatives: *chemical phobia.*
9.   Tells you that if you eat badly, you will be fine if you take a vitamin or vitamin and mineral supplement: *the sales pitch.*
10.   Recommends that everybody take vitamins or "health" foods or both: *the sales pitch.*
11.   Claims that "natural" vitamins are better than "synthetic" ones: *chemical phobia.*
12.   Promises quick, dramatic, miraculous cures: *the diet-cures-all-ills myth.*
13.   Uses testimonials and "case histories" to support claims: *the anecdotes-are-proof myth.*
14.   Offers you a vitamin that really is not: *the sales pitch.*
15.   Espouses the "conspiracy theory" and its twin, "the controversy claim": *the-medical-community-is-out-to-get-me claim* and the *my-claims-are-controversies-not-fakes myth.*
16.   Is legally belligerent: *the old I-shall-sue-to-get-attention trick.*

---

[1]Adapted from Herbert (1980).

STEP 5: WHOM TO TRUST

As a dietetic technician in an era marked by a simultaneous rise in nutrition awareness and food fraud, it is your responsibility to be able to inform the public accurately on current nutrition theory. It is important for you to be able to guide others away from health fraud, and to steer them to reliable sources of nutrition information. The most reliable resources for nutrition advice and diet therapy bear the following credentials:

○ Registered dietitians (R.D.), Registered Dietetic Technicians (D.T.R.), members of the American Dietetic Association (ADA), members of the American Institute of Nutrition (AIN), members of the American Society for Clinical Nutrition (ASCN), members of the Institute of Food Technology (IFT), Extension Food and Nutrition Specialists of the Cooperative Extension Service.

Some notable sources of questionable—possibly fraudulent—nutrition advice may bear the following "credentials":

○ Certified Nutritionist, Doctor of Naturopathy (N.D.), Certified Herbologist (C.H.), Registered Healthologist (R.H.), Nutrition Counselor (without appropriate educational credentials), Nutritionist (self-proclaimed, without appropriate educational credentials; in some states, use of this title is licensed to ensure professional acceptance).

If you or your patients encounter food fraud, you may want to contact one of the following agencies: Food and Drug Administration, Rockville, MD 20857; Federal Trade Commission, Bureau of Consumer Protection, 6th and Pennsylvania Ave. N.W., Washington, DC 20580; National News Council, One Lincoln Plaza, New York, NY 10023; Special Investigations Division, U.S. Postal Service, 1200 Pennsylvania Ave. N.E., Washington, DC 20260; American Medical Association, 535 N. Dearborn Street, Chicago, IL 60610; American Cancer Society, Committee on New or Unproven Methods of Treatment, 219 East 42nd Street, New York, NY 10017.

Exercise on Reliable Nutrition Information Sources

Appendix V includes an up-to-date list of recommended references on diet and health. Use the preceding information and the references in Appendix V to prepare a helpful handout for your patients; see the Sample Handout. Such information can help health-conscious individuals—including yourself—to avoid falling prey to the potential dangers of nutrition fraud.

Sample Handout

Recommended Sources of Nutrition Information

   I. *Credentials to Look for:* R.D., D.T.R., ADA, AIN, ASCN, IFT; "nutritionist" title requires information on educational background and professional affiliations.

  II. *Organizations:* Nonprofit; directed by persons with proper nutrition/medical credentials; offering sound health advice without use of scare tactics or questionable product/service promotion.

 III. *Books and Pamphlets:* American Dietetic Association. 1987. What You Should Know About Nutrition and Health. Chicago: ADA.
Brody, J. 1985. Jane Brody's Good Food Book. New York: W. W. Norton.
Connor, S., and Connor, W. 1986. The New American Diet. New York: Simon & Schuster.
Hamilton, E., Whitney, E., and Sizer, F. 1988. Nutrition: Concepts and Controversies, 4th Edition. St. Paul, MN: West Publishing Co.
Lindsay, A. 1988. The American Cancer Society Cookbook. New York: Hearst Books.
U.S. Department of Agriculture. 1985. Nutrition and Your Health: Dietary Guidelines for Americans. Washington, D.C.: Government Printing Office.

 IV. *Newsletters:* Environmental Nutrition, 2112 Broadway, Suite 200, New York, NY 10023.
Nutrition Clinics, George F. Stickley Co., 210 West Washington Square, Philadelphia, PA 19106.
Tufts University Diet & Nutrition Letter, P.O. Box 10948, Des Moines, IA 50940.

  V. *For Further Information:* State health departments, local health agencies, accredited colleges, hospitals, and medical schools with nutritionists can be excellent sources of reliable information.

STEP 6: POST-TEST ON NUTRITION FRAUD

There may arise a significant number of situations in which your expertise in nutrition will be called upon in order to answer certain questions or clear up specific misconceptions. Therefore, it is important for you to have a working knowledge of medically sound diet therapies and an up-to-date understanding of questionable diet "cures." Complete the post-test below for a general evaluation of your current level of understanding about some of the popular diet claims and the nutrition fads and frauds which entice the American public. Answers are given in the Answer Key. Remember that nutrition is a relatively new and ever-changing science, so it is essential for practitioners to constantly monitor both the latest health research and the newest diet "cures."

Indicate whether you think each of the following statements is true (T) or false (F).

_____ 1. The mass media—television, magazines, newspapers, etc.—can always be trusted to provide unbiased, factual nutrition information.

_____ 2. It is essential to try to examine impartially all sides of any nutrition controversy.

_____ 3. Most ailments can be cured by dietary manipulation alone.

_____ 4. "Vitamin" B_{15} is also known as pyridoxine.

_____ 5. Arthritis has been proven to be curable with the use of large daily doses of "vitamin" B_{15}.

_____ 6. Use of laetrile as a cancer treatment has caused fatal results.

_____ 7. It is advisable for individuals with serious illnesses to forgo conventional medical treatment to test out the newest dietary regimens.

_____ 8. There are no known dietary cures for arthritis, cancer, and a number of other degenerative diseases.

Select the answer that best completes the following statements:

_____ 9. A self-proclaimed "nutritionist" might have
(a) sent for "credentials" from a mail-order diploma mill. (b) products to sell which only offer unproven health claims. (c) testimonials and anecdotes rather than documented evidence to back up diet claims. (d) honest advice. (e) all of these.

_____ 10. Reliable nutrition information is generally given
(a) by R.D.s. (b) by word-of-mouth. (c) in professional journals. (d) a and c. (e) all of these.

REFERENCES

AMERICAN MEDICAL ASSOCIATION. 1979. Concepts of nutrition and health. J. Am. Med. Assoc. *242*, Nov. 23, 2335.

ARONSON, V. 1983. You can't tell a nutritionist by the diploma. FDA Consumer, Jul./Aug., 28.

BARRETT, S. 1980. The Health Robbers. Philadelphia: George F. Stickley Co.

HERBERT, V. 1980. Nutrition Cultism. Philadelphia: George F. Stickley Co.

Part III

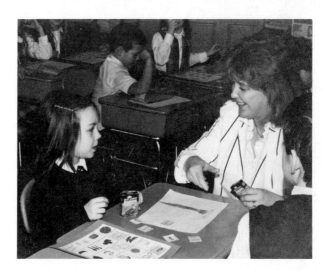

How Can You Counsel about the Different Stages of the Life Cycle?

From pre-birth until death, food is essential to life and proper nutrition helps to determine health status. During certain stages of the life cycle, special nutrition considerations are required. Without proper attention to diet, significant nutrition problems can occur during pregnancy and **lactation,** infancy and childhood, the teen years, and old age. (Post-adolescent adults who do not yet qualify for senior citizen benefits are certainly not immune to nutritional disorders, but they cannot be grouped together by need quite so conveniently). At all ages, the need for individualization in diet therapy is essential. Yet, there are certain special diet modifications to be aware of with patients at the vulnerable stages of life.

To be a successful dietetic technician in nutrition care, you should learn how to be an effective **nutrition counselor.** In order to do so, you must have an understanding of the relationship of food and human needs. It is important to be able to assess each patient's nutritional status, and to determine specific nutrition demands; individualized diet plans suiting lifestyle needs can then be developed.

Nowhere is the old adage "You can lead a horse to water, but you can't make him drink" truer than in consideration of dietary advice. Pregnant women, infants and children, teenagers, and older folks often have finicky appetites as well as special dietary needs. Part III may assist you in developing the required skills to be an effective nutrition counselor, so that you can help patients at all stages of the life cycle to optimize their own diets.

Note: Highly suggested as study aids are "Colorado's Self-Teaching Modules, Nos. 2 and 3," available from Nutrition Services, Office of Health Care Services, Colorado Department of Health, 4210 E. 11th Avenue, Denver, CO 80220.

lactation: Period of breastfeeding.

nutrition counselor: A trained professional who provides individualized guidance to assist individuals in modifying daily food consumption in order to meet specific health needs; diet counselor, or one who provides professional diet advice, diet plans, diet therapy.

Chapter Seven

Eating during Pregnancy and Lactation

CHAPTER BLUEPRINT

Step 1: Take the Pre-test on Pregnancy and Lactation Nutrition and participate in the assigned group discussion in order to begin to reflect on your own concepts about the role of nutrition during pregnancy and lactation.

Step 2: Examine the Nutrition Facts List on pregnancy and prepare the assigned handout.

Step 3: Read the Healthy? excerpt and participate in the group discussion.

Step 4: Read the materials and complete the list on Bottle vs. Breast; begin to formulate the suggested file.

Step 5: Examine the Pregnancy Guidelines and complete the role play assignment.

Step 6: Take the Post-test on Pregnancy and Lactation Nutrition to evaluate what you have learned from the information and activities provided in this chapter.

Step 7: Reexamine the Pre-test and make those alterations which you deem appropriate in consideration of the information you acquired from this chapter.

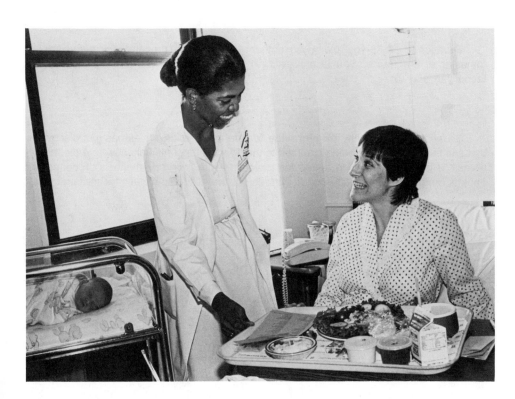

STEP 1: PRE-TEST ON PREGNANCY AND LACTATION NUTRITION

fetus: The unborn child from 3 months to birth (prior to that, the proper term is embryo).

Proper nutrition during pregnancy has been documented as one of the most important factors in determining the eventual outcome. Inadequate nutritional intake, including calories and specific nutrients, may result in insufficient weight gain, **fetal** malnutrition, prematurity, and/or low birth weight. Poor maternal nutrition has been associated with an increased incidence of prematurity, still birth, neonatal mortality, and fetal deformities. Like the physical, genetic, and psychological influences on pregnancy, diet is an essential health-contributing factor.

Lactation also mandates attention to nutrient intake. Although a poor diet does not have a significant effect on the nutritional composition of breast milk, the volume can be reduced and the health of the mother may be jeopardized. Obviously, careful selection of a variety of foods to form a well-balanced and calorically adequate diet is an important health concern for both mother and infant.

Pregnancy and Lactation Consultation Pre-test

As a practicing dietetic technician, it is important for you to have a clear understanding of your own philosophies as they relate to patient care. For each of the following sample situations, give your own best response as the assigned dietetics personnel: Elaborate on each situation to create a patient file and record your answer using the SOAP format (see Chapter 1, Step 6), indicating whether you would employ the assistance of other health professionals. Discuss your answers with classmates or co-workers. Do you think that future training and experience will alter your responses? You may want to reexamine your answers (see Step 7) after you have completed Chapter 7, and again once you have dealt with a number of real-life situations similar to the samples depicted.

Situation 1: An underweight 18-year-old female comes to the prenatal clinic. Her medical history reveals a recent significant weight loss, borderline anemia, and that she is in her second trimester of her first pregnancy. As the assigned dietetic technician, I would

Situation 2: A 35-year-old obese mother of two visits the prenatal clinic during her first trimester of pregnancy. She is requesting a weight loss diet. As the assigned dietetic technician, I would

primigravida: Woman in her first pregnancy.

Situation 3: A healthy **primigravida** female in her midtwenties has just discovered that she is pregnant after being admitted to the hospital for continual nausea. A diet history reveals a fast-paced lifestyle pattern as a working wife, with an emphasis on coffee and donuts, burgers and fries, and frozen entrees. As the assigned dietetic technician, I would

pancreatitis: Inflammation of the pancreas, acute or chronic, usually accompanied by jaundice.

Situation 4: A 30-year-old mother of four is admitted for **pancreatitis.** Although in the fifth month of pregnancy, she admits to drinking "a few cocktails" and to smoking "a pack or two" of cigarettes every day. As the assigned dietetic technician, I would

Situation 5: A healthy young mother has just given birth to her first child and is undecided as to whether she should breastfeed. Her husband is a successful lawyer who has encouraged her to take a leave of absence to stay at home with the new healthy and hungry baby. As the assigned dietetic technician, I would

STEP 2: NUTRITION FACTS

Perhaps more than at any other time during their lifetimes, pregnant women realize the importance of eating nutritiously and judiciously. As a dietetic technician involved in nutrition education, you may be able to take advantage of such motivation and provide your patients with important information. A successful pregnancy requires a sound dietary basis. It is your responsibility to assist nutritionally vulnerable mothers-to-be in understanding the dietary facts. The following Nutrition Facts List provides some of the most current diet-related information to include in counseling pregnant individuals.

Nutrition Facts List

1.   Since most Americans today realize that diet is one factor the pregnant woman is able to control, maternal nutrition is usually not ignored, yet few women understand the influence of food choices on the fetus; if diet is inadequate, mother and fetus compete for available nutrients, then both depend on the mother's reserves.

2.   During the first 2 months of pregnancy, a normal well-balanced diet should be sufficient; in the third month, daily caloric intake should be increased by 300 calories with an emphasis on high-protein and calcium-rich foodstuffs.

3.   During pregnancy, 75,000 calories—in addition to maternal requirements—are needed; the RDAs for the pregnant woman can be determined using Table 7.1.

4.   Weight should increase by 23 to 30 lb, primarily during the fifth to ninth month; pre-pregnancy weight and the number of pounds gained during pregnancy are two important factors in determining birth weight.

5.   The average birth weight is around 7 lb, the median weight gain is 29 lb; more weight is usually gained by younger, thinner, first-time mothers.

6.   Weight gain should approximate the pattern given in Fig. 7.1, with the total gain as follows:

Breast increase	1–3 lb
Blood increase	$4\frac{1}{2}$–5 lb
Maternal stores	4–8 lb
Placenta	1–2 lb
Amniotic fluid	2–3 lb
Fetus	$7\frac{1}{2}$–8 lb
Uterus increase	2–5 lb

amniotic fluid: Fluid in uterus in which the fetus floats, cushioned against injuries and maintained at a constant temperature.

Table 7.1   RDAs for Women

	Ages 19–22 yr	Ages 23–50 yr	Increase for pregnancy (+)	Increase for lactation (+)
Protein (g)	44	44	30	20
Vitamin C (mg)	60	60	20	40
Thiamin (mg)	1.1	1.0	0.4	0.5
Riboflavin (mg)	1.3	1.2	0.3	0.5
Niacin (mg)	14	13	2	5
Vitamin B_6 (mg)	2	2	0.6	0.5
Folacin (μg)	400	400	400	100
Vitamin B_{12} (μg)	3	3	1	1
Vitamin A (μg)	800	800	200	400
Vitamin D (μg)	7.5	5	5	5
Vitamin E (mg)	8	8	2	3
Calcium (mg)	800	800	400	400
Phosphorus (mg)	800	800	400	400
Magnesium (mg)	300	300	150	150
Iron (mg)	18	18	[a]	[a]
Zinc (mg)	15	15	5	10
Iodine (μg)	150	150	25	50

[a]Supplements of 30–60 mg/day are recommended to meet the increased needs of pregnancy and to replenish stores during the first few months after delivery.

CHART YOUR WEIGHT GAIN

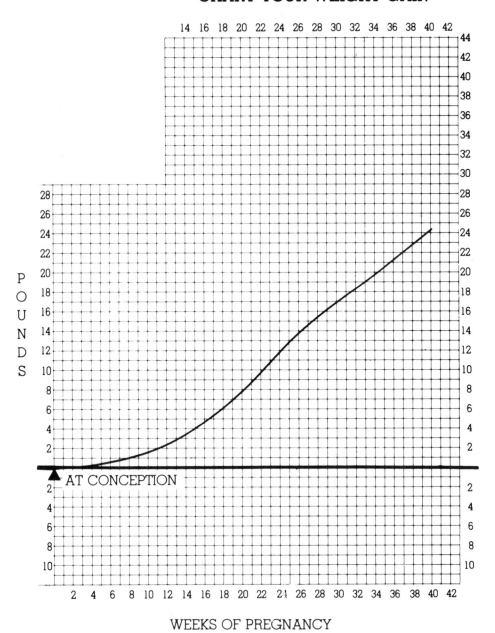

Fig. 7.1   Pregnancy weight gain chart. From Hess and Hunt (1987).

The physician should be called immediately if there is a sudden gain (2–5 lb in 1 week) or an inadequate gain (less than 2 lb/week during the third trimester).

    7.   The American College of Obstetricians and Gynecologists warns that any attempt to restrict the diet during pregnancy can jeopardize the fetus; overweight women should not try to reduce during pregnancy.

    8.   Eating for two does not mean two adults, so it is important for pregnant women to avoid the urge to overindulge.

postpartum: Occurring after childbirth.

    9.   **Postpartum** weight loss:

> ↓ 11 lb with delivery ($7\frac{1}{2}$ baby + $1\frac{1}{2}$ placental membranes + 2 amniotic fluid)
> ↓ 7 lb during next 2 weeks (accumulated fluids in tissue + uterus + breasts + blood volume)

↓ to normal weight by 6 months postpartum
↓ with lactation which requires ↑ 350–450 calories per day
↓ (without fads) by eating for one + exercising regularly
↓ by avoiding snacking during each feeding time

10.   If the pregnant woman is losing weight, fat stores are being broken down; this releases **ketone bodies,** causing an acidic environment which impairs fetal development and, during the third trimester, fetal brain development can be inhibited.

11.   It is now known that larger babies do not necessitate longer labor nor increased delivery risk for the infant (however, birth weight exceeding 10 lb may be indicative of maternal diabetes); women were once warned that excessive weight gain could cause **toxemia,** but are now informed that an inadequate gain can do so.

12.   Women with greater lean body weight as compared to fat stores also tend to have difficulty conceiving; women at less than 85%—or greater than 120%—of their proper weight are at increased nutritional risk upon conception.

13.   For the pregnant adolescent, the diet must meet the needs of both the growing, maturing mother and her fetus; more infants born to teens die, partially due to the fact that teens often enter pregnancy in a poor nutritional state.

14.   Teens tend to have low-birth-weight infants with greater chances for mental and physical handicaps and lesser chances for survival.

15.   Ages 20–29 are statistically the most successful years for pregnancy, yet 25% of the U.S. primigravida are under 20, and the 1980s have seen a 22% increase in births to women aged 35–39.

16.   A nutritionally adequate diet helps to prevent toxemia, premature birth, and infant death; proper diet—both prior to and during pregnancy—results in fewer labor complications, larger and healthier infants, faster maternal recovery, and greater chance for successful breastfeeding.

17.   The pregnant woman should follow a diet which supplies an increased amount of specific nutrients for the reasons shown in Table 7.2.

18.   Pre-pregnancy use of oral contraceptives can add to the elevated need for B vitamins, especially folacin and pyridoxine, so the physician may prescribe supplementation.

19.   During the third trimester, the fetus builds iron reserves for the first 3–4 months of life, so the premature infant may become iron deficient; since women in the childbearing years are often iron deficient, many enter pregnancy with low iron stores and may require supplementation.

20.   According to the National Research Council of the National Academy of Sciences, the use of multi-purpose nutrition supplements during pregnancy is merely for "insurance" purposes, but many physicians do prescribe specially formulated prenatal supplements.

21.   Drinking milk is the most efficient way to meet the increased need for calcium during pregnancy and, if vitamin D fortified, 1 quart/day can help provide both calcium and phosphorus which will be readily absorbed; supplementation with bone meal or **dolomite** can be dangerous and may cause lead poisoning.

Table 7.2   Increased Nutrients in Pregnant Woman's Diet

Nutrients	Reasons
Protein	Tissue growth (fetus) and maintenance (mother)
Calcium	Skeletal growth (fetus) and maintenance (mother)
Phosphorus	Skeletal and muscle growth (fetus)
Iron	Iron reserve (fetus) and anemia prevention (mother)
Iodine	**Thyroxine** for growth and development (fetus) and increased metabolism (mother)
Vitamin A	Cell integrity, bone and tooth formation (fetus)
B-complex	Caloric increase necessitates more B vitamins (mother)
Vitamin C	Tissue development (fetus) and iron absorption (mother)
Vitamin D	Assimilation of calcium and phosphorus (fetus)
Vitamin K	**Prothrombin** deficiency/**hemorrhagic disease of the newborn** prevention (fetus)
Water	Waste product excretion facilitation (from fetus via mother) and maintenance of expanded blood volume (mother)

ketone bodies: Group of chemical compounds produced during the oxidation of the fatty acids which accumulate during ketosis.

toxemia (eclamptogenic): Potentially fatal condition after twentieth week of pregnancy characterized by fluid retention, elevated blood pressure, nausea, fever, coma and seizures.

dolomite: A form of limestone marketed as a calcium supplement; may contain undesirably high quantities of lead and other potentially toxic metals.

thyroxine: Hormone produced by the thyroid gland.

prothrombin: Chemical which circulates in the bloodstream and produces the enzyme thrombin for clotting.

hemorrhagic disease of the newborn: Abnormal bleeding due to inadequate maternal prothrombin or delayed fetal synthesis of vitamin K; treated with administration of vitamin K.

edema: Excessive accumulation of fluids in body tissues.

22.   Fluoride is essential to help form strong teeth and bones, so if the local water supply is not fluoridated, the physician may prescribe a supplement.

23.   During pregnancy, blood volume increases by 33%, the water reserve in cells increases, and **edema** is common; use of diuretics is inadvisable and salt need not be restricted. Resting with the feet up, removing tight rings, and wearing comfortable shoes can help to minimize discomfort.

24.   Unless laboratory test results indicate a need, it is unnecessary to restrict dietary cholesterol intake during pregnancy; cholesterol is essential for hormone production (which is increased during pregnancy), and a link between cholesterol intake and health detriments during pregnancy has not been substantiated.

25.   Food cravings are a concern only if the budget becomes strained or the diet unbalanced; however, *pica* (craving for nonfood items such as dirt, clay, ice, or laundry starch) may indicate low iron stores. The medical implications of eating such nonfood items as charcoal, wall plaster, moth balls, and toilet-bowl fresheners include toxemia of pregnancy, congenital lead poisoning, and other serious pre- and post-natal disorders.

26.   Caffeine can stimulate unpleasant gastrointestinal (GI) disturbances, especially in the pregnant woman suffering from heartburn; decaffeinated products also contain certain acids which can cause GI distress. Although insufficient data is available on quantitative recommendations for caffeine use during pregnancy, research indicates that moderation during pregnancy is advisable.

27.   Alcohol intake during pregnancy is associated with *fetal alcohol syndrome* (see p. 100), threatening both the physical and mental health of the fetus, and can interfere with the nutrient intake of the pregnant woman. Just how nutritional deficiencies exacerbate the detrimental effects of alcohol intake is still under research. Most physicians recommend abstinence from alcohol during pregnancy.

28.   Pregnant women who smoke more than 10 cigarettes a day often deliver babies that are premature or small for gestational age because nicotine causes blood vessel constriction (which interferes with placental blood flow) and increases blood levels of carbon monoxide, resulting in a reduced fetal oxygen supply. Cigarette smoking is a *preventable* cause of low birth weight.

29.   Most drugs cross placental barriers and none have been proven to be totally safe for the growing fetus; nicotine, caffeine, and alcohol are considered drugs, as are vitamins and minerals in large dosages.

30.   The simplest method for balancing the diet during pregnancy is to select foods from the Basic Food Groups in the amounts outlined in Table 7.3 in the Sample Handout.

31.   Pregnancy can prove to be an appropriate time to improve the diets of the rest of the patient's family as well.

32.   It is essential for the pregnant woman who follows a vegetarian regime or has other dietary restrictions to obtain individualized nutrition counseling.

33.   Physicians and physical therapists can advise on desirable exercise techniques, both during and after pregnancy; it is unwise to participate in physical activities which hurt, require lying on the back (in late pregnancy, pressure from the heavy uterus can slow blood flow), or involve back arching (such as sit-ups).

34.   Nearly 60% of all pregnant women experience nausea of some kind during the first 2–3 months, which is often referred to as "morning sickness" (but can occur at any time of day or night); this is a common temporary symptom which usually diminishes by the time nutrient needs increase.

35.   Nausea occurs because the digestive process slows during early pregnancy so that less gastric juices are being produced; treatment basically consists of eating small, frequent meals with alternating solids and liquids while avoiding the high-fat, hard-to-digest foods.

36.   Some specific anti-nausea tips include the following: (a) A container of crackers, popcorn, or dry cereal next to the bed can enable the "morning sickness" sufferer to relieve nausea before arising. (b) Sudden movement can worsen nausea, so arising should be slow. (c) Coffee and cigarette smoking stimulate the acid secretion which aggravates nausea. (d) Individuals vary, and foods that might be craved by one person can make another ill.

37.   The physician should be contacted by those who are unable to keep down fluids, are vomiting more than twice daily, or are still experiencing "morning sickness" during the second trimester of pregnancy.

38.   Since hormonal changes during pregnancy slow intestinal muscle action, constipation can occur (and iron supplementation may contribute to the problem). Required dietary control includes the following: plenty of fluids, fiber-rich foodstuffs, and nature's own laxative—the prune.

39.   During the last trimester when the fetus is growing rapidly, the expanded uterus may press against the stomach, causing contents to return to the esophagus; the burning symptoms may be alleviated somewhat with these anti-heartburn tips: (a) Food intake should be divided into 4–6 small meals which are eaten slowly in a relaxed environment. (b) Spicy, high-fat, and rich foods, as well as caffeine, alcohol, and individually bothersome items, are to be avoided. (c) Food intake just prior to bed or nap time can cause symptoms. (d) Antacids should only be taken if prescribed by the attending physician.

40.   Toxemia occurs more frequently in the primigravida who (i) is under age 20 or over 35, (ii) suffers from diabetes, hypertension, or kidney disease, or (iii) is expecting twins. Although the cause has yet to be pinpointed, the well-known symptoms are as follows: (a) *pre-eclampsia*—edema especially noticeable in extremities, indicated in the third trimester by a gain in weight of over 2 lb in one week; requires bedrest, proper diet, and medical attention. (b) *eclampsia*—untreated pre-eclampsia can lead to blurred vision, headache, abdominal pain, and convulsion; requires immediate medical attention to prevent serious damage to both mother and fetus.

41.   Pregnancy and obesity are two contributing factors to the development of maturity-onset diabetes; 20–30% of women with gestational diabetes (glucose intolerance occurs during pregnancy but reverts to normal after delivery) develop permanent diabetes within 5 years. Thus, strict control of blood glucose levels is important for maternal health, while fetal mortality and neonatal hypoglycemia make maternal control imperative to infant health as well.

42.   Since most women with gestational diabetes are overweight, the dietary goal is proper weight gain (not loss) and maintenance of a fasting blood glucose below 100 mg/dL (milligrams glucose per deciliter of blood); insulin may be required, in addition to a well-balanced diet with limited intake of concentrated carbohydrates (more in Chapter 11).

Exercise Using the Nutrition Facts List

Using the preceding list, prepare a simplified one-page version to hand out to pregnant women receiving nutrition counseling. You may include graphics and/or use a poster format, if desired; see the Sample Handout. Show your handout in rough draft form to classmates or co-workers for constructive criticism on the overall design, content, and potential effectiveness for use in pertinent diet counseling situations. Then prepare a final version for version for your own future use as a practicing dietetic technician.

Sample Handout

Your *diet* plays an important role in your overall health status all of your life. During pregnancy, what you eat also affects your unborn child. This is one of the factors influencing the outcome of your pregnancy over which you do have some control. Thus, it is up to *you* to eat right—for both your own sake, and that of your baby.

Table 7.3 outlines the daily servings from each of the Basic Food Groups which you should include in your diet.

You are eating for two, but not two adults!

○   Milk is the best source of calcium, and provides phosphorus plus other nutrients as well. If you do not like milk, try low-fat yogurt and cheeses or add dried skim milk powder to casseroles and other foods.

○   Iron is better absorbed with vitamin C. Drink orange juice at meals, and take your iron supplement with grapefruit juice.

○ Ask your physician if your local water supply is fluoridated. If not, ask your physician about supplements.

○ Avoid food fads and mega-nutrients. Only take supplements if your physician prescribes them.

Table 7.3   Diet during Pregnancy[a]

Food group	No. daily servings
Fruits and vegetables	
Total	5 or more
Including vitamin C-rich	1 or more
Including green leafy or bright yellow	2
Breads and cereals	4 or more
Milk and cheeses	4 or more
Meats and alternates	3
Others	2 Tbsp oil or margarine
Water	8 or more cups

[a]Note: To meet the RDAs for pregnant girls aged 11 to 18, additional servings from the Basic Food Groups are required in order to supply adequate calories and nutrients for both maternal growth and pregnancy/lactation needs.

STEP 3: HEALTHY?

Much of the nutrition "information" currently available to the general public is based on myth and fallacy. When individuals who are at nutritional risk adopt misleading dietary advice, ill health—even death—can result. Pregnant women—like infants, children, older folks, and unhealthy individuals—have an elevated need for certain nutrients, so are more susceptible to both nutritional deficiencies and food faddism. Therefore, many unproven dietary claims are aimed at the nutritionally naive, yet health conscious pregnant woman.

As a practicing dietetic technician in nutrition care, it is your responsibility to help protect the pregnant woman (and her fetus) from falling prey to dangerous dietary claims. By educating the pregnant woman on the basics of normal nutrition and her own special needs during pregnancy, you can provide her with a sturdy foundation on which to base her dietary practices. Then, by warning her about the dangers of fad diets and mega-supplements, you can assist her in preserving her own health and promoting proper growth of the fetus.

Exercise on Nutrition Misinformation Aimed at Pregnant Women

Read Table 7.4 excerpted from Dr. Lendon Smith's "Foods for Healthy Kids" (1981) and answer the discussion questions below. Note that Smith's books often promote unproven nutrition concepts and "old wives' tales" or common misconceptions about dietary needs. Discuss your answers with classmates or co-workers.

Begin to scan the media—television, magazines, newspapers, billboards, books, leaflets, etc.—for misleading advertisements for dietary aids aimed at pregnant women. You might want to develop a file on nutrition misinformation to use in counseling pregnant women on proper diet versus food fads.

Helpful information for answering these questions appears in the Nutrition Facts List on pregnancy (Step 2) and in Parts I and II of this book.

1. Do you think that nuts, cheese, and high-protein foods are a wise choice for treatment of nausea? Why or why not?

2. Do you think that "nibbling on protein" is a sensible weight loss tip for an individual gaining undesirable poundage? Why or why not?

Table 7.4   Old Wives' Tales or Dangerous Nutrition Nonsense?[a]

Symptom or sign	Could lead to	To relieve, try this
Nausea and vomiting in early pregnancy	Exhaustion, malnutrition, seborrhea, **colic,** learning disabilities	B_6, nibbling on nuts, cheese, protein
Muscle cramps, backache	Painful delivery	Calcium, magnesium, manganese, potassium
Stretch marks	Stretch marks	Vitamins E, A, zinc
Gas	Discomfort	Change diet, acidophilus
Fatigue	Exhaustion, depression, inability to nurse	B complex, B_{12}, folic acid
Edema, swollen ankles	High blood pressure, toxemia	Protein diet, B_6, salt (fluid needed for nursing)
Headaches	Fatigue and depression	Nibbling on protein and vegetables, no sugar
Gaining too much	Fatigue (if due to unrefined carbohydrates)	Nibbling on protein and vegetables
Gaining too little	Undernourished baby	Add vitamins B, C, calcium, and minerals. May benefit from vitamin shots.
Food cravings Smoking Alcohol ingestion Drugs	Malnutrition	B complex (50–100 mg of each of B vitamins), calcium (2000 mg), magnesium (800–1000 mg), raw vegetables, seeds, nuts, brewer's yeast, kelp
Excessive intra-uterine activity	Allergic or hyperactive child	Stop milk and foods eaten daily. Use 4-day **rotation diet.** Add calcium.
Sinusitis, increase in allergies, rashes, wheezes	Allergic child	Plan to nurse; use calcium, extra vitamins C and B, pantothenic acid; eliminate milk

[a]From L. Smith. 1981. Foods for Healthy Kids. McGraw-Hill, New York.

colic: Intestinal spasms, often accompanied by abdominal pain, most common during the first 3 months of life.

rotation diet: Restrictive diet which allows a limited number of foods for several days, then alternates to allow a limited amount of different items for several days; used to try to pinpoint bothersome foods and specific food sensitivities.

3. Would the addition of vitamins and minerals alone to the diet promote desired weight gain? Why or why not?

4. Do you think that it is a wise idea to advise a pregnant woman to "stop milk" with "excessive intra-uterine activity?" Would the use of calcium supplements such as dolomite or bone meal be advisable substitutes for milk products? Explain your answers:

5. Have large supplemental doses of vitamins and minerals been documented as an important constituent of the diet program required for healthy pregnancy? for proper fetal growth and development? Briefly explain your viewpoint on mega-nutrient supplement usage during pregnancy:

STEP 4: BOTTLE VS. BREAST

One of the most important choices a mother-to-be must make regarding her newborn is whether to bottle feed or breastfeed. For those who are unable to breastfeed due to inadequate milk supply or other physical reasons, the decision to use infant formula requires further consideration in the selection of a satisfactory brand. Dietary patterns should differ for those mothers using infant formulas rather than breastmilk (see Table 7.1).

The advantages of human milk are undeniable, but when conditions make breastfeeding impossible, there are a number of commercial formulas which are quite comparable. Infant formulas are developed by copying nature as closely as possible, yet there *are* certain differences. Since mother/infant closeness is an important psychological component of child rearing, mothers of bottle-fed babies should be careful to practice the same handling and attention provided during breastfeeding.

It is important for the nutrition practitioners involved in pregnancy counseling to support the mothers-to-be in their feeding choices. As a dietetic technician in nutrition care, you can impart as much health information as possible, provide handouts and references, and assist in the decision-making process. Yet, the final decision belongs to the new mothers, and each should be encouraged to opt for the feeding method with which she will be most comfortable. After all, is it not better for infants to be held lovingly during bottle feeding, than to be subjected to maternal tension and anger at breastfeeding time?

Briefs on Baby Feeding

In counseling mothers-to-be you need to be well acquainted with the following facts:

○ An impaired *let-down reflex* can inhibit breastfeeding due to a psychosomatic reflex whereby suckling triggers milk to move back into the milk sinuses, and only *fore* milk is released, rather than the fat-rich *hind* milk. The problem can be caused by lack of self-confidence and anxiety.

○ As a safety feature, the RDAs for infants have been set slightly higher for certain nutrients than the amounts found in breast milk, since some nutrients are absorbed more efficiently from breast milk.

○ Due to immature enzyme systems, certain "unessential" amino acids may be required in the diets of premature infants (e.g., cystine and tyrosine), and low stores of vitamins and minerals can mean that special premature infant formulas plus supplementation (e.g., calcium, phosphorus, and vitamin D) are necessitated in the nonbreastfed.

○ Recent estimates indicate that over one-half of new mothers start out breastfeeding, and more than one-quarter are still breastfeeding when the child reaches 6 months of age.

○ Upon weaning to infant formula, it is important to use an iron-fortified product.

○ Breastfeeding in infancy seems to prevent hypercholesterolemia in adulthood, but research is still underway to establish the physiological explanation.

○ Recent research does not support the belief that a mother's intake of cow's milk will cause colic in the breastfed infant.

○ Dark-skinned infants who live in a cold climate may require vitamin D supplements if breastfed; if regular exposure to sun cannot be substituted for supplementation, care should be taken to prevent vitamin D overdose.

○ If the maternal diet is lacking in certain nutrients, the breast milk may also be low; a limited caloric intake by the mother can reduce breast milk volume.

○ Breastfeeding does not guarantee good health for the recipient, nor does bottle feeding mean poor health; if nutritional needs are met, both forms of feeding can prove healthful and satisfying—to infant and mother as well.

Suggested Readings on Pregnancy and Lactation Nutrition

AMERICAN ACADEMY OF PEDIATRICS. 1984. A Gift of Love: Breast Feeding. Elk Grove Village, IL: AAP.

AMERICAN DIETETIC ASSOCIATION. 1981. Handbook of Clinical Dietetics, p. A63. New Haven, CT: Yale University Press.

AMERICAN DIETETIC ASSOCIATION. 1986. Position of The American Dietetic Association: Promotion of breast feeding. J. Am. Dietet. Assoc. 86, Nov., 1580.

BARNESS, L. 1980. Infant feeding: Benefits of formulas. Professional Nutritionist 1, Summer, 4.

BRADY, M., et al. 1982. Formulas and human milk for premature infants: A review and update. J. Am. Med. Assoc. 80, Nov., 547.

EDITOR. 1988. Breast not necessarily best. Lancet 1, Mar. 19, 624.

FOMAN, S. 1986. Breast-feeding and evolution. J. Am. Dietet. Assoc. 86, Mar., 317.

GOLDFARB, J., and TIBBETTS, E. 1980. Breastfeeding Handbook: A Practical Reference for Physicians, Nurses and Other Health Professionals. Hillside, NJ: Enslow Publishing Co.

HESS, M., and HUNT, A. 1982. Pickles and Ice Cream, pp. 195–200. New York: McGraw-Hill.

LA LECHE LEAGUE INTERNATIONAL. 1986. The Womanly Art of Breastfeeding. Franklin Park, IL: LLLI.

NATIONAL DAIRY COUNCIL. 1980. Current infant feeding practices. Dairy Counc. Dig. 51, Jan./Feb., 1.

NEVILLE, M., and NEFERT, M. 1983. Lactation: Physiology, Nutrition, and Breast-feeding. New York: Plenum Press.

OLSON, C., and PSIAKI, D. 1980. Current Knowledge on Breastfeeding: A Review for Medical Practitioners. Ithaca, NY: Cornell University.

SAUNDERS, S., and CARROLL, J. 1988. Post-partum breast feeding support. J. Am. Dietet. Assoc. *88,* Feb., 213.

SHEARD, N., and WALKER, W. 1988. The role of breast milk in the development of the gastrointestinal tract. Nutrition Rev. *46,* Jan., 1.

SUCHOW, E. 1983. Feeding the premature infant. Environmental Nutr., Nov., 1.

TIBBETTS, E., and CADWELL, K. 1981. Opportunities for community health professionals to support breastfeeding. J. Nutr. Ed. *13,* Dec., 132.

WIDDERSON, E. 1987. Fetal and neonatal nutrition. Nutrition Today *22,* Sept./Oct., 16.

WOLMAN, P. 1984. Feeding practices in infancy and prevention of obesity in preschool children. J. Am. Dietet. Assoc., *84,* Apr., 436.

WORTH, C. 1983. Breastfeeding Basics. New York: McGraw-Hill.

Table 7.5 Bottle vs. Breast Chart

Bottle feeding pros	Breastfeeding pros
1. Breastfeeding is not always possible for new mothers.	1. Contains antibodies to protect against disease.
2. Bottle formulas are sterilized.	2. Human milk is bacteria-free, unexposed to external sources of contamination.
3. Convenient for working women.	3. Convenient.
4. Extra food for lactating mother is costly.	4. Economical.

Your Babyfeeding Pro/Con Chart (Continued from Table 7.5)

No.	Bottle feeding pros	Breastfeeding pros

Exercises on Bottle vs. Breast

1. After reading the preceding Briefs on Baby Feeding and several of the Suggested Readings, complete the chart following Table 7.5 by adding some pros and cons of your own. Try to list as many pros as possible for each choice. Use the chart to elaborate on baby feeding options. More and more contemporary women in our society are opting for breast-feeding, mainly due to the increased level of public interest in optimal health and well-being. Only 1% of those who attempt to breastfeed are unsuccessful. Unfortunately, many developing countries have seen a decline in the incidence of breastfeeding, partially due to massive advertising campaigns for infant formulas.

2. Those women who select to bottle feed their infants may require extended assistance in the selection and preparation of appropriate infant formulas. Women who choose to wean their infants from breast to bottle after only a few months may also need help in making selections from the various brands of infant formula currently available. Thus, it would be to your advantage to begin assembling a file on available formulas, ingredients, and costs to use in counseling mothers with questions on bottle feeding. You can collect materials from pharmaceutical companies, hospital pharmacy departments, and local obstetricians or pediatricians. Remember to keep your file updated so that the material you provide to others is current and accurate.

Side Note: Nutrition after Pregnancy

In order to provide continued counsel to new mothers, you need to be aware of the following facts.

○ Dietary needs of the lactating woman include an extra 350–450 calories per day with an emphasis on foods high in protein, calcium and phosphorus, iron, vitamins A and C, and the B-complex vitamins.

○ Supplements are usually not required since additional nutrient needs can be met by increasing the intake of milk, cheese, eggs, whole grain products, vegetables, and fruits including citrus.

○ Since the process of lactation utilizes a significant number of calories, adherence to the suggested dietary pattern will allow for gradual loss of excess weight (that is, unless high-calorie cravings of pregnancy continue and cause overindulgence).

○ Bottle-feeding mothers should diminish food intake to achieve a well-balanced diet at a caloric level appropriate for gradual loss of undesired weight.

○ Sufficient energy for mothering and nutritional adequacy for recovery are important to new mothers, so it is imperative that fad diets and low-calorie dieting are avoided; although some physicians recommend continued use of prenatal supplements (for "insurance" purposes), self-prescribed nutrients and mega-supplements are to be avoided.

○ Postpartum overweight and constipation can be reduced with generous intakes of fresh fruit and vegetables as low-calorie, high-fiber snacks; portion control can also assist weight loss endeavors.

○ Tending a newborn certainly requires significant energy output, but a program of regular exercise can further enhance weight loss, as well as help to tone muscle and reduce stress; it is important for the postpartum female to consult her physician prior to embarking on an exercise program.

STEP 5: PREGNANCY GUIDELINES

In order to be able to advise pregnant women on desirable dietary patterns, it is essential to have access to all of the hands-on material required for effective counseling sessions. It is also important to be able to record all of the pertinent information regarding each diet counseling session in the patient's medical charts. If you found it difficult to complete the Pre-test in Step 1, the information provided in the Suggested Readings and Counseling Guidelines should help to improve your confidence—and skills—regarding your counseling abilities.

This step includes suggested strategies to use in counseling pregnant women. The following references may prove helpful.

Suggested Readings on Nutrition and Pregnancy

ABEL, E. (Editor). 1981. Fetal Alcohol Syndrome. Boca Raton, FL: CRC Press.

AMERICAN DIETETIC ASSOCIATION. 1981. Assessment of Maternal Nutrition. Chicago: ADA.

BING, E., and COLEMAN, L. 1980. Having a Baby After Thirty. New York: Bantam.

COLORADO DEPARTMENT OF HEALTH. 1981. Colorado's Self-Teaching Modules, No. 4: Prenatal Nutrition. Denver: Nutrition Services, Office of Health Care Services, CDH.

EISENBERG, A., EISENBERG-MURKOFF, W., and EISENBERG-HATHAWAY, S. 1986. What to Expect When You're Expecting. New York: Workman.

HESS, M., and HUNT, A. 1987. Pickles and Ice Cream: The Complete Guide to Nutrition during Pregnancy. Winnetka, IL: Hess & Hunt, Inc.

HINTON, S., and KERWIN, D. 1982. Maternal, Infant, and Child Nutrition. Chapel Hill, NC: Health Sciences Consortium.

HOLLINGSWORTH, D. 1984. Pregnancy and Birth: A Management Guide. Baltimore, MD: Williams & Wilkins.

HOPE, J., and BRIGHT-SEE, E. 1982. Everywoman's Book of Nutrition. Toronto, Canada: McGraw-Hill Ryerson.

JOHNSTON, P. 1988. Counseling the pregnant vegetarian. Am. J. Clin. Nutr. 48, Sept. Supp., 901.

MARCH OF DIMES FOUNDATION. 1981. Working with the Pregnant Teenager: A Guide for Nutrition Educators. Washington, DC: Government Printing Office.

MARCH OF DIMES FOUNDATION. 1986. Nutrition and Adolescent Pregnancy: A Selected Annotated Bibliography. Washington, DC: Government Printing Office.

MILUNSKY, A., FRIEDMAN, E., and GLUCK, L. (Editors). 1982. Advances in Prenatal Medicine. New York: Plenum Press.

NATIONAL RESEARCH COUNCIL. 1982. Alternative Dietary Practices and Nutritional Abuses in Pregnancy. Washington, DC: National Academy of Sciences.

RITCHEY, S., and TAPER, J. 1983. Maternal and Child Nutrition. New York: Harper & Row.

ROSSETT, H. 1984. Alcohol and the Fetus: A Critical Perspective. New York: Oxford University Press.

SOCIETY FOR NUTRITION EDUCATION. 1982. Pregnancy and Nutrition (Annotated Bibliography). Oakland, CA: SNE.

SUTUR, C., and OTT, D. 1984. Maternal and infant nutrition recommendations: A review. J. Am. Dietet. Assoc. 84, May, 572.

VETTER, J. (Editor). 1981. Maternal Nutrition in Pregnancy: Eating for Two? New York: Academic Press.

WIC. 1988. The National WIC Evaluation. Am. J. Clin. Nutrition 48, Aug. Supp., 389.

WINICK, M. (Editor). 1985. Feeding the Mother and Infant. New York: John Wiley & Sons.

WINICK, M. 1986. Nutrition and Pregnancy. White Plains, NY: March of Dimes Foundation.

WORTHINGTON-ROBERTS, B. 1987. Nutritional support of successful reproduction: An update. J. Nutrition Ed. 19, Feb., 1.

WORTHINGTON-ROBERTS, B., VERMEERSCH, J., and WILLIAMS, S. 1985. Nutrition in Pregnancy and Lactation, 2nd Edition. St. Louis: C. V. Mosby Co.

For patient handouts:

Allegheny County Health Department, Nutrition Services, 3441 Forbes Avenue, Pittsburgh, PA 15213.

Health Sciences Consortium, 200 Eastown Drive, Suite 213, Chapel Hill, NC 27514.

March of Dimes Foundation, 1275 Mamoroneck Avenue, White Plains, NY 10605.

Ministry of Health, Nutrition Division, Province of British Columbia, Victoria, British Columbia, Canada.

For audiovisuals:

Great Expectations. Society for Nutrition Education, 1700 Broadway, Suite 300, Oakland, CA 94612.

Healthy Mother, Healthy Baby. Alfred Higgins Productions, 9100 Sunset Boulevard, Los Angeles, CA 90069.

Nutritional Management of High-Risk Pregnancy. Society for Nutrition Education, 1700 Broadway, Suite 300, Oakland, CA 94612.

Nutrition and Fitness in Pregnancy. Milner-Fenwick, Inc., 2125 Greenspring Drive, Timonium, MD 21093.

For further information:

American College of Obstetricians and Gynecologists, Resource Center, 600 Maryland Avenue SW, Suite 300E, Washington, DC 20024.

Family Service Association of America, 44 East 23rd Street, New York, NY 10010.

La Leche League International, PO Box 1209, Franklin Park, IL 60131.

Maternity Center Association, 48 East 92nd Street, New York, NY 10028.

National Maternal and Child Health Clearinghouse, 3520 Prospect Street NW, Washington, DC 20057.

Counseling Guidelines—Pregnancy

Table 7.6 outlines the steps for diet counseling during pregnancy. The following material gives the details of each step.

I.   Initial Session

I.   A.   General Guidelines

1.   Use Medical History Form to assess patient's nutritional status.

2.   Weigh patient and record on Weight Record. The graph is a helpful tool for visualization of weight status. Note: Consider as high risk the underweight woman who has not gained 10 lb by the fifth month of pregnancy.

3.   Instruct patient to maintain own Weight Record for visualization of weight gain pattern. Note: Weight gain of more than 6 lb/month is considered excessive.

4.   Assist patient in recording 24-hour recall of food intake using 24-Hour Recall Form. This will aid patient in keeping an accurate Food Intake Record.

5.   Instruct patient to keep daily Food Intake Record so that typical food intake patterns can be evaluated. Advise patient not to deviate from normal eating pattern. Stress the importance of recording food intake immediately after eating.

6.   Instruct patient to complete Diet History. This provides for a basic evaluation of food intake patterns. (Use Pre-test on Your Eating Habits from Chapter 2.)

7.   Record assessment and recommendation(s) using the SOAP method (See Chapter 1, Step 6) in Technician's Notes. This form can be kept in your files with a copy in the patient's medical records.

I.   B.   Patient Records

1. Medical History Form

Date _____ Referred by _____
Name _____ Date of birth _____
Address _____ Phone no. _____
Occupation _____ Hours per work week _____ Work phone no. _____
Educational background _____ Religious/ethnic background _____
Sex ____ Marital status _____
Household composition: Live alone _____ Spouse _____ Children/No. _____ Other: _____

General health status:

Physician _____ Address _____
Phone no. _____ Date of last visit _____
Expected delivery date: _____
Ambulatory care required? _____ If so, describe: _____
Neuromuscular problems? _____ If so, how is eating affected? _____
Visual/auditory problems? _____ If so, describe: _____
Chewing difficulties? _____ If so, describe: _____
Appetite typically good? _____ Fair? _____ Poor? _____
Digestion/elimination difficulties? _____ If so, describe: _____
Food intolerances? _____ If so, describe: _____
Other: _____

Diabetes? _____ If so, describe: _____
Hyperlipidemia? _____ If so, describe: _____
Hypertension? _____ If so, describe: _____
Anemia? _____ If so, describe: _____

History of smoking? _____
History of alcohol intake? _____
Other: _____

Height: ____ Weight ____ Frame ____
Triceps skinfold thickness _____ Mid-arm circumference _____
Mid-arm muscle circumference _____
Desired nonpregnant weight _____ Pre-gravid weight _____
Weight changes/problems? _____ If so describe: _____

Clinical signs of nutritional status:

Skin _____ Mouth _____
Hair _____ Eyes _____
Teeth _____ Other: _____

Lab data:

Blood pressure _____
CBC _____ Urine glucose _____ Urine acetone _____
Serum albumin _____
Other: _____

Pregnancy-related health problems:
Morning sickness? _____
Heartburn? _____
Edema? _____
Constipation? _____
Cravings? _____
Other: _____

Medications taken regularly: _____
Prescribed by: _____ Date(s) prescribed: _____
Nutrition supplements taken regularly: _____
Prescribed by: _____ Date(s) prescribed: _____
Special diet prescription: _____
Prescribed by: _____ Date(s) prescribed: _____
How closely is diet followed? Always adhered to ___ Sometimes ___ Rarely ___ Never ___

Type of housing: Room ___ Apartment ___ Home ___ Institution ___
Prepare own meals? ___ Dine out? Often (more than once a day) ___ Rarely ___
Food shopping done independently? ___ If not, describe required assistance: ___
_____
Eligible for food stamps? _____ If so, are they currently being used? ___
Cigarette smoker during pregnancy? ___ If so, how much: _____
Exercise regularly? _____ If so, describe: _____
    No. times per week _____ No. minutes per session _____

Comments: _____

2. Weight Record

Instruction: Slow steady weight gain is important during pregnancy. After initial weigh-in, continue to record weight on a weekly basis by drawing a line from the last weight to the new weight. Using this chart, visualization of weight gain pattern is facilitated. A regular time should be established for all weigh-ins.

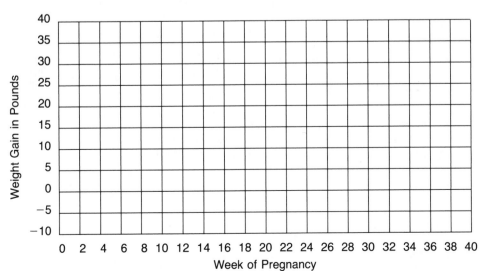

3. 24-Hour Recall Form

Date and time (over 24-hr period)	Food and amount	Where eaten[a]	Eaten with whom[b]	Associated activity[c]

[a]For example, at the kitchen table, at home—sitting at a desk, in a car, or at a restaurant.
[b]For example, with parents, friend(s), or spouse.
[c]For example, while studying, driving, talking, or watching TV.

I.   C.   Assignments

1. Food Intake Record

Date and time	Duration of meal (min)	Food and amount	Where eaten[a]	With whom	Associated activity[b]	Associated emotions[c]

[a]Such as work, restaurant, kitchen, living room.
[b]For example, watching television, reading, socializing, driving, talking on the phone, cooking.
[c]Attitude: bored, anxious, frustrated, depressed, happy, angry, tense, etc.

2. Diet History

Use the Pre-test from Chapter 2 (p. 30) to provide a record of typical foods eaten.

I.   D.   Technician's Notes

Patient: _____   Date: _____

S   (Subjective data—how patient feels):
O   (Objective data—physical measurements including diet/nutritional status):
A   (Assessment—acceptability of dietary progress/nutritional status):
P   (Plan—diet prescription and instruction):
Comments:

II.   Follow-up Session(s)

II.   A.   General Guidelines

1. Weigh patient and record on Weight Record.
2. Review assignments and discuss.
3. Individualize Personal Diet Plan and instruct patient in its use.
4. Assign Learning Assessment Quiz to evaluate the counseling process and to determine if additional counseling is needed.
5. Record assessment and recommendation(s) using the SOAP method in Technician's Notes. This form can be kept in your files with a copy in the patient's medical records.

II.   B.   Handouts

1. Personal Diet Plan

Name: _____

How to use diet plan:

1. Select a variety of foods from each of the Basic Food Groups.
2. Include the recommended number of servings from each Food Group. (See Table 7.3.)
3. Drink eight or more cups of fluid daily.
4. For aid in prevention of constipation, eat foods high in fiber (see list a) and drink plenty of liquids.
5. Choose foods high in folic acid and iron (see lists b and c).
6. Use calcium-dense foods (see list d) if unable to include the recommended number of servings from the Milk and Cheeses Group.
7. If morning sickness or heartburn occurs, modify food intake appropriately (see list e).

a. Foods high in fiber:

Whole grain breads and cereals
Bran products
Raw fruits, including skins and seeds
Dried fruits (Prunes and prune juice may act as laxatives.)
Vegetables, including skins and seeds (especially raw/lightly cooked)

b. Foods high in folic acid:

Organ meats
Legumes
Dark green leafy vegetables
Wheat germ, bran, brewer's yeast

c. Foods high in iron:

Meat, especially organ meats
Oysters, clams
Legumes
Whole grain and enriched breads and cereals
Dried fruits and their juices
Dark green leafy vegetables
Potato, sweet potato
Foods cooked in iron cookware

d. Calcium-dense foods:

Milk, cheese, and yogurt
Sardines, salmon (with bones)
Dark green leafy vegetables
Almonds
Soybeans, fortified soybean milk products
Milk-based foods, such as puddings, creamed soups, chowders, milkshakes, and creamed dishes
Dry powdered milk or cheese added to foods, such as milk (1 cup milk plus 2 Tbsp dried milk = 2 cups milk), sauces, mashed potatoes, extended meat dishes, and casseroles

e. Tips on relieving morning sickness and heartburn:

Divide food intake into five or six small meals.
Avoid fried and fatty foods.
Avoid spicy foods.
Sip fluids in between rather than during meals.
Eat crackers before arising.

2. Learning Assessment Quiz

Answer true (T) or false (F) to the following statements:

____ 1. Nutritional status prior to pregnancy has little effect on subsequent total growth.
____ 2. Weight gain during pregnancy should not exceed 15 lb.
____ 3. If overweight, it is a good idea to reduce or to minimize weight gain during pregnancy.
____ 4. Regular physical exercise is usually contraindicated during pregnancy.
____ 5. The use of drugs, alcohol, and nicotine during pregnancy should be discussed with the attending physician.
____ 6. Foods high in fiber should be avoided during pregnancy.
____ 7. Morning sickness may be alleviated by dividing daily food intake into two large meals.
____ 8. Salt must be restricted during pregnancy.
____ 9. Snacking should be avoided during pregnancy.
____ 10. Soups and juices contribute to fluid intake.

II. C. Technician's Notes

Patient: _____   Date: _____

S (Subjective data—how patient feels):
O (Objective data—physical measurements including diet/nutritional status):
A (Assessment—acceptability of dietary progress/nutritional status):
P (Plan—diet prescription and instruction):
Comments:

Pregnancy Counseling Role Playing

Keeping in mind the preceding Suggested Readings and Counseling Guidelines, participate in one or more of the following role play situations; elaborate on each situation to develop a patient/audience profile. Select different partners, either classmates or co-workers, for each situation. You may want to utilize your handout from Step 2 and your chart from Step 4 (Table 7.5). As a dietetic technician in nutrition care, do you consider yourself capable of conducting effective counseling sessions with pregnant women, including teenagers? Do you feel confident in your ability to assist in the choice of bottle or breastfeeding? Would you or your family be able to adhere to your nutrition guidelines during and after pregnancy?

Role Play Situation 1. A pregnant teenager in her second trimester is referred to you, a dietetic technician in an out-patient clinic, for diet counseling. Follow the guidelines to complete the charts and provide her with an individualized diet plan. Prepare a SOAP note for your department files with a copy to be sent to the referring physician.

Role Play Situation 2. A pregnant mother of two is referred to your community health clinic for diet counseling. She is in her third trimester and complains of bloatedness; she wants to halt her weight gain due to a strong fear of postpartum obesity. Follow the guidelines to complete the charts and provide her with an individualized diet plan. Prepare a SOAP note for your department files with a copy to be sent to the referring physician.

Role Play Situation 3. As a dietetic technician assigned to the maternity/pediatrics ward of a community hospital, you are responsible for conducting a weekly class on infant feeding. Prepare a class outline and present to the new mother(s). Prepare a SOAP note which could be recorded in the medical chart of each class attendant.

STEP 6: POST-TEST ON PREGNANCY AND LACTATION NUTRITION

In order to evaluate your understanding of diet in pregnancy, complete the Post-test below: Section I is the Learning Assessment Quiz for pregnant patients. (If the diet counselor is unable to complete this test successfully, how can the patient be expected to?) Section II incorporates much of the material from this chapter. Answers are given in the Answer Key. Will your pregnant patients succeed in "eating for two" in order to help support the development of a healthy fetus? Will they opt for the most desirable feeding practices to help ensure proper infant growth and health?

Section I: Complete the quiz from Pregnancy Guidelines given on p. 152. Check your answers with the Answer Key.

Section II: Indicate whether you think the following statements are true (T) or false (F). Check your answers with the Answer Key.

_____ 1. The fetus typically accounts for $7\frac{1}{2}$–8 lb of the weight gained during pregnancy.

_____ 2. Weight loss during pregnancy can cause fetal brain damage.

_____ 3. Excessive weight gain during pregnancy is currently believed to be the cause of toxemia.

_____ 4. Teenage females tend to deliver low-birth-weight infants.

_____ 5. There is no documented need for an increased fluid intake during pregnancy.

_____ 6. Nutrients tend to be absorbed more efficiently during pregnancy.

_____ 7. Dietary cholesterol should be restricted by pregnant women.

_____ 8. Mild nausea is common and temporary in the early stages of pregnancy.

_____ 9. Eclampsia can be treated at home by salt restriction.

_____ 10. Excessive intra-uterine activity can be safely and effectively treated by substituting dolomite or bone meal for milk and milk products.

_____ 11. Nutrients can be absorbed most efficiently from breast milk (vs. cow's milk and formulas).

_____ 12. All women should breastfeed or the psychological bonding between mother and child is impossible to create.

Select the answer which best completes the following statements and check your answers with the Answer Key.

_____ 13. The diet of the female in her third trimester of pregnancy should include
(a) 300 additional calories (above normal requirements). (b) a quart of milk (or an equivalent number of milk products such as yogurt and cheese). (c) extra servings of fruits and/or vegetables. (d) at least 8 cups of liquids. (e) all of these.

_____ 14. Nutritionally acceptable substitutes for breast milk include
(a) evaporated milk. (b) cow's milk. (c) infant formula. (d) goat's milk. (e) all of these.

_____ 15. An effective diet counseling session with a pregnant woman should include
(a) a medical history with evaluation of pre-pregnancy and current medical problems. (b) the establishment of present weight and desirable weight gain patterns. (c) an individualized diet plan. (d) tips on obtaining the best food sources of fiber, iron, and certain other nutrients. (e) all of these.

STEP 7: PRE-TEST (A RETAKE) ON PREGNANCY AND LACTATION NUTRITION

After reading this chapter and participating in the assigned activities, you may have acquired a significant amount of new information regarding diet in pregnancy and lactation. You should have profited also from the guidelines given on diet counseling for pregnant and lactating individuals. Therefore, you might want to reevaluate the responses you gave to the various sample situations depicted in Step 1. In light of the facts you have gathered throughout Chapter 7, make any revisions you deem necessary in your files. Explain each modification briefly below. Discuss your changes with classmates or co-workers. Do you think more revisions will become necessary as your experience as a practicing dietetic technician continues to expand?

Situation 1:

Situation 2:

Situation 3:

Situation 4:

Situation 5:

REFERENCE

HESS, M., and HUNT, A. 1987. Pickles and Ice Cream: A Complete Guide to Nutrition during Pregnancy. Winnetka, IL: Hess and Hunt, Inc.

Chapter Eight

The Growing Years—
Infancy through Teens

CHAPTER BLUEPRINT

Step 1: Take the Pre-test on the Growing Years to begin reflecting on your own understanding of the role of nutrition during the growing years.

Step 2: Examine the Nutrition Facts List on optimal diets for the growing years and prepare the assigned handout.

Step 3: Read the Healthy? materials and participate in the group discussion.

Step 4: Examine the Infancy Guidelines and complete the role play assignment.

Step 5: Examine the Childhood Guidelines and complete the role play assignment.

Step 6: Examine the Teen Guidelines and complete the role play assignment.

Step 7: Take the Post-test to evaluate what you have learned from the information and activities provided in this chapter.

Step 8: Reexamine the Pre-test (a Retake) and make those alterations which you deem appropriate in consideration of the information you acquired from this chapter.

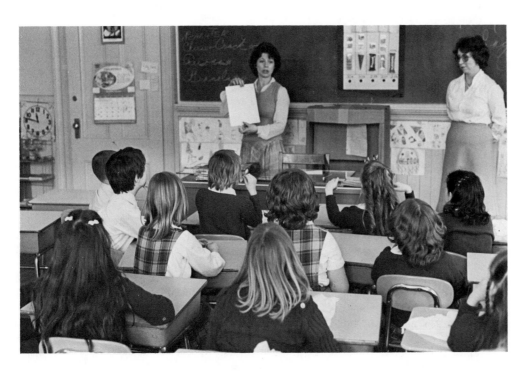

STEP 1: PRE-TEST ON THE GROWING YEARS

Adequate nutrition during the growing years, from birth to adulthood, is essential in facilitating proper growth and optimizing overall health. Inadequate nutritional intake, including calories and specific nutrients, may result in retarded physical and mental development, delayed sexual maturity, and increased susceptibility to ill health. Thus, parents should become well versed in the dietary basics, and nutrition education is best begun as early as possible.

As a practicing dietetic technician, it is important for you to have a clear understanding of your own philosophies as they relate to patient care. For each of the following sample situations, indicate your own best response as the assigned dietetic technician. Elaborate on each situation to develop a patient profile. Record your answer using the SOAP format (Chapter 1, Step 6) and indicate whether you would employ the assistance of other health professionals. Discuss your answers with classmates or co-workers. Do you think that future training and experience will alter your responses? You may want to reexamine your answers after you have completed this chapter (see Step 8), and again once you have dealt with a number of real-life situations similar to the samples depicted below.

Situation 1: A bottle-fed infant is brought into the out-patient nutrition clinic due to a diagnosis of iron-deficiency anemia. As the assigned technician, I would

Situation 2: A first grader who lives in your neighborhood is put on the Feingold Diet, a controversial additive-free regime, by his concerned mother. As a friend of the family and a knowledgeable dietetic technician, I would

Situation 3: A fourth-grade girl is hospitalized for a week with a fractured fibula. She refuses to eat anything green—except for green jelly beans. As the dietetic technician assigned to pediatrics, I would

Situation 4: A 16-year-old female is admitted with minor contusions and a concussion suffered during a fainting spell, the cause as yet undiagnosed. Her height is 5 ft 6 in. and her weight is 88 lb; she refuses both the meal trays and the required bed rest. As the assigned dietetic technician, I would

Situation 5: A 17-year-old boy is brought to the out-patient nutrition department because his parents are concerned about dramatic weight loss. A brief discussion with the boy reveals that he has been fasting to "make weight" for the upcoming wrestling season. As the assigned dietetic technician, I would

STEP 2: NUTRITION FACTS

Mothers are usually quite eager to provide their offspring with a total environment that is supportive of optimal health and growth. Oftentimes, a mother will put her child's needs before her own and make a sincere effort to acquire nutrition knowledge for the sake of the young one, despite a previous history of dietary indifference. Pre-schoolers, primary school children, and pre-adolescents can be taught how to balance their diets, either through direct nutrition education efforts or via their parents; setting a good example, nutritionally speaking—for teachers, parents, nutrition educators, and/or dietetics personnel—is one of the major factors in obtaining compliance from youngsters. Teenagers, too, can be a receptive audience for nutrition education, especially if their strong interest in good looks and physical prowess is capitalized on. The impact of peers—important from childhood on, usually peaking during the teen years—must also be considered in the evaluation of dietary intake, and can be used advantageously in the impartation of nutrition guidance.

Examine the following Nutrition Facts List, which provides some of the most current diet-related information to include in counseling youngsters (from infancy through the teens) and/or their parents, and complete the exercise that follows.

Nutrition Facts List

Infancy

1. Each infant or child is an individual, so flexibility in feeding schedules is important; feedings should be planned in accordance with individual growth and physical maturity, with gradual progression to self-feeding when the infant is ready.

2. At birth the stomach holds 1 Tbsp, at age one it holds around 1 cup, and the average adult can hold 2 qt.

3. Only in special circumstances (e.g., food allergy or metabolic disorder) is there a need for an infant to take nutrition supplements, and any such product should be prescribed by the pediatrician for treatment of a diagnosed deficiency.

4. Solids should not be introduced to the young infant because the immature digestive system is usually unable to handle foodstuffs until 6 months of age; protein and lactose can be digested properly, but starch cannot until—with age—enough **amylase** can be produced.

5. Until infants can open the mouth and lean forward to indicate desire, turn away their own heads to indicate "fullness," and are able to roll/push food to the back of the oral cavity and swallow, they are not physically ready for solid foods; by 6 months of age, most infants are physiologically capable of the proper handling of solid foods, and larger infants may be ready as early as 4 months of age.

6. Solid foods should not be introduced before 4–6 months of age as this can lead to overfeeding: cereals, fruits, and other solid foods provide more calories than an equivalent amount of milk, causing the infant to consume more calories in order to feel full. The extra calories are converted to fat at a time when fat-storage cells are multiplying and are susceptible to undesirable expansion in both number and size; this can mean more fat storage capacity throughout life.

7. Overfeeding in infancy can lead to overweight in later life.

8. Since obesity is far easier to prevent than it is to treat, the practice of overfeeding during infancy is best avoided.

9. Skim milk has significantly greater quantities of protein and sodium than does whole milk, but it lacks the essential fatty acid required for growth. Since it is less dense calorically, more must be consumed to satisfy needs, which can lead to an early overeating habit. Thus, most nutritionists warn against using the skimmed form until age five or so.

10. Feeding cow's milk to an infant prior to the first birthday is undesirable because (a) the protein content is significantly higher than in breast milk; (b) it is difficult to digest; (c) the curd results in heavy demands on the kidneys; (d) gastrointestinal bleeding can occur, resulting in anemia; and (e) there are definite nutritional drawbacks, including low iron and low vitamin C content (both of which are not readily absorbed), and fat which is saturated.

11. The infant's gastrointestinal tract is immature and highly sensitive to foreign proteins and textures, causing an increased likelihood for the development of food allergies upon early introduction of solids; oftentimes, reintroduction with advanced physical development will result in tolerance.

12. Egg whites are usually avoided until later in development since they commonly cause allergic response in a significant number of infants.

13. Those parents who believe that the feeding of solids to the 1-to-4-month-old infant will encourage a complete night's sleep (for everyone) should be informed that the excessive caloric intake may lead to digestive disturbances (with interrupted sleep).

14. Solid foods should be introduced gradually as the child gets older (Table 8.1), one new item per week, so that individual adverse reactions (vomiting, diarrhea, respiratory distress, or skin eruptions) can be identified. Iron-fortified, high-protein rice cereal is the best food to introduce first; after a month, strained fruits can be added one at a time, followed by strained vegetables, strained meats at 9 months of age, then on to junior foods, with table scraps after the first birthday.

amylase: Enzyme which breaks down starch, found in salivary and pancreatic secretions.

Table 8.1   Introduction of Solid Foods

Age (months)	Foods to add
0–1	Supplement(s) if formula is inadequate
1–2	Diluted orange juice if formula is inadequate
4–6	Iron-fortified rice cereal
6–7	Other high-protein iron-fortified cereals, strained vegetables, strained fruits, juices— one item introduced at a time
6–8	Protein foods (cheese, yogurt, fish, chicken, egg yolk, beans) in mashed form—one item introduced at a time
9	Meat, finely chopped or strained
More than 9	Cottage cheese, toast/zwieback, egg white

15.   Iron-fortified rice cereal is recommended as the first choice for cereal when adding solid foods to the diet, due to a greater probability for initial allergic-type reactions to wheat and corn products.

16.   It has been estimated that nearly one-third of infants under 1 year of age are iron deficient; breastfed infants may require iron supplementation once birth weight is doubled, whereas formulas should always be iron fortified and an iron-fortified cereal should be the first solid food used.

17.   Infants *not* fed solids after 6 months of age may suffer delay in growth; food given at this time and the associated eating experiences can have great impact on physical and emotional status at later stages of life. By 4–5 months of age, some infants are consuming caloric needs in three feedings, but many nutritionists encourage more frequent, smaller feedings; again, individuality demands flexibility in feeding patterns.

18.   Fluid intake is especially important during infancy, as the immature kidney must excrete larger amounts of water to properly eliminate wastes, while the rapid metabolism can cause dehydration; the infant must replace 10–15% of body weight as water every day (compared to 2–4% by the adult), so as the use of solid foods increases, water/fluids should be added to the diet.

19.   If the local water supply is not fluoridated, the pediatrician may prescribe a fluoride supplement.

20.   Well water can contain an excessively high concentration of nitrate, which can cause **methemoglobinemia** in infants under 6 months of age; county health departments may assist in well water analysis for prevention of this often fatal disease.

21.   Honey should be avoided during infancy because the **botulism** spores which may be present can germinate rapidly in the immature intestinal tract to form a poisonous toxin.

22.   Infant cult diets can result in serious health detriments, and patients should be so warned. (A recent example was a group in California who fed their infants a self-concocted composition of barley water, whole milk, and corn syrup or honey. The infants developed recurring infections, diarrhea, and vomiting. Fortunately, all symptoms were alleviated with the substitution of standardized formula.) Restrictive diets (e.g., low fat/low cholesterol regimes) can cause failure to thrive in infants.

23.   If evidence indicates that infants are not being fed either breast milk or commercial formula, it is essential that the diet be carefully analyzed.

24.   Comprehensive nutritional analysis of baby food can be obtained by using the figures given in the "Composition of Foods: Baby Foods—Raw, Processed, Prepared" (USDA 1978).

25.   The RDAs for infants (Table 8.2) merely serve as broad guidelines, whereas a better method for nutritional assessment is the use of height and weight charts; serious deviations from the norm may require interpretation by the pediatrician, but can be discovered by attentive parents.

26.   Food cannot and should not replace maternal attention; every whimper and cry is not a signal that the infant is hungry.

27.   When infants indicate that they have had enough, feeding should be halted immediately.

28.   An overdependence on milk and constant bottle sucking are undesirable and can lead to "milk anemia" (when milk replaces iron-rich foods with an intake exceeding 2½–3

methemoglobinemia: Blood disorder in which an altered form of hemoglobin is present due to toxic substances such as nitrate-contaminated water; may be an inherited condition.

botulism: Severe poisoning from food contaminated with the botulinus toxin produced by *Clostridium botulinum;* can result in paralysis and death.

Table 8.2   RDAs for Infants[a]

Nutrient	Age, 0–6 months	Age, 6–12 months
Calories	Weight (kg) × 115	Weight (kg) × 105
Protein (grams)	Weight (kg) × 2.2	Weight (kg) × 2
Vitamin C	35 mg	35 mg
Thiamin	0.3 mg	0.5 mg
Riboflavin	0.4 mg	0.6 mg
Niacin	6 mg	8 mg
Folacin	30 µg	45 µg
Vitamin B_6	0.3 mg	0.6 mg
Vitamin B_{12}	0.5 µg	1.5 µg
Vitamin A	420 µg (retinol equivalent)	400 µg (retinol equivalent)
Vitamin D	400 I.U.	400 I.U.
Vitamin E	3 mg (alpha tocopherol equivalent)	4 mg (alpha tocopherol equivalent)
Calcium	360 mg	540 mg
Phosphorus	240 mg	360 mg
Iron	10 mg	15 mg
Zinc	3 mg	5 mg
Magnesium	50 mg	70 mg
Iodine	40 µg	50 µg

[a] Adapted from Natl. Res. Council/Food and Nutr. Board (1980).

cups per day after the age of one), overweight (due to use of milk to reward, to halt crying, etc.) and a distorted jaw line.

29. Iron-deficiency anemia is the most common nutritional deficiency. It is widespread in poor countries due to the low intake of animal foods combined with a high intake of fiber—**phytic/oxalic acids** bind iron. In the industrialized countries, infants or youngsters often develop iron-deficiency anemia because of (a) prolongation of the milk-based diet; (b) dependence on nonnutritious foods after weaning; and (c) diminished appetite after age one with dependence on beverages and sweets.

30. It is important to ensure that the infant cereal used through the age of 18 months is iron fortified; after this, the diet should be varied, well balanced, and iron rich.

31. Commercial baby foods are convenient and nutritious, plus they are safe and sanitary if refrigerated immediately after opening; infants should not be fed out of jars unless leftovers are to be discarded since salivary enzymes cause product breakdown. Most products do not contain added salt and sugar, but all labels should be examined carefully.

32. Homemade infant food should be produced in small quantities under strict sanitary conditions and properly stored; there is no need for parents to add salt and sugar to appease their own palates. Infant use of canned products should be avoided, as some contain undesirably high contents of lead.

33. Infants have a keen sense of taste since they have taste buds on the insides of their cheeks and in their throats, as well as on their tongues (only those found on the tongue remain when older), so they tend to dislike strongly flavored and spicy foods.

34. Nonnutritive stimulation (visual, vocal, and physical) and avoidance of a negative attitude toward the overweight infant are essential for healthy emotional development; and parental example-setting is important.

35. Overweight infants tend to suffer from more illnesses, especially of the respiratory tract; fatter babies tend to be less active physically and sometimes eat less, while thinner infants exercise and eat more.

36. Overeaters should not face dietary restrictions, but slow down weight gain until growth catches up by using careful portion control and increasing exercise; between-meal snacks can consist of fruit and vegetable pieces with water substituted for milk and juice, and daily intake of concentrated fats and sweets can be controlled.

37. Severe dietary restriction during infancy may cause undesirable side effects, such as a reduction in the fat-free body tissues as well as body fat, growth inhibition, and the depletion of those energy reserves required for handling stress.

phytic acid: Chemical found in high-fiber foods which binds minerals (such as zinc), making them unavailable for absorption.

oxalic acid: Chemical found in certain foods (e.g., chard, rhubarb, spinach) which binds minerals (such as calcium), making them unavailable for absorption.

38.   Very little is known regarding the subtle long-term consequences of improper infant feeding practices, especially during the first 3 months of life, when the rates of physical growth and brain development are the most rapid of any time during the lifespan.

39.   Food is not just important for the nutrients provided, but for aid in proper emotional and physical development; suggested food-related behavior guidelines for parents of young children include the following: (a) food can be used as a learning tool, and eating times can contribute to proper development and behavior; (b) food textures can provide stimulation and information until eating utensils can be managed; (c) weaning from bottle to cup should be accomplished around the first birthday; (d) use of food as reward and denial of food as punishment is undesirable at all ages; (e) food refusal can be a demonstration of independence, and force-feeding is unwise; and (f) infants are born with an affinity for sweet-tasting foodstuffs.

40.   Parents should understand the importance of relaxation during an infant's feeding periods, as well as the desirable influence of maintaining a positive attitude during mealtimes.

41.   Bottle propping can cause *nursing bottle syndrome* in which milk or juice pools in the sleeping infant's mouth, causing rampant dental decay.

42.   Milk at mealtimes does not contribute significantly to dental decay; however milk at naptime or nighttime does contribute to decay because of diminished sucking and swallowing, minimal salivary flow, and the fact that teeth are in constant contact with stagnant milk. Prolonged sleep-sucking can cause decay to occur in breastfed infants as well.

43.   Studies indicate that breastfeeding may help to protect against dental decay due to the presence of **monolaurin,** but immunity from caries is not guaranteed.

44.   **Pedodontist** visits on a regular basis beginning at age three (or earlier)—in addition to use of fluoridated water or supplements, proper tooth brushing technique, avoidance of nursing bottle syndrome, and desirable dietary intake—can help to promote oral health.

45.   Although most inborn errors of metabolism are rare, **PKU** is relatively common and is detected at birth via regular hospital screening procedures; treatment begins immediately.

46.   Inborn errors of carbohydrate metabolism require dietary restriction of the offending sugar (e.g., fructose or lactose); although milk allergies do occur with some frequency, most are only temporary and disappear after several days. Soy-based formulas are used to replace milk for intolerant infants.

47.   Colic is believed to be caused by gas trapped by the infant's immature digestive system; specific foods consumed by lactating mothers have never been proved as contributory factors.

48.   Studies indicate that a relatively high cholesterol intake during infancy may assist the body to regulate cholesterol synthesis later in life. Since cholesterol is essential in the synthesis of bile acids and hormones, a low-cholesterol diet should not be followed by infants unless prescribed by the pediatrician to help treat a diagnosed disorder.

49.   Teething infants enjoy chewing on zwieback and dried toast, but care should be taken not to let these foods offset total dietary intake.

50.   After the first year of life, growth slows and appetite diminishes, so it is important for parents to avoid the urge to force-feed their finicky children. Food jags are normal and, unless the fixations continue for weeks, are best ignored. Refused vegetables can be incorporated into favored foods (e.g., carrot cake, zucchini bread, and spaghetti sauce with pureed vegetables).

Childhood

1.   Preschoolers are impressionable so are influenced by parental food likes and dislikes, as well as by the food habits of siblings.

2.   Parents should use growth charts to watch over the child's growth rate, and report any deviations from the norm to the pediatrician; although both growth rate and appetite diminish after the first birthday, total caloric requirements and nutrient needs continue to increase.

3.   The RDAs for growing children can be met with gradually increased portions of the recommended servings from the Basic Food Groups, divided into several daily meals and snacks.

monolaurin: Chemical derivative of lauric acid found in milk and in coconut and palm oils.

pedodontist: Dentist specializing in the treatment of children and teenagers.

PKU: Phenylketonuria, an inborn error of metabolism.

4. Children require the following: four servings from the Fruits and Vegetables Group; four servings from the Breads and Cereals Group; three servings from the Milk and Cheeses Group; and two servings from the Meats and Alternates Group. Yet, a *serving* is not equivalent to an adult serving, but should approximate 1 Tbsp per year of age (except milk, which should be consumed in cupfuls).

5. Until the third birthday, brain cell development continues to be intense, which makes adequate protein intake critical; muscular development, as the toddler begins to stand or walk and to participate in sports or games, adds to the importance of protein intake. Most children in our society are able to obtain an adequate amount of high-quality protein.

6. A deficiency of vitamins A and C in the toddler diet is readily corrected with the addition of fruits and vegetables, while a marginal intake of calcium is easily improved with adequate milk consumption. Adding pureed fruits or vegetables and dried skim milk powder to favorite foods (oatmeal–raisin cookies, vegetable–meat loaf, etc.) can help to improve the diets of finicky eaters.

7. Iron-fortified cereals can be used with "adult" hot cereals and baked goods to help prevent iron-deficiency anemia, which is especially common when routine screenings halt at age one.

8. Poor eating habits cannot be remedied by giving children nutrition supplements; vitamin/mineral preparations are drugs and require prescription by a physician.

9. Up until the age of two, babies are usually quite willing to try new foods, but this interest gradually decreases with age until the fourth birthday, then increases again until the sixth year; wasted food is usually inevitable and preferable to force-feeding.

10. Food jags are expected and, if treated calmly, usually run their own course. Table 8.3 lists some foods generally favored by children, but childhood dietary preferences are highly individualistic.

11. Growth spurts can cause simultaneous spurts in appetite as well as increased physical activity.

12. Dietary deficiencies—especially at 10 months, $2\frac{1}{2}$ years, and 5 years of age—can be detrimental to proper tooth enamel development; a well-balanced diet and adequate dental care should begin in early childhood.

13. Dental caries is the most prevalent disease for all age groups beyond infancy, afflicting over 95% of all pre-adult Americans; the average American has 8 or 9 decayed or filled teeth by 17 years of age.

14. Despite claims to the contrary, there is no need for total elimination of sugar from the diets of children; sound meals with occasional sweets for dessert—immediately followed by proper tooth brushing—are not apt to damage oral health, whereas frequent snacking on sticky sweets may contribute to dental decay. Note that dried fruits (such as raisins, dates, prunes, and figs) are high in sugar and have retention qualities so are not good snack choices. Note: Recent research indicates that unsweetened carbohydrate foodstuffs may also be cariogenic (Schachtele 1982).

15. Ingestion of fluoridated water (or a prescribed supplement in areas without an

Table 8.3 Children's Dietary Preferences by Categories[a]

Favorite foods	Preschool (%)	Elementary (%)	Disliked foods	Preschool (%)	Elementary (%)
Meats	39	52	Cooked vegetables	50	48
Snack items	17	4½	Mixed dishes, casseroles	14	11
Dairy foods	11	4½	Meat	9	8
Mixed dishes	11	20	Liver	7	12
Breads, cereals	5½	4½	Raw vegetables	5	6
Desserts	5½	9	Cottage cheese	3½	1½
Fruits	5½	—	Fish	3½	6
Vegetables	5½	4½	Fruit	3½	1½
			Eggs	2	5
			Milk	2	1½

[a] Adapted from Beyer and Morris (1974).

adequate supply) may reduce the incidence of dental caries up to 60% and decrease premature tooth loss up to 75%. The extent of dental caries is declining in this country, primarily due to the increased use of fluoridated water and toothpastes.

16.   The same suggestions for prevention or treatment of overweight infants are applicable to the pre-school years, with the emphasis on slowed weight gain rather than weight loss; it is important to obtain the advice of a physician prior to undertaking any weight control program during the growing years.

17.   The offspring of obese parent(s) are more likely to become overweight as well, again illustrating the importance of the parental example.

18.   Obesity can begin to develop during childhood after a traumatic event such as moving, hospitalization, or parental death or separation. Thus, it is essential for parents to monitor the eating and exercise patterns of their children.

19.   The main cause of obesity in children is not overeating but underactivity; acceptable dietary alterations during childhood include use of skim or low-fat milk, moderation in fatty meats and sweets, and limited snacks of the low-calorie variety.

20.   A family history of hypercholesterolemia may warrant the monitoring of cholesterol levels in both blood and diet during childhood; it is important to avoid severe fat restriction, but the amount and type of fats in the diet can be regulated at this time.

21.   School athletics sometimes lead to bizarre diets, and it is essential for proper growth and development to ensure the schoolchild avoids crash weight loss programs and other diet fads.

22.   Heat stroke can be fatal, and is a serious threat to school-age athletes who fail to replenish lost fluids; it is important for sports-minded children to understand that thirst is *not* the best indicator of the need for water, and that it is essential to consume plenty of fluids with exercise.

23.   The National School Lunch Act stipulates that every public school must make nutritionally adequate lunches available to children. School lunches are required to supply one-third of the RDAs for calories and certain nutrients, with recent changes in the regulations designed to reduce wastage. School lunches are required to include milk (skim or low-fat), a protein-rich food, vegetables, fruits, and grains.

24.   Parents of schoolchildren who repeatedly fail to consume breakfast may check to see if the school provides an acceptable breakfast program, or prepare appealing home-made morning meals in advance (such as easy-to-heat mini-pizzas, peanut butter and banana sandwiches, and other nontraditional breakfast foods).

25.   Breakfast is an important component of the day for everyone, especially school-children; studies have demonstrated that breakfast skippers are more careless and inattentive in the late morning than are their nutritionally satisfied peers, and that schoolwork can be improved significantly with the inclusion of breakfast every day. Unfortunately, children omit breakfast more often than any other meal.

26.   Since the average American child spends more time in front of the television set than in school, it is important for parents and nutrition educators to recognize the significant impact of viewing habits on between-meal snacking and obesity. Concerned adults can minimize children's TV viewing hours, combat food advertising propaganda with fact, and expose hidden messages.

27.   Pre-schoolers are usually open to nutrition education endeavors, and this can be a good time to encourage the development of positive attitudes regarding food and health.

28.   Teachers actually have "prime time" that can be used for the purpose of providing nutrition education. Nutrition education programs can be increased in effectiveness if parents are involved. It is also important for school foodservice personnel to impart a positive attitude regarding meals.

29.   By the time a child enters elementary school, a firm foundation for lifelong eating habits has usually been established. However, school opens the doors to independent thinking, rebellion, and peer pressure which can lead to significant dietary changes.

30.   Patient, consistent parental discipline can help children avoid the development of undesirable eating habits. Suggestions are as follows: (a) Quiet time before meals can help to relax children, and those who are easily distracted from eating by others may want to begin meals alone before others are seated. (b) Mealtimes should be happy times. (c) Foods served should be easily handled by children and served in small portions. (d) Meals should be served at regular times, with nutritious snacks as needed. (e) Children should be

allowed to assist in the preparation and planning of meals. (f) Children should not be allowed to use food, eating, or not eating to get attention.

31.   It is essential for parents to realize that most children are not—and need not be—nutritionally perfect, but can be encouraged to make wise food decisions to provide themselves with varied, well-balanced diets.

32.   Worried parents may want to attempt to maintain a diet diary for a week or so in order to determine just what their children are eating; many times, overly concerned parents discover that their children are obtaining diets approaching or surpassing the RDAs for their age group.

33.   School-aged children are quite capable of making decisions which will or will not support good health.

34.   During the pre-puberty period, diet is especially important, as nutrient stores are formed to meet the requirements of the adolescent growth spurt; calcium intake often cannot meet the increased demands of the teen years, so the creation of dense calcium stores is essential prior to adolescence.

35.   As the pre-adolescent enters the teens, there occurs a significantly increased need for calories and nutrients due to heightened growth patterns and hormonal changes. Yet, this is the very time period when most children gravitate away from sound nutrition practices. Biases often develop, and the childhood interest in eating and nutrition is transformed into the common teen obsession with looks and physique.

Teens

1.   During the teen years, dietary habits may be impossible for parents to control, as pre-adults begin to assert maturity and emulate their peers via new eating patterns.

2.   The teen years are filled with changes as children develop into adults and face a variety of problems with physical, emotional, educational, and nutritional impacts; peer pressure becomes very strong, while teens attempt to establish their own beliefs and ideals. As lifestyle habits develop, the teen years serve as the last opportunity to develop healthy eating patterns before adulthood, when major changes are usually far more difficult to make.

3.   Popular concerns for most teens are centered around their own individual physical and emotional self-image and include body weight, skin problems, use of cigarettes and/or drugs, and alcohol intake.

4.   The adolescent growth spurt usually begins as early as age 10 or 11 in females, peaking at age 12, with completion around age 15; in males, the spurt begins at age 12 or 13, peaks at 14, and is not usually complete until age 19.

5.   The need for protein is high due to continued growth, yet the extra calcium intake required at this time may be overlooked—teenage females especially tend to eliminate milk drinking. Teens may attempt vegetarian/semivegetarian lifestyles, and anemia due to iron-deficiency is relatively common during the teen years.

6.   Teens often skip breakfast, an important meal for school-goers. For those who also skimp on lunch, the day's nutritional requirements may not be met. Nutritious snacks can help to replenish low nutrient intakes and allay fatigue. The typical teenager obtains around one-quarter of the day's total caloric intake from snacks, and most studies indicate that snack choices tend to be nutritionally as well as calorically significant.

7.   Failure to meet the increased nutritional requirements of rapid growth and tissue development can lead to delayed sexual maturation and reduction in ultimate overall size.

8.   During adolescence, height typically increases around 15%, and weight nearly doubles. Body composition changes, with males depositing proportionately more lean body tissue and skeletal mass, females more fat. Males, however, do not begin the adolescent growth spurt until 2 years later than their female counterparts, so the inactive boy may become overweight before the increase in height trims him down.

9.   One-fifth of all American teenagers are overweight, yet their average caloric intakes are below recommended levels; this trend (i.e., eating less than in the past but growing fatter) can be correlated with a simultaneous reduction in the level of physical activity.

10.   Obesity can adversely affect college admission, elicit job discrimination, interfere with social progress, and limit choice of mate. It is increasingly difficult for teens to remain slim these days due to lifestyle patterns that encourage lack of physical activity, use of

ineffective reducing diets, overeating to relieve familial tensions and other daily stresses, and peer/environmental pressures to indulge in high-calorie foodstuffs.

11.   Dieting per se should not begin until growth is complete. Even though highly restrictive diets are quite dangerous, "crash" programs are popular with teens (especially females) who seek quick results.

12.   Dieting is also a social event of sorts, serving as a source of intimate conversation, a means for attracting attention, and a game for teens to play: try a new diet, test one's "will power," discuss the diet with friends, and compare notes. Only when dieting becomes an obsession does the diagnosis of anorexia nervosa become a possibility.

13.   Anorexia nervosa is a serious health problem which commonly afflicts teenage females (less than 10% of victims are male) and is characterized by the following symptoms: (a) Despite extreme thinness, an inappropriate body image causes self-denial of the existing emaciated state. (b) Despite prolonged starvation, hunger is denied. (c) Despite frantic exercise (to further weight loss) and minimal energy intake, fatigue is denied.

14.   Many teens of normal body weight (for height and age) consider themselves to be overweight; recent estimates indicate that one third of all teenage girls are on a diet, and an even greater number are dissatisfied with their present weights. This trend is due to the current thin-is-in fashions, the emulation of diet-conscious mothers, as well as the natural pubertal fat distribution (onto hips, thighs, and breasts) which triggers a lifelong compulsion to get rid of normal female fat deposits.

15.   Anorexia nervosa is a psychological disorder which manifests itself as a proposed loss of appetite with stringent dieting to the point of starvation, emaciation, even death. Victims are typically academically successful, well-liked, "good girls."

16.   Anorexia nervosa usually begins in a relatively harmless way with a self-imposed diet to lose a few pounds, sometimes unnecessarily, but continues up to and beyond a loss of 25% total body weight. The typical anorexic is preoccupied with food, yet refuses to eat. The death rate for this disease used to be over 10%, but has dropped due to success in treatment modes.

17.   Victims of anorexia nervosa usually require psychiatric care, yet many first need to be hospitalized in order to counteract progressive malnutrition. Behavioral programs appear to be the most effective method of treatment—including the reteaching of eating behaviors, readjustment of body image, and psychotherapy to uncover personality factors which may have led to the onset of destructive dieting.

18.   Table 8.4 illustrates some of the differences between the behavioral characteristics which identify normal weight reduction activity and those which may be indicative of anorexia nervosa.

19.   Physical symptoms of anorexia include (a) wasted muscle tissue; (b) arrested sexual development; (c) drying/yellowing skin (from accumulated carotene released from body fat); (d) loss of health and texture in hair; (e) growth of **lanugo** hair; (f) pain upon touch; (g) decreased blood pressure and metabolic rate; (h) anemia(s); (i) severe sleep disturbances; and (j) constipation.

lanugo: Fine downy hairs which cover the body.

20.   Bulimics are also phobic about fatness, but participate in episodes of overeating followed by starvation, self-induced vomiting, and/or laxative abuse to avoid weight gain; some use diuretics as well. Up to 50,000 calories at one sitting may be ingested, and such binges can occur at a rate of ten episodes a day. The problem may begin with dieting and/or anorexia, and become a gorging–purging compulsion once the body's hunger cues are confused.

21.   Physical side effects of bulimia include tooth decay with enamel erosion, gastrointestinal disturbances, skin problems, muscle spasms, glandular swelling, hair loss, dehydration, heart **arrhythmias,** and serious organ damage. Yet, because most bulimics are highly secretive and drastic weight loss is uncommon, the disorder may be difficult to diagnose.

arrhythmia: Irregular heart beat.

22.   Once considered to be a rare disorder, bulimia now afflicts an estimated 1% of American females aged 12 to 25. Due to the national preoccupation with thinness and increasing emotional pressures for young women, bulimic symptoms may now occur in as many as one out of every five college coeds.

23.   *Acne vulgaris* often occurs during puberty, when the sebaceous glands increase in size, become more active, and secrete more oil which collects in the pores; here, infection with normal skin bacteria causes the notorious pimples. The condition may become chronic with scarring, or exist as an occasional aggravation. The most successful treatments (for

Table 8.4   Behavioral Characteristics of Dieters

Anorexic dieter	Normal dieter
1. Diets to weight far below that desired.	1. May never lose enough weight to reach desired goal.
2. Is mildly overweight, if overweight at all, before dieting.	2. Is mildly or seriously overweight.
3. Is extremely sensitive to remarks made about weight.	3. May be slightly sensitive about weight.
4. Has no apparent appetite.	4. May have appetite under control, but it can re-emerge full force at any time.
5. Refuses to eat or avoids food.	5. Enjoys looking at and eating food; is easily tempted.
6. Lets minor fluctuations in weight interfere with normal activities.	6. May wear clothes that hide extra weight, so as not to interfere with social life.
7. Is preoccupied with weight; enjoys dieting and being thin.	7. Dislikes dieting and often feels angry for having to diet.
8. Indulges in food rituals; cuts food into little pieces, moves food around the plate, and pretends to be eating; may hoard food instead of eating.	8. Enjoys food and never hoards food; will only cut and eat food methodically if on a behavior modification program.
9. Exercises and moves constantly, sometimes at a frantic pace.	9. Avoids extremes of exercise.
10. Will vomit and take diuretics and laxatives to induce weight loss.	10. Rarely vomits or uses laxatives.
11. Has **amenorrhea.**	11. Has normal menstruation.
12. Is a perfectionist.	12. May be neat or sloppy.
13. Expresses much concern for order.	13. Is orderly or even somewhat haphazard about lifestyle and appearance.
14. Feels better the more skeletonlike in appearance.	14. Does not desire an overly thin appearance.

amenorrhea: Lack of menstruation.

less serious disorders not requiring dermatological treatment) now known usually include one of the following: (a) benzoyl peroxide; (b) sulfur; (c) resorcinol; (d) salicylic acid; and (e) topical retinoic acid.

24.   Vitamin A taken orally in large doses is toxic, and will cause side effects far more dangerous than acne.

25.   *No* foods have proven to be directly correlated to acne. However, caffeine usage may aggravate existing acne (hence, the condemnation of chocolate and cola), alcohol intake can cause inflammatory skin reactions, and large amounts of iodide may cause dermatological irritation. A well-balanced diet, regular exercise, proper rest, and exposure to fresh air are the best prescriptions for preventing unruly skin.

26.   An increasing number of teens are becoming addicted to cigarette smoking, partly due to peer pressure and widespread advertising directed at young audiences.

27.   Although heavy cigarette smoking does diminish somewhat the blood level of vitamin C, there is usually no need for supplementation; the important health considerations of cigarette smoking are not nutritional, but respiratory and cardiovascular—and recent research indicates possible correlations between cigarette smoking and cancer of the esophagus, bladder, and colon.

28.   Regular use of marijuana can result in characteristic physical effects—including altered taste sensations ("the munchies" may be partially due to an enhanced enjoyment of sweets)—yet prolonged use does not seem to lead to weight gain.

29.   If the use of marijuana escalates into "hard" drug experimentation/addiction, nutritional and health effects become pronounced, as indicated by the following characteristics: (a) Money is spent on drugs in place of nutritious foodstuffs. (b) Interest in food is entirely overlooked during "highs." (c) Illness (due to improper self-health care) ensues, with increased nutritional demands.

30. Recent estimates indicate that around 50% of all seventh graders in this country have tried alcohol, and 90% of all seniors have done so; around 90% of college students currently admit to using alcohol, of which 5–10% will experience related complications of a serious nature and more than 8% will become either "problem" drinkers or alcoholics as adults. Alcohol may replace more nutritious foods causing dietary deficiencies and impairing growth.

31. It is essential for most teenagers to have an emulative role model—rock star, TV hero, parent, teacher, coach, or professional athlete—yet the nutrition educator is better able to steer interested teens down factual nutrition pathways.

32. Many teens fall prey to nutrition nonsense due to a desire for physical perfection which surpasses scientific fact and overlooks biological reality. Many ignore the warnings of well-meaning nutrition counselors, and listen instead to self-proclaimed "nutritionists" with unrealistic diet fads and costly, yet appealing, diet cures and claims.

Exercise Using the Nutrition Facts List

Using the preceding Nutrition Facts List, prepare a simplified one-page version for use as a patient handout for either the mothers of infants, young children and their parents, or teenagers. You may include graphics and/or a poster, if desired; a sample handout for teenage girls is shown. Show your handout in rough draft form to classmates or co-workers for constructive criticism on the overall design, content, and potential effectiveness for use in pertinent diet counseling situations. Then prepare a final version for your own future use as a practicing dietetic technician. You may decide to prepare several handouts aimed at the different age groups, or share those prepared by your classmates or co-workers, in order to be better prepared for diet counseling with growing individuals who vary in their nutritional needs.

Sample Handout for Teenage Girls

Spot the signs of anorexia nervosa listed in Table 8.5 before it is too late!

Table 8.5 Symptoms of Anorexia Nervosa

Physical symptoms	Behavioral symptoms	Psychological symptoms
Excessive thinness	Poor sleeping habits[a]	Denial of thinness
Loss of body weight (up to or beyond 25% of former body weight)	Constant "dieting" behaviors[a]	Denial of loss of weight
	Avoidance of situations which may tempt eating[a]	Denial of hunger[a]
Wasted muscle tissue	Indulgence in food rituals	Denial of fatigue[a]
Constant body movement (exercise, fidgeting, pacing)	Food hoarding behaviors[a]	Preoccupation with food, dieting, body size[a]
Arrested sexual development	Self-induced vomiting after eating[a]	Extreme sensitivity about body image[a]
Amenorrhea	Excessive use of laxatives[a]	
Drying, yellowing skin and unhealthy hair		Excessive fear of becoming overweight[a]
Lanugo hair on body		Extreme orderliness, perfectionism
Decreased blood pressure		
Decreased metabolic rate		
Constipation[a]		
Pain upon touch		
Anemia		

[a]Also a symptom of bulimia, the binge–purge behavior disorder.

STEP 3: HEALTHY?

Much of the diet advice currently advocated to the public is based on nutrition myths and misinformation. When individuals who are at nutritional risk adopt such dietary advice, ill health—even death—can result. Infants, children, and teenagers need increased nutrition and can serve as prime targets for diet faddism. Thus, a host of unsupported dietary claims are aimed at these nutritionally naive, vulnerable, and susceptible subpopulations.

Suggested Readings on Diet and Hyperactivity

AMERICAN COUNCIL ON SCIENCE AND HEALTH. 1982. Food Additives and Hyperactivity. New York: ACSH.

BOCK, A. 1982. Food Allergy: A Primer for People. Denver: AJ Publishing.

BRENEMAN, J. 1984. Basics of Food Allergy. Springfield, IL: Charles C. Thomas.

FEINGOLD, B. 1974. Why Your Child is Hyperactive. New York: Random House.

INSTITUTE OF FOOD TECHNOLOGISTS. 1976. Diet and Hyperactivity: Any Connection? Chicago: IFT.

NATIONAL ADVISORY COMMITTEE ON HYPERKINESIS AND FOOD ADDITIVES. 1975. Report of the NACHFA to The Nutrition Foundation. New York: The Nutrition Foundation.

NATIONAL ADVISORY COMMITTEE ON HYPERKINESIS AND FOOD ADDITIVES. 1977. Statement Summarizing Research Findings on the Issue of the Relationship Between Food Additive–Free Diets and Hyperkinesis in Children. New York: The Nutrition Foundation.

NATIONAL ADVISORY COMMITTEE ON HYPERKINESIS AND FOOD ADDITIVES. 1981. Final Report of the NACHFA. New York: The Nutrition Foundation.

NATIONAL DAIRY COUNCIL. 1981. Diet and human behavior. Dairy Counc. Dig. *52,* May/Jun., 13.

NUTRITION AND HEALTH ASSOCIATION. 1983. Nutrition and Behavior, I and II. Tallahassee, FL: Nutrition and Health Association.

STARE, F., and ARONSON, V. 1982. Dear Dr. Stare: What Should I Eat? pp. 48–51. Philadelphia: George F. Stickley Co.

STARE, F., WHELAN, E., and SHERIDAN, M. 1980. Diet and hyperactivity: Is there a relationship? Pediatrics *65,* Oct., 521.

STEVENS, G., STEVENS, L., and STONER, R. 1977. How to Feed Your Hyperactive Child. New York: Doubleday & Co.

For further information:

American Council on Science and Health, 1995 Broadway, New York, NY 10023.
Feingold Association of the U.S., PO Box 6550, Alexandria, VA 22306.
Nutrition and Health Associates, PO Box 11102, Tallahassee, FL 32302.
The Nutrition Foundation, 1126 16th Street NW, Washington, DC 20036.

The Feingold Diet

The Feingold diet was developed by the late Benjamin Feingold, M.D., who claimed that 50% of the hyperactive children who follow an additive-free diet will calm down; two thirds of these children will calm down dramatically (Feingold 1975). Feingold diet proponents believe that some children are highly sensitive to food additives and to the salicylates found naturally in certain fruits and vegetables; they believe that the food "allergy" response is exhibited as hyperactive behavior. Despite the popularity of this theory, large-scale research studies have repeatedly failed to demonstrate a significant correlation between food additives and behavior. The preceding Suggested Readings provide information on both sides of this controversial topic.

Exercise on Food Faddism

As a practicing dietetic technician in nutrition care, it is your responsibility to help protect the growing infant, child, pre-teen, and teenager from falling prey to dangerous dietary claims. You can read some of the preceding Suggested Readings on Diet and Hyperactivity and answer the following Questionnaire in order to focus on one of the many diet fads popular with young people and their parents. Discuss your answers with classmates or co-workers. Begin to scan the media for misleading advertisements for dietary aids aimed at children and teens. Also, begin to collect advertisements and information from various newspapers, magazines, and books on dieting, over-the-counter diet aides, and special weight loss foods and/or programs.

Questionnaire on Diet and Hyperactivity

1. Do you think that food additives are harmful to most consumers? Explain your viewpoint:

2. In consideration of the research results, do you think that the Feingold Diet is an effective method of treatment for hyperactivity? Explain your answer:

3. Do you consider the Feingold Diet to be well balanced? If not, outline the possible nutritional disadvantages of long-term adherence.

4. Do you think it would be practical for schoolchildren to follow the Feingold Diet? List some of the restricted foods which might prove difficult to eliminate from a child's diet:

5. Why do *you* think the Feingold Diet appears to be successful for some, and is supported by the families of so many hyperactive children?

STEP 4: INFANCY GUIDELINES

In order to be able to advise pregnant women and/or new mothers as to the most desirable dietary patterns for their infants, it is essential to have access to all of the hands-on material required for effective counseling sessions. It is also important to be able to record all of the pertinent information regarding each counseling session in the patients' medical charts. If you found it difficult to complete the Pre-test in Step 1, some of the information provided below should help to improve your confidence—and skills—regarding your counseling abilities.

This step includes suggested strategies to use in counseling patients on proper nutrition for infants from birth to 1 year of age. Note that the sessions may apply to either the breastfed or bottle-fed infant. Any reference to *patient* applies to the infant's mother. The following references may prove helpful.

Suggested Readings on Infant Nutrition

AMERICAN ACADEMY OF PEDIATRICS. 1980. On the feeding of supplemental foods to infants. Pediatrics *65,* Jun., 1178.

AMERICAN ACADEMY OF PEDIATRICS. 1985. Pediatric Nutrition Handbook. Elk Grove Village, IL: AAP.

ARNEIL, G., and METCOFF, J. (Editors). 1985. Pediatric Nutrition. Stoneham, MA: Butterworth Publishers.

BAKER, S., and HENRY, R. 1986. Parents' Guide to Nutrition: Healthy Eating from Birth through Adolescence. Reading, MA: Addison-Wesley.

BEATON, G. 1985. Nutritional needs during the first year of life: Some comments and perspectives. Pediat. Clin. North Amer. *32,* Apr., 275.

COLORADO DEPARTMENT OF HEALTH. 1981. Colorado's Self-Teaching Modules, No. 5: Preschool/Childhood Nutrition. Denver: Nutrition Services, Office of Health Care Services, CDH.

DURRELL, D. 1984. The Critical Years: A Guide for Dedicated Parents. Oakland, CA: New Harbinger Publications.

ENDRES, J., and ROCKWELL, R. 1980. Food, Nutrition, and the Young Child. St. Louis: C. V. Mosby Co.

FOMAN, S. 1974. Infant Nutrition. Philadelphia: W. B. Saunders.

GRAND, R., SUTPHEN, J., and DIETZ, W. 1987. Pediatric Nutrition: Theory and Practice. Stoneham, MA: Butterworth Publishers.

HINTON, S., and KERWIN, D. 1982. Maternal, Infant, and Child Nutrition. Chapel Hill, NC: Health Sciences Consortium.

HOWARD, R., and WINTER, H. (Editors). 1984. Nutrition and Feeding of Infants and Toddlers. Boston: Little, Brown & Co.

NATIONAL DAIRY COUNCIL. 1986. Nutrition controversies relative to infants and children. Dairy Counc. Dig. 57, Jul/Aug., 21.

OLSON, R. (Editor). 1988. Parental health beliefs may cause failure to thrive. Nutrition Rev. 46, Jun., 217.

PIPES, P. 1985. Nutrition in Infancy and Childhood, 3rd Edition. St. Louis: C. V. Mosby Co.

PUGLIESE, M., et al. 1987. Parental health beliefs as a cause of nonorganic failure to thrive. Pediatrics 80, Aug., 175.

RICHEY, S., and TAPER, J. 1983. Maternal and Child Nutrition. New York: Harper & Row.

ROSS LABORATORIES. 1976. Growth Charts: Boys/Girls Birth to 36 Months. Columbus, OH: Ross Laboratories.

SATTER, E. 1986. Child of Mine: Feeding with Love and Good Sense. Palo Alto, CA: Bull Publishing Co.

SATTER, E., and DYKSTAL, V. 1983. Feeding Your Infant and Toddler. Madison, WI: Infant Nutrition Publications, Jackson Clinic.

SUSKIND, R. (Editor). 1981. Textbook of Pediatric Nutrition. New York: Raven Press.

TSANG, R., and NICHOLS, B. 1988. Nutrition During Infancy. Philadelphia: Hanley & Belfus.

U.S. DEPARTMENT OF AGRICULTURE. 1978. Composition of Foods—Baby Foods—Raw, Processed, Prepared, USDA Handbook No. 8-3. Washington, DC: Government Printing Office.

U.S. DEPARTMENT OF AGRICULTURE, 1981. What Shall I Feed My Baby? A Month-by-Month Guide, Publication No. 1281. Washington, DC: Government Printing Office.

U.S. DEPARTMENT OF HEALTH AND HUMAN SERVICES. 1978. National Center for Health Statistics Growth Curves for Children: Birth–18 Years, Publication No. PHS 78-1650. Washington, DC: Government Printing Office.

WHITE, A. 1983. The Total Nutrition Guide for Mother and Baby. New York: Ballantine.

WINICK, M. (Editor). 1985. Feeding the Mother and Infant. New York: John Wiley & Sons.

For patient handouts and infant formula handbooks:

Allegheny County Health Department, Nutrition Services, 3441 Forbes Avenue, Pittsburgh, PA 15213.

Mead Johnson and Co., 2404 Pennsylvania Avenue, Evansville, IN 47721.

Ross Laboratories, 625 Cleveland Avenue, Columbus, OH 43216.

For audiovisuals:

Feeding Skills—Your Baby's Early Years. Churchill Films, 662 North Robertson Boulevard, Los Angeles, CA 90069.

First Foods. Society for Nutrition Education, 1700 Broadway, Suite 300, Oakland, CA 94612.

Foods for Baby—When? What? How? Allegheny County Health Department, Nutrition Services, 3441 Forbes Avenue, Pittsburgh, PA 15213.

No Better Gift. Society for Nutrition Education. 1700 Broadway, Suite 300, Oakland, CA 94612.

For further information:

American Academy of Pediatrics, PO Box 1034, Evanston, IL 62004.

American College of Obstetricians and Gynecologists, Resource Center, 600 Maryland Avenue SW, Suite 300E, Washington, DC 20024.

Health Sciences Consortium, 200 Eastowne Drive, Suite 213, Chapel Hill, NC 27514.

La Leche League International, PO Box 1209, Franklin Park, IL 60131.

National Maternal and Child Health Clearinghouse, 3520 Prospect Street NW, Washington, DC 20057.

Counseling Guidelines—Infants

Table 8.6 outlines the steps for diet counseling with the mothers of infants. The following material gives the details of each step.

I. Initial Session

I. A. General Guidelines

1. Use Medical Histories Form to assess nutritional status.

2. *Breastfed infant:* (a) Assist patient in recording 24-hour recall of own food intake, using 24-Hour Recall Form. This will aid patient in keeping an accurate Food Intake Record.

Table 8.6 General Outline for Infant Counseling

I. Initial Session
  A. General Guidelines
  B. Patient Records
    1. Medical Histories Form
    2. 24-Hour Recall Form
  C. Assignments
    1. Food Intake Record
    2. Diet History
    3. Infant Diet History
  D. Technician's Notes
II. Follow-up Session(s)
  A. General Guidelines
  B. Handouts
    1. Personal Diet Plan
    2. Infant Growth Chart
    3. Guide to Adding Foods to Infant Diet
    4. Hints for Feeding Overweight Infants
    5. Learning Assessment Quiz
  C. Technician's Notes

(b) Instruct patient to keep daily Food Intake Record so that typical food intake patterns can be evaluated. Advise patient not to deviate from normal eating pattern. Stress the importance of recording food intake immediately after eating. (c) Instruct patient to complete Diet History. This provides for a basic evaluation of patient food intake patterns. (Use Pre-test from Chapter 2.) (d) Instruct patient to complete Infant Diet History. This provides for a basic evaluation of infant's food intake patterns.

Bottle-fed infant: (a) Assist patient in recording 24-hour recall of infant's food intake, using 24-Hour Recall Form. This will aid in keeping an accurate Food Intake Record for the infant. (b) Instruct patient to keep infant's daily Food Intake Record until next session so that typical food intake patterns can be evaluated. (c) Instruct patient to complete Infant Diet History. This provides for a basic evaluation of infant's food intake patterns.

3. Record assessment and recommendation(s) using the SOAP method (see Chapter 1, Step 6) in Technician's Notes. This form can be kept in your files with a copy in the patient's medical records.

I. B. Patient Records

1. Medical Histories Form

Date _____ Referred by _____

Name of infant _____ Date of birth _____ Sex _____

Pediatrician _____ Address _____

Phone no. _____ Date of last visit _____

General health status:

Ambulatory care required? _____ If so, describe: _____

Neuromuscular problems? _____ If so, how is eating affected? _____

Visual/auditory problems? _____ If so, describe: _____

Feeding difficulties? _____ If so, describe: _____

Appetite typically good? _____ fair? _____ poor? _____

Digestion/elimination difficulties? _____ If so, describe: _____

Food intolerances? _____ If so, describe: _____

Inborn error(s)? _____ If so, describe: _____

Other: _____

Length _____ Weight _____ Triceps skinfold thickness _____

Birth weight _____ Birth length _____ Head circumference _____

Chest circumference ____ Growth abnormalities/problems? _____

Gestational period: No. weeks _____ Small for date? _____ Premature? _____

Clinical signs of nutritional status:

Skin _____ Mouth _____

Hair _____ Eyes _____

Teeth _____ Other: _____

Lab findings: _____

Immunizations: _____

Medications: _____

Prescribed by: _____ Date(s) prescribed: _____

Vitamin/mineral supplements: _____

Prescribed by: _____ Date(s) prescribed: _____

Name of mother _____ Date of birth _____

Address _____ Phone no. _____

Occupation _____ Hours per work week _____ Work phone no. _____

Educational background _____ Religious/ethnic background _____

Marital status _____

Household composition: Live alone _____ Spouse _____ Children/No. _____

Other: _____

General health status (briefly describe):

Overweight? _____

Diabetes? _____

Anemia? _____

History of cigarette smoking? _____

History of alcohol intake? _____

Other: _____

Height _____ Weight _____ Frame _____ Pre-gravid weight _____

Triceps skinfold thickness _____ Mid-arm circumference _____

Mid-arm muscle circumference _____

Weight changes/problems? _____ If so, describe: _____

Clinical signs of nutritional status:

Skin _____ Mouth _____

Hair _____ Eyes _____

Teeth _____ Other: _____

Lab data:

Blood pressure _____

CBC _____

Serum albumin _____

Other: _____

Medications taken regularly: _____

Prescribed by: _____ Date(s) prescribed: _____

Nutrition supplements taken regularly: _____

Prescribed by: _____ Date(s) prescribed: _____

Special diet prescription: _____

Prescribed by: _____ Date of prescription: _____

How closely is diet followed? Always adhered to __ Sometimes __ Rarely __ Never __

Type of housing: Room _____ Apartment _____ Home _____ Institution _____

Prepare own meals? _____ Dine out: Often (more than once a day) _____ Rarely _____

Food shopping done independently? _____ If not, describe required assistance: _____

_____

Eligible for food stamps? _____ If so, are they currently being used? _____

Cigarette smoker? _____ If so, how much: _____

Exercise regularly? _____ If so, describe: _____

   No. times per week _____ No. minutes per session _____

Comments: _____

2. 24-Hour Recall Form

Date	Time	Food and amount

I. C. Assignments

1. Food Intake Record

Date and time	Duration of meal (min)	Food and amount

2. Diet History

Use the Pre-test from Chapter 2 (p. 30) to provide a record of typical foods eaten.

3. Infant Diet History

Water Intake: ____ oz/day
Breastfed: Yes ____ No ____
Bottle Fed: Yes ____ No ____
Type of Formula: Name _____ No. calories/oz ____
Feeding intervals: No. feedings/day ____ Times _____
Total Daily Intake: No. oz/feeding ____ Total no. oz ____

Describe introduction of solid food by considering the following: Juices, cereals, crackers, breads, egg yolk, fruits, vegetables, meats, egg white, and puddings.

Introduction of Solid Food

Time of introduction	Brand and type of food	Frequency of use	Acceptance[a]

[a]Excellent, good, fair, poor.

I. D. Technician's Notes

Patient: _____   Date: _____

S (Subjective data—how patient feels):
O (Objective data—physical measurements including diet/nutritional status):
A (Assessment—acceptability of dietary progress/nutritional status):
P (Plan—diet prescription and instruction):
Comments:

II. Follow-up Session(s)

II. A. General Guidelines

1. Review assignments and discuss.

2. Individualize Personal Diet Plan and instruct patient in its use.

3. Instruct patient to maintain Infant Growth Chart for better visualization of the pattern of weight gain. (A copy may be maintained by the counselor if desired.)

4. Use Guide to Adding Foods to Infant Diet to aid patient in proper infant feeding practices.

5. Use Hints for Feeding Overweight Infants to aid patients with overweight infants.

6. Assign Learning Assessment Quiz to evaluate counseling process and to determine if additional counseling is needed.

7. Record assessment and recommendation(s) using the SOAP method in Technician's Notes. This form can be kept in your files with a copy in the patient's medical records.

II. B. Handouts

1. Personal Diet Plan

Name: _____

How to use diet plan:

1. *Breastfed infant* (see Table 8.7): Select foods from all food groups. Include the recommended number of servings for lactation. At least 8 cups of fluid per day are recommended.
    Bottle-fed infant (see Table 8.8): Select formula which meets recommended nutrient composition, unless otherwise advised. The Infant's Feeding Pattern chart (Table 8.9) may be useful as a guide.

2. The nutrients low in breast milk or formulas may be prescribed by the physician as *supplements* for the infant (see Table 8.10).

3. Table 8.11 indicating Daily Protein and Calorie Allowances for infants may be useful as a guide.

Table 8.7 Breastfed Infant: Mother's Lactation Needs

Food group	No. of servings/day
Milk and cheeses	4
Meats and alternates	3
Fruits	2 (at least one citrus or good source Vitamin C)
Vegetables	2 (dark green and yellow often)
Breads and cereals	4

Table 8.8 Bottle-fed Infant: Recommended Formula Composition[a]

Nutrient	% of total calories
Protein	7–16
Carbohydrate	35–65
Fat	30–55

[a]Formula concentration should not exceed 1 calorie/milliliter.

Table 8.9 Infant's Feeding Pattern

Age in months	No. feedings/day	Amount/feeding (oz)
0–4	6–15	2–6 to 6–7
4–6	4–5	6–8
6–9	3–4	6–8
9–12	4	6

Table 8.10 Supplements for Infants

Type of feeding	Nutrients needed: Fluoride[a]	Iron[b]	Vitamin C	Vitamin D
Breast milk	×	×		×
Evaporated milk formula (fortified with vitamin D)	×	×	×	
Commercial formula (fortified with iron and vitamins C and D)	×			

[a]Depending on fluoride content of area water supply.
[b]Provide supplement at 2 or 4 months of age depending on gestational age of infant at birth.

Table 8.11 Daily Protein and Calorie Allowances

	Birth–6 mo	6–12 mo
Protein	1 gram/lb	0.9 gram/lb
Calories	53 calories/lb	48 calories/lb

2. Infant Growth Chart

Record infant's size on a monthly basis by drawing a line from the last length–weight to the new length–weight. Using Fig. 8.1, it is possible to compare the infant's size to the reference norm (Ross Labs 1976). Any rapid changes in growth may warrant physician consultation.

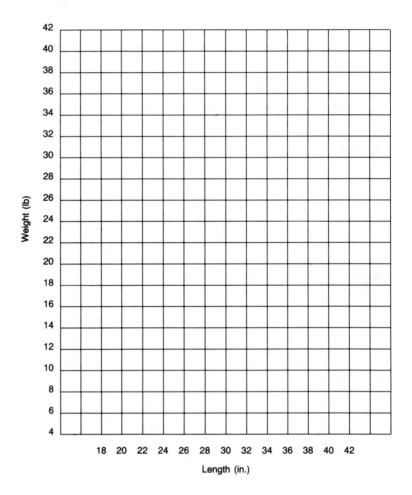

Fig. 8.1   Infant growth chart.

3. Guide to Adding Foods to Infant Diet

Table 8.12 gives guidelines for what and how much solid food should be added to an infant's diet.

4. Hints for Feeding Overweight Infants

○   Do not feed infant skim or low-fat milk.
○   Do not feed infant more than 32 oz of formula daily, but not less than 26 oz.
○   Avoid force-feeding; let infant dictate needs.
○   Avoid feeding high-calorie foods such as: fatty foods; fatty meats; gravies or rich sauces; rich or high-sugar desserts (e.g., puddings, ice cream, sweetened gelatins); foods seasoned with bacon, butter, lard, margarine, salt pork, or other fats.
○   Be careful to avoid weight *loss:* Allow proper growth via increased height.
○   Ensure proper growth for height with pediatrician; use growth charts for guidelines.

Table 8.12 Adding Foods to Infant Diet

Age	Foods and amounts
0–4 months	2–3 oz of formula or breast milk per feeding, with gradual increases
4–5 months	1 tsp iron-fortified rice cereal mixed with formula, gradually increasing to 2 Tbsp, 1–2 times per day
5–6 months	4 Tbsp infant cereals (introducing one cereal at a time is essential—wait 1 month before trying each new type of cereal)
6 months	4 oz fruit juice (noncitric)
	1 tsp plain strained vegetable, gradually increasing to 2–3 Tbsp daily (introducing one at a time, starting with the milder varieties such as carrots, squash, and peas)
	1–2 Tbsp fruit, strained (introducing one at a time, starting with the milder varieties such as applesauce and banana)
	1–2 Tbsp meats, pureed/strained
12 months	Milk/formula—weaning to cup
	4 oz fruit juice plus 2+ Tbsp raw fruit
	4+ Tbsp chopped or mashed vegetables
	4+ Tbsp cereal
	2+ Tbsp meat/beans, ground or finger food
	Egg yolk

5. Learning Assessment Quiz

Give to new mothers after nutrition counseling sessions.
Answer true (T) or false (F) to the following statements:

—— 1. Bottle feeding guards against overfeeding.
—— 2. Use of skim milk in bottle feeding is an acceptable practice.
—— 3. The nutritional status of a mother has little effect on her breastfed infant.
—— 4. Formula-fed infants require extra supplementation with vitamin D.
—— 5. Iron deficiency is common among children between 6 months and 2 years of age.
—— 6. Solid foods should be introduced as early as possible.
—— 7. If a food is rejected, it should be retried as early as possible.
—— 8. Snack feeding should be avoided.
—— 9. Salt should be added to most homemade baby foods.
—— 10. Following an acute illness, an infant's intake of food and beverage should be sharply decreased.
—— 11. One good method for calming an infant is the use of a pacifier dipped in honey.
—— 12. Cow's milk should be introduced by 2 months of age.
—— 13. Nursing bottle syndrome results from constant and prolonged exposure of teeth to milk or fruit juice and can lead to serious tooth decay.

II. C. Technician's Notes

Patient: _____   Date: _____

S (Subjective data—how patient feels):
O (Objective data—physical measurements including diet/nutritional status):
A (Assessment—acceptability of dietary progress/nutritional status):
P (Plan—diet prescription and instruction):
Comments:

Infant Nutrition Counseling Role Playing

Keeping in mind the preceding Suggested Readings and Counseling Guidelines, participate in one or more of the following role play situations; elaborate on each situation to develop a patient and audience profile. Select different partners, either classmates or co-workers, for each situation. You may want to utilize your handout from Step 2. As a dietetic technician in nutrition care, do you consider yourself to be capable of conducting effective counseling sessions with the mothers of infants? Would you or your family be able to adhere to your nutrition guidelines during infant feeding practices?

Role Play Situation 1.   A lactating young mother from a lower class neighborhood wants to start feeding solid foods to her 6-month-old daughter. She is referred to you, a dietetic technician in an out-patient clinic, for diet counseling. Follow the guidelines to complete the charts, and provide her with an individualized diet plan for her infant. Prepare a SOAP note for the departmental files with a copy to be sent to the referring pediatrician.

Role Play Situation 2.   The mother of an underweight 8-month-old baby—who has finally begun to thrive and will soon be discharged—requests dietary advice for her infant. As a dietetic technician assigned to the pediatrics ward, follow the guidelines to complete the charts and provide the mother with an individualized diet plan for her baby. Prepare a SOAP note which could be recorded in the infant's medical chart.

Role Play Situation 3.   The nutritionists in the public health department where you are employed are planning a workshop for new mothers on the prevention of childhood obesity. As one of the speakers, prepare an outline on one aspect of the subject to present to the mothers' group. Prepare a brief written report on the workshop (attendance, response, use of visual aids, suggestions for revisions, etc.) for insertion in departmental files.

STEP 5: CHILDHOOD GUIDELINES

In order to be able to assist growing children and their anxious parents in adopting desirable dietary patterns, it is essential to have access to all of the hands-on material required for effective counseling sessions. It is also important to be able to record all of the pertinent information regarding each counseling session in the patient's medical charts. If you found it difficult to complete the Pre-test in Step 1, some of the information provided below should help to improve your confidence—and skills—regarding your counseling abilities.

This step includes suggested strategies for use with young patients requiring nutrition counseling and their parents. The following references may prove helpful.

Suggested Readings on Child Nutrition

AMERICAN ACADEMY OF PEDIATRICS. 1983. Toward a prudent diet for children. Pediatrics *71,* Jan., 78.
AMERICAN ACADEMY OF PEDIATRICS. 1985. Pediatric Nutrition Handbook. Elk Grove Village, IL: AAP.
AMERICAN ACADEMY OF PEDIATRICS. 1986. Prudent life-style for children: Dietary fat and cholesterol. Pediatrics *78,* Sept., 521.
APPLEBAUM, G. 1982. School lunch: Changes and challenges. Nutrition News *45,* Feb., 1.
ARNEIL, G., and METCOFF, J. 1985. Pediatric Nutrition. Stoneham, MA: Butterworth Publishers.
BAKER, S., and HENRY, R. 1986. Parents' Guide to Nutrition: Healthy Eating from Birth through Adolescence. Reading, MA: Addison-Wesley.
CEREAL INSTITUTE, 1976. A Complete Summary of the Iowa Breakfast Studies. Chicago: Cereal Institute.
CLANCY-HEPBURN, K., HICKEY, A., and NEVILL, G. 1974. Children's behavioral responses to TV food advertisements. J. Nutr. Educ. *6,* Jul.–Sept., 93.
COLORADO DEPARTMENT OF HEALTH. 1981. Colorado's Self-Teaching Modules, No. 7: Dental Nutrition. Denver: Nutrition Services, Office of Health Care Services, CDH.
COTUGNA, N. 1988. TV ads on Saturday morning children's programming: What's new? J. Nutr. Educ. *20,* Jun., 125.
DIETZ, W., and GORTMAKER, S. 1985. Do we fatten our children at the television set? Obesity and television viewing in childhood. Pediatrics *75,* May, 807.
ENDRES, J., and ROCKWELL, R. 1980. Food, Nutrition, and the Young Child. St. Louis: C. V. Mosby Co.
FOMAN, S., and ANDERSON, T. (Editors). 1972. Practices of Low-Income Families in Feeding Children with Particular Attention to Cultural Subgroups. Washington, DC: Government Printing Office.
FOMAN, S., et al. 1976. Nutritional Disorders of Children: Prevention, Screening, and Follow-up, Publication No. HSA 76-5612. Washington, DC: Government Printing Office.
GRAND, R., SUTPHEN, J., and DIETZ, W. 1987. Pediatric Nutrition: Theory and Practice. Stoneham, MA: Butterworth Publishers.

HANNING, R., and ZLOTKIN, S. 1985. Unconventional eating practices and their health implications. Pediat. Clin. North Amer. *32,* Apr., 429.

HINTON, S., and KERWIN, D. 1982. Maternal, Infant, and Child Nutrition. Chapel Hill, NC: Health Sciences Consortium.

HOWARD, R., and WINTER, H. 1984. Nutrition and Feeding of Infants and Toddlers. Boston: Little, Brown & Co.

HURLEY, L. 1980. Developmental Nutrition. Englewood Cliffs, NJ: Prentice-Hall.

KELTS, D., and JONES, E. 1984. Manual of Pediatric Nutrition. Boston: Little, Brown & Co.

LABERT-LAGACÉ, L. 1982. Feeding Your Child. New York: Beaufort Books.

LANSKY, V. 1988. Fat-Proofing Your Children . . . So That They Never Become Diet-Addicted Adults. New York: Bantam.

MCWILLIAMS, M. 1980. Nutrition for the Growing Years, 3rd Edition. New York: John Wiley & Sons.

MEAD JOHNSON AND CO. 1978. Growth Charts with Reference Percentiles for Boys and Girls. Evansville, IN: Mead Johnson and Co.

NATIONAL DAIRY COUNCIL. 1986. The role of diet and nutrition in oral health. Dairy Counc. Dig. *57,* May/Jun., 15.

NATIONAL DAIRY COUNCIL. 1988. Nutrition and the school-age child. Dairy Counc. Dig. *59,* Mar./Apr., 7.

NATOW, A., and HESLIN, J. 1984. No-Nonsense Nutrition for Kids. New York: McGraw-Hill.

NIELSON, A. C. 1985. Nielson Report on Television. Chicago: A. C. Nielson Co.

PEAVY, L., and PAGENKOPF, A. 1980. Grow Healthy Kids. New York: Grosset & Dunlop.

PIPES, P., 1985. Nutrition in Infancy and Childhood, 3rd Edition. St. Louis: C. V. Mosby Co.

RITCHEY, S., and TAPER, J. 1983. Maternal and Child Nutrition. New York: Harper & Row.

SATTER, E. 1986. Child of Mine: Feeding with Love and Good Sense. Palo Alto, CA: Bull Publishing Co.

SATTER, E. 1987. How to Get Your Kid to Eat . . . But Not Too Much. Palo Alto, CA: Bull Publishing Co.

SUSKIN, R. (Editor). 1981. Textbook of Pediatric Nutrition. New York: Raven Press.

For patient handouts:

Energize at Sunrise. Kellogg's Nutritional Education Units, PO Box 5012, Kalamazoo, MI 49003.

Peanut Butter and Pickles. Office of Education, Humboldt County, 901 Myrtle Avenue, Eureka, CA 95501.

Super Heroes Super Health Cookbook—Good Foods Kids Can Make Themselves. 1981. New York: Warner Books.

For audiovisuals:

Diet Counseling for Preventive Dentistry. Health Sciences Consortium, 200 Eastowne Drive, Suite 213, Chapel Hill, NC 27514.

Nutrition for Teachers: Preschool and Elementary Grades. Pennsylvania State University, Audiovisual Services, Keller Building, University Park, PA 16802.

SHAPEDOWN for Children. PO Box 26427, San Francisco, CA 94126.

You're in Charge: Nutrition for Preschool Children. Society for Nutrition Education, 1700 Broadway, Suite 300, Oakland, CA 94612.

For further information:

Allegheny County Health Department, Nutrition Services, 3441 Forbes Avenue, Pittsburgh, PA 15213.

American Academy of Pediatrics, PO Box 1034, Evanston, IL 60204.

March of Dimes Foundation, 1275 Mamoroneck Avenue, White Plains, NY 10605.

Mead Johnson and Co., 2404 Pennsylvania Avenue, Evansville, IN 47721.

National Maternal and Child Health Clearinghouse, 3520 Prospect Street NW, Washington, DC 20057.

Office of Child Development, Office of Education/Public Health Service, 9000 Rockville Pike, Bethesda, MD 20014.

Table 8.13 General Outline for Counseling Children

I. Initial Session
  A. General Guidelines
  B. Patient Records
    1. Medical Histories Form
    2. 24-Hour Recall Form
  C. Assignments
    1. Food Intake Record
    2. Diet History
  D. Technician's Notes
II. Follow-up Session(s)
  A. General Guidelines
  B. Handouts
    1. Cariogenic Food Evaluation Chart
    2. Personal Diet Plan
    3. Good Eating Checklist
  C. Technician's Notes

Counseling Guidelines—Children

Table 8.13 outlines the steps for nutrition counseling with children. The following material gives the details of each step. For young children, parents should be involved in counseling sessions and may maintain or assist with patient records and assignments.

I.   Initial Session

I.   A.   General Guidelines

1. Use Medical Histories Form to assess patient's nutritional status.
2. Assist patient in recording 24-hour recall of food intake using 24-Hour Recall Form. This will aid patient in keeping an accurate Food Intake Record.
3. Assist patient to keep daily Food Intake Record so that typical food intake patterns can be evaluated. Instruct patient not to deviate from normal eating patterns. Stress the importance of recording food intake immediately after eating.
4. Instruct patient to complete Diet History. This provides for a basic evaluation of food intake patterns. (Use Pre-test from Chapter 2.)
5. Record assessment and recommendation(s) using the SOAP method in Technician's Notes. This form can be kept in your files with a copy in the patient's medical records.

I.   B.   Patient Records

1. Medical Histories Form

Date _____ Referred by _____

Name _____ Date of birth _____

Address _____ Phone no. _____

Sex _____ No. of siblings _____ Age span _____

Pediatrician _____ Address _____

Phone no. _____ Date of last visit _____

Dentist _____ Address _____

Phone no. _____ Date of last visit _____

General health status:

Ambulatory care required? ____ If so, describe: _____

Neuromuscular problems? ____ If so, how is eating affected? _____

Visual/auditory problems? ____ If so, describe: _____

Eating difficulties? ____ If so, describe: _____

Appetite typically good? _____ fair? _____ poor? _____

Digestion/elimination difficulties? ____ If so, describe: _____

Food intolerances? ____ If so, describe: _____

Dental caries? ____ If so, describe extent:_____

Other: _____

Height _____ Weight _____ Frame _____

Triceps skinfold thickness _____ Mid-arm circumference _____

Mid-arm muscle circumference _____

Weight changes/problems? ____ If so, describe: _____

Clinical signs of nutritional status:

Skin _____ Mouth _____

Hair _____ Eyes _____

Teeth _____ Other: _____

Lab findings: _____

Immunizations: _____

Medications: _____

Prescribed by: _____ Date(s) prescribed: _____

Nutrition supplements: _____

Prescribed by: _____ Date(s) prescribed: _____

Special diet prescription: _____

Prescribed by: _____ Date(s) prescribed: _____

Name of mother _____ Date of birth _____

Address _____ Phone no. _____

Occupation _____ Hours per work week _____ Work phone no. _____

Educational background _____ Religious/ethnic background _____
Marital status _____
Household composition: Live alone _____ Spouse _____ Children/No. _____
Other: _____

General health status (briefly describe):

Overweight? _____
Diabetes? _____
Anemia? _____
History of cigarette smoking? _____
History of alcohol intake? _____
Other: _____

Height ____ Weight ____ Frame ____
Triceps skinfold thickness _____ Mid-arm circumference _____
Mid-arm muscle circumference _____
Weight changes/problems? ____ If so, describe: _____

Clinical signs of nutritional status:

Skin _____ Mouth _____
Hair _____ Eyes _____
Teeth _____ Other: _____

Medications taken regularly: _____
Prescribed by: _____ Date(s) prescribed: _____
Nutrition supplements taken regularly: _____
Prescribed by: _____ Date(s) prescribed: _____
Special diet prescription: _____
Prescribed by: _____ Date of prescription: _____
How closely is diet followed? Always adhered to ___ Sometimes ___ Rarely ___ Never ___

Type of housing: Room ____ Apartment ____ Home ____ Institution ____
Prepare own meals? ____ Dine out: Often (more than once a day) ____ Rarely ____
Food shopping done independently? ____ If not, describe required assistance: _____
_____
Eligible for food stamps? ____ If so, are they currently being used? _____
Cigarette smoker? ____ If so, how much: _____
Exercise regularly? ____ If so, describe: _____
     No. times per week ____ No. minutes per session _____

Comments: _____

2. 24-Hour Recall Form

Date	Time	Food and amount

I. C. Assignments

1. Food Intake Record

Date and time	Duration of meal (min)	Food or amount	Where[a]	With whom	Associated activity[b]	Associated emotions[c]

[a]Such as school, restaurant, kitchen, living room.
[b]For example, watching television, reading, talking.
[c]Attitude: bored, anxious, frustrated, depressed, happy, angry, tense, etc.

2. Diet History

Use the Pre-test from Chapter 2 (p. 30) to provide a record of typical foods eaten.

I. D. Technician's Notes

Patient: _____   Date: _____

S (Subjective data—how patient feels):
O (Objective data—physical measurements including diet/nutritional status):
A (Assessment—acceptability of dietary progress/nutritional status):
P (Plan—diet prescription and instruction):
Comments:

II. Follow-up Session(s)

II. A. General Guidelines

1. Review assignments and discuss.
2. To analyze patient's Food Intake Record, assist patient in circling all foods with high cariogenic potential, and use Cariogenic Food Evaluation Chart to identify the following as possible problem areas: specific day(s), specific meal(s), snacking, and/or physical form of sweets. Note that the potential acid production is only an estimate, as foods vary in their actual cariogenic potentials depending on the physical form and the individual consumer.
3. Individualize Personal Diet Plan and instruct patient in its use.
4. Using Food Intake Record and Good Eating Checklist, assist patient in a general evaluation of nutrient intake.
5. Instruct patient to self-evaluate adherence to Personal Diet Plan and development of good eating habits through continued use of Food Intake Record, Cariogenic Food Evaluation Chart, and Good Eating Checklist.
6. Record assessment and recommendation(s) using the SOAP method in Technician's Notes. This form can be kept in your files with a copy in the patient's medical records.

II. B. Handouts

1. Cariogenic Food Evaluation Chart

Instructions: Total the number of circled items (foods with high cariogenic potential) on Food Intake Record for each meal and/or snack. Transfer each number to the appropriate column on this chart. Determine total/meal, total/day, total liquids/week, total solids/week, and grand total. To calculate the potential acid production in minutes, use the following formulas:

Total/meal × 20 min = Potential acid production/meal (in min): _____
Total/day × 20 min = Potential acid production/day (in min): _____
Grand total × 20 min = Potential acid production/week (in min): _____

Physical form of sweets eaten	Day 1				Day 2				Day 3				Day 4				Day 5				5-day total
	B	L	D	S	B	L	D	S	B	L	D	S	B	L	D	S	B	L	D	S	
Liquid[a]																					
Solid[b]																					
Total/meal																					
Total/day																					

Grand total _____

Key: B = Breakfast   L = Lunch   D = Dinner   S = Snack
[a]Liquid = Sweets such as fruit drinks, soft drinks, and coffee sweetened with sugar.
[b]Solid = Sweets such as sugar-coated cereals, pastries, dried fruits, and sugared gum.

2. Personal Diet Plan

Name: _____

How to use diet plan:

1. Select a variety of foods from each of the Basic Food Groups.
2. Include the recommended number of servings from each Food Group.
3. Incorporate snacks such as those included in the Acceptable Snacks list (Table 8.14).
4. Limit intake of foods with high cariogenic potential, such as those included in the Foods to Minimize list (Table 8.15).

Table 8.14   Children's Acceptable Snacks

Food group	Acceptable snacks[a]
Fruits and vegetables	Raw fruits, unsweetened fruit juices Raw vegetables, juices
Breads and cereals	Crackers, toast, pretzels, popcorn, muffins, unsweetened cereals
Milk and cheeses	Milk, cheese, plain yogurt
Meats and alternates	Cold meats, peanut butter, cottage cheese
Others	Pizza, tacos, sandwiches

[a]Brush your teeth after *any* snack, as new evidence indicates that nonsugary foods also may cause tooth decay.

Table 8.15   Foods to Minimize in Children's Diets

Pastries and pies	Sherbet	Popsicles
Doughnuts	Sweetened	Caramel popcorn
Sweet rolls	yogurt	Candied apples
Cakes, rich	Puddings	Marshmallows
Cookies, frosted	Gelatin,	Dried fruits, bite-size fruits[a]
Candy, especially bite-size[a]	flavored	Fruits in syrup
	Jams	Sugar-coated cereals
Mints, cough drops	Jellies	Cereals containing more than 15% sugar
Sugared gum	Syrups	
Fruit drinks	Sugars	Hot dogs, small tubular-
Soft drinks	Honey	shaped foods, and nuts[a]

[a]Be careful to chew foods thoroughly to avoid choking!

3. Good Eating Checklist

Instructions: Using Food Intake Record, total the number of daily servings from each Food Group and transfer to this chart. Evaluate by comparison to Recommended Daily Servings (RDSs).

Day	No. of servings/Food Group					
	Fruits	Vegetables	Grains	Milk	Meat	Others
1						
2						
3						
4						
5						
RDSs	2	2	4	3	2	—

II. C. Technician's Notes

Patient: _____   Date: _____

S (Subjective data—how patient feels):
O (Objective data—physical measurements including diet/nutritional status):
A (Assessment—acceptability of dietary progress/nutritional status):
P (Plan—diet prescription and instruction):
Comments:

Child Nutrition Counseling Role Playing

Keeping in mind the preceding Suggested Readings and Counseling Guidelines, participate in one or more of the following role play situations; elaborate on each situation to develop a patient/audience profile. Select different partners, either classmates or co-workers, for each situation. You may want to utilize your handout from Step 2. As a dietetic technician in nutrition care, do you consider yourself to be capable of conducting effective counseling sessions with growing children and their concerned parents? Would your siblings, children, or other family members be able to adhere to your nutrition guidelines during child feeding practices?

Role Play Situation 1. A 2-year-old (who had accompanied a parent seeking dental care) is referred to you, a dietetic technician working in a large dental clinic, for diet counseling. His teeth show rampant decay, and he is sucking on a honey-dipped pacifier. Follow the guidelines to complete the charts and provide the parents of this child with an individualized diet plan. Prepare a SOAP note which could be recorded in the child's dental chart.

Role Play Situation 2. A slightly overweight 6-year-old (post-appendectomy) is about to be discharged from the pediatrics ward where you are the assigned dietetic technician. The physician requests a weight control plan. Follow the guidelines to complete the charts and provide the child (and parents) with an individualized diet plan. Prepare a SOAP note which could be recorded in the child's medical chart.

Role Play Situation 3. The dietary department of the hospital where you are employed as a dietetic technician has been requested by the local school department to give a presentation on fluoridation for an upcoming Parent–Teachers Association meeting. As one of the speakers, prepare an outline on the benefits of fluoridation for children to present to the PTA. Prepare a brief written report on the meeting (attendance, response, use of visual aids, questions, suggestions for revisions, etc.) for insertion in departmental files.

STEP 6: TEEN GUIDELINES

In order to be able to assist teenagers in developing desirable dietary patterns and avoiding dangerous fads, it is essential to have access to all of the hands-on material required for effective counseling sessions. It is also important to be able to record all of the pertinent information regarding each counseling session in the patients' medical charts. If you found it difficult to complete the Pre-test in Step 1, some of the information provided below should help to improve your confidence—and skills—regarding your counseling abilities.

This step includes suggested strategies for use with teenage clients requiring nutrition counseling. The following references may prove helpful.

Suggested Readings on Adolescent Nutrition

BAKER, S., and HENRY, R. 1986. Parents' Guide to Nutrition: Healthy Eating from Birth Through Adolescence. Reading, MA: Addison-Wesley.

BLINN, L. 1983. Your Nutrition. Cincinnati: South-Western Publishing Co.

BRUCH, H. 1978. The Golden Cage: The Enigma of Anorexia Nervosa. Cambridge, MA: Harvard University Press.

BRUCH, H. 1988. Conversations with Anorexics. New York: Basic Books.

BRUMBERG, J. 1988. Fasting Girls. Cambridge, MA: Harvard University Press.

COLORADO DEPARTMENT OF HEALTH. 1981. Colorado's Self-Teaching Modules, No. 6: Adolescent Nutrition. Denver: Nutrition Services, Office of Health Care Services, CDH.

IKEDA, J. 1987. Winning Weight Loss for Teens. Palo Alto, CA: Bull Publishing Co.

MAHAN, L., and REES, J. (Editors). 1984. Nutrition in Adolescence. St. Louis: Times Mirror/Mosby.

MARCH OF DIMES FOUNDATION. 1986. Nutrition and Adolescent Pregnancy: A Selected Annotated Bibliography. Washington, DC: Government Printing Office.

MELLIN, L. 1987. SHAPEDOWN for Adolescents. San Francisco: Balboa Publishers.

NATIONAL DAIRY COUNCIL. 1987. Adolescent nutrition: Issues and challenges. Dairy Counc. Dig. 58, Jul./Aug., 19.

RYE, J., ROSANDER, K., and LAQUATRA, I. 1981. Nutrition in a Changing World: A Curriculum for Junior High Health. University Park, PA: Pennsylvania State University.

SACKER, I., and ZIMMER, M. 1987. Dying to Be Thin. New York: Warner Books.

STARE, F., and ARONSON, V. 1985. Food for Today's Teens. Philadelphia: George F. Stickley Co.

U.S. DEPARTMENT OF AGRICULTURE. 1981. Working with the Pregnant Teenager: A Guide for Nutrition Educators. Washington, DC: Government Printing Office.

U.S. DEPARTMENT OF HEALTH AND HUMAN SERVICES. 1978. National Center for Health Statistics Growth Curves for Children: Birth–18 Years, Publication No. PHS 78-1650. Washington, DC: Government Printing Office.

WINICK, M. 1982. Adolescent Nutrition. New York: John Wiley & Sons.

For patient handouts (including games and workbooks):

Health Education Services, Food and Nutrition Catalog, 10,000 Culver Boulevard, PO Box 802, Culver City, CA 90230.

For audiovisuals:

Anorexia Nervosa. Soundwords, 56-11 217 Street, Bayside, NY 11364.

Diets for All Reasons. Churchill Films, 662 North Robertson Boulevard, Los Angeles, CA 90069.

Eating for the Health of It. Dairy Council, Inc., 12450 North Washington, Thornton, CO 80241.

Eating on the Run. Alfred Higgins Productions, 9100 Sunset Boulevard, Los Angeles, CA 90069.

Nutrition for Your Busy Lifestyle. National Dairy Council, 6300 North River Road, Rosemont, IL 60018.

The Fast Food Phenomenon. Nutrition Resource Center, Pennsylvania State University, University Park, PA 16802.

The Great American Eating Scene. Dairy Council, Inc., 12450 North Washington, Thornton, CO 80241.

Counseling Guidelines—Teens

Table 8.16 outlines the steps for nutrition counseling for teenagers. The following material gives the details of each step.

I. Initial Session

I. A. General Guidelines

1. Use Medical History Form to assess patient's nutritional status.
2. Assist patient in recording 24-hour recall of food intake using 24-Hour Recall Form. This will aid in keeping an accurate Food Intake Record.
3. Assign patient to keep daily Food Intake Record so that typical food intake patterns can be evaluated. Instruct patient not to deviate from normal eating patterns. Stress the importance of recording food intake immediately after eating.
4. Instruct patient to complete Diet History. This provides for a basic evaluation of food intake patterns. (Use the Pre-test from Chapter 2.)
5. Record assessment and recommendation(s) using the SOAP method in Technician's Notes. This form can be kept in your files with a copy in the patient's records.

I. B. Patient Records

1. Medical History Form

Date _____ Referred by _____

Name _____ Date of birth _____

Address _____ Phone no. _____

Sex _____ No. of siblings _____ Age span _____

Pediatrician _____ Address _____

Phone no. _____ Date of last visit _____

Dentist _____ Address _____

Phone no. _____ Date of last visit _____

General health status:

Ambulatory care required? ____ If so, describe: _____

Neuromuscular problems? ____ If so, how is eating affected? _____

Visual/auditory problems? ____ If so, describe: _____

Eating difficulties? ____ If so, describe: _____

Appetite typically good? _____ fair? _____ poor? _____

Digestion/elimination difficulties? ____ If so, describe: _____

Food intolerances? ____ If so, describe: _____

Dental caries? ____ If so, describe extent:_____

Other: _____

Height _____ Weight _____ Frame _____

Triceps skinfold thickness _____ Mid-arm circumference _____

Mid-arm muscle circumference _____

Weight changes/problems? ____ If so, describe: _____

Clinical signs of nutritional status:

Skin _____ Mouth _____

Hair _____ Eyes _____

Teeth _____ Other: _____

Lab data:

Blood pressure _____

CBC _____

Serum albumin _____

Other: _____

Medications taken regularly: _____

Prescribed by: _____ Date(s) prescribed: _____

Nutrition supplements taken regularly: _____
Prescribed by: _____ Date(s) prescribed: _____
Special diet prescription: _____
Prescribed by: _____ Date of prescription: _____
How closely is diet followed? Always adhered to ___ Sometimes ___ Rarely ___ Never ___

Type of housing: Room ____ Apartment ____ Home ____ Institution ____
Prepare own meals? ____ Dine out: Often (more than once a day) ____ Rarely ____
Food shopping done independently? ____ If not, describe required assistance: _____
_____
Eligible for food stamps? ____ If so, are they currently being used? _____
Cigarette smoker? ____ If so, how much: _____
Exercise regularly? ____ If so, describe: _____
    No. times per week ____ No. minutes per session _____

Name of mother _____ Date of birth _____
Address _____ Phone no. _____
Occupation _____ Hours per work week ____ Work phone no. _____
Educational background _____ Religious/ethnic background _____
Household composition: Live alone ____ Spouse ____ Children/No. ____ Other: ____
Comments: _____

2. 24-Hour Recall Form

Date	Time	Food and amount

I. C. Assignments

1. Food Intake Record

Date and time	Duration of meal (min)	Food or amount	Where[a]	With whom	Associated activity[b]	Associated emotions[c]

[a]Such as school, restaurant, kitchen, living room.
[b]For example, watching television, reading, talking.
[c]Attitude: bored, anxious, frustrated, depressed, happy, angry, tense, etc.

2. Diet History

Use the Pre-test from Chapter 2 to provide a record of typical foods eaten.

I.   D.   Technician's Notes

Patient: _____   Date: _____

S   (Subjective data—how patient feels):
O   (Objective data—physical measurements including diet/nutritional status):
A   (Assessment—acceptability of dietary progress/nutritional status):
P   (Plan—diet prescription and instruction):
Comments:

II.   Follow-up Session(s)

II.   A.   General Guidelines

1. Review assignments and discuss.
2. Individualize Personal Diet Plan and instruct patient in its use.
3. Using Food Intake Record and Good Eating Checklist, assist patient in a general evaluation of nutrient intake.
4. Instruct patient to self-evaluate adherence to Personal Diet Plan and development of good eating habits through continued use of Food Intake Record and Good Eating Checklist.
5. Record assessment and recommendation(s) using the SOAP method in Technician's Notes. This form can be kept in your file with a copy in the patient's medical records.

II.   B.   Handouts

1. Personal Diet Plan

Name: _____

How to use diet plan:

1. Select a variety of foods from each of the Basic Food Groups.
2. Include the recommended number of servings from each Food Group.
3. Incorporate snacks such as those included in the Acceptable Snacks list (Table 8.17).
4. Limit intake of foods with high cariogenic potential, such as those included in the Foods to Minimize list (Table 8.18).
5. Avoid becoming overweight or underweight by controlling portion sizes and exercising regularly.

Table 8.17   Teenagers' Acceptable Snacks

Food group	Acceptable snacks[a]
Fruits and vegetables	Raw fruits, unsweetened fruit juices Raw vegetables, juices
Breads and cereals	Crackers, toast, pretzels, popcorn, muffins, unsweetened cereals
Milk and cheeses	Milk, cheese, plain yogurt
Meats and alternates	Cold meats, peanut butter, cottage cheese, nuts
Others	Pizza, tacos, sandwiches

[a]Brush your teeth after *any* snack, as new evidence indicates that nonsugary foods may also cause tooth decay.

Table 8.18   Foods to Minimize in Teens' Diets

Pastries and pies	Sherbet	Popsicles
Doughnuts	Sweetened yogurt	Caramel popcorn
Sweet rolls	Puddings	Candied apples
Cakes, rich	Gelatin, flavored	Marshmallows
Cookies, frosted	Jams	Dried fruit rolls
Candy	Jellies	Fruits in syrup
Mints, cough drops	Syrups	Sugar-coated cereals
Sugared gum	Sugars	Cereals containing
Fruit drinks	Honey	more than 15% sugar
Soft drinks		

2. Good Eating Checklist

Instructions: Using Food Intake Record, total the number of daily servings from each Food Group and transfer to this chart. Evaluate by comparison to Recommended Daily Servings (RDSs).

Day	No. of servings/Food Group					
	Fruits	Vegetables	Grains	Milk	Meat	Others
1						
2						
3						
4						
5						
RDSs	2	2	4	4	2	—

II. C. Technician's Notes

Patient: _____   Date: _____

S (Subjective data—how patient feels):
O (Objective data—physical measurements including diet/nutritional status):
A (Assessment—acceptability of dietary progress/nutritional status):
P (Plan—diet prescription and instruction):
Comments:

Teen Nutrition Counseling Role Playing

Keeping in mind the preceding Suggested Readings and Counseling Guidelines, participate in one or more of the following role play situations; elaborate on each situation to develop a patient/audience profile. Select different partners, either classmates or co-workers, for each situation. You may want to utilize your handout from Step 2. As a dietetic technician in nutrition care, do you consider yourself capable of conducting effective counseling sessions with teenagers in need of nutrition guidance? Would you, your teenage friends, or any other teens be able to adhere to your dietary advice?

Role Play Situation 1.   A low-income family sends their two overweight teenage girls to the nutrition clinic where you are employed. Their physician has advised obtaining a weight control plan. Follow the guidelines to complete the charts and provide the teens with individualized diet plans. Prepare a SOAP note for each girl for your department files with copies to be sent to their physician.

Role Play Situation 2.   As a member of the adolescent health care team for a large private psychiatric hospital, you are responsible for providing diet counseling to recovering anorexics. Follow the guidelines to complete the charts and provide an underweight 16-year-old female with an individualized diet plan. Prepare a SOAP note which could be recorded in the patient's chart.

Role Play Situation 3.   A high school physical education class requests a presentation of "Nutrition for Athletics" to be given by the dietetics department of the hospital where you are employed. As one of the speakers, prepare an outline on one aspect of sports nutrition for teenagers to present to the high school class. Prepare a brief written report on the lecture (use of visual aids, class response, questions raised, suggestions for revision, etc.) for insertion in departmental files.

STEP 7: POST-TEST ON THE GROWING YEARS

In order to evaluate your understanding of dietary needs during the growing years, complete the Post-test below. Section I includes the Learning Assessment quiz for new parents. (If the diet counselor is unable to complete this test successfully, how can the patient be expected to?) Section II incorporates much of the material from this chapter. Will your patients succeed in attaining a healthy diet pattern conducive to proper growth and development? Will they avoid detrimental and dangerous dietary fads?

Section I. Complete the quiz on infant feeding from Infancy Guidelines (p. 175). Check your answers with the Answer Key.

Section II. Indicate whether the following statements are true (T) or false (F). Check your answers with the Answer Key.

_____ 1. Infants under the age of one should not be given cow's milk.
_____ 2. Children should not switch to skim milk until around the age of five.
_____ 3. The first solid food should be introduced at 3 months of age.
_____ 4. The best solid food to introduce first in the diet is iron-fortified wheat cereal.
_____ 5. Infants should be fed according to a rigid schedule which gradually diminishes to three feedings per day.
_____ 6. There is no need for concern regarding dental decay until the toddler period.
_____ 7. Colic is caused by the drinking of cow's milk by a lactating mother.
_____ 8. Cholesterol intake should be modified routinely beginning at age one.
_____ 9. Appetite—like growth—tends to diminish in intensity after the first birthday.
_____ 10. Growing children should eat as much as their parents with an additional serving of milk.
_____ 11. Food jags are normal and, if ignored, usually disappear without serious health damage.
_____ 12. To avoid dental decay, children should not include any sugar in their diets.
_____ 13. Overweight children should go on low-calorie diets.
_____ 14. Breakfast skippers are often less attentive in school.
_____ 15. Only a very small percentage of teens today are overweight.
_____ 16. Anorexia nervosa can prove to be fatal.
_____ 17. Bulimia is easily identified due to the emaciated state of most victims.
_____ 18. Overweight teens, like obese individuals at any age, are usually more sedentary than their normal weight peers.
_____ 19. Acne can be treated safely and successfully with self-prescribed doses of oral vitamin A.
_____ 20. The best method for counseling teens on improving dietary habits is to scare them into submission.

Select the answer which best completes the following statements. Check your answers with the Answer Key.

_____ 21. The Feingold Diet eliminates the intake of
(a) oranges. (b) certain vegetables. (c) synthetic food colors. (d) synthetic food flavors. (e) c and d. (f) all of these.
_____ 22. Documented evidence indicates that the Feingold Diet is
(a) effective in eliminating hyperactive behavior in the majority of afflicted children. (b) of questionable value for the majority of cases of hyperactivity. (c) a well-balanced, practical, and psychologically positive diet for children of all ages.
_____ 23. Acceptable snack foods for children and teens (from a dental standpoint) include
(a) popcorn. (b) raisins. (c) pretzels. (d) a and c. (e) all of these.
_____ 24. The safest, most effective method for weight control during the growing years includes
(a) increased physical activity. (b) a low-calorie diet. (c) both of these.

STEP 8: PRE-TEST (A RETAKE) ON THE GROWING YEARS

After reading this chapter and participating in the assigned activities, you may have acquired a significant amount of new information regarding nutritional needs for the growing years from infancy through the teens. You should also have profited from the guidelines provided on diet counseling for infants, children, and teenagers. Therefore, you might want to reevaluate the responses you gave for the various sample situations depicted in Step 1. In light of the facts you have gathered throughout this chapter, make any revisions you deem necessary in your files. Explain each modification briefly. Discuss your changes with classmates or co-workers. Do you think more revisions will become necessary, as your experience as a practicing dietetic technician continues to expand?

Situation 1:

Situation 2:

Situation 3:

Situation 4:

Situation 5:

REFERENCES

BEYER, R., and MORRIS, P. 1974. Food attitudes and snacking patterns of young children. J. Nutr. Educ. *6,* Oct.–Dec., 131.

FEINGOLD, B. 1975. Hyperkinesis and learning disabilities linked to artificial food flavors and colors. Amer. J. Nursing *75,* May, 797.

NATIONAL RESEARCH COUNCIL/FOOD AND NUTRITION BOARD. 1980. Recommended Dietary Allowances, 9th Edition. Washington, DC: National Academy of Sciences.

ROSS LABORATORIES. 1976. Growth Charts: Boys/Girls from Birth to 36 Months. Columbus, OH: Ross Laboratories.

SCHACHTELE, C. 1982. Changing perspectives on the role of diet in dental caries formation. Nutr. News *45,* Dec., 13.

U.S. DEPARTMENT OF AGRICULTURE. 1978. Composition of Foods: Baby Foods—Raw, Processed, Prepared, USDA Handbook No. 8-3. Washington, DC: Government Printing Office.

Chapter Nine

Adult and Geriatric Nutrition

CHAPTER BLUEPRINT

Step 1: Take the Pre-test on Adult and Geriatric Nutrition to begin to reflect on your own understanding of the role of nutrition in the later years.

Step 2: Examine the Nutrition Facts List on adult and geriatric nutrition and prepare the assigned handout.

Step 3: Read the suggested readings on Eating for One and complete the accompanying assignment.

Step 4: Read the suggested readings on Fad Diets and complete the discussion questions.

Step 5: Examine the Normal Adult Nutrition Guidelines and complete the role play assignment.

Step 6: Examine the Geriatrics Guidelines and complete the role play assignment.

Step 7: Take the Post-test to evaluate what you have learned from the information and activities provided in this chapter.

Step 8: Reexamine the Pre-test (a Retake) and make those alterations which you deem appropriate in consideration of the information you acquired from this chapter.

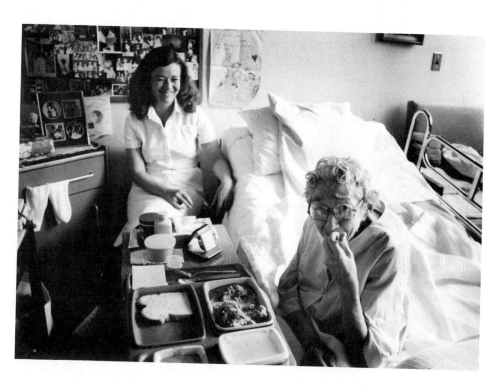

STEP 1: PRE-TEST ON ADULT AND GERIATRIC NUTRITION

Although adulthood and the elderly years are not usually thought of as periods of physical growth, the adult mind and body do develop and change in many ways. Health care is essential during this time in order to prevent chronic disease and enhance both the length and quality of life. Inadequate dietary intake may result in a shortened lifespan without the attainment of optimal levels of psychological and physiological health. As in the earlier years, it is important for an adult to become skilled at balancing his/her diet to ensure adequate nutritional status throughout life.

As a practicing dietetic technician, it is important for you to have a clear understanding of your own philosophies as they relate to patient care. For each of the following sample situations, indicate your own best response as the assigned dietetic technician; elaborate on each situation to develop a patient profile.

Record your answers using the SOAP format (see Chapter 1, Step 6) and indicate whether you would employ the assistance of other health professionals. Discuss your answers with classmates or co-workers. Do you think that future training and experience will alter your responses? You may want to reexamine your answers after you have completed Chapter 9, and again once you have dealt with a number of real-life situations similar to the samples that follow.

Situation 1:   An underweight middle-aged woman with diagnosed depression and a developing problem with alcohol abuse is referred to the out-patient nutrition clinic for diet counseling and aid in weight gain. As the assigned dietetic technician, I would

Situation 2:   A slightly overweight male in his early fifties who attends a departmental workshop on "Diet for Health and Longevity" asks for some suggestions for an increased lifespan. As a dietetic technician assisting in the conduction of the workshop, I would

Situation 3:   A friend of the family in her early thirties has decided to use oral contraceptives and is wondering whether there are any dietary changes she should consider. As a practicing dietetic technician, I would

Situation 4:   An elderly male is losing weight and refusing most meal trays. As a dietetic technician at the nursing home where he is living, I would

Situation 5:   An elderly female is new to the Meals-on-Wheels program and is markedly overweight. As the dietetic technician assisting the individuals included in this dietary program, I would

STEP 2: NUTRITION FACTS

By the time an individual reaches adulthood, lifestyle patterns are usually ingrained and it can be difficult to alter typical habits, including levels of physical activity and individual dietary intakes. Although many of today's consumers are more interested in and informed about health maintenance than the adults of a generation or two ago, the motivation to lead a healthy life and the knowledge required to do so are often lacking. Especially as aging progresses and social isolation increases, diet dwindles in overall quality for many individuals—and the physical and psychological ailments that accompany poor nutrition can contribute to failing health. To improve significantly the quality of life, optimal health is a must. Nutrition and diet play an integral role in the attainment and maintenance of good health—at any age. No one is ever too old for dietary self-improvement. The following Nutrition Facts List provides some of the most current diet-related information to include in counseling both individuals in their middle years and the aged.

Nutrition Facts List

Middle Years

1.   The adult years can be considered simply as a continuum of the earlier years with different physical and psychological influences on nutritional status and overall health, including the stresses of aging.

2.   Employment can influence dietary patterns due to hectic schedules, cocktail parties and business lunches, business trips, etc. Homemakers can also suffer nutrition imbalances due to erratic meal patterns, too much readily accessible food, and familial stresses.

3.   The financial burden of rearing a family can have a negative effect on the food budget.

4.   The traditional family dinner has gradually been replaced by solitary snacking and frequent dining out, so a well-balanced evening meal is no longer the norm.

5.   Many of the health problems commonly affecting the adult population can be controlled by the individual: the risks for developing a number of diseases can be significantly lowered by making simple decisions regarding cigarette smoking, alcohol use, physical activity, seat belt usage, weight control, dietary composition, and periodic screening for ailments such as high blood pressure and cancer.

6.   Upon reaching adulthood, growth is complete, the basal metabolic rate is slowing—after age 25, caloric needs decrease around 5% every decade—and the level of physical activity usually declines. Thus, energy intake should be reduced or weight gain will ensue. Activity levels can be increased, the amount and type depending on past fitness and present tolerance.

7.   Although not exclusively a female disorder, obesity is a more frequent problem in women: 12% of American women in their twenties, 20% of those aged 35 to 44, and nearly one half of those reaching their fifties are obese. This trend can also be seen in other developed countries.

8.   Although sometimes blamed for weight gain, oral contraceptives are usually only responsible for temporary fluid retention.

9.   It is estimated that around 10 million American women now use oral contraceptives, which can affect the disposition of carbohydrate, protein, fat, vitamins, and minerals. It appears that only certain women are vulnerable to nutritional depletion and the effects differ with each individual, but it is usually the water-soluble vitamins that are depleted.

10.   The body is sometimes able to adapt to the metabolic effects of oral contraceptives, and it is not possible to predict the nutritional consequences unless the user's dietary intake and nutritional status are analyzed.

11.   **Megaloblastic anemia** can occur in those users of oral contraceptives who are at nutritional risk due to (a) a diet low in folic acid, (b) an excessive alcohol intake, (c) the use of certain anticonvulsant medications, (d) the presence of malabsorption syndromes, and (e) a pregnancy immediately following the discontinuance of oral contraceptives.

megaloblastic anemia: Blood disorder characterized by the presence of abnormally large, immature red blood cells known as *megaloblasts.*

12.   Since some nutrients are better absorbed with use of oral contraceptives while others are utilized less efficiently, regular over-the-counter multiple vitamin/mineral supplements may be inappropriate.

13.   Oral contraceptive users may be at increased nutritional risk (see Table 9.1), whereas those using the **IUD** may become iron deficient due to increased blood losses with menstruation.

IUD: Intrauterine contraceptive device consisting of a coil or loop which, when inserted in the uterus, interferes with the implantation of a fertilized ovum (egg); may be left in place for up to a year, but undesirable side effects can occur.

14.   Although the potential for nutritional side effects does exist, the typical oral contraceptive user has a lower nutritional risk than women with inadequate diets and those with repeated pregnancies.

15.   According to recent research, **fibrocystic breast disease** is probably not associated with consumption of the methylxanthines (chemical compounds known as caffeine, theophylline, and theobromine) found in coffee, tea, chocolate, cola, and some over-the-counter medications. However, some individuals do find that symptoms disappear with dietary change.

fibrocystic breast disease: Condition in which a number of small sacs of fluid, surrounded by fibrous thickened tissue, appear in the breasts.

16.   Caffeine is a drug. In assessing the diet, the intake of caffeine-containing products needs to be taken into consideration, especially if typical use is regular and excessive.

17.   Use of prescription drugs often leads to abuse. Since there has yet to be a drug developed which has no side effects, the hundreds of millions of prescriptions written each

Table 9.1   Nutritional Implications of Oral Contraceptive Use

Nutrient	Possible alterations with use of oral contraceptives
Carbohydrate	Elevated blood glucose.
Protein	Elevated plasma **albumin**. Increased **tryptophan** and **nicotinic acid**.
Fat	Elevated blood triglycerides. Elevated blood cholesterol in those with Type II **hyperlipoproteinemia**.
Vitamin C	Decreased blood levels.
Riboflavin	Decreased blood levels, which can lead to **glossitis**.
Vitamin B$_6$	Decreased blood levels, which can lead to abnormal tryptophan metabolism, depression.
Folacin	Decreased blood levels, which can lead to megaloblastic anemia.
Vitamin B$_{12}$	Decreased blood levels, which can lead to anemia.
Vitamin A	Increased blood levels.
Iron	Increased blood levels.
Zinc	Decreased blood levels.
Copper	Increased blood levels.

albumin: Protein widely distributed in plant and animal tissue (e.g., serum albumin in blood, lactalbumin in milk, ovalbumin in egg white).

tryptophan: An essential amino acid.

nicotinic acid: Alternate term for niacin, also known as the antipellagra principle of the B-complex.

hyperlipoproteinemia: Increased amounts of cholesterol, phospholipid, and/or triglycerides in the blood, bound to plasma proteins and classified into five types.

glossitis: Inflammation of the tongue.

hyperlipidemia: Excessive amounts of fats in the blood.

year for mind-altering drugs are often accompanied by health ills with specific nutritional implications (see Appendix IV).

18.   Prolonged use of many prescription medications can result in nutrient depletion, especially in an alcohol user or a person who takes an excessive amount of laxatives. It is important for adults to avoid unnecessary prescriptions, limit multiple drug regimens if possible, and understand the nutritional effects of drug use.

19.   The nutritional implications of alcohol use are the same for the adult drinker as for the teen: daily consumption of large amounts of alcohol adds calories and depletes nutrients. Proper nutrition can assist the drinker in handling alcohol, but cannot protect against the damage incurred by heavy drinking. Alcohol abuse can cause **hyperlipidemia,** cancers, diseases of the gastrointestinal tract, pancreas/liver damage, muscular disorders, brain/heart damage, behavioral abnormalities, psychiatric diseases, and other ills.

20.   At birth, life expectancy is now more than 25 years longer than it was in 1900 but, at age 45, the American male has an increased life expectancy of only 5 years. The prevention of contagious disease has improved significantly, but current treatment for chronic disease has not.

21.   Parkinson's disease occurs most frequently in late middle age; the incurable, progressive degeneration of the central nervous system can create, among other problems, feeding difficulties and constipation. Those treated with levodopa must limit the intake of vitamin B$_6$, including supplements which contain the vitamin.

22.   More than one half of the deaths in this country can be attributed to coronary artery disease and stroke, but the gradual decline over the past decade accounts for much of the drop in the overall mortality rate. This trend should continue with improvements in the detection/control of high blood pressure, a reduction in cigarette smoking, an increase in exercise and fitness, stress management, and desirable dietary alterations.

23.   Maintenance of a well-balanced diet during adulthood can help to meet nutritional requirements and maintain health in the later years.

Elderly Years

1.   Our fastest growing "minority" is the over-fifty age group. In 1900, those aged 65 and over represented 4% of the American population, and now represent more than 11%.

2.   Although long life is certainly desirable, the quality of life may be even more important. Aging does not mean incapacitation, and performance is enhanced by remaining or becoming fit.

3.   Nutrition for the elderly is basically the same as it is during other stages in the life cycle, but some specific needs are distinctly different.

4.   Aging begins at the time of conception and continues all throughout the life span. As aging progresses, cell metabolism decreases and cells are lost. The rate of nerve impulse transmission slows, protein tissue begins to be replaced by adipose (even in the normal weight individual), and the senses are dulled.

5.   It is only a social fact that age 65 begins senior citizenry, since there is no uniform biological decline in physical/psychological function which begins at this time.

6.   The diets of the elderly population are more likely than those of younger persons to be inadequate, due in part to ill health: 80% of the elderly population suffer from one or more chronic conditions.

7.   The major factor affecting dietary balance is income, making an adequate budget or use of available food programs (Food Stamps, Supplemental Security Income, Title VII Nutrition) essential for attaining a desirable nutritional status (Watkin 1983).

8.   Grocery shopping can be difficult for aged persons if supermarkets are inaccessible and unaffordable. Home delivery and supermarket busing can help to solve this problem.

9.   Dental disease is common in the elderly due to the gradual loss of teeth plus poor oral hygiene. Swallowing becomes more difficult due to reduced salivary flow, and dentures can hamper chewing. Reduction in the number of taste buds interferes with taste, and ill-fitting dentures can interfere even further with eating pleasure.

10.   Gum disease increases in incidence with age, affecting 90% of those aged 65–74.

11.   American citizens over the age of 65 often fail to include enough iron, vitamins A and C, and calcium in their diets and tend to rely too much on foods high in simple carbohydrates, saturated fats, and/or sodium.

12.   The RDAs for several nutrients [see National Research Council/Food and Nutrition Board (1980)] are given for the single age group of "51-plus" (with different calorie levels for ages 51–75 and for 76-plus), yet there are significant differences between individuals that occur as aging progresses. Research into aging and the nutritional implications was minimal until the societal and governmental impact of this expanding population were realized during the 1980s.

13.   Although most of the major studies (DHHS 1972; DHHS 1975; USDA 1972) of the elderly population do not reveal typical dietary intakes significantly below the RDAs for most nutrients, these surveys usually fail to include individuals who are institutionalized—it is these persons who are more likely to suffer from malnutrition (Natow and Heslin 1980). Also, studies indicate that the elderly tend to underreport large food intakes and overreport smaller meals in order to appear nutritionally sound (Natow and Heslin 1980).

14.   Unless prescribed by the physician, there is no need to take vitamin/mineral supplements. Elderly individuals vulnerable to "health" food claims should be warned that there exists no dietary fountain of youth.

15.   To offset the catabolic processes of aging, adequate protein (same as adult RDA) is required, but elderly persons may not eat meat due to budgetary constraints and chewing difficulties; the use of alternatives such as cheese, eggs, peanut butter, and tofu should be encouraged.

16.   The elderly are at nutritional risk for developing iron-deficiency anemia, as dietary intake tends to be inadequate and absorption is diminished due to reduced gastric acid secretion; absorption of vitamin B_{12} may also be decreased due to a reduction in the presence of the **intrinsic factor.** Inexpensive, chewable sources of iron and B_{12} should be included in the diet; if necessary, the physician may advise supplementation.

intrinsic factor: Substance present in gastric juice which aids in the absorption of vitamin B_{12}.

17.   Daily ingestion of mineral oil as a laxative can cause deficiencies in the fat-soluble vitamins; fiber-rich foods and prune juice make wiser choices for those elderly persons suffering from constipation. An increased intake of fluids and daily exercise can also be helpful.

18.   Constipation is a frequent problem for the elderly, especially in the bed-ridden, and is caused by lack of adequate fiber and fluids, decrease in intestinal muscle tone, laxative abuse, insufficient food intake, medical problems, and/or certain medications. Intestinal gas is also a common problem as intestinal motility is slowed and gas is trapped; treatment includes the selective elimination of foods from the individual diet—in order to discover those items causing symptoms—and replacement with nutritionally equivalent foods, as well as education on eating slowly to minimize the swallowing of air.

19.   Psychological factors associated with poor dietary intake in the elderly include diminished self-worth, relocation or death of family and friends resulting in loss of emotional support, isolation and loneliness, lack of socialization and stimulation, as well as fear of death.

20.   Solitary dining can be emotionally depressing, and familial death and separation can further diminish appetite.

21.   Home-delivered Meals-on-Wheels and congregate (group) meals programs—organized by councils on aging, anti-poverty groups, hospitals, churches, and volunteer clubs—provide meals which meet one third of the RDAs. The nutrition education component emphasizes those nutrients/foods apt to be lacking in the elderly individual's diet, and discusses meal planning, budgeting, and cooking for one.

22.   Cooking for one (or two) requires knowledge of budgeting, marketing, food storage and preparation techniques, as well as the use of imagination to avoid mono-diets based on very few foods (e.g., tea and toast) or irregular meals. Suggestions to give elderly persons seeking to improve their food attitudes should include the following: (a) Use foods which vary in texture if taste sensations are dulled. (b) Drink a small glass of wine before dinner to stimulate appetite. (c) Divide food intake into five or six small meals/snacks and eat at regular times. (d) Avoid repetition of the same food/flavor/color/texture at meals. (e) Chop, grind, or blenderize foods that are difficult to chew, or mash them; use baby foods only if they are enjoyed. (f) Share foods or meals with others and dine out occasionally; be sure to take advantage of senior citizen discounts. (g) Take a daily walk. (h) Eat slowly, chew thoroughly, and drink plenty of fluids. (i) Eat a well-balanced diet that is both nutritious and tasty.

23.   In planning menus for the elderly, it is important to consider individual likes and dislikes. Breakfast is typically favored by the aged, so can be well suited to nutritional needs. Influencing factors such as ethnic background, religion, and social class need to be considered in menu planning, as should long-held beliefs about home remedies.

24.   Dietary habits develop gradually over time, and rapid changes can prove threatening. Dietary patterns may represent security for some elderly persons. Condescension is an undesirable attitude for those attempting to provide elderly persons with dietary assistance.

25.   Chronic diseases common in the elderly include obesity, diabetes, atherosclerosis, hypertension, arthritis, and orthopedic disorders. The most prevalent health conditions which afflict today's elderly include arthritis, auditory/visual impairments, hypertension, and heart disease. Each ailment can affect nutritional status, but dietary intervention is geared towards overall health maintenance rather than cure of long-held disabilities. After age 65, few people are free of illness or impairment, with about half reporting a resultant limitation on activity.

26.   With increasing amounts of time on their hands after retirement, elderly individuals may begin to overeat and nibble on snack foods, or they may lose their appetites. Many benefit by finding new hobbies and increasing physical activity.

27.   Especially for women after age 60, typical energy intake of elderly individuals tends to be low. This allows for nutritional inadequacies and can result in the onset of diet deficiency diseases.

28.   Undesirable weight loss can be reversed simply by increasing caloric intake. Aged persons are often overwhelmed when faced with large servings, making frequent smaller meals/snacks preferable—with or without supplemental products such as shakes or puddings.

29.   Elderly individuals commonly suffer from varying degrees of maldigestion/malabsorption due to (a) diminished **hydrochloric acid,** enzymes, and/or bile salts; (b) bacterial overgrowth in the small intestine (due to decreased acidity); (c) reduction in the number of functioning intestinal **villi,** with decreased absorption capabilities; (d) infections, **enteritis,** parasitic infestation; (e) localized surgery; (f) removal of part or all of the stomach or small intestine; (g) drug effects; and (h) individual intolerances.

30.   The reduced secretion of bile with aging causes lowered tolerance for fatty foods and an increased tendency for the development of **gallstones.**

31.   **Hiatus hernia** is common in the aged, and can be treated by provision of small, nonspicy meals; antacids may be prescribed, some of which provide significant amounts of calcium.

32.   For most individuals, blood pressure increases with age, but this is variable and individualistic; sodium may need to be restricted and weight loss may be required. Hyperlipidemia is not considered to be as influential a risk factor as in the younger years, but it is best to prevent the onset early in life rather than to try to treat the problem in later years.

33.   Specific foods do not cause arthritis or increase joint inflammation (except in **gout**), but diet therapy is a consideration in the following: (a) Sufferers of rheumatoid arthritis are

hydrochloric acid: Highly acidic constituent of gastric juice which aids in digestion.

villi: Threadlike hairs which line the gastrointestinal tract, increasing surface area and assisting nutrient absorption.

enteritis: Inflammation of the mucous tissues of the small intestine.

gallstone: Stonelike mass which forms in the gallbladder or bile ducts, composed of cholesterol, bilirubin, and protein; presence of stone(s) is condition known as *cholelithiasis.*

hiatus (or **hiatal**) **hernia:** Protrusion of a portion of the stomach through the diaphragm.

gout: Acute and chronic condition in which excessive amounts of uric acid appear in the blood and may be deposited in joints and other tissues; due to metabolic disorder involving purines.

often underweight, and might require increased calcium intakes. (b) Sufferers of osteo-arthritis may need to lose weight. (c) Sufferers of gout may need to lose weight and limit the dietary intake of fat, alcohol, and foods high in **purines.**

34.   Osteoporosis is a skeletal disorder with a decrease in the amount of bone which can lead to fractures, immobilization, and inactivity; symptoms appear far more frequently in females, and causative factors may include improper diet, lack of physical activity, hormonal imbalances, kidney dysfunction (calcium is not conserved or bone is increasingly resorbed), and defective intestinal absorption of certain nutrients. Treatment includes an adequate calcium intake, the development of proper muscle tone, increases in physical activity and dietary/sunlight sources of vitamin D, and sufficient intake of vitamin C and fluoride; dietary surveys have indicated deficiencies in calcium and vitamin D plus high intakes of **phosphate** in symptomatic osteoporotic females.

35.   The incidence of skin breakdown increases with age, due mainly to prolonged immobilization; **decubitus ulcers** occur more commonly in obese and underweight indi-viduals, with anemia and dehydration acting to worsen the condition. If the patient's nutri-tional status is poor, dietary improvement can aid in wound healing.

36.   Over 85% of the elderly population take prescription drugs, and the elderly are particularly susceptible to drug reactions and to food–drug interactions. Caffeine intake can hinder sleep and affect certain drug actions. Alcohol is detrimental if abused, but can be used in small quantities to stimulate appetite and enhance socialization as long as the concurrent use of medication(s) is also considered.

37.   Malnutrition in the elderly handicapped person living independently can be a problem, but may be solved with the use of convenience products, self-help eating devices, and architectural household changes.

38.   Nutritional assessments with the elderly should include medical history, diet histo-ry, 24-hour recall, food intake records, anthropometric measurements, physical exam for clinical signs of poor nutrition, and biochemical data in order to determine the potential for nutritional risk. Body weight alone is the most useful measurement tool. Laboratory data should include measurements for hemoglobin, plasma ascorbate, serum protein, and possi-ble elevations in vitamins A, D, and E due to oversupplementation.

39.   Elderly individuals who are institutionalized are greatly influenced by their en-vironment. Upgrading their overall nutritional status will improve their health. Some common examples of positive steps for institutional foodservices include the following: (a) Food is made fresh; the time period between preparation, cooking, and serving is short. (b) Meal-time is leisurely and foodservice is personal; independent dining facilities are available. (c) Foodservice and dining atmosphere are attractive. (d) Food is appetizing in appearance, texture, and flavor. (e) Hot foods are served hot and cold foods are served cold. (f) Menu is varied, using few institution and convenience foods but relying heavily on home-cooked products. (g) Diner's individual input is considered; the specifics of modified diets are kept on record. (h) Portion size is variable with provision for individual needs. (i) Assistance for feeding is available. (j) Weight fluctuations are noted. (k) Daily stimulation is available so that interest in eating, appetite, mood, and the resulting dietary intake are healthy.

40.   Nutritional deficiencies are one of the many causes of apparent, treatable **senility** —as well as drug interactions, depression, metabolic disorders, certain tumors, alcohol toxicity, sensory deprivation, anemia, and chronic infections.

41.   Nutrition educators should be aware of those changes which accompany aging that can affect learning: vision, audition, memory, motivation, and health status may influ-ence learning skills.

42.   Although nutrition education is essential for the young since dietary habits are not yet ingrained, modifications are possible at any stage of the life cycle.

43.   Psychological and nutritional preparation for the later years begins early in life; an individual who has remained lean, eaten a wide variety of foods, and kept physically active is most able to handle the changes and stresses of aging.

purines: End products of the digestion of certain dietary proteins that break down into uric acid; also manufactured by the body.

phosphate: Chemical important in main-taining the acid–base balance of the blood; used as a food additive.

decubitus ulcer: Open sore due to pres-sure exerted on the body, particularly the but-tocks, from confinement to bed or chair.

senility: Loss of mental and/or physical control associated with old age and due to gradual body deterioration.

Exercise on Nutrition Facts

Using the preceding list, prepare a simplified one-page version to hand out to either adults on normal diets or to the elderly. You may include graphics and/or use a poster format as desired; see the Sample Handout. Show your handout in rough draft form to classmates or co-workers for constructive criticism on the overall design, content, and potential effectiveness for use in pertinent diet counseling situations. Then prepare a final version for your own future use as a practicing dietetic technician. You may decide to prepare several handouts aimed at different ages, or share those prepared by classmates or co-workers, in order to be better prepared for diet counseling with adults of all ages and with specific nutritional needs.

Sample Handout

Basic Food Groups

Select a variety of foods from the different food groups (see Table 9.2) to include in your daily diet.

Table 9.2   Basic Food Group Requirements

Food group	No. servings daily
Fruits and vegetables	4 or more
Breads and cereals	4 or more
Milk and cheeses	3–4 (skim or low fat)
Meats and alternates	2 (lean)
Others	Moderate amounts

Nutrition and Your Health: Dietary Guidelines for Americans[1]

1. *Eat a variety of foods.*   Include selections of fruits; vegetables; whole grain and enriched breads, cereals, and grain products; milk, cheese, and yogurt; meats, poultry, fish and eggs; and legumes (dried peas and beans).
2. *Maintain a reasonable weight.*   To improve eating habits eat slowly, prepare small portions, and avoid second helpings. To lose weight increase physical activity, eat less fat and fatty foods, eat less sugar and sweets, and avoid too much alcohol.
3. *Avoid too much fat, saturated fat, and cholesterol.*   Choose lean meat, fish, poultry, dried beans and peas as your protein sources. Moderate your use of eggs and organ meats (such as liver). Limit your intake of butter, cream, hydrogenated margarines, shortenings, coconut oil, and foods made from such products. Trim excess fat off meats. Broil, bake, or boil rather than fry. Read labels carefully to determine both amount and types of fat contained in food.
4. *Eat foods with adequate starch and fiber.*   To eat more complex carbohydrates daily, substitute starches for fats and sugars and select foods which are good sources of fiber and starch, such as whole grain breads and cereals, fruits and vegetables, beans, peas, and nuts.
5. *Avoid too much sugar.*   Use less of all sugars, including white sugar, brown sugar, raw sugar, honey, and syrups. Eat less of foods containing these sugars such as candy, soft drinks, ice cream, cakes, and cookies. Select fresh fruits or fruits canned without sugar or in light syrup rather than heavy syrup. Read food labels for clues on sugar content—if the names sucrose, glucose, maltose, dextrose, lactose, fructose, or syrups appear first, then there is a large amount of sugar. Remember, how often you eat sugar is as important as how much sugar you eat.
6. *Avoid too much sodium.*   Learn to enjoy the unsalted flavors of foods. Cook with only small amounts of added salt. Add little or no salt to food at the table. Limit your intake of salty foods such as potato chips, pretzels, salted nuts and popcorn, condiments (soy sauce, steak sauce, garlic salt), pickled foods, and cured meats. Read food labels carefully to determine the amounts of sodium in processed foods and snack items.
7. *If you drink alcohol, do so in moderation.*

[1]From USDA (1980).

STEP 3: EATING FOR ONE

All too many individuals living alone adopt a bland, repetitious, and not very nutritious dietary pattern such as the following:

Breakfast: Tea and toast, or coffee and Danish
Lunch: Soup and crackers, or coffee and a sandwich
Dinner: Beans and franks, or hamburger and fries
Snack(s): Cookies and tea, or chips and beer

Adherence to such menus is sometimes due to the existing social situation since living alone does not inspire most people to create varied and exciting meals for themselves. Older individuals are unable to get out to shop due to lack of transportation and/or physical impairment. Those living on fixed incomes may find food costs prohibitive. Dentures, if improperly fitted, can transform eating into an unpleasant, even painful experience. And many people, of all ages, simply do not like to bother with meal preparation.

Granted, the current level of scientific knowledge about the nutritional requirements for people over age 65 is incomplete. Yet, numerous studies of diet and health in the elderly have identified the major nutrition factors to be dealt with. For adults and the aged, a healthy diet is quite simple to obtain with some basic nutrition knowledge, an idea of individual needs, and the desire to make the necessary dietary changes—for life.

Exercise on Eating for One

Read some of the Suggested Readings that follow and examine the recipes in the cookbooks and cooking pamphlets. Then devise your own menu for a week of well-balanced meals and snacks that might appeal to a healthy adult or elderly individual living alone who has a diminished appetite. You may want to review the nutrition information provided in Step 2 to keep in mind the important guidelines for planning menus for adults/elderly individuals.

Compare your menus with classmates or co-workers, and devise several collective menu plans; cooperation with other members of the health care team can result in the development of varied, appetizing menus which may be accepted by even the most finicky, nonhearty, disinterested eater who is living alone.

Suggested Readings on Eating for One

ALLEN, F. 1986. Eating Well in a Busy World. Berkeley, CA: Ten Speed Press.
ARONSON, V., and STARE, F. 1986. Rx: Executive Nutrition. Hanover, MA: The Christopher Publishing House.
EISENBERG, A., EISENBERG, H., and EISENBERG, S. 1982. The Special Guest Cookbook. New York: Beaufort Books.
FOOD AND DRUG ADMINISTRATION. 1983. Making Food Dollars Count. Pueblo, CO: Consumer Information Center.
FOOD AND DRUG ADMINISTRATION. 1985. Diet and the Elderly. Pueblo, CO: Consumer Information Center.
FRIEDMAN, S., STEINHEBER, F., and LASS, A. 1980. The Doctors' Guide to Growing Older. New York: New American Library.
GOODMAN, H., and MORSE, B. 1982. Just What the Doctor Ordered. New York: Holt, Rinehart & Winston.
JESTER, P. 1986. Age Buster Cookbook. Des Moines, IA: Creative Foods Ltd.
KOMARANSKY, Z., and LACKNEY, L. 1984. The World's Most Convenient Diet. Chicago: Turnbull & Willoughby.
LONG, P. 1986. The Nutritional Ages of Women. New York: Macmillan.
NATOW, A., and HESLIN, J. 1983. Nutrition for the Prime of Your Life. New York: Macmillan.
OSBORNE, K. 1985. Do Cook for One! Seattle, WA: K-D Enterprises.
PRUDDEN, B. 1986. Bonnie Prudden's After Fifty Fitness Guide. New York: Ballantine.
STARE, F., and ARONSON, V. 1985. Food for Fitness After Fifty. Philadelphia: George F. Stickley Co.
WILSON, J. 1987. Eating Well When You Just Can't Eat the Way You Used To . . . The Over 50 Cookbook. New York: Workman.

For cooking pamphlets:

Cooking for One: In the Senior Years. New York State College of Human Ecology, Cornell University, Ithaca, NY 14850.

Eats in My Room. Department of Social and Health Services, Health Services Division, PO Box 1788, Olympia, WA 98504.

Senior Citizens Cook Alone—And Like It. Senior Citizens, Inc., 147 East Street, Ithaca, NY 14850.

Single Burner Chef Cookbook. New Hampshire Network, PO Box 2, Durham, NH 03824.

STEP 4: HEALTHY PLUS?

Much of the dietary information currently available to the general public is based more on marketing strategy than on nutrition fact. When individuals who are at nutritional risk—the undernourished, the elderly, and those on medications and suffering from illnesses—adopt the dietary advice of self-proclaimed nutritionists, the side effects can prove damaging, even fatal. The elderly often are more susceptible to health hoaxes owing to their natural desire to stay young—and alive—for as long as possible. Thus, many unproven dietary claims are aimed at those seeking the mythical Fountain of Youth.

As a practicing dietetic technician in nutrition care, it is your responsibility to help protect both the adult and the elderly populations from falling prey to dangerous dietary claims. By educating the mature public on the basics of normal nutrition and their own special needs, you can provide them with a sturdy foundation on which to base their individual dietary practices. Then, by warning them about the dangers of fad diets and mega-supplements, you can assist the public to preserve and/or improve upon their individual states of overall health—and to save money, as well.

Exercise on Fad Diets

Read some of the articles from the following Suggested Readings on Fad Diets and Professional Critiques and answer the Discussion Questions that follow. Discuss your answers with classmates or co-workers. Also, begin to scan the media—television, magazines, newspapers, billboards, books, leaflets, etc.—for misleading advertisements for dietary aids specifically aimed at today's older population. You may want to begin to develop a file on nutrition misinformation to use in counseling aging individuals susceptible to the barrage of misleading dietary advice currently marketed to the nutritionally naive public.

Suggested Readings on Fad Diets and Professional Critiques

AMERICAN COUNCIL ON SCIENCE AND HEALTH. 1981. Book Review: Dr. Atkins' Nutrition Breakthrough. ACSH News and Views, Nov./Dec., 7.

AMERICAN MEDICAL ASSOCIATION. 1974. A Critique of Low-Carbohydrate Ketogenic Weight Reduction Regimens. Chicago: AMA.

ATKINS, R. 1981. Dr. Atkins' Nutrition Breakthrough. New York: William Morrow & Co.

BARRETT, S. 1982. The legacy of Adelle Davis. Environmental Nutrition, Nov., S-3.

BERGER, S. 1987. How to Be Your Own Nutritionist. New York: William Morrow & Co.

BERLAND, T. 1986. Rating the Diets. New York: Signet Books.

CALIFORNIA DIETETIC ASSOCIATION. 1987. Popular Diets: How They Rate. Santa Monica, CA: Los Angeles District California Dietetic Association.

COWLEY, D., and SIZER, F. 1987. Fad Diets: Fact *and* Fiction? Nutrition Clin. 2, Jun., 1.

DAVIS, ADELLE. Any book.

DE BOER, J., et al. 1986. Adaptation of energy metabolism in overweight women. Am. J. Clin. Nutr. *44,* Nov., 585.

DIAMOND, H., and DIAMOND, M. 1985. Fit for Life. New York: Warner Books.

DIAMOND, H., and DIAMOND, M. 1987. Fit for Life II: Living Health. New York: Warner Books.

FISHER, M., and LACHANCE, P. 1985. Nutrition evaluation of published weight-reducing diets. J. Am. Dietet. Assoc. *85,* Apr., 450.

GRINKER, J. 1973. Behavioral and metabolic consequences of weight reduction. J. Am. Dietet. Assoc. *62,* Jan., 30.

HARRIS, L. (Editor). Current Diet Reviews. Box 1914, Rialto, CA 92376.

KATAHN, M. 1986. The Rotation Diet. New York: W. W. Norton.

MAZEL, J. 1981. The Beverly Hills Diet. New York: Macmillan.

MIRKIN, G., and SHORE, R. 1981. The Beverly Hills Diet: Dangers of the newest weight loss fad. J. Am. Med. Assoc. 245, Jun. 5, 2239.

PEARSON, D., and SHAW, S. 1982. Life Extension: A Practical Scientific Approach. New York: Warner.

ROCK, C., and COULSTON, A. 1988. Weight control approaches: A review by the California Dietetic Association. J. Am. Dietet. Assoc. 88, Jan., 44.

SOCIETY FOR NUTRITION EDUCATION. 1986. Book review: Fit for Life. J. Nutr. Educ. 18, Jun., 136.

SOCIETY FOR NUTRITION EDUCATION. 1986. Rotation Diet review. J. Nutr. Educ. 18, Dec., 280.

SOCIETY FOR NUTRITION EDUCATION. 1988a. Book review: Fit for Life II. J. Nutr. Educ. 20, Apr., 98.

SOCIETY FOR NUTRITION EDUCATION. 1988b. Book review: How to Be Your Own Nutritionist. J. Nutr. Educ. 20, Apr., 97.

SOCIETY FOR NUTRITION EDUCATION. 1988c. Book review: The 35-Plus Diet for Women. J. Nutr. Educ. 20, Apr., 100.

SPODNICK, J., and GIBBONS, B. 1987. The 35-Plus Diet for Women. New York: Harper & Row.

SUBCOMMITTEE ON HEALTH AND LONG-TERM CARE, SELECT COMMISSION ON AGING. 1984. Quackery: The $10 Billion Scandal, House Document No. 98-262. Washington, DC: Government Printing Office.

WILLIS, J. 1985. Diet books sell well but . . . . FDA Consumer, Mar., 14.

YETIV, J. 1986a. A Review of "Life Extension." In Popular Nutritional Practices: A Scientific Appraisal, pp. 82–101. Toledo, OH: Popular Medicine Press.

YETIV, J. 1986b. Beverly Hills Diet (critique). In Popular Nutritional Practices: A Scientific Appraisal, p. 278. Toledo, OH: Popular Medicine Press.

Discussion Questions on Fad Diets

1. Briefly describe the nutritional deficits and potential side effects of Dr. Atkins' diet (and other low-carbohydrate regimens):

2. Briefly describe the nutritional drawbacks associated with the Beverly Hills Diet, and the Fit for Life programs (and other food combining diets):

3. Briefly describe the metabolic consequences of the 35-Plus Diet and the Rotation Diet (and other low-calorie diets):

4. List some of the nutrition fallacies proposed by Adelle Davis; describe the more recent dietary controversies of Dr. Berger:

5. Briefly describe one of the latest fad diets and the nutritional and health implications for adherents:

6. What would you advise a friend who had decided to try one of the fad diets described in questions 1–5?

STEP 5: NORMAL ADULT NUTRITION GUIDELINES

In order to be able to advise normal, healthy adults on the development of desirable dietary patterns, it is essential to have access to all of the hands-on material required for effective counseling sessions. It is also important to be able to record all of the pertinent information regarding each counseling session in the patient's medical charts. If you found it difficult to complete the Pre-test in Step 1, some of the information provided below should help to improve your confidence—and skills—regarding your counseling abilities.

This step includes suggested counseling strategies to use with healthy adults. Use the references on normal nutrition included in Appendix V. The following references on counseling may also prove helpful.

Suggested Readings on Counseling

AMERICAN DIETETIC ASSOCIATION. 1978. ADA Patient Care Audit: Quality Assurance Procedure Manual for Dietitians. Chicago: ADA.

ARONSON, V., FITZGERALD, B., and HEWES, L. 1990. Guidebook for Nutrition Counselors, 2nd Edition. Englewood Cliffs, NJ: Prentice-Hall.

BARTLEY, K. 1986. Dietetic Practitioner Skills. New York: Macmillan.

BERNSTEIN, L. (Editor). 1985. Interviewing: A Guide for Health Professionals. Norwalk, CT: Appleton-Century-Crofts.

D'ANDREA, V., and SALOVEY, P. 1983. Peer Counseling: Skills and Perspectives. Palo Alto, CA: Science and Behavior Books.

DANISH, S., D'ANGELLI, A., and HAVER, A., 1980. Helping Skills: A Basic Training Program. New York: Human Sciences Press.

DIKOVICS, A. 1987. Nutritional Assessment: Case Study Methods. Philadelphia: George F. Stickley Co.

DOWNEY, M., and HALFORD, B. 1982. Nutrition Counseling. Boston: Joselin Diabetes Center.

EGAN, G. 1982. The Skilled Helper. Monterey, CA: Brooks/Cole Publishing Co.

GARRETT, A. 1972. Interviewing: Its Principles and Methods. New York: Family Service Association of America.

HOLLI, B., and CALABRESE, R. 1986. Communication and Education Skills: The Dietitian's Guide. Philadelphia: Lea & Febiger.

IOWA RESEARCH CLINIC. 1981. Intensive Workshop on Nutrition Counseling Manual. Iowa City: Iowa Research Clinic.

JASMUND, J. 1981. The Diet History: A Tool and a Process. East Lansing, MI: Michigan State University Press.

KRALL, E., DWYER, J., and COLEMAN, K. 1988. Factors influencing the accuracy of dietary recall. Nutrition Res. 8, Jul., 829.

LOWENSTEIN, M., et al. 1986. Integrating diet therapy and dietary counseling: An alternative education technique. J. Am. Dietet. Assoc. 86, Jan., 44.

NATIONAL INSTITUTES OF HEALTH. 1984. Building Nutrition Counseling Skills. Washington, DC: Government Printing Office.

PURKEY, W. W. 1987. The Inviting Relationship: An Expanded Perspective for Professional Counseling. Englewood Cliffs, NJ: Prentice-Hall.

SCHILLER, M. 1988. Ethical issues in nutrition care. J. Am. Dietet. Assoc. 88, Jan., 13.

SNETSELAAR, L., et al. 1981. Model workshops on nutrition counseling. J. Am. Dietet. Assoc. 79, Dec., 678.

SOCIETY FOR NUTRITION EDUCATION. 1988. Nutrition Information Resources for Professionals. Oakland, CA: SNE.

VICKERY, C., and HODGES, P. 1986. Counseling strategies for dietary management: Expanded possibilities for effecting behavior change. J. Am. Dietet. Assoc. 86, Jul., 924.

For audiovisual:

Studies of the Patient Perspective, Viewpoint: Nutrition. American Association of Diabetes Educators, 500 North Michigan Avenue, Suite 1400, Chicago, IL 60611.

Counseling Guidelines—Normal Adults

Table 9.3 General Outline for Adult Counseling

I. Initial Session
  A. General Guidelines
  B. Patient Records
    1. Medical History Form
    2. 24-Hour Recall Form
  C. Assignments
    1. Food Intake Record
    2. Diet History
  D. Technician's Notes
II. Follow-up Session(s)
  A. General Guidelines
  B. Handouts
    1. Personal Diet Plan
    2. Good Eating Checklist
    3. Learning Assessment Quiz
  C. Technician's Notes

Table 9.3 outlines the steps for diet counseling with healthy adults. The following material gives the details of each step.

I.   Initial Session

I.   A.   General Guidelines

1. Use Medical History Form to assess patient's nutritional status.

2. Assist patient in recording 24-hour recall of food intake using 24-Hour Recall Form. This will aid in keeping an accurate Food Intake Record.

3. Assign patient to keep daily Food Intake Record so that typical food intake patterns can be evaluated. Instruct patient not to deviate from normal eating patterns. Stress the importance of recording food intake immediately after eating.

4. Instruct patient to complete Diet History. This provides for a basic evaluation of food intake patterns. (Use Pre-test from Chapter 2.)

5. Record assessment and recommendation(s) using the SOAP method (see Chapter 1, Step 6) in Technician's Notes. This form can be kept in your files with a copy in the patient's medical records.

I. B. Patient Records

1. Medical History Form

Date _____ Referred by _____

Name _____ Date of birth _____

Address _____ Phone no. _____

Occupation _____ Hours per work week _____ Work phone no. _____

Educational background _____ Religious/ethnic background _____

Sex _____ Marital status _____

Household composition: Live alone _____ Spouse _____ Children/No. _____

Other: _____

General health status:

Physician _____ Address _____

Phone no. _____ Date of last visit _____

Ambulatory care required? _____ If so, describe: _____

Neuromuscular problems? _____ If so, how is eating affected? _____

Visual/auditory problems? _____ If so, describe: _____

Chewing difficulties? _____ If so, describe: _____

Appetite typically good? _____ fair? _____ poor? _____

Digestion/elimination difficulties? _____ If so, describe: _____

Food intolerances? _____ If so, describe: _____

Other: _____

Height _____ Weight _____ Frame _____

Triceps skinfold thickness _____ Mid-arm circumference _____

Mid-arm muscle circumference _____

Weight changes/problems? _____ If so, describe: _____

Clinical signs of nutritional status:

Skin _____ Mouth _____

Hair _____ Eyes _____

Teeth _____ Other: _____

Lab data:

Blood pressure _____

CBC _____

Serum albumin _____

Other: _____

Medications taken regularly: _____

Prescribed by: _____ Date(s) prescribed: _____

Nutrition supplements taken regularly: _____

Prescribed by: _____ Date(s) prescribed: _____

Special diet prescription: _____

Prescribed by: _____ Date of prescription: _____

How closely is diet followed? Always adhered to ___ Sometimes ___ Rarely ___ Never ___

Type of housing: Room _____ Apartment _____ Home _____ Institution _____

Prepare own meals? _____ Dine out? Often (more than once a day) _____ Rarely _____

Food shopping done independently? _____ If not, describe required assistance: _____

Eligible for food stamps? _____ If so, are they currently being used? _____

Cigarette smoker? _____ If so, how much: _____

Exercise regularly? _____ If so, describe: _____

No. times per week _____ No. minutes per session _____

Comments: _____

2. 24-Hour Recall Form

Date	Time	Food and amount

I. C. Assignments

1. Food Intake Record

Date	Time	Food/Amount	Where[a]	With whom	Associated activity[b]

[a]Such as work, restaurant, kitchen, living room.
[b]For example, watching television, reading, socializing, driving, talking on the phone, cooking.

2. Diet History

Use the Pre-test from Chapter 2 (p. 30) to provide a record of typical foods eaten.

I. D. Technician's Notes

Patient: _____   Date: _____

S   (Subjective data—how patient feels):
O   (Objective data—physical measurements including diet/nutritional status):
A   (Assessment—acceptability of dietary progress/nutritional status):
P   (Plan—diet prescription and instruction):
Comments:

II. Follow-up Session(s)

II. A. General Guidelines

1. Review assignments and discuss dietary patterns with patient.
2. Individualize Personal Diet Plan and instruct patient in its use.
3. Using Food Intake Record and Good Eating Checklist, assist patient in a general evaluation of nutrient intake.
4. Instruct patient to self-evaluate adherence to Personal Diet Plan and development

of good eating habits through continued use of Food Intake Record and Good Eating Checklist.

5. Assign Learning Assessment Quiz to evaluate counseling process and to determine if additional counseling is needed.

6. Record assessment and recommendation(s) using the SOAP method in Technician's Notes. This form can be kept in your files with a copy in the patient's medical records.

II. B. Handouts

1. Personal Diet Plan

Name: _____

How to use diet plan:
1. Select a variety of foods from each of the Basic Food Groups.
2. Include the recommended number of servings from each Food Group.
3. Drink 6–8 cups of fluid daily.
4. For aid in prevention of constipation, eat foods *high in fiber* and drink plenty of liquids.
5. For females, foods *high in iron* may need to be included in the diet to avoid anemia.

Table 9.4 gives the daily nutritional needs for a normal adult.

Table 9.4   Adult Nutritional Needs

Food group (number of servings per day)

Fruits and vegetables (4; 1 citrus or good source of vitamin C; dark green or bright
   yellow vegetable several times a week)
Breads and cereals (4)
Milk and cheeses (3)
Meats and alternates (2)

Foods high in fiber

Whole grain breads and cereals
Raw fruits, including skins and seeds
Dried fruits (prunes and prune juice may act as laxatives)
Vegetables, including skins and seeds (especially raw/lightly cooked)
Bran products
Popcorn, nuts, seeds

Foods high in iron

Meat, especially organ meats
Oysters, clams
Legumes
Whole grain and enriched breads and cereals
Dried fruits and their juices
Dark green leafy vegetables
Potato, sweet potato
Foods cooked in iron cookware

2. Good Eating Checklist

Instructions: Using Food Intake Record, total the number of daily servings from each Food Group and transfer to this chart. Evaluate by comparison to Recommended Daily Servings (RDSs).

Day	No. of servings/Food group					
	Fruits	Vegetables	Grains	Milk	Meat	Others
1						
2						
3						
4						
5						
RDSs	2	2	4	3	2	—

3. Learning Assessment Quiz

Answer true (T) or false (F) to the following statements:

_____ 1. No single food contains all the nutrients required for proper growth and health.
_____ 2. Protein is the principle source of energy for the body.
_____ 3. All nutrients required by the body can be provided by food.
_____ 4. Vitamins and minerals are good sources of energy for the body.
_____ 5. Fat provides more calories per gram than either protein or carbohydrate.
_____ 6. Bread and potatoes should be avoided during a weight loss program.
_____ 7. Sherbet provides calories and a good variety of nutrients.
_____ 8. As caloric requirements decrease, nutrient needs lessen as well.
_____ 9. All chemicals must be listed on food labels.
_____ 10. "Light" foods are always low in caloric content.
_____ 11. Additives are dangerous to health because they are chemicals.
_____ 12. Natural and synthetic vitamin supplements are of equal nutritional value.

II. C. Technician's Notes

Patient: _____   Date: _____

S (Subjective data—how patient feels):
O (Objective data—physical measurements including diet/nutritional status):
A (Assessment—acceptability of dietary progress/nutritional status):
P (Plan—diet prescription and instruction):
Comments:

Adult Nutrition Counseling Role Playing

Keeping in mind the preceding Suggested Readings and Counseling Guidelines, participate in one or more of the following role play situations. Elaborate on each situation to create a patient/audience profile. Select different partners for each situation, either classmates or co-workers. You may want to utilize your handout from Step 2. As a dietetic technician in nutrition care, do you consider yourself capable of conducting effective counseling sessions on normal adult nutrition? Would you or other adults in your family be able to adhere to your nutrition guidelines for balancing the diet?

Role Play Situation 1. As a dietetic technician in a large teaching hospital, you are often required to provide normal nutrition counseling for interested patients who are being discharged. Follow the guidelines to complete the charts and provide one such healthy 45-year-old male (postoperative for minor prostate surgery) with an individualized diet plan. Prepare a SOAP note which could be recorded in the patient's medical chart.

Role Play Situation 2. As a dietetic technician assigned to the obstetrics—gynecology out-patient clinic, you are required to provide nutrition counseling to oral contraception (O.C.) users. Follow the guidelines to complete the charts and provide one such healthy 32-

year-old female with an individualized diet plan. You might want to prepare a table of possible dietary modifications for O.C. users to consider (see Nutrition Facts List and Table 9.1 in Step 2). Prepare a SOAP note which could be recorded in the patient's medical chart.

Role Play Situation 3. As a dietetic technician in a public health department, you are assisting in the development of a workshop entitled "For Adults Only: Optimizing Nutrition." Prepare an outline on one aspect of normal adult nutrition (e.g., weight control, cardiovascular risk factors, balancing the diet, nutrition nonsense, or use of alcohol) and present it to the audience. Prepare a brief written report on the workshop (visual aids used, audience response, questions asked, suggestions/revisions for other workshops, etc.) for insertion in departmental files.

STEP 6: GERIATRICS GUIDELINES

In order to be able to advise elderly individuals on the development of desirable dietary patterns, it is essential to have access to all of the hands-on material required for effective counseling sessions. It is also important to be able to record all of the pertinent information regarding each counseling session in the patient's medical charts. If you found it difficult to complete the Pre-test in Step 1, the following information should help to improve your self-confidence and competence as a counselor.

This section includes suggested counseling strategies to use with the elderly. The following references may prove helpful.

Suggested Readings on Geriatric Nutrition

ALBANESE, A. 1980. Nutrition for the Elderly. New York: Alan R. Liss, Inc.

AMERICAN DIETETIC ASSOCIATION. 1985. Food Sensitivity Series: Lactose Intolerance. Chicago: ADA.

AMERICAN DIETETIC ASSOCIATION. 1987. Aging, Nutrition, and Fitness. Chicago: ADA.

AMERICAN DIETETIC ASSOCIATION. 1987. Position of The American Dietetic Association: Nutrition, aging, and the continuum of health care. J. Am. Dietet. Assoc. 87, Mar., 344.

ARMBRECHT, H., PENDERGAST, J., and COE, R. (Editors). 1984. Nutritional Intervention in the Aging Process. New York: Springer-Verlag.

BURDMAN, G. 1986. Healthful Aging. Englewood Cliffs, NJ: Prentice-Hall.

CHARNOFF, R. 1987. Aging and Nutrition. Nutrition Today 22, Mar./Apr., 4.

COX, E., and SANDBERG, J. 1985. Nutrition and the Elderly: A Selected Annotated Bibliography for Nutrition and Health Professionals. Washington, DC: Government Printing Office.

FANELLI, M. 1987. The ABC's of nutritional assessment in older adults. J. Nutr. Elderly 6, Spring, 33.

FELDMAN, E. (Editor). 1983. Nutrition in the Middle and Later Years. Littleton, MA: Wright-PSG.

HSU, J., and DAVIS, R. (Editors). 1981. Handbook of Geriatric Nutrition: Principles and Applications for Nutrition and Diet in Aging. Park Ridge, NJ: Noyes Publications.

HUTCHINSON, M., and MUNRO, H. 1986. Nutrition and Aging. Orlando, FL: Academic Press.

IMERSHEIN, N. 1986. A bologna sandwich for Evelyn: A case report. J. Nutr. Elderly 6, Winter, 53.

MACARTHUR-BOYER, L. 1987. Nutritional Care of the Elderly in the Long-Term Care Facility: The Components and Process of Nutritional Assessment. Available from the author at 3747 East Green Street, Pasadena, CA 91107.

MUNROE, H. 1984. Nutrition and the elderly: A general overview. J. Amer. Coll. Nutr. 3, 3, 341.

NATIONAL DAIRY COUNCIL. 1988. Nutrition and aging. Dairy Counc. Dig. 59, Jul./Aug., 19.

NATOW, A., and HESLIN, J. 1986. Nutritional Care of the Older Adult. New York: Macmillan.

NOTELOVITZ, M., and WARE, M. 1982. Stand Tall! The Informed Woman's Guide to Preventing Osteoporosis. Gainesville, FL: Triad Publishing Co.

OLSON, R. (Editor). 1988a. Diet and the maintenance of mental health in the elderly. Nutrition Rev. 46, Feb., 79.

OLSON, R. (Editor). 1988b. Diet, exercise, and chronic disease patterns in older adults. Nutrition Rev. 46, Feb., 52.

OLSON, R. (Editor). 1988c. Practical nutrition for the elderly. Nutrition Rev. 46, Feb., 83.

ORDY, J., HARMAN, D., and ALFIN-SLATER, R. 1984. Nutrition in Gerontology. New York: Raven Press.

ROE, D. 1984. Drugs and Nutrition in the Geriatric Patient. New York: Churchill Livingstone.

ROE, D. 1987. Geriatric Nutrition. Englewood Cliffs, NJ: Prentice-Hall.

ROSOVSKI, S., and NELSON, M. 1985. Nutrition for the Elderly. New York: Brookdale Institute on Aging, Columbia University.

SCHLENKER, E. 1984. Nutrition in Aging. St. Louis: C. V. Mosby Co.

SKALKA, P. 1984. The American Medical Association Guide to Health and Well-Being After Fifty. New York: Random House.

STARE, F., and ARONSON, V. 1985. Food for Fitness After Fifty. Philadelphia: George F. Stickley Co.

TREBELLA, N. 1982. Behavior Modification for Weight Control in the Elderly. Colorado Springs, CO: Acacia Nutrition Program.

U.S. CONGRESSIONAL SELECT COMMITTEE ON AGING. 1982. Directory of State and Area Agencies on Aging. Washington, DC: Government Printing Office.

VIRGINIA COUNCIL ON HEALTH AND MEDICAL CARE. 1981. Nutrition Education for the Elderly. Richmond, VA: VCHMC.

WATKIN, D. 1983. Handbook of Nutrition, Health, and Aging. Park Ridge, NJ: Noyes Publications.

WATSON, R. 1985. Handbook of Nutrition in the Aged. Boca Raton, FL: CRC Press.

WILLIAMS, S., and WORTHINGTON-ROBERTS, B. 1988. Nutrition Throughout the Life Cycle. St. Louis: Times Mirror/Mosby.

YOUNG, E. 1986. Nutrition, Aging, and Health. New York: Alan R. Liss, Inc.

For journal subscriptions:

Aging. Government Printing Office, Washington, DC 20402.

Current Literature on Aging. National Council on Aging, 1828 L Street NW, Washington, DC 20036.

Journal of Gerontology. Gerontological Society of America, 1411 K Street NW, Suite 300, Washington, DC 20005.

Journal of Nutrition for the Elderly. Haworth Press, 75 Griswold Street, Binghamton, NY 13904.

For audiovisuals:

Be Well: Health in the Later Years. Churchill Films, 662 North Robertson Boulevard, Los Angeles, CA 90069.

Food: More for Your Money. Alfred Higgins Productions, 9100 Sunset Boulevard, Los Angeles, CA 90069.

Help Yourself to Better Health. Society for Nutrition Education, 1700 Broadway, Suite 300, Oakland, CA 94612.

Spice of Life. Dairy Council of Greater Metropolitan Washington, Inc., Bethesda, MD 20892.

For further information:

American Association of Retired Persons, 1225 Connecticut Avenue NW, Washington, DC 20036.

American Dietetic Association Gerontological Nutrition Practice Group, 216 West Jackson Boulevard, Chicago, IL 60606.

Gerontological Society of America, 1411 K Street NW, Suite 300, Washington, DC 20005.

Grey Panthers, 3700 Chestnut Street, Philadelphia, PA 19104.

National Association of Area Agencies on Aging, 600 Maryland Avenue SW, Suite 208, Washington, DC 20024.

National Clearinghouse on Aging, 330 Independence Avenue NW, Washington, DC 20201.

National Council of Senior Citizens, 925 15th Street NW, Washington, DC 20005.

National Institute on Aging, National Institutes of Health, Bethesda, MD 20892.

Counseling Guidelines—Geriatrics

Table 9.5 General Outline for Geriatric Counseling

I. Initial Session
   A. General Guidelines
   B. Patient Records
       1. Medical History Form
       2. 24-Hour Recall Form
   C. Assignments
       1. Food Intake Record
       2. Diet History
   D. Technician's Notes
II. Follow-up Session(s)
   A. General Guidelines
   B. Handouts
       1. Personal Diet Plan
       2. Good Eating Checklist
   C. Technician's Notes

Table 9.5 outlines the steps for diet counseling for the elderly. The following material gives the details of each step.

I. Initial Session

I. A. General Guidelines

1. Use Medical History Form to assess patient's nutritional status.

2. Assist patient in recording 24-hour recall of food intake using 24-Hour Recall Form. This will aid in keeping an accurate Food Intake Record.

3. Assign patient to keep daily Food Intake Record so that typical food intake patterns can be evaluated. Instruct patient not to deviate from normal eating patterns. Stress the importance of recording food intake immediately after eating.

4. Instruct patient to complete Diet History. This provides for a basic evaluation of food intake patterns. (Use Pre-test from Chapter 2.)

5.   Record assessment and recommendation(s) using the SOAP method in Technician's Notes. This form can be kept in your files with a copy in the patient's medical records.

I. B. Patient Records

1. Medical History Form

Date _____ Referred by _____
Name _____ Date of birth _____
Address _____ Phone no. _____
Occupation _____ Hours per work week _____ Work phone no. _____
Educational background _____ Religious/ethnic background _____
Sex ____ Marital status _____
Household composition: Live alone _____ Spouse _____ Children/No. _____
Other: _____

General health status:

Physician _____ Address _____
Phone no. _____ Date of last visit _____
Ambulatory care required? _____ If so, describe: _____
Neuromuscular problems? _____ If so, how is eating affected? _____
Visual/auditory problems? _____ If so, describe: _____
Chewing difficulties? _____ If so, describe: _____
Appetite typically good? _____ fair? _____ poor? _____
Digestion/elimination difficulties? _____ If so, describe: _____
Food intolerances? _____ If so, describe: _____
Other: _____

Height _____ Weight _____ Frame _____
Triceps skinfold thickness _____ Mid-arm circumference _____
Mid-arm muscle circumference _____
Weight changes/problems? _____ If so, describe: _____

Clinical signs of nutritional status:

Skin _____ Mouth _____
Hair _____ Eyes _____
Teeth _____ Other: _____

Lab data:

Blood pressure _____
CBC _____
Serum albumin _____
Other: _____

Medications taken regularly: _____
Prescribed by: _____ Date(s) prescribed: _____
Nutrition supplements taken regularly: _____
Prescribed by: _____ Date(s) prescribed: _____
Special diet prescription: _____
Prescribed by: _____ Date of prescription: _____
How closely is diet followed? Always adhered to ___ Sometimes ___ Rarely ___ Never ___

Type of housing: Room _____ Apartment _____ Home _____ Institution _____
Prepare own meals? _____ Dine out? Often (more than once a day) _____ Rarely _____
Food shopping done independently? _____ If not, describe required assistance: _____
_____

Eligible for food stamps? _____ If so, are they currently being used? _____
Cigarette smoker? _____ If so, how much: _____
Exercise regularly? _____ If so, describe: _____
   No. times per week _____ No. minutes per session _____

Comments: _____

2. 24-Hour Recall Form

Date	Time	Food and amount

I. C. Assignments

1. Food Intake Record

Date	Time	Food/Amount	Where[a]	With whom	Associated activity[b]

[a]Such as work, restaurant, kitchen, living room.
[b]For example, watching television, reading, socializing, driving, talking on the phone, cooking.

2. Diet History

Use the Pre-test from Chapter 2 (p. 30) to provide a record of typical foods eaten.

I. D. Technician's Notes

Patient: _____   Date: _____

S   (Subjective data—how patient feels):
O   (Objective data—physical measurements including diet/nutritional status):
A   (Assessment—acceptability of dietary progress/nutritional status):
P   (Plan—diet prescription and instruction):
Comments:

II. Follow-up Session(s)

II. A. General Guidelines
1. Review assignments and discuss dietary patterns with patient.
2. Individualize Personal Diet Plan and instruct patient in its use.
3. Using Food Intake Record and Good Eating Checklist, assist patient in a general evaluation of nutrient intake.

4. Instruct patient to self-evaluate adherence to Personal Diet Plan and development of good eating habits through continued use of Food Intake Record and Good Eating Checklist.
5. Record assessment and recommendation(s) using the SOAP method in Technician's Notes. This form can be kept in your files with a copy in the patient's medical records.

II. B. Handouts

1. Personal Diet Plan

Name: _____

How to use diet plan:

1. Select a variety of foods from each of the Basic Food Groups.
2. Include the recommended number of servings from each Food Group.
3. Drink 6–8 cups of fluid daily.
4. For aid in prevention of constipation, eat foods *high in fiber* and drink plenty of liquids.
5. Choose foods *high in iron.*

Table 9.6 gives the daily nutritional needs for a healthy elderly individual.

Table 9.6   Geriatric Nutritional Needs

Food group (number of servings per day)

　Fruits and vegetables (4; 1 citrus or good source of vitamin C; dark green or bright
　　yellow vegetable several times a week)
　Breads and cereals (4)
　Milk and cheeses (3–4)
　Meats and alternates (2)

Foods high in fiber

　Whole grain breads and cereals
　Raw fruits, including skins and seeds
　Dried fruits (prunes and prune juice may act as laxatives)
　Vegetables, including skins and seeds (especially raw/lightly cooked)
　Bran products
　Popcorn, nuts, seeds

Foods high in iron

　Meat, especially organ meats
　Oysters, clams
　Legumes
　Whole grain and enriched breads and cereals
　Dried fruits and their juices
　Dark green leafy vegetables
　Potato, sweet potato
　Foods cooked in iron cookware

2. Good Eating Checklist

Instructions: Using Food Intake Record, total the number of daily servings from each Food Group and transfer to this chart. Evaluate by comparison to Recommended Daily Servings (RDSs).

Day	No. of servings/Food group					
	Fruits	Vegetables	Grains	Milk	Meat	Others
1						
2						
3						
4						
5						
RDSs	2	2	4	3–4	2	—

II.   C.   Technician's Notes

Patient: _____   Date: _____

S   (Subjective data—how patient feels):
O   (Objective data—physical measurements including diet/nutritional status):
A   (Assessment—acceptability of dietary progress/nutritional status):
P   (Plan—diet prescription and instruction):
Comments:

Geriatric Nutrition Counseling Role Playing

Keeping in mind the preceding Suggested Readings and Counseling Guidelines, participate in one or more of the role play situations; elaborate on each situation to create a patient/audience profile. Select different partners, either classmates or co-workers, for each situation. You may want to utilize your handout from Step 2. As a dietetic technician in nutrition care, do you consider yourself capable of conducting effective counseling sessions with geriatric patients? Would elderly family members or friends be able to follow your nutrition guidelines for balancing the diet during the "golden years"?

Role Play Situation 1.   As a dietetic technician in a large nursing home, you are responsible for providing nutrition counseling to the residents. Follow the guidelines to complete the charts and provide one 82-year-old male (arthritic, bed-ridden) with an individualized diet plan. Prepare a SOAP note which could be recorded in the patient's medical chart.

Role Play Situation 2.   As a dietetic technician in a small community hospital, you are responsible for a discharge diet for a 68-year-old female with osteoporosis, as requested by her physician. Follow the guidelines to complete the charts, and provide her with an individualized diet plan. Prepare a SOAP note which could be recorded in the patient's medical chart.

Role Play Situation 3.   A senior citizen congregate feeding site has contacted the dietetics department of the hospital where you are currently employed. Prepare an outline for a talk on "Cooking for One" to present to the elderly audience. Prepare a brief written report on the mealtime talk (visual aids used, audience response, questions asked, suggestions/revisions for other talks to elderly groups, etc.) for insertion in departmental files.

STEP 7: POST-TEST ON ADULT AND GERIATRIC NUTRITION

In order to evaluate your understanding of adult dietary needs, complete the Post-test below: Section I is the Learning Assessment Quiz on normal adult nutrition. (If the diet counselor is unable to complete this test successfully, how can the patient be expected to?) Section II incorporates much of the material from this chapter. Answers are given in the

Answer Key at the back of the book. Will your adult patients be able to balance their diets so that they can enter into "the golden years" in glowing health? Will your elderly patients also be able to eat properly in order to ensure adequate nutritional status during the later years?

Section I: Complete the Learning Assessment Quiz in Step 5: Normal Adult Nutrition Guidelines on p. 206. Check your answers with the Answer Key.

Section II: Indicate whether you think the following statements are true (T) or false (F). Check your answers with the Answer Key.

_____ 1. After age 25, the metabolic rate slows so that caloric needs are gradually reduced.

_____ 2. Obesity is more common in adult males than females.

_____ 3. Users of oral contraceptives should routinely take an over-the-counter multiple vitamin/mineral supplement.

_____ 4. Caffeine is a drug, and some users exhibit physical and/or psychological side effects.

_____ 5. Elderly people who live alone tend to rely on high-protein foods for most of their daily caloric intake.

_____ 6. Dietary fat intake need not be modified by most elderly individuals.

_____ 7. The elderly are at nutritional risk for developing iron-deficiency anemia.

_____ 8. Use of supplements in large doses will postpone aging and promote good health.

_____ 9. Mineral oil is a nutritionally undesirable choice for use as a laxative.

_____ 10. Hiatus hernia, common in the aged, is best treated by using a high-protein diet consumed in three meals.

_____ 11. With osteoporosis, the chemical makeup rather than the amount of bone is altered, causing a weakened skeletal structure.

_____ 12. Drug interactions occur more frequently in the elderly.

Select the answer which best completes the following statements. Check your answers with the Answer Key.

_____ 13. Foods rich in folic acid—important for some users of oral contraceptives—include
(a) liver. (b) enriched breads. (c) most soups. (d) crackers. (e) all of these.

_____ 14. Foods high in fiber—to help prevent constipation, common in the later years—include
(a) bran cereal. (b) whole grains. (c) sautéed vegetables. (d) dried fruits. (e) all of these.

_____ 15. Foods which are a good source of iron—to help those at risk for developing iron-deficiency anemia—include
(a) sweet potato. (b) clams. (c) dried beans. (d) enriched breads. (e) all of these.

_____ 16. Calcium-rich products—which may play an important role in the prevention of osteoporosis—include
(a) lean meats. (b) milk and milk products. (c) liver. (d) eggs. (e) all of these.

STEP 8: PRE-TEST (A RETAKE) ON ADULT AND GERIATRIC NUTRITION

After reading this chapter and participating in the assigned activities, you may have acquired a significant amount of new information on nutrition for adulthood and the elderly years. You should also have profited from the guidelines provided for counseling on normal and geriatric nutrition. Therefore, you might want to reevaluate the responses you gave for the various sample situations depicted in Step 1. In light of the facts you have gathered throughout this chapter, make any required revisions below. Discuss your changes with classmates or co-workers. Do you think more revisions will become necessary as your experience as a practicing dietetic technician continues to expand?

Situation 1:

Situation 2:

Situation 3:

Situation 4:

Situation 5:

REFERENCES

NATIONAL RESEARCH COUNCIL/FOOD AND NUTRITION BOARD. 1980. Recommended Dietary Allowances, 9th Edition. Washington, DC: National Academy of Sciences.

NATOW, A., and HESLIN, J. 1980. Geriatric Nutrition, pp. 33–34. Boston: CBI Publishing Co.

U.S. DEPARTMENT OF AGRICULTURE. 1972. Household Food Consumption Survey, 1965–1966. Washington, DC: Agriculture Research Service Reports.

U.S. DEPARTMENT OF AGRICULTURE. 1980. Nutrition and Your Health: Dietary Guidelines for Americans, 1st Edition. Washington, DC: U.S. Department of Health and Human Services.

U.S. DEPARTMENT OF HEALTH AND HUMAN SERVICES. 1972. Ten States Nutrition Survey, 1968–1970, Publication No. HSM 72-8130-34. Atlanta, GA: Center for Disease Control.

U.S. DEPARTMENT OF HEALTH AND HUMAN SERVICES. 1975. Anthropometric and Clinical Findings, Preliminary Findings of the first Health and Nutrition Examination Survey (HANES), 1971–1972, Publication No. HRA 75-1229. Washington, DC: Government Printing Office.

WATKIN, D. 1983. Handbook of Nutrition, Health, and Aging, pp. 211–217. Park Ridge, NJ: Noyes Publications.

Part IV

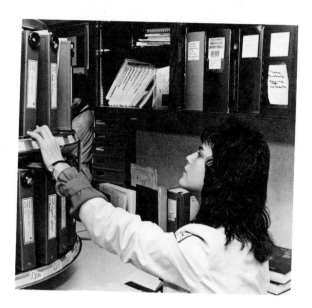

How Can You Counsel about Diet in Disease?

Effective nutrition education of patients afflicted by a variety of diet-related disorders can become a confusing and overwhelming burden to even the most skilled dietetic technician. It is a time-consuming task to collect and organize the most current diet therapy information available, and it is taxing to then devise pertinent materials for patient education. As a nutrition educator—in the hospital, clinic, or community setting—you will be most effective and feel least burdened by having at your fingertips all of the hands-on materials you will require for complete diet counseling sessions.

In assisting the dietitian(s) to manage and educate patients on various diets, it is imperative that you determine the patient's nutritional status, medical history, and diet history. Prescribed diets need to be explained so that patients understand not only *what* a diet entails, but also *why* a diet is important. Thus, the dietetic technician must develop a working knowledge of diet therapy: the components of determining and making required dietary modifications, the reasoning behind such changes, and the how-tos for the successful education and motivation of others. So, as an integral member of the health care team, it is your responsibility to contribute to the development of appropriate diet plans and to assist with compliance.

Since every institution is different in construct, each dietary department devises its own particular methods of operation including specific **menu cycles,** diet plans, etc. Therefore, it is important to realize that Part IV includes sample forms and outlines that may differ from those you will encounter in your own field experiences and employment settings. Yet, by familiarizing yourself with the designs and practicing the implementation of the given samples, you can become skilled in effective diet counseling techniques. Also, the chapter contents may be incorporated into patient education materials that you can utilize throughout your career as a dietetic technician and effective counselor on diet in disease.

menu cycle: Preplanned schedule of daily meals, organized to avoid repetition and to maximize preparation, ordering, inventory, and nutritional adequacy.

Chapter Ten

Overweight and Underweight

CHAPTER BLUEPRINT

Step 1: Take the Pre-test on Weight and participate in the assigned activities in order to examine your own body image and possible prejudices against those of abnormal weight.

Step 2: Examine the Overweight Causes and Effects Facts List and prepare the assigned handout.

Step 3: Examine the Underweight Causes and Effects Facts List and prepare the assigned handout.

Step 4: Read the materials on Fads and Facts and complete the accompanying assignment.

Step 5: Examine the Weight Loss Guidelines and complete the role play assignment.

Step 6: Examine the Weight Gain Guidelines and complete the role play assignment.

Step 7: Take the Post-test on Weight to evaluate what you have learned from the information and activities provided in this chapter.

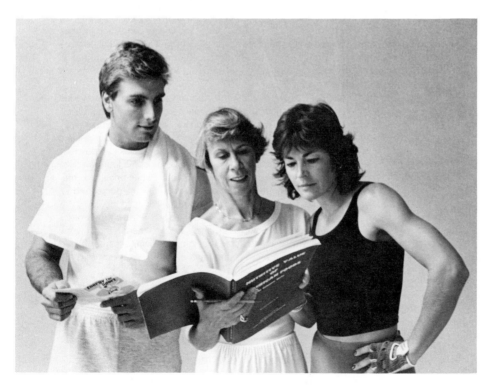

STEP 1: PRE-TEST ON WEIGHT

Feeding The Hungry Heart: Feeling Fat[1]

Dr. Colby was tall, with stiff gray hair and a head that wobbled when he walked. He thought I was too fat. He told me that a lot, but especially each June, when I had to go to him for my camp physical.

On the day before the physical, our maid, Ann, would spend the afternoon with me as I stepped in and out of steamy baths, trying to melt the pounds away. After each bath I'd weigh myself, with Ann putting her head over my shoulder to peer at the scale. "A few more pounds," I'd tell her, "and I'll be okay." So we'd draw another bath and she would sit with me as the beads of perspiration formed on my face and my fingertips grew shriveled. When I couldn't stand the heat anymore, we'd leave the bathroom and spend the next hour or so doing exercises on the pink shag carpet in my bedroom. Ann watched Jack LaLanne on television every morning, so she was well versed in the latest and most uncomfortable calisthenics for waist, hips and thighs.

Every visit was the same. I'd have to take off all my clothes except my panties. He'd poke me with his fingers, then use a stethoscope, and finally he'd ask me to get on the scale. Heart pounding, I'd put one foot and then the other on the cool gray slab. He'd push up the scale weights notch after notch, past 60, 70, 80, until finally the pointer stopped wobbling. He'd grimace; I'd cringe. He'd start talking in steel-laced sentences: "You've gained too much weight. It's just not pretty to be fat, not pretty at all. You don't want to walk around feeling ugly, now do you? None of the boys will like you. Look at Nancy [his daughter], how thin Nancy is. Why don't you be like her? You're too fat, Geneen, too fat. Fat is disgusting."

I look now at pictures of myself from those years—when I was eight to around fourteen or fifteen: me in a ballet recital wearing a blue tutu, me on the front lawn playing volleyball, me in my first formal dress—pink and glittering and wire-mouthed. I looked like everyone else, with a body like most of the other girls. Not scrawny, not lanky, but certainly not fat.

Being and/or Feeling Fat: Dieting[2]

I am fifteen. My mother picks me up at the bus station; it is the end of the summer, and I have just spent eight weeks at camp, linking braces with Mark Gold and not giving a thought to the ropes and ropes of licorice from the canteen that I ate every day. I am in love; my mother says I am fat. She says that she herself is also fat and so is my cousin Laura. My mother makes phone calls. Two days later the three of us are standing in front of a doctor who claims he can help us lose weight. He weighs us, takes our blood pressure, listens to our beating hearts, and injects something into our arms with what sounds like a staple gun. We don't ask him what's in the shot. We are mute, passive, obedient. He tells us in a German accent not to eat between meals. "Even if you eat a hot fudge sundae," he says, "do it at the end of a meal. Never, never anything in between."

He sends us to the front desk. A plump nurse named Cathy with purple eyelids and a scarlet mouth is seated in front of a row of Tupperware containers, each filled with a different size and color of pill. To her right is a phone, to her left a typewriter. I am dazed by the sight; I count the containers—sixteen in all. Such lovely colors. I like the emerald green best. One at a time we walk up to the desk. She looks at the chart the doctor has made out, takes out a small white envelope, and counts fourteen pills, two a day for a week. She gives my mother yellow ones, Laura white ones, and me, passion-pink pills. She charges my mother $50 for each of us to see the doctor and $7 per week's supply. Wishing us luck, she smiles sweetly and walks us to the door. We leave, clutching our envelopes. I have no idea what is in the pills or how they work. I ask no questions. All I want is to lose weight. "It's magic," I tell my friend Lizzy a week later. "I've lost six pounds!" Lizzy, wanting some magic of her own, uses her allowance that she's been saving for three months and pays a visit to the doctor and the plump nurse.

Lizzy and I compare notes daily. I settle on a diet of no breakfast, Grape-Nuts for lunch, and half a cup of applesauce for dinner. Lizzy prefers one hot fudge sundae a day. We both take the pills religiously. We continue to lose weight. Seventeen pounds

[1]Adapted from G. Roth, 1982, pp. 32–33.
[2]Adapted from G. Roth, 1982, pp. 64–66. Reprinted with permission of Bobbs-Merrill Co., an imprint of Macmillan.

and two months later I am still taking the pills, but no more weight is coming off. I complain to Cathy, the nurse, whom I see weekly; the doctor seems to be either out of town or in business meetings. I don't miss him. Cathy upgrades me to the next level of pills—the emerald-green lovelies.

But something is happening that I don't understand. I am edgy and tense; I can't sleep at night. Same with Lizzy. And now with Rebecca, with whom Lizzy has shared the magic. Having our own phones, we spend the hours from midnight to dawn whispering complaints about our bodies. We think the nervousness could be from the pills, but we don't know; besides, we don't want to risk the possibility of going off them. They have become our gateway to thinness and therefore to our happiness.

In college I call Cathy long distance. I send her a check; she sends me the pills. She thinks maybe I should upgrade my dose in order to lose more weight. (I am not fat, but I think I am huge.) So I graduate to big red capsules. Eventually—I can't remember how—I stop.

But it is only to go on to the next diet and the next. Protein with ketchup for breakfast, lunch and dinner; two bananas a day; the mistake of fried chicken for every meal. Stillman's, Atkins', Weight Watchers, until I become a vegetarian and food-combining expert. I stop the intake of all protein; I eat only raw food. I fast on water for days at a stretch. I become anorectic and drop to ninety-two pounds: my friends call me "Bones."

Although it is often unnecessary and usually futile, many individuals spend their lives in relentless pursuit of the "perfect" physique. Dieting has reached epidemic proportions, and an increasing number of individuals with eating disorders are seeking professional help. The majority of people with eating problems are women, but the number of overweight men in our society has increased, and some underweight males—usually teenagers—are receiving dietary assistance as well.

As a dietetic technician in nutrition care, you will encounter a significant proportion of patients who need to reduce body weight. You may also need to counsel individuals requiring dietary changes to induce body weight gain. It is essential for a diet counselor to be empathetic, and to avoid the adoption of a condescending or scolding attitude. Thus, you need to examine your self-image regarding your own body size, and utilize honest insight to uncover any personal biases you may have against those of abnormal body weight.

Do the exercise given below and complete the accompanying questionnaire. Be as honest as possible. Is your own body image accurate? Are you able to be impartial in your assessment of the body size of others? Do you have certain biases which might undermine the success of your diet counseling sessions with overweight individuals? Or with underweight patients? Discuss your responses to the activity and the questionnaire with classmates or co-workers, and devise some possible methods for overcoming any existing weight biases.

Exercise on Your Own Body Image[1]

1. Obtain three blank sheets of paper ($8\frac{1}{2}$ in. × 11 in.) and a felt-tip marker; title the sheets Them, Me, and Me-2.
2. Select a peer partner and quickly sketch each other's figure on the Them sheet; make your drawing a simple outline of the body shape.
3. On the Me sheet, sketch your own figure as you picture yourself; again, make your drawing a simple outline of the body shape.
4. Use a mirror to examine carefully your body image. Then, on the Me-2 sheet, draw another outline of your figure as you see it.
5. Give your Them sheet to the individual you sketched.
6. Compare the three drawings of your body image and briefly summarize your reactions:

---

[1]Note: Recommended as a teaching tool is Marcia Mills' 1984 edition of "Body Image Questionnaire," Community Diet Counseling Service, 100 Eastowne Dr., Suite 202, Chapel Hill, NC 27514 (available as worksheets and slides).

Questionnaire on Body Weight Biases

1. An extremely obese young female is sitting in a restaurant eating an ice cream sundae. Your reaction is

2. An overweight middle-aged businessman squeezes into an overcrowded elevator and is blocking your exit. You are thinking

3. Your neighbor is obese, her husband is moderately overweight, and their children are all becoming fat. At the neighborhood block party, you watch this family stuff themselves with food and drink. You are thinking

4. At the supermarket, you examine the contents of the shopping cart belonging to an overweight individual: chips, soft drinks, frozen french fries, cookies, sour cream, bacon, hot dogs, canned hash, etc. Your reaction is

5. Your friend's young relative is markedly underweight and appears thinner every time you see her. Your friend complains of her own inability to shed a few pounds and expresses envy for the "willpower" of her young relative. Your response is

6. A very thin male jogs by your house every morning. Whenever you see this fat-less figure running by, your reaction is

STEP 2: OVERWEIGHT FACTS

A threat to physical and emotional well-being, obesity is best treated by prevention. However, for a significant segment of the population, excess poundage has already accumulated, and education on safe and effective procedures for weight loss and maintenance is required. It is your responsibility to assist patients who need to reduce body weight to do so—gradually, using a nutritionally sound diet program. The following Overweight Causes and Effects Facts List provides some of the most current diet-related information to include in counseling overweight individuals.

Overweight Causes and Effects Facts List

1. Obesity is defined as an accumulation of body fat in excessive proportion to total body mass, usually 20% or more above the age/sex/height-related norms.
2. The overweight individual—usually 10–20% above the desirable range—is not necessarily obese, as the composition of the weight may be due to bone mass or muscle tissue.
3. Although obesity and overweight are not synonymous terms, most individuals who are 20% or more overweight are in fact obese.
4. America has become an overweight nation permeated with stressful social pressures to attain and maintain acceptable body weight. Yet, effective preventive measures are scarce.
5. The American attitude toward excessive body weight is moralistic, and society tends to view this condition as a manifestation of lack of willpower, weak personality structure, and gluttonous self-indulgence. This bias also pervades the medical community and consequently can hamper treatment. Excess body fat is also a social stigma which can ostracize the afflicted and lead to overeating for emotional stimulation.
6. Since the beginning of the nineteenth century, there has been a gradual shift away from the admiration for plumpness towards a view of excess weight as an abnormality.
7. Americans waste over $15 billion annually on unsuccessful attempts to shed unwanted poundage via "dietetic," "light," "low-calorie," and artificially sweetened products, health spas, appetite suppressants, diets, and devices for spot reduction.
8. A certain amount of body fat is important for insulation of the body from heat, cold, and mechanical shock, to serve as an energy supply when glycogen reserves are depleted

and food intake is delayed, and for protection against environmental stresses. However, in a society where food is readily available, excess fat is unnecessary.

9.   Overweight afflicts 10% of all American schoolchildren, 15% of those under age 30, and 25 to 30% of the adult population, with certain subgroups displaying a markedly elevated incidence (e.g., lower socioeconomic classes, blacks, Mexican-Americans, Native Americans, and Eskimos).

10.   The prevalence of obesity increases rapidly after age 25, and by age 50–59, one third of American males are at least 20% overweight, as are one-half of the females.

11.   An individual who was lean at age 25 can be overweight at 65 without gaining a single pound: with aging, body composition changes and physical activity usually diminishes, muscles become smaller, bones are less dense, and fat stores increase.

12.   Food is widely used for nonnutritive purposes, especially in a culture where food is abundant.

13.   Food and emotions are tightly and complexly interrelated. Diet promoters take advantage of human nature by appealing to the common desire to believe that food/diet can quickly and painlessly guarantee love, beauty, youth, and long life—or immortality.

14.   Environmental factors associated with overweight include the availability of food, socioeconomic status, cultural/ethnic considerations, social and occupational customs, daily activity patterns—which currently emphasize sedentary work, labor-saving devices, spectator sports, and increased use of elevators, automobiles, and other forms of passive travel.

15.   The typical overweight individual suffers from a mild personality disorder characterized by anxiety and depression, neurotic eating behaviors, and hypersensitivity to environmental eating cues; the body serves as a target for unresolved psychological problems, and reduction of anxiety via overeating becomes a habit.

16.   Hilde Bruch, a noted researcher on eating disorders, has divided the overweight population into three main groups with the following characteristics: (a) normal psychological make-up but overweight due to physical structure; (b) psychological problems, personality disorders, and abnormal family transactions resulting in "developmental" obesity; and (c) psychological problems stemming from a traumatic experience, with overeating used as a shield against deeper depression.

17.   The results rather than the causes of obesity include depression, anxiety, and low self-esteem.

18.   Overweight persons often use food as a means for self-reward or self-punishment and to manipulate others.

19.   Diagnosis of obesity can be conducted by use of (a) growth charts for infants, children, and adults; (b) examination of physical appearance; (c) skinfold thickness with pinch test or **calipers;** (d) height/weight tables (based on weights associated with the lowest mortality rates); and (e) body composition measurements (which estimate body fat versus mass, but are expensive, time consuming, and usually restricted to metabolic research).

calipers: Instrument for measuring the diameter of solids such as skinfolds.

20.   Skinfold thickness can be measured at the triceps on the back of the arm, at the angle of the **scapula,** and over the lower abdomen above the **iliac crest;** the triceps are the easiest to measure, and may be the most accurate representation of total body fatness.

scapula: Shoulder blade.

21.   New height/weight charts were published in 1983 with elevated allowances for weight ranges. The proposed changes met with much criticism (most nutritionists advocate that any overall increase in weight should occur only as muscle mass upon training). Since there exist no clear-cut criteria for defining body frame as small, medium, or large, height/weight tables can provide only a general indication of whether body weight is appropriate for height and frame. The charts from 1959 are still preferred by most health professionals (see Table 10.1).

iliac crest: Hip bone, or upper portion of widest section of the pelvis.

22.   In February of 1985, a National Institutes of Health conference on the health implications of obesity advised that any amount of excess weight is deleterious. The panel concluded that body weight 20% or more above desirable is a serious risk, and for those with other risk factors (i.e., high blood pressure, elevated blood lipids, and diabetes) even 5 to 10 extra pounds can prove dangerous. Excess *fat* is of more concern than *overweight* due to well-developed muscle tissue (see Table 10.2). Location of excess fat is an important predictor for obesity-associated health hazards: excess abdominal fat poses more risk for disease than does fat in the thighs and legs.

Table 10.1   Desirable Weight Charts[a]

| Desirable weights for women, age 25 and over | | | | | Desirable weights for men, age 25 and over | | | | |
| Height with shoes (2-in. heels) | | Small frame | Medium frame | Large frame | Height with shoes (1-in. heels) | | Small frame | Medium frame | Large frame |
Feet	Inches				Feet	Inches			
4	10	92–98	96–107	104–119	5	2	112–120	118–129	126–141
4	11	94–101	98–110	106–122	5	3	115–123	121–133	129–144
5	0	96–104	101–113	109–125	5	4	118–126	124–136	132–148
5	1	99–107	104–116	112–128	5	5	121–129	127–139	135–152
5	2	102–110	107–119	115–131	5	6	124–133	130–143	138–156
5	3	105–113	110–122	118–134	5	7	128–137	134–147	142–161
5	4	108–116	113–126	121–138	5	8	132–141	138–152	147–166
5	5	111–119	116–130	125–142	5	9	136–145	142–156	151–170
5	6	114–123	120–135	129–146	5	10	140–150	146–160	155–174
5	7	118–127	124–139	133–150	5	11	144–154	150–165	159–179
5	8	122–131	128–143	137–154	6	0	148–158	154–170	164–184
5	9	126–135	132–147	141–158	6	1	152–162	158–175	168–189
5	10	130–140	136–151	145–163	6	2	156–167	162–180	173–194
5	11	134–144	140–155	149–168	6	3	160–171	167–185	178–199
6	0	138–148	144–159	153–173	6	4	164–175	172–190	182–204

[a]Prepared by Metropolitan Life Insurance Company. Derived primarily from data of the Build and Blood Pressure Study. 1959. Society of Actuaries.

Table 10.2   Percentage of Body Fat

| Athletes | | Nonathletes | | |
Male	Female	Male	Female	Category
6	16	12	22	Lean
7–15	17–23	13–21	23–28	Acceptable
15+	23+	21+	28+	Overweight
10–12	18–20	13–15	23–25	Ideal

23.   Although the overall mechanism for the development of obesity seems simple (i.e., imbalance in energy intake versus energy expenditure), the underlying causes are complex, multifactorial, and incompletely understood.

24.   Although several strains of animals have demonstrated obesity as an inherited trait, this pattern has yet to appear in humans. However, genetic factors may play a role in the development of obesity; identical twins raised separately tend to have similar body weights, more so than fraternal twins—even when raised together. Lifestyle and food attitudes are also likely to influence the familial weight pattern.

25.   Somatotype can also play an important role in body weight: it is unusual for an ectomorph to become obese, and the probability that endomorphs will avoid obesity is low unless preventive methods are employed early in life (see Chapter 3, Table 3.1).

26.   The few types of obesity caused by **hypothyroidism** will respond to hormonal treatment. Most endocrine abnormalities associated with excess body fat appear to be due to rather than a cause of obesity, and the symptoms diminish or disappear with weight loss.

27.   The complex physiology of hunger and satiety are not yet completely understood, but lack of adequate physical activity is believed to be the major factor contributing to the widespread incidence of obesity in the United States today. Evidence indicates that the overweight do not routinely eat significantly more than their leaner peers, but may be significantly less active.

28.   Excess amounts of fat are stored in the adipose tissue cells of the body. The adipose cell theory proposes that overfeeding at critical time periods causes **hyperplasia** of adipose tissue, producing an increased number of adipose cells with an increased capacity

hypothyroidism: Condition in which insufficient amounts of the thyroid hormone thyroxine are secreted, causing reduced basal metabolic rate.

hyperplasia: Increase in tissue size due to formation and growth of new cells.

for fat storage. Weight loss later in life can empty these cells of stored adipose but will not reduce the number present, and this predisposes the individual to easy weight gain.

29.   Individuals with an abnormally large number of fat cells may be abnormally hungry, despite reduced body size and weight loss, so might be unable to overcome the urge to overeat.

30.   The adipose cell theory has been confirmed in rats, but has received strong criticism. More recent evidence indicates that the critical time period for adipose cell proliferation may not be limited to infancy, but may continue throughout adolescence into adulthood; weight status during adolescence may be a more accurate prediction for adult weight than is infant weight. However, prevention of obesity should begin at birth and continue throughout the life cycle.

31.   The obese individual is more likely to develop diabetes, heart disease, high blood pressure, arthritis, gallbladder disorders, respiratory ailments, fertility/pregnancy problems, abnormal skin conditions, varicose veins, and decreased life expectancy. Obesity, like cigarette smoking and a sedentary lifestyle, can contribute to the aging process.

32.   The overall death rate of the overweight is over 50% above that of the normal weight population.

33.   Life expectancy may be shortened by 1% for every 1% over Desirable Weight; in rats, lifespan can be increased 10% above the norm for those kept 10% below the normal body weight.

34.   For obese individuals, complications are more common during acute illness and following accidents, general anesthesia, and surgery.

35.   Maturity-onset diabetes occurs four times more often in overweight persons, and around three quarters of those afflicted with this type of diabetes are obese.

36.   Enlarged fat cells become resistant to insulin so that excess glucose remains in the blood, stimulating the insulin-producing cells to secrete more insulin; this leads to a greater degree of fat storage, whereas weight loss will restore insulin levels to normal. Enlarged fat cells may also be less sensitive to other hormones which promote fat breakdown.

37.   Successful treatment of obese individuals requires a significant investment of time for both the overweight patient and members of the health care team.

38.   A multidisciplinary approach—including nutritionist, physician, nurse, psychologist, exercise physiologist, and social worker—which avoids oversimplicity can prove effective, whereas simplified treatment programs typically fail to achieve long-term results.

39.   Health professionals can best assist overweight patients by setting an example that can be emulated.

40.   Treatment of overweight individuals should also include significant others (e.g., spouse, parents, siblings, and children) in order to prevent sabotage and encourage support.

41.   It is important to expose individual rationalizations for being overweight and to dispel diet myths. For example, *cellulite* is medically nonexistent; the term merely refers to normal adipose fat localized in the buttocks and thighs that can only be eradicated with exercise and weight loss. As aging progresses, **collagen** becomes less elastic and adipose forms pockets that pucker more readily; thus, it may be more difficult for older individuals to rid themselves of "cellulite," but treatment modes are the same: proper diet and exercise.

collagen: Fibrous protein of the connective tissue including bones, ligaments, cartilage, and skin.

42.   Treatment of obesity is often unsuccessful due to a noncompliant personality and resistance to change; old patterns can provide positive reinforcement and alleviate anxieties. The inability to "go cold turkey" and abstain from all food results in an ever-threatening temptation to overindulge.

43.   It is important to evaluate the chances for successful treatment; the potential for success may diminish with (a) early weight problems leading to serious obesity; (b) a history of repeated dieting failures and large swings in body weight; (c) individuals expecting "magical" results from diet gimmicks; (d) individuals who place the responsibility on others; and (e) individuals who search for a cure for obesity rather than self-control for weight maintenance.

44.   Medications used in treating obese patients will suppress appetite, cause diuresis, provide bulk to diminish hunger, or increase the metabolic rate; the ill effects caused by **amphetamines** and the potential for addiction appear to outweigh the positive effects (i.e., diminished appetite), while diuretics only cause temporary loss of body fluids, not fat

amphetamine: Addictive drug which stimulates the central nervous system; used in the treatment of certain types of depression, narcolepsy, hyperactivity, and for appetite control.

(and can lead to dangerous side effects from electrolyte imbalance and dehydration). The natural bulk of fibrous food is preferable to drugs, and thyroid-type/metabolism-stimulating medications should only be used to treat a diagnosed imbalance.

45. No known drug is both safe and effective in treating obesity, and many are hazardous. In fact, the only effective appetite suppressant for which tolerance does not develop over time is cigarette smoking, an obviously unwise method to aid in weight loss.

46. As a last resort, hospitalization with long-term fasting can help to decrease weight dramatically while protecting dieters from hurting themselves due to dangerous side effects—including irritability, depression, aggressiveness, paranoia, liver enzyme alterations, potassium losses, ketosis, **hyperuricemia,** dehydration, even death.

hyperuricemia: Excessive amounts of uric acid in the blood.

47. Surgery is usually reserved for the morbidly obese: **jejunoileal bypass** is associated with a significant mortality rate, diarrhea/**steatorrhea** with mineral losses are common, and liver damage occurs; side effects can only be reversed by **reanastamosis**.

jejunoileal bypass: Surgical procedure in which the jejunum and ileum (of the small intestine) are shunted to decrease the total absorptive area and reduce total caloric absorption.

48. Surgery for weight loss purposes is a radical approach, and the intestinal bypass is no longer considered by the medical and nutrition communities to be an advisable treatment mode. Gastric stapling—which reduces the size of the stomach by closing off a portion of it—is safer, but also has postoperative risks and can be sabotaged by the patient who chooses to constantly eat small amounts of food. Even less effective is the cosmetic surgery to remove fat from beneath the skin: *lipectomies* have had temporary success at best. Before undergoing weight loss surgery, obese individuals should obtain a second opinion from another physician.

steatorrhea: Fatty stools.

reanastamosis: Surgical reconnection of two bodily structures (e.g., two sections of the intestines).

49. Jaw wiring restricts obese patients to a liquid diet sipped through a straw. Once the jaw is unwired, however, new eating habits must be adopted to maintain weight loss.

50. The concept of lifelong maintenance of a reasonable weight through proper diet and regular exercise should be introduced early in weight therapy, and patients need to accept the responsibilities involved.

51. Self-imposed diets and "yo-yo" dieting behaviors should be discouraged. Repeated attempts at low-calorie dieting will cause the body's metabolic rate to drop, resulting in weight plateaus and more efficient storage of caloric intake as body fat.

52. The best method for boosting a slowed metabolism is the adoption of a regular exercise program. Exercise will enhance loss of body fat while building lean body tissue and assisting with appetite control.

53. It is essential for anyone planning to embark on a weight loss program to first consult a physician.

54. Encouraging patients on weight loss programs to sign a contract may enhance feelings of commitment (see Weight Control Contract that follows).

55. Although the scale only serves as a gauge—since weight measured is body mass (not fat) and fluctuates due to a variety of influencing factors—it is the most accessible method for determining gains and losses. Weigh-ins should be limited to once a week, preferably without clothing and immediately upon arising.

56. The Prader-Willi syndrome is characterized by feeding difficulties in infancy, followed by very rapid weight gain and obesity in early childhood. Intelligence may range from severely delayed to near normal, **hypotonia** and slowed motor development cause inactivity, and linear growth is slackened; satiety awareness is absent, so that the children gorge, hoard, even steal food, and may consume inedible items.

hypotonia: Loss of muscle tone.

57. Treatment of the Prader-Willi syndrome includes environmental control, caloric/dietary intake to allow for linear growth, and familial support. Early intervention may prevent obesity and can result in higher IQ; difficulties in control multiply with aging, as autonomy increases and time away from home allows for unobserved overeating episodes.

58. Is it not ironic that fat members of developed countries may die due to overnutrition/excess caloric intake, while starvation is the major cause of death in underdeveloped nations?

Exercise on Counseling the Overweight

Keeping in mind the preceding Overweight Causes and Effects Facts List, which provides some of the most current diet-related information to include in counseling overweight individuals, prepare a simplified version for use as a patient handout. You may include graphics and/or use a poster format, if desired; see the Sample Handout. Show your handout in rough draft form to classmates or co-workers for constructive criticism on the overall design, content, and potential effectiveness for use in pertinent diet counseling situations. Then prepare a final version for your own future use as a practicing dietetic technician.

Sample Handout

Weight Control Contract

I, _____, on this date of _____, do hereby pledge to attempt a gradual weight loss by adherence to a sensible, lowered-calorie diet plan and a regular exercise program. In this way, I can alter my lifestyle to improve my nutritional status, physical appearance, self-esteem, and overall health. I am doing so for my own sake, and plan on a lifetime of sensible eating and regular exercise.

Signed: _____

Individuals each develop their own eating behaviors due to varied backgrounds, environments, and emotions. Food usually means much more than a way to satisfy physical hunger. Thus, it is important to utilize habit awareness and insight in order to control eating behaviors and alter undesirable food habits. The following tips may assist you in doing so.

1.   Choose desirable alternatives to food for use as a reward. For example, reward yourself with a new article of clothing after a difficult week, or treat yourself to a new movie upon achieving success in weight loss endeavors.

2.   Leave one bite on your plate at each meal or snack—resist the temptation to "clean the plate"; also, avoid the urge to encourage others to eat against their will. In order not to waste food, ask for or give yourself smaller servings.

3.   Whenever you are eating, ask yourself whether it is by your own choice, or triggered by someone, someplace, or some event from your past. For example, do you really want to overindulge on Thanksgiving every year, just because you always have?

4.   Avoid letting the *sight* of food trigger you to eat unless you are *physically* hungry. Close your eyes and pass by the ice cream parlor.

5.   Avoid letting the *smell* of food trigger you to eat unless you are *physically* hungry. Stand up straight, hold your breath, and pass by the bakery.

6.   Avoid letting things in the environment trigger you to eat unless you are *physically* hungry. Try not to fantasize about food; instead, fantasize about all of the future improvements in your body, health, diet, and self-esteem.

7.   Eat only when you are *physically* hungry, not just because it is "time to eat." If you are not hungry at noon, wait until a bit later to eat, and if you are full after dinner, skip your evening snack.

8.   Make eating a sole activity. When you have a meal or snack, sit down and enjoy it; do *not* read, watch TV, talk on the phone, etc., until you have finished eating. You may find yourself eating *less* and enjoying it *more.*

9.   Select alternative outlets for emotions and avoid the kitchen when your emotions are stirred. Get a dart board, a close friend, a counselor, or go for a brisk walk when problems arise—and work them out, if possible.

10.   Whenever tempted to eat instead of undertaking a necessary task, ask yourself this: "Will I simply delay the undesirable activity or avoid it altogether if I eat?" Then either *do* the task or *do not* do it; eating is not going to help either way.

11.   Avoid running to the kitchen whenever others stir up your emotions. Instead, develop alternate places to seek refuge, such as a local park, a health club, or a friend's house. It is amazing how much insight can be gained during a few hours of absence from a problem person.

12.   Before embarking on a frustrating safari in search of that unknown something to eat, stop and reflect. By taking some time to determine just what your needs are, you can then identify exactly what might satisfy these needs. You may even choose not to eat at all.

STEP 3: UNDERWEIGHT FACTS

Below-normal body weight is usually not a threat to overall health. However, thin individuals often want to increase their weight in order to round out body curves or build up muscles. Individuals suffering from anorexia nervosa need to be encouraged to gain weight and improve overall health. It is your responsibility to assist those seeking or requiring weight gain to be able to do so—gradually, using a nutritionally sound diet program. The following Underweight Causes and Effects Facts List provides some of the most current diet-related information to include in counseling underweight individuals.

Underweight Causes and Effects Facts List

1. Millions of Americans are members of the commonly overlooked minority in our diet-crazed society for whom gaining weight is a losing battle.

2. Some of the common causes for underweight include disease, poor and erratic eating habits, malabsorption of food, starvation, and anorexia; influential factors include heredity, hunger and satiety irregularities, psychological factors, and familial patterns.

3. Underweight patients at high risk for developing malnutrition due to physiological or psychological conditions (e.g., anorexia, a digestive problem, trauma, or a debilitating disease) may require a high-calorie, high-protein diet to promote weight gain and tissue repair.

4. Underweight individuals may develop decreased resistance to infection and disease.

5. Underweight individuals may tire easily, often feel chilled, weak, and nervous, but generally tend to be in good health.

6. Although underweight can occur in any age or sex group, it is a common problem for the elderly (see Chapter 9) and teenagers (see Chapter 8).

7. Underweight individuals tend to eat slowly, linger over their food, avoid between-meal snacking, take small portions, and include less sweets and fatty foods in their diets.

8. The underweight individual attempting to gain weight needs to adjust slowly to increased quantities of food, with well-balanced meals and snacks suitable to personal tastes and tolerances. Commercial supplemental formulas can also help to increase caloric and nutrient intake.

9. The strategy for increasing body weight centers on the use of foods that are high in calories but low in volume (e.g., nutritious milkshakes, liberal servings of grains and starchy vegetables, cheeses and lean meats, nuts and nut butters). The higher calorie foods from each of the Basic Food Groups should be emphasized at each meal, and snacking can become a regular part of the daily menu pattern.

10. As in weight loss, plateaus can be expected during weight gain; feelings of discouragement and hopelessness may be alleviated with increased physical exercise and involvement in outside interests.

11. Underweight individuals tend to have fewer adipose cells and a keen sense of satiety; some are cigarette smokers or excessive exercise enthusiasts, and many have high-strung personalities which can cause fidgety behavior and poor sleeping habits.

12. The underweight individual embarking on a weight gain plan should consult a physician in order to rule out any possible underlying medical problems.

13. The major difference which distinguishes underweight from anorexia nervosa is that the latter entails self-induced starvation. If untreated, anorexia nervosa can lead to brain damage and death. Fortunately, current strategies for treatment are proving effective and recovery is possible.

14. Anorexia nervosa can be identified upon loss of 25% or more of body weight, whereas underweight is defined as more than 10% below normal levels (see Table 10.1).

15. Weight gain, like weight loss, is gradual, so weekly rather than daily weigh-ins are more practical and less discouraging. Treatment should include regular but not excessive exercise and adequate rest.

16. It is important for underweight individuals to understand that body weight is less important than physical fitness, good health, and self-respect.

Exercise on Counseling the Underweight

Keeping in mind the preceding Underweight Causes and Effects Facts List, which provides some of the most current diet-related information to include in counseling under-weight individuals, prepare a simplified version for use as a patient handout. You may include graphics and/or use a poster format, if desired; see the Sample Handout. Show your handout in rough draft form to classmates or co-workers for constructive criticisms on the overall design, content, and potential effectiveness for use in pertinent diet counseling situations. Then prepare a final version for your own future use as a practicing dietetic technician.

Sample Handout

Table 10.3 gives valuable tips for underweight individuals.

Table 10.3 High-Calorie Diet Tips

Basic food group	Add to recommended daily servings[a]
Fruits and vegetables	May be sweetened or in sauces or dressings.
	Drink juices instead of water.
Grains	Include liberal amounts, including pastas, dried beans and peas, potatoes and starchy vegetables.
Milk and dairy	Stir skim milk powder into milk, eggnogs, drinks, or mix into casseroles, meatloaf, pudding, etc.
	Add cheeses to mixed dishes, sprinkle on casseroles, melt in sandwiches.
	Include ample amounts of milk and cheeses, yogurt, ice cream, cottage cheese, custards and pudding.
Meats and alternates	Include generous portions of lean choices and dried beans and peas. Snack on dried meats, chunks of cheese, chicken, turkey, etc.
	Use nuts, nut butters, and seeds as snacks.
	Make omelets with lean meats and cheeses.
Others	Use moderate amounts of fats, sweets, and alcoholic beverages to help increase caloric intake.

[a]Note: Commercial supplements may be used to provide between-meal calories.

STEP 4: FADS AND FACTS

The diet business is currently a multibillion dollar industry with plans for expansion. Yet, less than 10% of those attempting to shed unwanted poundage are able to do so and successfully maintain the loss. Clearly, if the magic cure for obesity had been discovered, the overweight segment of our population would be shrinking in number rather than swelling in size. Popular weight loss fads and gimmicks change regularly, but are typically based on the same central theme: rapid loss of fat without effort, hunger, or feelings of deprivation. Although this concept defies the laws of nature, and despite the fact that many dieters are well aware that weight loss requires eating properly and exercising regularly, a growing number of overweight individuals continue to fall prey to misleading dietary claims.

Although underweight individuals do not represent as large a market for the diet busi-ness, they do tend to spend a significant amount of money on useless "weight gain" powders, bust developers, and muscle-building supplements. Although many realize the uselessness of such products in that they know that weight gain requires eating well and building up with exercise, underweight individuals often opt for miracle cures—just in case one might work. Anorexics may develop compulsive dieting behaviors after trying a popular fad diet.

As a practicing dietetic technician in nutrition care, it is your responsibility to help protect weight-conscious individuals from the potential damages to overall health and financial status posed by fad diet plans. By educating on the basics of sound dieting practices, you can provide the background information required for safe and effective weight control. Then, by warning against useless and potentially dangerous fad diets and weight control gimmickry, you can help dieters to avoid unnecessary loss of money and motivation. Repeated diet failures—like any defeat—can cause depression and destroy feelings of self-worth, whereas the successful loss of poundage on a sensible diet plan can markedly improve self-image. For the underweight individual seeking to gain weight, a sensible diet program—without repeated failure due to use of ineffective gimmicks—can also help to achieve both physical fitness and improved self-confidence.

Exercises on Diet Fads and Facts

After reading some of the Suggested Readings on Fad Diets and Professional Critiques beginning on page 200, spend some time in the diet/health section of a local bookstore. Then make an outline that lists the different types of fad diets and weight loss/gain gimmicks currently available. Prepare a brief oral presentation on one of these fads, and present to classmates or co-workers: describe the gimmick, discuss any associated claims, explain why the product would prove ineffectual, and include a display of advertisements (or a sample if possible). Also, begin to scan the media—television, magazines, newspapers, billboards, books, leaflets, etc.—for misleading advertisements for dietary aids aimed at the overweight or underweight individual. You might want to expand your file on fad diets and body weight mythology for use in counseling those seeking to lose or gain poundage—safely and successfully.

STEP 5: WEIGHT LOSS GUIDELINES

Today's typical American is fatter than ever before. There are some 80 million overweight individuals living in this country. The weight loss business is a booming industry, yet less than 10% of those attempting to lose weight are successful in attaining and maintaining their desired weights. Obviously, our current methods for shedding unwanted poundage are not solving the problem.

In the past, the prescription of a low-calorie diet was the only medically acceptable method for treating obesity. Yet, during the last few decades, the public has been assaulted by an endless succession of diets, plus an array of other weight loss techniques including belts and machines, surgery and drugs, hypnosis and psychotherapy, "fat farms" and injections. Diet has remained the key factor in weight loss programs, yet it has become obvious that low-calorie diets rarely result in successful, long-term loss of excess body weight. Research indicates that the *only* effective method for weight loss and lifelong weight control is adoption of a sensible, nutritionally adequate diet plan and participation in a regular exercise program.

Weight control will continue to be a national obsession for aesthetic reasons, if not for health purposes. While most reports in the literature indicate poor results for weight loss programs, it *is* possible to achieve safe, successful, and permanent control of body weight. The practical treatment of overweight requires a long-term program combining individualized diet plans with factual health education and aid in lifestyle modification. Therefore, it is essential for the program to meet the following criteria:

1. There is skilled, well-trained professional leadership.
2. A physical and psychological assessment of program participants is conducted by professionals.
3. The program incorporates economic, emotional, social, and other individualistic lifestyle factors.
4. There is an understanding by professionals and participants that weight control is a long-term commitment requiring motivation, endurance, persistence, and skill.

The most successful type of weight control program to date is referred to as the "Three-Prong Program." Although more follow-up research is still needed, this approach appears to be the most effective, healthy, and practical treatment for overweight. Such programs, conducted on an individual basis and/or in group settings, include the following components:

1. a well-balanced diet plan
2. a program of regular physical exercise
3. modification of eating and exercise habits

The most successful diet plan is low enough in caloric content to allow for gradual loss of body fat, yet adequate in nutritional value and psychologically satisfying for the dieter. The lowest caloric level which can allow for these two factors is 1200 calories per day with additional calories to meet the individual's age, sex, size, and weight goal requirements. The diet plan should be based on the Basic Food Groups and include a wide variety of different foods in moderate amounts. Individual likes and dislikes must be incorporated into the diet plan, and the meal pattern should be fitted to the lifestyle of the dieter.

A regular program of physical activity should be adopted by the dieter. The program may consist of simply a brisk daily walk, or it can include jogging, swimming, bicycling, group sports, or a combination of activities. Daily activity is emphasized, both to aid in caloric expenditure and to tone and strengthen muscles. The psychological benefits of exercise are also essential to the success of the program, and vigorous physical activity can help to diminish appetite as well.

Behavior modification for dieters includes learning to restructure the environment by changing food and exercise habits, developing alternative responses to situations that lead to overeating, adapting to the reality of the postdiet condition, and accepting new lifestyle patterns both physically and psychologically. Many different techniques can be employed to assist with behavioral change. Again, individualization of treatment is essential. Also, regular assessments of the patient's understanding of and compliance with the treatment plan are important.

In order to be able to advise overweight individuals on weight loss techniques, it is essential to have access to all of the hands-on material required for effective counseling sessions. It is also important to be able to record all of the pertinent information regarding each diet counseling session in the patient's medical charts. The information in the following Suggested Readings and Counseling Guidelines should help to improve your confidence—and skills—regarding your counseling abilities.

This step includes suggested counseling strategies for use with patients requiring weight control. A weight loss program may be contraindicated in certain medical conditions. Patients should have their physician's permission to undertake a weight loss program. The following references may prove helpful.

Suggested Readings for Sensible Weight Control

ALLSEN, P. 1984. Fitness for Life. Dubuque, IA: William C. Brown Co.

AMERICAN DIETETIC ASSOCIATION. 1986. The American Dietetic Association's Nutrition Recommendations for Women. J. Am. Dietet. Assoc. *86,* Dec., 1663.

ARONSON, V. 1987. Thirty Days to Better Nutrition. Englewood Cliffs, NJ: Prentice-Hall.

BLONZ, E., and STERN, J. 1981. Obesity and fad diets. In Controversies in Nutrition, L. Ellenbogen (Editor), pp. 105–124. New York: Churchill Livingstone.

BOYLE, P., STORLIEN, L., and KEESEY, R. 1978. Increased efficiency of food utilization following weight loss. Physiology and Behavior *21,* 2, 261.

BRAY, G. 1980. Comparative Methods of Weight Control. Westport, CT: Food and Nutrition Press.

BROWNELL, K. 1984. The psychology and physiology of obesity: Implications for screening and treatment. J. Am. Dietet. Assoc. *84,* Apr., 406.

BROWNELL, K. 1985. The LEARN Program for Weight Control. Philadelphia: University of Pennsylvania.

BROWNELL, K. 1987. Obesity and weight control: The good and bad of dieting. Nutrition Today *22,* Jun., 4.

CALIFORNIA DIETETIC ASSOCIATION. 1987. Popular Diets: How They Rate. Santa Monica, CA: Los Angeles District California Dietetic Association.

CONN, H., DEFELICE, E., and KUO, P. (Editors). 1983. Health and Obesity. New York: Raven Press.

CORBIN, C. and LINDSEY, R. 1984. The Ultimate Fitness Book. Champaigne, IL: Leisure Press.

DEBOER, J., et al. 1986. Adaptation of energy metabolism in overweight women to low energy intake. Amer. J. Clin. Nutr. *44,* Nov., 585.

ENVIRONMENTAL NUTRITION. 1982. EN's Ready-Reference Guide to Weight Control. EN, 2112 Broadway, Suite 200, New York, NY 10027.

FERGUSON, J. 1988. Habits Not Diets, 2nd Edition. Palo Alto, CA: Bull Publishing Co.

FRANKLE, R., and YANG, M. 1988. Obesity and Weight Control. Rockville, MD: Aspen Publishers.

GARNER, D., et al. 1980. Cultural expectations of thinness in women. Psychol. Reports *47,* 3, 483.

GREENWOOD, M. R. C. (Editor). 1983. Obesity. New York: Churchill Livingstone.

GROSSMAN-MCKEE, D. 1987. Eating confidence questionnaire. Bariatrician, Spring, 25.

HOLLI, B. 1988. Using behavior modification in nutrition counseling. J. Am. Dietet. Assoc. *88,* Dec., 1530.

IKEDA, J. 1987. Winning Weight Loss for Teens. Palo Alto, CA: Bull Publishing Co.

JOHNSON, W. (Editor). 1987. Treating and Preventing Obesity: Advances in Eating Disorders. Greenwich, CT: JAI Press.

KALLEN, D., and SUSSMAN, M. (Editors). 1984. Obesity and the Family. New York: Haworth Press.

KANO, S. 1985. Making Peace with Food: A Step-by-Step Guide to Freedom from Diet-Weight Conflicts. Allston, MA: Amity Publishing Co.

KATCH, F., and MCARDLE, W. 1988. Nutrition, Weight Control, and Exercise, 2nd Edition. Philadelphia: Lea & Febiger.

KEYS, A. 1950. The Biology of Human Starvation. Minneapolis, MN: University of Minnesota Press.

MACDONALD, D., BUCKLE, R., and BERARDI, R. (Editors). 1983. Nutrition and Fitness Manual: A Summary of Research and Resources. Toronto, Ont.: Nutrition Information Service, Ryerson Polytechnical Institute.

MACKENZIE, M. 1983. Fear of Fat: The Politics of Body Size. New York: Columbia University Press.

MARVINNEY, S., and FAINE, M. (Editors). 1985. The Role of Nutrition and Exercise in Health. Seattle: University of Washington.

MILLS, M. 1984. Body Image Questionnaire. Chapel Hill, NC: Community Diet Counseling Service.

MIRKIN, G. 1983. Getting Thin. Boston: Little, Brown & Co.

NATIONAL DAIRY COUNCIL. 1988. Weight control: New findings. Dairy Counc. Dig. *59,* May/Jun., 13.

NATIONAL INSTITUTES OF HEALTH CONSENSUS DEVELOPMENT CONFERENCE. 1985. Health Implications of Obesity. Bethesda, MD: NIH.

POLIVY, J., and HERMAN, C. P. 1983. Breaking the Diet Habit. New York: Basic Books.

POLIVY, J., and HERMAN, C. P. 1985. Dieting and binging: A causal analysis. Amer. Psychol. *42* Feb., 193.

ROSS, S. 1987. Adult learning theory: Application to weight management. Nutrition News *50,* Apr., 6.

SCHULZ, L. 1986. Obese, overweight, desirable, ideal: Where to draw the line? J. Am. Dietet. Assoc. *86,* Dec., 1666.

SIMONSON, M. 1982. An overview: Advances in research and treatment of obesity. Food/Nutr. News, Mar./Apr., 1.

STEFFEE, W. 1982. The medical syndrome of obesity. Primary Care *9,* Sept., 581.

STUART, R., and JACOBSON, B. 1987. Weight, Sex, and Marriage: A Delicate Balance. New York: W. W. Norton.

STUNKARD, A. (Editor). 1980. Obesity. Philadelphia: W. B. Saunders Co.

STUNKARD, A., and STELLAR, E. (Editors). 1984. Eating and Its Disorders. New York: Raven Press.

TREBELLA, N. 1982. Behavior Modification for Weight Control in the Elderly. Colorado Springs, CO: Acacia Nutrition Program.

WEIGLEY, E. 1984. Average? Ideal? Desirable? A brief overview of height-weight tables in the U.S. J. Am. Dietet. Assoc. *84,* Apr., 417.

WEINSIER, R., et al. 1984. Recommended therapeutic guidelines for professional weight control programs. Amer. J. Clin. Nutr. *40,* Oct., 865.

WILMORE, J. 1986. Sensible Fitness. Champaigne, IL: Leisure Press.

WING, R., and JEFFERY, R. 1979. Outpatient treatments of obesity: A comparison of methodology and clinical results. Intl. J. Obesity *3,* 3, 261.

WINICK, M. (Editor). 1986. Nutrition and Exercise. New York: John Wiley & Sons.

For journal subscriptions:

Bariatrician. American Society of Bariatric Physicians, 7430 East Caley Avenue, Suite 210, Englewood, CO 80111.

Current Diet Review. Box 1914, Rialto, CA 92376.

International Journal of Eating Disorders. John Wiley & Sons, 605 Third Avenue, New York, NY 10158.

International Journal of Obesity. John Libbey & Co., 80–84 Bondway, London, England SW8 1SK.

International Obesity Newsletter. Route 1, Box 6A, Hettinger, ND 58639.

For audiovisuals:

Calorie Comparison Charts. Nutrition Graphics, PO Box 1527, Corvallis, OR 97339.

Fad Diet Circus. Sterling Educational Films, 241 East 34th Street, New York, NY 10016.

Food Sense—Part V: Reducing Diets. Nutrition Resource Center, Pennsylvania State University, University Park, PA 16802.

For Tomorrow We Shall Diet. Churchill Films, 662 North Robertson Boulevard, Los Angeles, CA 90069.

Good Loser: The Weight Control Game. Didactron, Inc., PO Box 1501, Ann Arbor, MI 48109.

Lifesteps: Weight Management Program. National Dairy Council, 6300 North River Road, Rosemont, IL 60018.

Nutrition for the Overweight. Milner-Fenwick, Inc., 2125 Greenspring Drive, Timonium, MD 21093.

Overweight: How Did I Get This Way? Milner-Fenwick, Inc., 2125 Greenspring Drive, Timonium, MD 21093.

Overweight: What Can I Do About It? Milner-Fenwick, Inc., 2125 Greenspring Drive, Timonium, MD 21093.

Shaping Up. The Polished Apple, 3742 Seahorn Drive, Malibu, CA 90265.

Sizing Up a Weight Loss Program. San Mateo County Health Department Health Services, 225 West 37th Avenue, San Mateo, CA 94403.

Winding Your Weight Down. Nutrition Counsultant Services of Houston, University Bank Plaza Building, 5615 Kirby Drive, Suite 512, Houston, TX 77005.

For further information:

American Alliance for Health, Physical Education, Recreation, and Dance, 1900 Association Drive, Reston, VA 22091.

American Society of Bariatric Physicians, 7430 East Caley Avenue, Suite 210, Englewood, CO 80111.

Food and Nutrition Health Catalog, Health Education Services, 10,000 Culver Boulevard, PO Box 802, Culver City, CA 90230.

Lowfat Lifeline, Dept. 301, 52 Condolea Court, Lake Oswego, OR 97035.

President's Council on Physical Fitness and Sports, 450 5th Street NW, Suite 7103, Washington, DC 20001.

Counseling Guidelines—Weight Loss

Table 10.4 outlines the steps for diet counseling for weight loss. The following material gives the details of each step.

Table 10.4 General Outline for Weight Loss Counseling

I. Initial Session
   A. General Guidelines
   B. Patient Records
      1. Medical History Form
      2. Weight Chart
      3. 24-Hour Recall Form
   C. Assignments
      1. Food Intake Record
      2. Activity Record
      3. Diet History
   D. Technician's Notes
II. Follow-up Sessions
   A. General Guidelines
   B. Handouts
      1. Personal Diet Plan
      2. Tip Sheets
      3. Learning Assessment Quiz
   C. Technician's Notes

I. Initial Session

1. A. General Guidelines

1. Use Medical History Form to assess patient's nutritional status.

2. Weigh patient and record on Weight Chart. The chart is a helpful tool in visualization of patient's weight status.

3. Assist patient in recording 24-hour recall of food intake using 24-Hour Recall Form. This will aid in keeping an accurate Food Intake Record.

4. Instruct patient to keep daily Food Intake Record so that typical food intake patterns can be evaluated. Advise patient not to deviate from his/her normal eating pattern, so that the cues which lead to inappropriate eating behavior can be pinpointed. Stress the importance of recording food intake and associated activity immediately after eating.

5. Instruct patient to keep Activity Record in order to provide comparison of patient's conception of own activity with actual activity level. Advise patient not to deviate from normal activity pattern. This form can be utilized continually to emphasize the importance of regular physical activity.

6. Instruct patient to complete Diet History. This provides for a basic evaluation of food intake patterns, influences on eating behavior, success/failure of previous dieting, and motivation for weight loss. (Also use Pre-test from Chapter 2.)

7. Record assessment and recommendation(s), using the SOAP method in Technician's Notes. This form can be kept in your files with a copy in the patient's medical records.

I. B. Patient Records

1. Medical History Form

Date _____ Referred by _____

Name _____

Address _____ Date of birth _____

_____ Phone no. _____

Occupation _____ Hours per work week ____ Work phone no. _____

Educational background _____ Religious/ethnic background _____
Sex ____ Marital status ____
Household composition: Live alone ____ Spouse ____ Children/No. ____
Other: _____

General health status:

Physician _____ Address _____
Phone no. _____ Date of last visit _____
Ambulatory care required? ____ If so, describe: _____
Neuromuscular problems? ____ If so, how is eating affected? _____
Visual/auditory problems? ____ If so, describe: _____
Chewing difficulties? ____ If so, describe: _____
Appetite typically good? _____ fair? _____ poor? _____
Digestion/elimination difficulties? ____ If so, describe: _____
Food intolerances? ____ If so, describe: _____
Hypertension? ____ If so, describe: _____
Hyperlipidemia? ____ If so, describe: _____
Diabetes? ____ If so, describe: _____
Arthritis/gout? ____ If so, describe: _____
Gallbladder disorder? ____ If so, describe: _____
Thyroid disorder? ____ If so, describe: _____
Other: _____

Height _____ Weight _____ Frame _____
Triceps skinfold thickness _____ Mid-arm circumference _____
Mid-arm muscle circumference _____
Weight changes/problems? ____ If so, describe: _____

Clinical signs of nutritional status:

Skin _____ Mouth _____
Hair _____ Eyes _____
Teeth _____ Other: _____

Lab data:

Blood pressure _____ EKG _____ Exercise stress test _____
Cholesterol _____ Triglycerides _____ Lipoprotein profile _____
Fasting blood glucose _____ CBC _____
Serum T_3 _____ Serum T_4 _____ PBI _____
Other: _____

Medications taken regularly: _____
Prescribed by: _____ Date(s) prescribed: _____
Nutrition supplements taken regularly: _____
Prescribed by: _____ Date(s) prescribed: _____
Special diet prescription: _____
Prescribed by: _____ Date of prescription: _____
How closely is diet followed? Always adhered to ____ Sometimes ____ Rarely ____ Never ____

Type of housing: Room _____ Apartment _____ Home _____ Institution _____
Prepare own meals? _____ Dine out? Often (more than once a day) _____ Rarely _____
Food shopping done independently? ____ If not, describe required assistance: _____

Eligible for food stamps? _____ If so, are they currently being used? _____
Cigarette smoker? _____ If so, how much: _____
Exercise regularly? _____ If so, describe: _____
  No. times per week _____ No. minutes per session _____

Comments: _____

2. Weight Chart

Starting weight _____   Reasonable weight _____

Date	No. weeks on diet	Weight	Comments

3. 24-Hour Recall Form

Date and time (over 24-hr period)	Food and amount	Where eaten[a]	Eaten with whom[b]	Associated activity[c]

[a]For example, at the kitchen table, at home—sitting at a desk, in a car, or at a restaurant.
[b]For example, with parents, friend(s), or spouse.
[c]For example, while studying, driving, talking, or watching TV.

I. C. Assignments

1. Food Intake Record

Date and time	Duration of meal (min)	Food and amount	Where eaten[a]	With whom	Associated activity[b]	Associated emotions[c]

[a]Such as work, restaurant, kitchen, living room.
[b]For example, watching television, reading, socializing, driving, talking on the phone, cooking.
[c]Attitude: bored, anxious, frustrated, depressed, happy, angry, tense, etc.

2. Activity Record

Instructions: Record those physical activities which were sustained for at least 20 minutes.

Date and time	Type of activity	Duration

3. Diet History

First use the Pre-test from Chapter 2 (p. 30) to provide a record of foods typically consumed. Then have patient complete the following questionnaire.

1. What are your reasons for seeking weight loss?

2. Were you an overweight infant? ____ child? ____ adolescent? ____
3. List any relatives who are/have been overweight:
4. Do any of the following people influence your dieting/weight?
   Spouse _____ Children _____
   Parent(s) _____ Friend(s) _____
   Other: _____
5. Indicate previous dieting methods:

Weight loss program	Inclusive dates	Maximum weight loss

Weight Watchers
Diet Workshop
T.O.P.S.
Mail order diet
Formula diet
Diet pills/injections
Medically prescribed
Self-imposed
Psychotherapy
Hypnosis
Behavior modification
Popular diet in magazine/book
   (list types): _____
   _____
   _____
   _____
   _____
 	
Other: _____
_____
_____
_____		

6. How often does "binge" eating occur? _____
7. Describe how you feel after finishing most meals/snacks (e.g., sleepy, uncomfortable, full, dissatisfied, satisfied):
8. Why do you think you have a weight problem?

I. D. Technician's Notes

Patient: _____   Date: _____

S (Subjective data—how patient feels):
O (Objective data—physical measurements including diet/nutritional status):
A (Assessment—acceptability of dietary progress/nutritional status):
P (Plan—diet prescription and instruction):
Comments:

II. Follow-up Sessions

II. A. General Guidelines

1. Weigh patient and record on Weight Chart.
2. Review assignments and discuss; analyze patient's Food Intake Record and Activity Record. Remember to give praise often and to avoid overemphasis on wrong behaviors. Emphasize change in behavior rather than loss of weight.
3. Aid patient in determining a realistic weight goal by using insurance company actuarial tables, skinfold thicknesses, and/or the following formulas: for women of medium build, use 100 lb for first 5 ft of height plus 5 lb for each additional inch; for men of medium build, use 106 lb for first 5 ft of height plus 6 lb for each additional inch; for those with small builds, subtract 10% and for those with large frames, add 10%. Make long-term goal realistic by dividing into short-term goals; patients should not strive to lose more than 10% of body weight in a 6-month period.
4. Using Activity Record, determine if patient's activity level is sedentary, moderate, or strenuous.
5. Determine desired daily caloric intake level by using the following formulas: If activity level is sedentary, multiply desired weight by thirteen; if moderate, multiply by fifteen; if strenuous, multiply by twenty. Subtract the number of calories which would lead to desired weekly weight loss. (Note: 3500 calories = 1 lb.)
6. Individualize a diet plan using Personal Diet Plan and instruct patient on its use.
7. Provide Tip Sheets on dieting for at-home and dining out guidelines.
8. Assign Learning Assessment Quiz to evaluate counseling process and to determine the additional counseling strategies which will be required.
9. Instruct patient to continue to maintain daily Food Intake Record and Activity Record.
10. Record assessment and recommendation(s) using the SOAP method in Technician's Notes. This form can be kept in your files with a copy in the patient's medical records.

II. B. Handouts

1. Personal Diet Plan

Name _____

Daily caloric allowance _____

How to use diet plan:
1. Use Basic Diet Plan (Table 10.5) for the foundation of the Personal Diet Plan.

Table 10.5   Basic Diet Plan (1200 cal)[a]

List	Food group	Servings
A	Fruits	3
B	Vegetables	3
C	Grains	4
D	Milk	4
E	Meat	3
F	Fats	3

[a]Added calories (determined individually):
1200 calories + ____ = Daily Caloric Allowance.

2.   Determine Daily Caloric Allowance (see item 5 of General Guidelines) by adding calories to the Basic Diet Plan that will promote a $\frac{1}{2}$–1-lb weight loss per week.

3.   Add Food Group Servings to build up caloric intake to approximate individual Daily Caloric Allowance. (Note that a daily intake of less than 1200 calories will eventually lower metabolic rate and halt weight loss.)

4.   Use Food Group Lists (Table 10.6) to determine appropriate food choices.

5.   Devise a sample Meal Pattern to use as a guide in planning daily food intake.

Meal Pattern[a]

Eating time	Number of servings					
	Fruits	Vegetables	Grains	Milk	Meat	Fats
Breakfast						
Snack						
Lunch						
Snack						
Supper						
Snack						

[a]To be determined individually.

2. Tip Sheets

Tips for home

1.   Eat slowly—to make small amounts more satisfying:
     Put down silverware between mouthfuls.
     Chew food thoroughly, and swallow before taking another mouthful.
     Take time out from eating to socialize or rest; learn to relax during meals.
     Remember that it takes the body at least 20 minutes to respond to a feeling of fullness.

2.   Reduce external food cues:
     Use smaller plates.
     Keep serving dishes away from the table.
     Keep all food in kitchen only, out of sight, and as far out of reach as possible.
     Store foods in opaque containers so that food is less visible.
     Plan to avoid having leftovers, and freeze any you may have immediately.
     Keep only allotted snack items on hand; avoid purchasing tempting or problem foods.
     Enter kitchen only at mealtimes.
     Be aware of visual stimuli, such as gourmet magazines, tempting television commercials, etc.

Table 10.6 Food Group Lists

List A: Fruits (approximate calories per serving = 60)

Fruit	Amount	Fruit	Amount
Apple	½ med	Kiwi	1 med
Applesauce	½ cup	Kumquat	2 lg
Apricots, fresh	2	Mango	½ sm
Apricots, dried	4 halves	Melon:	
Banana	½ small	Cantaloupe	¼ sm
Berries:		Casaba	⅛ sm
Blackberries	½ cup	Honeydew	⅛ sm
Blueberries	½ cup	Watermelon	1 cup
Boysenberries	½ cup	Nectarine	1 sm
Cranberries	1 cup	Orange	1 sm
Raspberries	½ cup	Papaw	1 lg
Strawberries	¾ cup	Papaya	¾ cup
Cherries	10 lg	Passion fruit	1 med
Dates	2	Peach	1 med
Fig, fresh or dried	1	Pear	½ med
Fruit cocktail	½ cup	Persimmon	1 med
Grapefruit	½	Pineapple	½ cup
Grapes	12	Plantain	⅓ sm
Juices:		Plums	2 med
Apple	⅓ cup	Prunes	2 med
Cider	⅓ cup	Quince	⅓ cup
Cranberry	¼ cup	Raisins	2 Tbsp
Grape	¼ cup	Tangerine	1 med
Grapefruit	½ cup	Tangelo	1 med
Nectar	⅓ cup		
Orange	½ cup		
Papaya	⅓ cup		
Pineapple	⅓ cup		
Prune	¼ cup		

Note: Fruits and juices should be fresh, dried, canned, or frozen without added sugar.

List B: Vegetables (approximate calories per ½ cup serving = 25)

Alfalfa sprouts	Eggplant	Rhubarb
Artichoke	Greens:	Rutabaga
Asparagus	Beet	Sauerkraut
Bamboo shoots	Chard	Scallions
Bean sprouts	Collard	Squash
Beans, green or wax	Dandelion	Patty pan
Beets	Kale	Scallop
Broccoli	Mustard	Summer
Brussels sprouts	Spinach	Zucchini
Cabbage	Turnip	Tomatoes
Carrots	Kohlrabi	Tomato juice
Cauliflower	Leeks	Turnip
Celery	Mushrooms	Vegetable juice cocktail
Chayote	Okra	Water chestnuts
Chinese pea pods	Onions	
Cucumber	Pepper, green or red	

The following vegetables may be eaten in unlimited amounts:

Chicory	Endive	Parsley
Chinese cabbage	Escarole	Radishes
Cilantro	Lettuce	Watercress

Note: Starchy vegetables are included with *Grains*.

Table 10.6 (*Continued*)

List C: Grains (approximate calories per serving = 80)

Kind	Amount
Breads	
Any, average slice	1 slice
Bagel	½ small
Biscuit, 2 in. (omit 1 Fat serving)	1
Breadcrumbs, dry	3 Tbsp
Cornbread, 2 in. × 2 in. × 1 in. (omit 1 Fat serving)	1
English muffin	½
Hamburger bun	½
Hotdog roll	½
Muffin, 2 in. (omit 1 Fat serving)	1
Pancake, 5 in. × ½ in. (omit 1 Fat serving)	1
Pizza crust	1/7 med pie
Roll, hard	1 sm
Roll, plain small	1
Taco shell	1
Tortilla, 6 in.	1
Waffle, 5 in. × ½ in. (omit 1 Fat serving)	1
Cereals	
Barley	1½ Tbs
Bran, unprocessed	¼ cup
Cereal, cooked	½ cup
Cereal, dry	¾ cup
Cereal, puffed	1 cup
Chow mein noodles (omit 1 Fat serving)	½ cup
Cornmeal, dry	2 Tbsp
Cornstarch	2 Tbsp
Cracked wheat, dry (bulgur)	2 Tbsp
Flour	2½ Tbsp
Grits, cooked	½ cup
Kasha, dry (buckwheat groats)	2 Tbsp
Pasta, cooked (macaroni, noodles, spaghetti)	½ cup
Popcorn, cooked (without added fat)	3 cups
Rice or barley, cooked	½ cup
Wheat germ	¼ cup
Crackers	
Arrowroot	3
Butter type, round (omit 1 Fat serving)	5
Chips (omit 2 Fat servings)	15
Matzo, 6 in. sq	½
Melba toast	4
Oyster	20
Pretzels, stick type	20
Pretzels, twisted	6
Rye wafers, 2 in. × 3½ in.	3
Saltines	6
Soda, 2½ in. sq	4
Wheat wafers, 2 in. sq	3
Legumes	
Baked beans (without added fat)	¼ cup
Dried beans, cooked (red, soy, white)	½ cup
Dried peas, cooked (blackeye, cow, split)	½ cup
Lentils, cooked	½ cup
Starchy vegetables	
Corn	⅓ cup
Corn on the cob	1 sm
Lima beans	½ cup
Mixed (carrots, limas, and peas)	½ cup
Parsnips	⅔ cup
Peas, green	½ cup
Potato, white	1 sm
Potato, white, mashed	½ cup
Potatoes, french-fried (omit 1 Fat serving)	8
Pumpkin	¾ cup
Winter squash	½ cup
Yam or sweet potato	¼ cup

(*continued*)

Table 10.6 (*Continued*)

List D: Milk and dairy (approximate calories per serving = 90)

Kind	Amount
Skim or nonfat milk	1 cup
99% fat-free milk (omit ½ Fat serving)	1 cup
98% fat-free (low-fat) milk (omit 1 Fat serving)	1 cup
Whole milk (omit 2 Fat servings)	1 cup
Goat's milk (omit 2 Fat servings)	1 cup
Low-fat buttermilk (omit 1 Fat serving)	1 cup
Whole milk buttermilk (omit 2 Fat servings)	1 cup
Canned, evaporated skim milk	½ cup
Canned, evaporated whole milk (omit 2 Fat servings)	½ cup
Nonfat dry milk powder	⅓ cup
Whole milk powder (omit 2 Fat servings)	⅓ cup
Low-fat yogurt, unflavored (omit 1 Fat serving)	1 cup
Whole milk yogurt, unflavored (omit 2 Fat servings)	1 cup
Cheese, low-fat:	
St. Ortho Swiss, skim milk cheeses	1½ oz
Sapsago	4 Tbsp
Cheese, medium-fat:	
Edam, skim American, skim mozzarella	1 oz
Cheese, high-fat: (omit ½ Fat serving)	
American, brick, cheddar, provolone, Romano, Swiss	1 oz
Parmesan	4 Tbsp

List E: Meat

Low-Fat: (approximate calories per serving = 55)

Kind	Amount
Beef	
Chuck (all cuts except ground), dried beef, flank steak (sirloin, tenderloin), plate skirt steak, round (all cuts except ground), tripe	1 oz
Cheese	
Cottage, dry or low-fat	¼ cup
Ricotta-part skim, St. Ortho Swiss, special dietary low-fat cheeses	1 oz
Sapsago	3 Tbsp
Fish	
Any, fresh or frozen	1 oz
Fish or shellfish, canned	¼ cup
Sardines, drained	3 med
Shellfish, fresh or frozen	1 oz
Frog	1 oz
Lamb (all cuts except breast and ground)	1 oz
Pork	
Leg (fresh ham—all cuts, smoked ham—all cuts)	1 oz
Poultry (without skin)	
Chicken (including liver), hen (Cornish, Guinea), pheasant, turkey (including liver)	1 oz
Rabbit	1 oz
Veal (all cuts except breast and ground)	1 oz
Venison	1 oz
Meat alternatives	
[a]Dried beans, cooked (red, soy, white)	¼ cup
[a]Dried peas, cooked (blackeye, cow, split)	¼ cup
[a]Lentils, cooked	¼ cup
[a]Peanut butter (omit 2½ Fat servings)	2 Tbsp
Textured vegetable protein	2 Tbsp
[a]Tofu (soybean curd)	2½ oz

[a]Incomplete protein sources.

List E (continued)

Medium-fat (approximate calories per serving = 75)

Kind	Amount
Beef	
Canned corned beef, loin (porterhouse, T-bone, top loin), rib (eye steak, roast, steak), tongue	1 oz
Cheese	
Cottage, creamed	¼ cup
Farmers', neufchatel, processed spread, skim American, skim mozzarella	1 oz
Organ meats	
Heart, kidney, liver, sweetbreads	1 oz
Pork	
Canadian bacon, ham (boiled, canned, country-style), loin (all chops, blade roast, rib half or whole, sirloin cutlets or ribs, top loin roast), shoulder arm picnic, smoked pork shoulder (picnic, roll)	1 oz

High-fat (approximate calories per serving = 100)

Kind	Amount
Beef	
Brisket, ground beef (all commercial), tongue	1 oz
Cheese	
American, blue-roquefort, brick, camembert, cheddar, colby, limburger, Parmesan, provolone, Romano, Swiss, processed cheese	1 oz
Cold cuts	1 oz
Frankfurter	1 oz
Lamb	
Breast, ground	1 oz
Pork	
Deviled ham, ground, loin (back ribs, country pork), spareribs	1 oz
Poultry	
Capon, duck (domestic), goose	1 oz
Sausage	1 oz
Veal	
Breast, ground	1 oz

Notes: All canned fish should be packed in water.
Meats should be *well* trimmed of all visible fat.
To minimize fat content, request that beef be ground *after* trimmed of all visible fat.
Bake, boil, broil, or roast without added fats.
All cold cuts, frankfurters, and sausages contain less protein per serving than other meat items.
Indicated serving sizes refer to weights after cooking.

List F: Fats (approximate calories per serving = 45)

Kind	Amount
Avocado, 4 in.	⅛
Bacon, crisp	1 strip
Bacon fat	1 tsp
Butter	1 tsp or 1 pat
Chocolate, unsweetened	2 tsp or ⅓ oz
Coconut, dried	2 Tbsp
Coconut milk	4 tsp
Cocoa, dry powder	3 Tbsp
Cream	
Half and half	3 Tbsp
Heavy	1 Tbsp
Heavy, whipped	2 Tbsp
Light	2 Tbsp
Nondairy	3 Tbsp
Sour	2 Tbsp
Cream cheese	1 Tbsp
Lard	1 tsp

(*continued*)

Table 10.6 (*Continued*)

List F (continued)

Kind	Amount
Margarine	1 tsp
Margarine, low-calorie	2 tsp
Mayonnaise	1 tsp
Mayonnaise, low-calorie	2 tsp
Nuts	
Almonds, whole	10
Macadamia, whole	3
Peanuts: Spanish (whole), Virginia (halves)	20
Pecans, large	2
Pistachios	20
Others	6
Oil	1 tsp
Olives	5 sm
Salad dressing	
Blue cheese or roquefort	2 tsp
French	1 Tbsp
Italian	2 tsp
Mayonnaise-type	1 Tbsp
Russian	2 tsp
Thousand island	2 tsp
Salt pork	$\frac{3}{4}$ in. cube
Tartar sauce	1 Tbsp

Note: Read labels to determine appropriate serving sizes for low-calorie salad dressings.

Low-calorie items (approximate calories negligible—reasonable amounts may be included)

Bouillon, without fat	Lime
Club soda	Mineral water
Cereal beverages	Mustard
Coffee	Pickles, unsweetened (sour or dill)
Gelatin, sugar-free or unflavored	Soft drinks, sugar-free
Gum, sugar-free	Spices
Herbs	Tea
Horseradish	Vinegar
Lemon	

Alcoholic beverages

To determine the caloric content, use the following formula: $0.8 \times$ proof $\times$ ounces = calories.
Count each 45 calories of an alcoholic beverage as 1 Fat serving.
Note that dry wines or low-calorie beers are better choices than sweet wines or regular beers and ales.
Liqueurs and sweetened mixers contain considerable amounts of sugar.

Eat only at predetermined habitual eating places.
Avoid other activities while eating; remove television, magazines, newspapers, phone, etc., from habitual eating places.
3. Increase daily activity:
Develop a daily pattern of sustained exercise.
Walk more; park car further from destination, get off public transportation a few stops before destination, use stairs instead of elevators, walk whenever feasible.
Learn to enjoy physical activities such as bicycling, swimming, jogging, tennis, etc.
4. Engage in alternate activities in response to eating cues:
Develop new hobbies.
Enjoy activities away from home.
Turn to pleasurable activities, such as reading, napping, phoning friends, etc.
Accomplish household tasks such as letter writing, room rearrangement, gardening, etc.
5. Consider the following additional tips:
Do not skip meals.
If hungry before mealtime, have a small snack such as raw vegetable sticks or yogurt.
Start meals off with salad or other nutritious bulky filler.

Shopping and cooking tips

1. Plan ahead:
Plan menus in advance, using appropriate references.
Prepare several meals in advance and freeze them in partitioned containers.
Plan portion-controlled meals to avoid leftovers.
Establish regular meal times.
Make a shopping list and adhere to it.
Choose and modify recipes carefully to limit calories and maximize nutritional values.
Never shop when hungry.
2. Employ sound nutrition principles while shopping:
Read labels carefully to check for ingredients, serving size, and nutrient and caloric contents.
Be wary of "dietetic" and "light" foods.
Purchase nutritious low-fat snack items.
Avoid spontaneous purchase of items not included on shopping list; resist familial persuasions.

3. Eliminate excess fat-calories in cooking:
    Broil, boil, bake, or roast meat/poultry/fish without added fat.
    Remove all visible fat, including skin, from meat and poultry.
    Use rack when roasting meat/poultry/fish.
    Some fat may be skimmed from meat juices, soups, and stews after refrigeration.
    Steam or simmer, do not fry; use nonstick cooking utensils.
    Use seasonings, vinegar, and lemon in cooking.
    Use water-packed tuna, juice/water-packed fruit, skim milk, and skim milk products.
    Allow butter/margarine to soften so that spreading is easier and a lesser amount can be used.
    Become familiar with low-fat cooking methods, such as cuisine minceur and wok cookery.
4. Reduce food cues during meal preparation and clean up:
    Elicit help from others so that food contact is lessened; request presence of others to reduce boredom, loneliness, and tediousness associated with preparation and clean up.
    Avoid nibbling during meal preparation (chew sugarless gum).
    In order to facilitate immediate storage of leftovers after dining, ready storage containers prior to mealtime.
    Request that others clear table and store leftovers.

Dining out tips

1. Avoid overindulgence on holidays and when dining out:
    Eat a small, nutritious snack before leaving home to avoid dining out when ravenous.
2. Always plan ahead:
    Determine wisest menu selections before leaving home.
    Explain diet to others to elicit their support.
    Bring along low-calorie dressings.
3. Minimize intake of rich foods:
    Order first to avoid the influence of others.
    Instead of ordering alcoholic beverages, select unsweetened juices, ice water, or club soda garnished with fruit wedges.
    To avoid overeating bread and butter, request that salad be served immediately; request salad dressing on the side.
    Request that meats and vegetables be prepared without added breading, sauces, or fats; avoid escalloped, creamed, au gratin, fried, sautéed, and marinated dishes.
    Request that meat/fish salads be served with mayonnaise on the side.
    Select the less rich desserts such as angel food cake or fresh fruit.
    Instead of overeating large portions, bring some home in a "doggie bag."
    Steer clear of high-fat snack items at parties by minimizing time spent near food.
    Do not submit to the social pressures to overindulge in food and drink.

3. Learning Assessment Quiz

Answer true (T) or false (F) to the following statements:

____ 1. There are more calories in a medium-sized baked potato than in a 2-oz serving of roast beef.
____ 2. Grapefruit contains an enzyme that burns fat in the body.
____ 3. Exercise increases the appetite of the sedentary individual.
____ 4. On a low-calorie diet, bread and potatoes are forbidden.
____ 5. An ideal weight loss program is a high-protein, low-carbohydrate diet.
____ 6. If you are at a reasonable weight, you can be assured that your nutrient intake is adequate.
____ 7. Many sources of protein are also high in fat.
____ 8. As much protein as desired may be consumed without contributing to weight gain.
____ 9. Skim milk is a good alternative to whole milk as a source of calcium.
____ 10. Toast contains significantly fewer calories than bread.
____ 11. Unsweetened fruit juices do not contain calories.
____ 12. In order to cut down on calories, substitute honey for sugar.
____ 13. Margarine has fewer calories than butter.
____ 14. A high level of mental activity, such as studying, utilizes a large number of calories.

_____ 15. Nuts and seeds are low-fat snack items.
_____ 16. Fresh fruits and vegetables are always higher in nutrients than frozen produce.
_____ 17. Sorbitol is a calorie-free sweetener.
_____ 18. Use of diuretics results in loss of water, not loss of fat.
_____ 19. Excess weight is rarely due to hypothyroidism.
_____ 20. The stomach shrinks in size during dieting.

II. C. Technician's Notes

Patient: _____   Date: _____

S (Subjective data—how patient feels):
O (Objective data—physical measurements including diet/nutritional status):
A (Assessment—acceptability of dietary progress/nutritional status):
P (Plan—diet prescription and instruction):
Comments:

Weight Loss Counseling Role Playing

Keeping in mind the preceding Suggested Readings and Counseling Guidelines, participate in the following role play situations; use the sample menu (Fig. 10.1) as a teaching aid. Select different partners, either classmates or co-workers, for each situation and elaborate on each role play situation to develop a patient/audience profile. You may want to use your handout from Step 2. Use the SOAP method to record in each patient's medical chart.

As a dietetic technician in nutrition care, do you consider yourself capable of conducting effective counseling sessions with overweight individuals? Would you or your family be able to adhere to your nutrition guidelines in order to achieve and maintain a reasonable weight? Do you need to do so?

Role Play Situation 1.   An overweight 6-year-old boy is referred to you, a dietetic technician on the pediatrics ward of a teaching hospital, for a discharge diet. Follow the guidelines to complete the charts and provide the patient with an individualized diet plan. Prepare a SOAP note which could be recorded in the patient's medical chart. (*Note:* The boy has been immobilized with a broken **tibia**.)

tibia: Inner, larger leg bone below the knee.

Role Play Situation 2.   An overweight female neighbor seeks your advice informally as to a reliable weight loss program. Briefly draw up a SOAP note regarding your interchange which—if she had been your patient—could be recorded in her medical chart.

Role Play Situation 3.   The weight control clinic where you are employed is conducting a weekend workshop for newcomers. Using the Tip Sheets (pp. 236, 239–240), prepare a brief handout for the audience. Present the handout as part of a short talk on "Dieting as a Weigh of Life." Complete a written summary on the presentation for insertion in the clinic files.

Role Play Situation 4.   Devise several different weight control situations in order to practice calculating various meal patterns and planning accompanying menus. See Fig. 10.1. Repeat with various caloric levels until you feel comfortable with calorie-controlled meal and menu planning.

STEP 6: WEIGHT GAIN GUIDELINES

Underweight can be both nutritionally threatening and psychologically upsetting. Thus, if a patient needs and wants to gain weight in order to attain and maintain a reasonable weight, it is essential to devise an individualized, appetizing, and well-balanced diet plan. Daily activity should be encouraged, to derive both physical and psychological benefits. Meals should be pleasurable, and special dietary supplements can provide additional calories and nutrients if necessary. Regular assessments of the patient's understanding of and compliance with the treatment plan are important. If anorexia nervosa and/or bulimia are diagnosed, special medical/psychological treatment is essential for recovery.

In order to be able to assist underweight individuals seeking to gain weight, it is

Name _____ Room _____
Diet **Calorie controlled** _____

Breakfast Please circle your selections below

Fruits and juices	Cereals	Entrees	Breads	Miscellaneous
Orange juice	Cream of wheat	Bacon	Bran muffin	Salt
Grapefruit juice	Grits	Sausage	Corn muffin	Pepper
Prune juice ¼ cup	Oatmeal	Scrambled egg	Plain muffin	Sugar substitute
Apple juice ⅓ cup	Cornflakes	Poached egg	English muffin	Butter
Cranberry juice LC	Rice Krispies	Egg substitute	White toast	Margarine
Grapefruit sections LC	Special K	Pancakes	Wheat toast	Lemon
Stewed prunes LC	Puffed rice	French toast	Rye toast	Dietetic jelly
Banana ½	Puffed wheat	Omelet of the Day		Dietetic syrup
	Shredded wheat			
	All Bran			
	Bran Flakes			

Beverages			
Coffee		Whole milk	
		4 oz. whole milk	
Tea	Cream	Skim milk	
Decaffeinated coffee	Nondairy creamer	4 oz. skim milk	

LC = Low Calorie

Name _____ Room _____
Diet **Calorie controlled** _____

Luncheon Please circle your selections below

Appetizers	Vegetables
Apple juice	Whipped potato
Cranberry juice LC	Baked potato
Tomato juice	Noodles
Fruit cup LC	Rice
Consomme/chicken/beef	Broccoli
Chicken noodle soup	Corn
Vegetable soup	Spinach
Cream of tomato soup	Carrots
Cream of chicken soup	Green beans
Soup du jour	Beets
	Peas
	Squash

Entrees	Salads and dressings
Tomato with:	
Chicken salad, ½ cup	Lettuce/tomato
Tuna salad, ½ cup	Tossed greens
Cottage cheese, ½ cup	Lettuce wedge
Egg salad, ½ cup	Cole slaw
Chef's bowl/meat & cheese	Salad special
Cottage cheese & fruit	Mayonnaise
Roast beef sandwich	French LC
Sliced turkey sandwich	Italian LC
Tuna salad sandwich	Oil & vinegar
Chicken salad sandwich	Lemon and vinegar
Egg salad sandwich	Sour cream
Tuna noodle casserole	
Turkey/gravy/dressing	Desserts
Roast beef au jus	Unsweetened peaches
Macaroni and cheese	Unsweetened fruit cocktail
Scrod	Unsweetened baked apple
Ham/plain	Unsweetened pears
Steak/mushrooms	Unsweetened apricots
Chicken/cranberry LC	Unsweetened applesauce
Grilled cheese/dill pickle	Fresh fruit
Veal/gravy	Sunshine cup
Pork chop/plain	Ice cream
Shell macaroni	Orange sherbet
Beefburger or cheeseburger	Raspberry sherbet
(dill pickles)	Gelatin LC
Salisbury/gravy	Custard LC
Chef's special if allowed	Angel cake

Breads		Miscellaneous
White	Dinner Roll	Salt
Wheat	Crackers	Pepper
Rye		Sugar substitute
		Butter
Beverages		Margarine
Coffee		Lemon
Tea		Dietetic jelly
Decaffeinated coffee		Mustard
Cream		Catsup LC
Nondairy creamer		Relish LC
Whole milk		
4 oz. whole milk		
Skim milk		
4 oz. skim milk		

LC = Low Calorie

Name _____ Room _____
Diet **Calorie controlled** _____

Dinner Please circle your selections below

Appetizers	Vegetables
Apple juice	Whipped potato
Cranberry juice LC	Baked potato
Tomato juice	Noodles
Fruit cup LC	Rice
Consomme/chicken/beef	Broccoli
Chicken noodle soup	Corn
Vegetable soup	Spinach
Cream of tomato soup	Carrots
Cream of chicken soup	Green beans
Soup du jour	Beets
	Peas
	Squash

Entrees	Salads and dressings
Tomato with:	
Chicken salad, ½ cup	Lettuce/tomato
Tuna salad, ½ cup	Tossed greens
Cottage cheese, ½ cup	Lettuce wedge
Egg salad, ½ cup	Cole slaw
Chef's bowl/meat & cheese	Salad special
Cottage cheese & fruit	Mayonnaise
Roast beef sandwich	French LC
Sliced turkey sandwich	Italian LC
Tuna salad sandwich	Oil & vinegar
Chicken salad sandwich	Lemon and vinegar
Egg salad sandwich	Sour cream
Tuna noodle casserole	
Turkey/gravy/dressing	Desserts
Roast beef au jus	Unsweetened peaches
Macaroni and cheese	Unsweetened fruit cocktail
Scrod	Unsweetened baked apple
Ham/plain	Unsweetened pears
Steak/mushrooms	Unsweetened apricots
Chicken/cranberry LC	Unsweetened applesauce
Grilled cheese/dill pickle	Fresh fruit
Veal/gravy	Sunshine cup
Pork chop/plain	Ice cream
Shell macaroni	Orange sherbet
Beefburger or cheeseburger	Raspberry sherbet
(dill pickles)	Gelatin LC
Salisbury/gravy	Custard LC
Chef's special if allowed	Angel cake

Breads		Miscellaneous
White	Dinner Roll	Salt
Wheat	Crackers	Pepper
Rye		Sugar substitute
		Butter
Beverages		Margarine
Coffee		Lemon
Tea		Dietetic jelly
Decaffeinated coffee		Mustard
Cream		Catsup LC
Nondairy creamer		Relish LC
Whole milk		
4 oz. whole milk		
Skim milk		
4 oz. skim milk		

LC = Low Calorie

Fig. 10.1 Controlled-calorie menu.
© The Seiler Corporation. Reprinted by permission.

essential to have access to all of the hands-on material required for effective counseling sessions. It is also important to be able to record all of the pertinent information regarding each diet counseling session in the patient's medical charts. The information provided below should help to improve your confidence—and skills—regarding your counseling abilities.

This step includes suggested counseling strategies for use with patients requiring weight gain. Those patients with diagnosed eating disorders need specific medical/psychological support of professionals trained to counsel in this area. The following references may prove helpful in identifying individuals requiring referral for anorexia nervosa and/or bulimia treatment.

Suggested Readings on Eating Disorders

AGRAS, W. 1987. Eating Disorders. New York: Pergamon Press.

AMERICAN COLLEGE OF PHYSICIANS. 1986. Position paper on eating disorders: Anorexia nervosa and bulimia. Ann. Internal Med. *105*, Nov., 790.

AMERICAN DIETETIC ASSOCIATION. Position of The American Dietetic Association: Nutrition intervention in the treatment of anorexia nervosa and bulimia nervosa. J. Am. Dietet. Assoc. *88*, Jan., 68.

AMERICAN PSYCHIATRIC ASSOCIATION. 1987. Diagnostic and Statistical Manual of Mental Disorders, 3rd Edition. Washington, DC: APA.

ANDERSEN, A. 1985. Practical Comprehensive Treatment of Anorexia Nervosa and Bulimia. Baltimore: Johns Hopkins University Press.

ANDERSEN, A. 1988. Anorexia nervosa: Who are you? Where are you? Mayo Clinic Proc. *63*, May, 511.

BOSKIND-WHITE, M., and WHITE, W. 1987. Bulimarexia: The Binge-Purge Cycle, 2nd Edition. New York: W. W. Norton.

BROWNELL, K., and FOREYT, J. (Editors). 1986. Handbook of Eating Disorders. New York: Basic Books.

BRUCH, H. 1973. Eating Disorders. New York: Basic Books.

CHERNIN, K. 1981. The Obsession: Reflection on the Tyrannies of Slenderness. New York: Harper & Row.

CHERNIN, K. 1985. The Hungry Self. New York: Harper & Row.

CRISP, A. 1980. Anorexia Nervosa: Let Me Be. Philadelphia: Grune & Stratton.

DALLY, P. 1980. Obesity and Anorexia Nervosa: A Question of Shape. London, England: Faber & Faber.

EMMETT, S. 1985. Theory and Treatment of Anorexia Nervosa: Biomedical, Sociocultural, and Psychological Perspectives. New York: Brunner/Mazel.

GARNER, D. 1980. Cultural expectations of thinness in women. Psychol. Reports *47*, Oct., 481.

HASKEW, P., and ADAMS, C. 1984. When Food is a Four-Letter Word: Programs of Recovery from Anorexia, Bulimia, Bulimarexia, Obesity, and Appetite Disorders. Englewood Cliffs, NJ: Prentice-Hall.

HUSE, D., and LUCAS, A. 1983. Dietary treatment of anorexia nervosa. J. Am. Dietet. Assoc. *83*, Dec., 687.

KEYS, A. 1950. The Biology of Human Starvation. Minneapolis: University of Minnesota Press.

KIRKLEY, B. 1986. Bulimia: Clinical characteristics, development, and etiology. J. Am. Dietet. Assoc. *86*, Apr., 468.

KOLODNEY, N. 1987. When Food's a Foe. Boston: Little, Brown & Co.

LEVENKRON, S. 1982. Treating and Overcoming Anorexia Nervosa. New York: Warner Books.

NATIONAL DAIRY COUNCIL. 1985. Eating disorders. Dairy Council Digest *56*, Jan./Feb., 1.

NEUMAN, P., and HALVORSON, P. 1983. Anorexia Nervosa and Bulimia: A Handbook for Counselors and Therapists. New York: Van Nostrand Reinhold.

PALLA, B., and LITT, I. 1988. Medical complications of eating disorders. Pediatrics *81*, May, 613.

ROTH, G. 1982. Feeding the Hungry Heart. New York: Bobbs-Merrill Co.

SCHWARTZ, H. 1986. Never Satisfied: A Cultural History of Diets, Fantasies, and Fat. New York: Macmillan.

STORY, M. 1986. Nutrition management and dietary treatment of bulimia. J. Am. Dietet. Assoc. *86*, Apr., 517.

STUNKARD, A., and STELLAR, E. 1984. Eating and Its Disorders. New York: Raven Press.

YATES, W., and SIELENI, B. 1987. Anorexia and bulimia. Primary Care *14*, Dec., 737.

For journal subscription:

International Journal of Eating Disorders. John Wiley & Sons, 605 Third Avenue, New York, NY 10158.

For audiovisuals:

Dieting: The Danger Point. CRM/McGraw-Hill Films, PO Box 641, Del Mar, CA 92014.
Diet unto Death: Anorexia Nervosa. ABC Wide World of Learning, 1330 Avenue of the Americas, New York, NY 10019.
Fear of Fat: Dieting and Eating Disorders. Churchill Films, 662 North Robertson Boulevard, Los Angeles, CA 90069.
Portraits of Anorexia. Churchill Films, 662 North Robertson Boulevard, Los Angeles, CA 90069.

For further information:

American Anorexia/Bulimia Association, Inc., 133 Cedar Lane, Teaneck, NJ 07666.
Anorexia Nervosa and Associated Disorders, PO Box 271, Highland Park, IL 60035.
Anorexia Nervosa and Related Eating Disorders, Inc. (ANRED), PO Box 5102, Eugene, OR 97405.
National Anorexia Aid Society, Inc., PO Box 29461, Columbus, OH 43229.

Counseling Guidelines—Weight Gain

Table 10.7 General Outline for Weight Gain Counseling

I. Initial Session
   A. General Guidelines
   B. Patient Records
      1. Medical History Form
      2. Weight Chart
      3. 24-Hour Recall Form
   C. Assignments
      1. Food Intake Record
      2. Activity Record
      3. Diet History
   D. Technician's Notes
II. Follow-up Session(s)
   A. General Guidelines
   B. Handouts
      1. Personal Diet Plan
      2. Tip Sheets
   C. Technician's Notes

Table 10.7 outlines the steps for diet counseling for weight gain. The following material gives the details of each step.

I. Initial Session

I. A. General Guidelines

1. Use Medical History Form to assess patient's nutritional status.

2. Weigh patient and record on Weight Chart. The chart is a helpful tool in visualization of weight status.

3. Assist patient in recording 24-hour recall of food intake using 24-Hour Recall Form. This will aid patient in keeping an accurate Food Intake Record.

4. Instruct patient to keep daily Food Intake Record so that typical food intake patterns can be evaluated. Advise patient not to deviate from his/her normal eating pattern. Stress the importance of recording food intake and associated activity immediately after eating.

5. Instruct patient to keep Activity Record. Advise patient not to deviate from normal activity pattern.

6. Instruct patient to complete Diet History. This provides for a basic evaluation of patient's food intake patterns. (Use Pre-test from Chapter 2.)

7. Record assessment and recommendation(s) using the SOAP method in Technician's Notes. This form can be kept in your files with a copy in the patient's medical records.

I. B. Patient Records

1. Medical History Form

Date _____ Referred by _____

Name _____ Date of birth _____

Address _____ Phone no. _____

Occupation _____ Hours per work week ____ Work phone no. _____

Educational background _____ Religious/ethnic background _____

Sex ____ Marital status ____

Household composition: Live alone ____ Spouse ____ Children/No. ____

Other: _____

General health status:

Physician _____ Address _____

Phone no. _____ Date of last visit _____

Ambulatory care required? ____ If so, describe: _____

Neuromuscular problems? ____ If so, how is eating affected? _____

Visual/auditory problems? ____ If so, describe: _____

Chewing difficulties? ____ If so, describe: _____

Appetite typically good? _____ fair? _____ poor? _____

Digestion/elimination difficulties? ____ If so, describe: _____

Food intolerances? ____ If so, describe: _____

Hypertension? ____ If so, describe: _____

Hyperlipidemia? ____ If so, describe: _____

Diabetes? _____ If so, describe: _____

Arthritis/gout? _____ If so, describe: _____

Gallbladder disorder? _____ If so, describe: _____

Thyroid disorder? _____ If so, describe: _____

Other: _____

Height _____ Weight _____ Frame _____

Triceps skinfold thickness _____ Mid-arm circumference _____

Mid-arm muscle circumference _____

Weight changes/problems? _____ If so, describe: _____

Clinical signs of nutritional status:

Skin _____ Mouth _____

Hair _____ Eyes _____

Teeth _____ Other: _____

Lab data:

Blood pressure _____ EKG _____ Exercise stress test _____

Cholesterol _____ Triglycerides _____ Lipoprotein profile _____

Fasting blood glucose _____ CBC _____

Serum T_3 _____ Serum T_4 _____ PBI _____

Other: _____

Medications taken regularly: _____

Prescribed by: _____ Date(s) prescribed: _____

Nutrition supplements taken regularly: _____

Prescribed by: _____ Date(s) prescribed: _____

Special diet prescription: _____

Prescribed by: _____ Date of prescription: _____

How closely is diet followed? Always adhered to ___ Sometimes ___ Rarely ___ Never ___

Type of housing: Room _____ Apartment _____ Home _____ Institution _____

Prepare own meals? _____ Dine out? Often (more than once a day) _____ Rarely _____

Food shopping done independently? _____ If not, describe required assistance: _____

_____

Eligible for food stamps? _____ If so, are they currently being used? _____

Cigarette smoker? _____ If so, how much: _____

Exercise regularly? _____ If so, describe: _____

 No. times per week _____ No. minutes per session _____

Comments: _____

2. Weight Chart

Starting weight _____   Reasonable weight _____

Date	No. weeks on diet	Weight	Comments

3. 24-Hour Recall Form

Date and time (over 24-hr period)	Food and amount	Where eaten[a]	Eaten with whom[b]	Associated activity[c]

[a]For example, at the kitchen table, at home—sitting at a desk, in a car, or at a restaurant.
[b]For example, with parents, friend(s), or spouse.
[c]For example, while studying, driving, talking, or watching TV.

I.   C.   Assignments

1. Food Intake Record

Date and time	Duration of meal (min)	Food and amount	Where eaten[a]	With whom	Associated activity[b]	Associated emotions[c]

[a]Such as work, restaurant, kitchen, living room.
[b]For example, watching television, reading, socializing, driving, talking on the phone, cooking.
[c]Attitude: bored, anxious, frustrated, depressed, happy, angry, tense, etc.

2. Activity Record

Date and time	Type of activity	Duration

3. Diet History

Use the Pre-test from Chapter 2 (p. 30) to provide a record of typical foods eaten.

I. D. Technician's Notes
Patient: _____   Date: _____

S (Subjective data—how patient feels):
O (Objective data—physical measurements including diet/nutritional status):
A (Assessment—acceptability of dietary progress/nutritional status):
P (Plan—diet prescription and instruction):
Comments:

II. Follow-up Session(s)

II. A. General Guidelines
1. Weigh patient and record on Weight Chart.
2. Review assignments and discuss; analyze patient's Food Intake Record and Activity Record and remember to praise patient often and to avoid overemphasis on wrong behaviors. Emphasize change in behavior rather than weight gain.
3. Aid patient in determining a realistic weight goal by using insurance company actuarial tables, skinfold thicknesses, and/or the following formulas: For women of medium build, use 100 lb for first 5 ft of height plus 5 lb for each additional inch; for men of medium build, use 106 lb for first 5 ft of height plus 6 lb for each additional inch; for those with small builds, subtract 10% and for those with large builds, add 10%.
4. Using Activity Record, determine if patient's activity level is sedentary, moderate, or strenuous.
5. Determine desired daily caloric intake level by using the following formulas: If activity level is sedentary, multiply desired weight by 13; if moderate, multiply by 15; if strenuous, multiply by 20. Add the number of calories which would lead to desired weekly weight gain. (Note: 3500 calories = 1 lb.)
6. Individualize a diet plan and instruct patient in its use. (Use the handout Personal Diet Plan on pp. 236–238 with modifications for weight gain).
7. Provide Tip Sheets for at-home and dining out guidance.
8. Instruct patient to continue to keep daily Food Intake Record and Activity Record.
9. Record assessment and recommendation(s) using the SOAP method in Technician's Notes. This form can be kept in your files with a copy in the patient's medical records.

II. B. Handouts

1. Personal Diet Plan

Use the Personal Diet Plan handout form given on pp. 236–238.

2. Tip Sheets

Tips for home

1. Eat regular meals at predetermined times:
Avoid erratic eating schedules by planning menus and mealtimes in advance.
Include three or more meals daily, plus planned snacks.
Follow a nutritious diet plan composed of well-balanced meals and snacks.
2. Include several snacks daily:
Choose foods to suit personal tastes.
Try to include larger portions than normal.
Include high-calorie, low-volume items (e.g., cheese, nuts, peanut butter, and ice cream) as well as ample complex carbohydrates (e.g., potatoes and pastas).
Try various commercial supplements or whip up blenderized "thickshakes."
3. Eat slowly and learn to enjoy food:
Put down silverware between bites.

Chew food thoroughly.

Make dining atmosphere as pleasurable and non-stressful as possible.

Relax during meals.

4. Increase daily activity:

Develop a regular daily pattern of some type of exercise(s).

Learn to enjoy physical activities, such as bicycling, jogging, and tennis.

Avoid excessive exercise which might defeat weight gain attempts.

5. Consider the following additional tips:

Avoid skipping meals.

Eat moderate amounts of desserts, sweets, and other high-calorie foods—but not to the exclusion of more nutritious fare.

Keep nutrient-rich snacks on hand, within easy reach.

Shopping and cooking tips

1. Plan ahead:

Plan menus in advance for meals and snacks.

Prepare shopping lists from the planned menus.

Shopping when hungry can add to food appeal.

2. Employ sound nutrition principles while shopping:

Read labels carefully to check for ingredients, nutrients, and calories.

Purchase nutritious snack foods.

3. Add calories during food preparation:

Dried skim milk powder can be added to casseroles, puddings, meatloaf, and other recipes.

Toppings such as wheat germ, seeds, and nuts can be sprinkled on cereals, casseroles, etc.

Add yogurt to fruit, or serve with sauces.

Melt cheese on vegetables, or serve with sauces.

Breads—including muffins, bagels, and quick breads—can be topped with peanut butter, cream cheese, and/or melted cheese.

Potatoes and their skins can be topped with melted cheese, blue cheese, or Parmesan cheese.

Nutritious desserts include homemade fruit pies, oatmeal and peanut butter cookies, and ice cream.

Dining out tips

1. Plan ahead:

Determine nutritious menu selections from favorite restaurants.

Fast food fare is often high in fat-calories, but certain selections are more nutritious than others.

Avoid spoiling the appetite by unplanned snacking or nibbling before dining out.

2. Maximize caloric intake:

Alcoholic beverages contribute calories and may stimulate the appetite, but overindulgence has the opposite effect.

Avoid filling up on soups or bread and butter (or salad bar) so the complete meal can be enjoyed.

Relax—and enjoy the meal.

Have dessert on occasion.

Stand near the party food at social gatherings and indulge in the more nutritious choices.

3. Make dining out as pleasurable as eating at home—or more so.

II. C. Technician's Notes

Patient: _____   Date: _____

S (Subjective data—how patient feels):

O (Objective data—physical measurements including diet/nutritional status):

A (Assessment—acceptability of dietary progress/nutritional status):

P (Plan—diet prescription and instruction):

Comments:

Breakfast

Name _____ Room _____
Diet **Regular**—plus extra calories _____

Please circle your selections below

Fruits and juices
Orange juice
Grapefruit juice
Prune juice
Apple juice
Cranberry juice
Grapefruit sections
Stewed prunes
Banana

Beverages
Coffee
Tea
Decaffeinated coffee
Cocoa

Cereals
Cream of wheat
Grits
Oatmeal
Cornflakes
Rice Krispies
Special K
Puffed rice
Puffed wheat
Shredded wheat
All Bran
Bran Flakes
Cream
Nondairy creamer

Entrees
Bacon
Sausage
Scrambled egg
Poached egg
Egg substitute
Pancakes
French toast
Omelet of the Day

Whole milk
4 oz. whole milk
Skim milk
4 oz. skim milk

Breads
Apple muffin
Blueberry muffin
Bran muffin
Corn muffin
Plain muffin
Danish pastry
Doughnut
White toast
Wheat toast
Rye toast

Miscellaneous
Salt
Pepper
Sugar
Sugar substitute
Butter
Margarine
Lemon
Jelly
Pancake syrup

Name _____ Room _____
Diet **Regular**—plus extra calories _____

Luncheon

Please circle your selections below

Appetizers
Apple juice
Cranberry juice
Tomato juice
Fruit cup
Consomme/chicken/beef
Chicken noodle soup
Vegetable soup
Cream of tomato soup
Cream of chicken soup
Soup du jour

Entrees
Tomato with:
  Chicken salad
  Tuna salad
  Cottage cheese
  Egg salad
Chef's bowl/meat & cheese
Fruit and cottage cheese
Roast beef sandwich
Sliced turkey sandwich
Tuna salad sandwich
Chicken salad sandwich
Egg salad sandwich
Sandwich special
Peanut butter & jelly sandwich
Tuna noodle casserole
Turkey/gravy/dressing
Roast beef au jus
Chicken a la king/toast
Macaroni and cheese
Scrod
Ham/pineapple
Steak/mushrooms
Chicken/cranberry
Fish/chips
Veal parmesan
Grilled cheese/pickle
Veal/gravy
Pork chop/applesauce
Shell macaroni
Beefburger/cheeseburger
Salisbury/gravy
Chef's special

Breads
White   Rye   Dinner Roll
Wheat   Crackers

Beverages
Coffee
Tea
Decaffeinated coffee
Cocoa
Cream
Nondairy creamer
Whole milk
4 oz. whole milk
Skim milk
4 oz. skim milk

Vegetables
Whipped potato
Baked potato
Oven-browned potato
Noodles
Rice
Broccoli
Corn
Carrots
Green beans
Beets
Peas
Squash

Salads and dressings
Lettuce/tomato
Tossed greens
Lettuce wedge
Cole slaw
Mayonnaise
French dressing
Italian dressing
Thousand island dressing
Creamy Italian
Oil & vinegar
Sour cream

Desserts
Peaches
Fruit cocktail
Baked apple
Pears
Apricots
Applesauce
Fresh fruit
Dessert of the day
Sugar cookies
Oatmeal cookies
Cupcake
Apple pie
Cheesecake
Shortcake/topping
Chocolate pudding/topping
Butterscotch pudding/
  topping
Tapioca/topping
Ice cream
Orange sherbet
Raspberry sherbet
Gelatin
Custard
Eclair
Angel cake

Miscellaneous
Salt   Lemon
Pepper   Jelly
Sugar   Mustard
Sugar substitute Catsup
Butter   Relish
Margarine

Name _____ Room _____
Diet **Regular**—plus extra calories _____

Dinner

Please circle your selections below

Appetizers
Apple juice
Cranberry juice
Tomato juice
Fruit cup
Consomme/chicken/beef
Chicken noodle soup
Vegetable soup
Cream of tomato soup
Cream of chicken soup
Soup du jour

Entrees
Tomato with:
  Chicken salad
  Tuna salad
  Cottage cheese
  Egg salad
Chef's bowl/meat & cheese
Fruit and cottage cheese
Roast beef sandwich
Sliced turkey sandwich
Tuna salad sandwich
Chicken salad sandwich
Egg salad sandwich
Sandwich special
Peanut butter & jelly sandwich
Tuna noodle casserole
Turkey/gravy/dressing
Roast beef au jus
Chicken a la king/toast
Macaroni and cheese
Scrod
Ham/pineapple
Steak/mushrooms
Chicken/cranberry
Fish/chips
Veal parmesan
Grilled cheese/pickle
Veal/gravy
Pork chop/applesauce
Shell macaroni
Beefburger/cheeseburger
Salisbury/gravy
Chef's special

Breads
White   Rye   Dinner Roll
Wheat   Crackers

Beverages
Coffee
Tea
Decaffeinated coffee
Cocoa
Cream
Nondairy creamer
Whole milk
4 oz. whole milk
Skim milk
4 oz. skim milk

Vegetables
Whipped potato
Baked potato
Oven-browned potato
Noodles
Rice
Broccoli
Corn
Carrots
Green beans
Beets
Peas
Squash

Salads and dressings
Lettuce/tomato
Tossed greens
Lettuce wedge
Cole slaw
Mayonnaise
French dressing
Italian dressing
Thousand island dressing
Creamy Italian
Oil & vinegar
Sour cream

Desserts
Peaches
Fruit cocktail
Baked apple
Pears
Apricots
Applesauce
Fresh fruit
Dessert of the day
Sugar cookies
Oatmeal cookies
Cupcake
Apple pie
Cheesecake
Shortcake/topping
Chocolate pudding/topping
Butterscotch pudding/
  topping
Tapioca/topping
Ice cream
Orange sherbet
Raspberry sherbet
Gelatin
Custard
Eclair
Angel cake

Miscellaneous
Salt   Lemon
Pepper   Jelly
Sugar   Mustard
Sugar substitute Catsup
Butter   Relish
Margarine

Fig. 10.2 Menu for weight gain.
© *The Seiler Corporation. Reprinted by permission.*

Weight Gain Counseling Role Playing

Keeping in mind the preceding Suggested Readings and Counseling Guidelines, participate in the following role play situations; use the sample menu (Fig. 10.2) as a teaching aid. For each situation select different partners, either classmates or co-workers, and elaborate on each role play situation to develop a patient profile. You may want to use your handout from Step 3. Use the SOAP method to record in each patient's medical chart.

As a dietetic technician in nutrition care, do you consider yourself capable of conducting effective counseling sessions with individuals seeking to gain weight? Would you or your family be able to adhere to your nutrition guidelines in order to attain and maintain a reasonable weight? Do you need to do so?

Role Play Situation 1.   As a dietetic technician on the adolescent ward of a community hospital, your newest patient is a teenaged male recovering from **mononucleosis.** He is discouraged with his low body weight and asks for assistance in "building up." Follow the guidelines to complete the charts and provide an individualized diet plan. Prepare a SOAP note which could be recorded in the patient's medical chart.

mononucleosis: Abnormally elevated level of a certain type of white cells (mononuclear leukocytes) in the blood; infectious mononucleosis is a viral condition characterized by swollen glands and spleen, fever, and sore throat.

Role Play Situation 2.   You have long suspected a distant female friend to be suffering from bulimia, and she finally approaches you for help. As a practicing dietetic technician in a large metropolitan hospital, you refer her to a specialist in your department and become a supportive member of the assigned health care team. Follow the guidelines to complete the charts and prepare the initial SOAP note for departmental files.

Role Play Situation 3.   An elderly widow is hospitalized after a minor injury, but her body weight is noted to be seriously low. As the dietetic technician assigned to develop the in-house diet, follow the guidelines to complete the charts (incorporating dietary supplements) in order to devise an individualized diet plan to meet her nutritional needs. Prepare a SOAP note which could be included in the patient's medical chart.

Role Play Situation 4.   Devise several different situations for weight gain counseling in order to practice calculating various meal patterns and planning accompanying menus. See Figure 10.2. Repeat with various caloric levels until you feel comfortable with high-calorie meal and menu planning.

STEP 7: POST-TEST ON WEIGHT

In order to evaluate your understanding of weight control and the most effective weight loss/maintenance/gain techniques, complete the Post-test below. Section I is the Learning Assessment Quiz provided for overweight patients. (If the diet counselor is unable to complete this test successfully, how can the patient be expected to?). Section II incorporates much of the material from this chapter. Answers are given in the Answer Key at the end of the book. Will your overweight patients be able to attain reasonable weights successfully? Will your underweight patients be able to do so as well? Will they opt for the "Three-Prong Program" to safely and effectively maintain a body weight which is reasonable and supportive of optimal health?

Section I: Complete the Learning Assessment Quiz (pp. 240–241) from Step 5: Weight Loss Guidelines. Check your answers with the Answer Key.

Section II: Indicate whether you think the following statements are true (T) or false (F). Check your answers with the Answer Key.

_____   1.   Obesity is defined as an accumulation of body fat in an amount elevating weight 10% above the norm.

_____   2.   Overweight individuals always have an overabundance of adipose.

_____   3.   Low-calorie diets (i.e., under 1200 calories per day) slow metabolism and hinder weight loss efforts.

_____   4.   Overeating is considered to be the major factor contributing to contemporary American obesity.

_____   5.   The adipose cell theory, although unproven, supports the need for early intervention in weight control.

_____ 6. Maturity-onset diabetes occurs more often in the overweight.

_____ 7. Cellulite can be removed with special spot-reducing agents.

_____ 8. Early intervention treatment of the Prader-Willi syndrome can reduce the severity of mental and physical side effects.

_____ 9. Underweight is defined as body weight less than 5% below Desirable Weight levels.

_____ 10. The dietary strategy for increasing body weight focuses on high-protein foods consumed in three large meals.

_____ 11. Underweight individuals are usually indistinguishable from those with anorexia nervosa.

_____ 12. Those seeking to gain weight should avoid physical exercise.

_____ 13. The safe and effective weight control/loss/gain plan includes a wide variety of foods in the amounts required to achieve weight goals.

_____ 14. Bulimia is often a secretive and difficult to detect eating disorder.

Select the answer which best completes the following statements and check your answers with the Answer Key.

_____ 15. The "three prong program" is based on
(a) a well-balanced, calorie-controlled diet. (b) regular daily exercise. (c) appropriate alterations in eating and exercise behaviors. (d) all of these.

_____ 16. The most sensible—and nutritionally inadequate—food group to eliminate during weight loss is the
(a) fruits and vegetables group. (b) breads and cereals group. (c) milk and cheeses group. (d) meat and alternates group. (e) others (fats, sweets, alcoholic beverages) group. (f) all of these.

REFERENCES

MILLS, M. 1984. Body Image Questionnaire. Chapel Hill, NC: Community Diet Counseling Service.
ROTH, G. 1982. Feeding the Hungry Heart. New York: Bobbs-Merrill Co.

Chapter Eleven

Diabetes

CHAPTER BLUEPRINT

Step 1: Take the Pre-test on Diabetes and participate in the assigned group discussion.
Step 2: Examine the Juvenile-Onset Facts List and prepare the assigned handout.
Step 3: Examine the Maturity-Onset Facts List and prepare the assigned handout.
Step 4: Read the Hypoglycemia Facts List and the Suggested Readings; then prepare the assigned handout.
Step 5: Examine the Diabetes Guidelines and complete the role play assignment.
Step 6: Take the Post-test on Diabetes to evaluate what you have learned from the information and activities provided in this chapter.

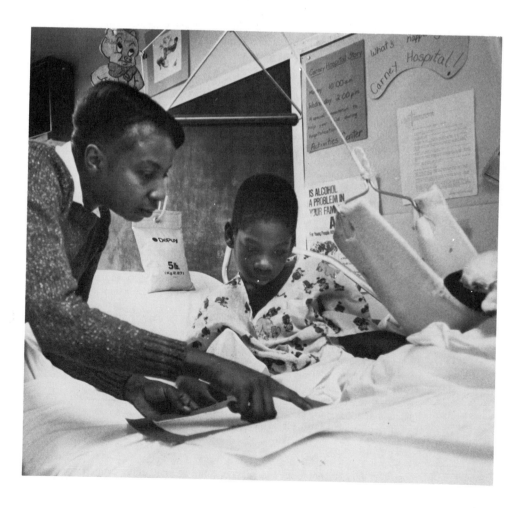

STEP 1: PRE-TEST ON DIABETES

Diabetes Club at Union Hospital[1]

Union Hospital is a 210-bed community health care center located 12 miles north of Boston which serves a population of 240,000. For the past five years, Union has pursued the concept of preventive medicine through education and is currently recognized as a geographic leader in this field. As part of the hospital's overall commitment to improving the general health and well-being of its community members, a club for patients with diabetes was established in the winter of 1979.

The authors, a nutritionist and a nurse educator, have offered a variety of community health education programs covering topics of interest and need determined by the utilization of a community assessment.

The assessment, which compared national, regional Health Systems Agency (HSA) and local morbidity and mortality statistics, indicated that Union patients with diabetes spend the most days hospitalized, and that diabetes is the seventh cause of mortality locally, regionally, and nationally.

On the basis of this information, the Diabetes Club was designed with three main components: (a) An educational format with specified topics based both on current diabetic teaching strategies and the club members' perceived needs; (b) a social context for peer support and information exchange; and (c) an opportunity to make educated choices about diabetes, its management, and lifestyle requirements.

Each club member is given an assessment questionnaire asking for basic demographic data and current diabetic management procedures. Vital signs and height and weight are recorded and documented for later comparison, and a pre-test is administered to determine basic knowledge of diabetes, its causes, symptoms, complications, and treatment. At the end of the program, the assessment questionnaire and test are again administered to measure changes in knowledge and self-management techniques. Also, physical measurements are again made.

Meetings are held once a month for two hours at Union Hospital. Printed materials on diabetes and on the monthly scheduled topic are made available, and blood pressure screenings are provided for interested members and their guests. Sessions focus on issues such as stress reduction, exercise, diabetic management, and related health strategies.

Two of the Diabetes Club meetings each year are conducted by the community health education nutritionist. Both of these diet meetings are conducted informally. The first quarter hour is devoted to the club agenda and social interactions, and the final quarter hour is left open for chatting and for private discussions with the nutritionist. Club members may ask questions or add personal comments at any time during these meetings. One meeting focuses on the diet for patients with diabetes, including a discussion of philosophy, goals, and current ideologies. The next meeting looks at diet and disease, with a discussion of obesity, heart disease, and the possible roles of food fat, sugar, salt, and fiber in today's degenerative diseases.

During the first diet meeting, discussion focuses on the recent changes in the structure of the diet for patients with diabetes. The myth of carbohydrates as "enemies" is disposed of; the importance of invisible and visible fats is emphasized; and the new **Exchanges** are explained. Methods for simplification of label interpretation and recipe modification are illustrated. Handouts discuss Exchange values, reading labels, modifying recipes, and nutritious snacks. Snacks are provided by the nurse educator and the nutritionist; club members take turns in contributing acceptable snacks for later club meetings. Recipes and pertinent nutrition information for all snacks are provided to club members at each meeting.

Other handouts made available to the group provide tips for dining out, shopping and cooking, and other suggestions relating to nutrition and diabetes.

The second diet meeting involves more member participation. After a brief explanation of the role of nutrition in selected degenerative diseases, discussion is steered toward the emotional aspects of diet and diabetes. Members express personal experiences and their individual feelings of guilt, deprivation, depression, and isolation. Common fears about the results of various dietary indiscretions are exposed, as are the frustrations that accompany dietary rigidity.

One club member who successfully lost more than 100 pounds and maintained

Exchanges: Food portion system devised by the American Diabetes Association in which items with similar nutrient values and caloric contents are interchangeable; used in diabetic diets and weight loss regimens, and with certain other conditions requiring strict diet planning.

[1]Schutt and Aronson, 1980. Reprinted by permission from Journal of the American Dietetic Association.

the loss for more than a year shared her diet routine and the accompanying problems with the group. She was given a standing ovation for her determination and visible success. Other members have complained of personal experiences with incomplete or nonexistent diet instructions. Interested club members are told about available nutrition counseling services in the area.

It has become obvious that diet is not only one of the most important roads to success for the diabetic, but is also one of the major avenues of discouragement and self-destruction. Through education, open discussion, and peer support, club members are able to realize that they are not alone in their feelings of despair. The Diabetes Club offers patients with diabetes the opportunity to increase their own education about the disease, and enables them to expose and explore their own disease-related emotions. It is hoped that, by identifying and sharing insights and experiences, each member of Union Hospital's Diabetes Club can better smooth the road toward successful control of his/her disease.

Being diagnosed as diabetic can prove to be one of the more traumatic experiences of a lifetime. Learning to take care of overall health and to take control over the disease can mean the difference between debilitation and good health, suffering and well-being, self-pitying depression and psychological wellness. It may appear to be easier to opt for despair and immobility, but the long-term results of positive attitude and motivation to change can include improved health and increased longevity.

Complete the questionnaire below, and discuss your answers with classmates or co-workers. As a dietetic technician in nutrition care, it is important for you to understand the psychological impact of diabetes and to develop a working knowledge of the associated physical factors and dietary implications.

Diabetes Questionnaire

1. You have just been diagnosed as diabetic and must learn to self-administer insulin and readjust diet/activity patterns. Describe your initial reaction:

2. Your spouse has just been diagnosed as diabetic, and requests your assistance in insulin administration and dietary modifications. Briefly explain how you would help him/her—physically and psychologically—to manage the disease:

3. Your 8-year-old child has just been diagnosed as a juvenile diabetic. Briefly explain how you would help him/her—physically and psychologically—to manage the disease:

4. A newly diagnosed diabetic teenager adamantly refuses to follow the diet prescription because she "feels like a weirdo." Briefly describe your response as a member of the attending health care team:

5. A middle-aged diabetic admits that he has not been adhering to his diet plan because he "likes to have a few beers with the boys." Briefly describe your response as a member of the attending health care team:

6. What role would a psychologist play as part of the overall framework of a Diabetes Club (similar to the one described in the preceding report)?

STEP 2: JUVENILE-ONSET DIABETES

In most developed Western societies, less than 10% of all diabetics are afflicted with the more severe form called juvenile-onset (or Type I), while the majority have the milder (Type II) maturity-onset type. Those suffering from the former type require strict control and may suffer from serious complications. Often young when the disease is discovered, juvenile-onset diabetics require special attention to ensure proper physical and psychological health.

The following Juvenile-Onset Facts List provides some of the most current diet-related information to include in counseling individuals with insulin-dependent diabetes.

Juvenile-Onset Facts List

1. Diabetes is a chronic systemic disease characterized by disorders of (a) the metabolism of insulin, carbohydrate, fat, and protein; and (b) the structure and function of blood vessels. The early signs are due to metabolic disorders and later complications are caused by the **microangiopathic** changes in the blood vessels.

2. Diabetes is a chronic metabolic disorder which gives rise to (a) **hyperglycemia;** (b) **glycosuria;** (c) increased protein **catabolism;** (d) ketosis; and (e) acidosis.

3. The four stages of diabetes are diagnosed using results of the **glucose tolerance test (GTT), fasting blood sugar measurement (FBS),** and the **cortisone glucose tolerance test (CGTT),** and are as follows: (a) prediabetes; (b) subclinical diabetes; (c) latent diabetes; and (d) overt diabetes. Prediabetes is without symptoms; subclinical and latent diabetes may have symptoms difficult to detect without laboratory testing, and clinical symptoms are typically observable only in the overt stage (see Table 11.1).

4. *Primary* diabetes is due to genetic causes, while *secondary* diabetes may be caused by an endocrine disorder (e.g., pituitary gland or adrenal gland), pancreatic destruction, or stress reactions such as infections, surgery, pregnancy, drug therapies (e.g., thiazide diuretics or cortisone), low carbohydrate intake, and starvation.

5. Diabetes is not one, but several disorders; the predominant type is noninsulin dependent or *maturity-onset* diabetes (Type II), with the insulin-dependent and chromium deficiency types occurring less frequently.

6. *Juvenile-onset* (Type I) diabetes usually appears suddenly during childhood or puberty with the distinguishing symptoms of **polyphagia, polydipsia, polyuria, nocturia,** and uncontrolled levels of blood glucose. Even small changes in insulin dosage or exercise and the onset of infection or stress can cause great fluctuations in blood glucose levels and the undesirable physical effects.

7. Juvenile-onset diabetes requires insulin therapy since afflicted individuals have little or no endogenous insulin.

8. The severe metabolic abnormalities associated with this form of diabetes include severe hyperglycemia, ketonemia, ketoacidosis, coma, and death. Serum lipid abnormalities are also common.

9. The discoveries of insulin and antibiotics have led to a lengthened life expectancy for diabetics, but vascular and neural complications are common (e.g., degeneration of the **retina** can lead to blindness, and renal failure and cardiovascular disorders occur more frequently and at a younger age).

10. The juvenile-onset diabetic requires exogenous insulin because the beta (β) cells of the islets of Langerhans found in the pancreas have become **hyalinized,** replaced by fiber, and unable to produce insulin; oral hypoglycemic agents are insufficient since the pancreatic cells can no longer be stimulated to produce insulin. Individualization of drug/insulin therapy can be a lengthy process to be conducted with the patient, primary care physician, and health care team (see Table 11.2 for insulin types).

microangiopathy: Disorder involving the small blood vessels.

hyperglycemia: Excessive level of glucose in the blood.

glycosuria: Abnormally high content of glucose in the urine.

catabolism: Destructive metabolism in which complex substances become simpler and energy is released.

glucose tolerance test (GTT): Used to measure body's ability to metabolize carbohydrates; standard test administers 100 g of glucose to fasting patient with blood/urine samples taken beforehand, after $\frac{1}{2}$ hour, then at hourly intervals for 4–5 hours.

fasting blood sugar measurement (FBS): Used to determine blood level of glucose in fasting state, usually following several days of adherence to a high-carbohydrate diet.

cortisone glucose tolerance test (CGTT): Cortisone acetate is administered several times prior to the standard GTT.

polyphagia: Excessive food ingestion.

polydipsia: Excessive thirst.

polyuria: Excessive urination.

nocturia: Excessive urination at night.

retina: Innermost layer of the eyeball which is sensitive to light and responsible for color vision.

hyalinize: Convert into glasslike collagen material.

Table 11.1 Classifying Diabetes

Lab test[a]	Prediabetes	Subclinical diabetes	Latent diabetes	Overt diabetes	Secondary diabetes
Fasting blood glucose	Normal	Normal	Normal	Increased	Increased
Glucose tolerance test	Normal	Normal; abnormal during pregnancy and stress	Abnormal	Abnormal	Abnormal
Cortisone glucose tolerance test	Normal	Abnormal	Abnormal	Abnormal	Abnormal

[a]Note: A 2-hour **postprandial** blood glucose level of greater than 120 mg/dL (deciliter) for those aged 20–40, or greater than 160 mg/dL for those over 40 is indicative of diabetes. Normalization is defined as within the 60–160 mg/dL range.

postprandial: Following a meal.

Table 11.2 Insulin Action

Type of insulin	Acting time	Time of onset (hours)	Peak effect (hours)	Duration of action (hours)
Crystalline (regular)	Short	$\frac{1}{2}$	2–4	6–8
Semi-lente (amorphous zinc)	Short	1	3–6	12
Globin zinc	Intermediate	2–4	6–8	18
Lente (combination of 30% semi-lente and 70% ultra-lente)	Intermediate	1–2	10–16	24
NPH (neutral protamine–hagedorn) or isophane	Intermediate	1–2	10–16	23
Protamine zinc (PZI)	Long	4–6	16–24	24–36
Ultra-lente	Long	5–8	20–26	36

11. An abnormally high sugar content in the blood creates the perfect breeding ground for bacteria. Since the cells are poorly nourished, infection sets in and injuries are unable to heal properly. Thus, the juvenile-onset diabetic who is not in good control is susceptible to serious infection and poor recovery from wounds.

12. Ketosis or acidosis occurs when the body utilizes fats for energy and, since fat cannot be metabolized completely when used in this way, acidic breakdown products called ketones accumulate in the blood; this disturbs the body's normal acid–base balance leading to coma and, if untreated, death.

13. Some fatty acids that are incompletely oxidized are excreted in the urine; acetone results in a positive Acetest, an indication that diabetes is out of control.

14. The four major treatment strategies for diabetes are the following; the first three may require a decrease in body fat:

a. Improve glucose tolerance and decrease insulin resistance.
b. Regulate glycemia, including the prevention of hypoglycemia.
c. Prevent or reduce the complications of diabetes including vascular problems, **neuropathy,** cataracts, ketosis.
d. Manage other complications such as pregnancy, renal failure, and hypertension.

neuropathy: Any disorder(s) of the peripheral (noncentral) nervous system.

15. Diabetics should eat only those foods allowed on their individualized diet plans and in the prescribed amounts: if more is eaten than needed, a shortage of insulin will result, causing acidosis; when too little is eaten, the excess insulin leads to insulin shock.

16. Diet should be adjusted to the amount of insulin available, used to prevent the spillage of sugar into the urine, and controlled to keep blood sugar levels normal; the diet should also allow for good health and normal physical activity.

17. The dietary habits of the diabetic infant should not differ from the normal infant until the age of 2 years.

18. The Wetzel, Iowa, or Stuart growth charts can be used to determine desirable weights for diabetic children.

19. For children, adolescents, and pregnant clients, the Recommended Dietary Allowances can be used as a guideline in estimating caloric and nutrient requirements, and the diet can be adjusted accordingly.

20. Caloric and nutrient requirements of the diabetic child are usually high in the initial phase of dietary treatment due to depleted nutritional stores.

21. During prepubescent growth, insulin requirements may gradually increase. After puberty, insulin and caloric requirements decrease and must be adjusted to prevent excess weight gain.

22. For the insulin-dependent juvenile diabetic, consistency in meal times and content should be stressed.

23. Self-responsibility should be encouraged in the diabetic child.

24. Parents should avoid excessive pampering and coddling of the diabetic child; there is no need for guilt feelings concerning the child's disease. Parents should not punish the diabetic child for dietary indiscretions; a simple explanation of the importance of proper management is usually sufficient.

25. Appropriate school lunch selections can be made by evaluation of menus in advance.

26.   Careful selection of a diabetic summer camp can provide the child with significant learning experiences amongst peers. Local diabetic associations usually can provide camp information.

27.   Parents of the diabetic child should take advantage of the professional guidance offered by local counseling services (e.g., diabetes clubs, diabetes clinics, and American Diabetes Association chapters).

28.   The basic nutritional requirements of the diabetic are similar to those of the normal individual, yet the diabetic must be particularly careful to make appropriate food choices. Diet is an integral part of a comprehensive health care program which includes periodic medical examinations, regular exercise, avoidance of cigarette smoking, and careful attention to personal hygiene for prevention of infection.

29.   The diet plan is designed to help prevent the metabolic disorders of diabetes, to reduce the risk factors associated with cardiovascular disease, and to reduce the risk of other complications.

30.   An important objective of diabetic care is the attainment of a reasonable weight through a calorically controlled and nutritionally balanced diet; excess body fat decreases glucose tolerance and increases insulin resistance, heightening the demand on the pancreas for insulin. Drug therapy does not eliminate the need for proper control of diet and weight.

31.   The occurrence of hyperglycemia and hypoglycemia should be minimized; feasting and fasting must be avoided to prevent rapid swings in blood glucose levels. Complex carbohydrates are preferable since simple carbohydrates are absorbed rapidly and are associated with hyperglycemic peaks.

32.   The composition of carbohydrates (i.e., whole grain vs. processed) and of meals (i.e., mixed with protein/fat vs. mostly carbohydrates) will affect blood glucose levels as well. Nutrition counseling can provide information on the "glycemic index" of foods, that is, the timing and effect on blood glucose of carbohydrates to be included in the diet. Certain fibers may help to improve carbohydrate metabolism (e.g., soluble fibers in oat bran and legumes).

33.   Individualization is important and, since insulin needs are always changing, constant adjustments are required to maintain diabetic control.

34.   Insulin and food intake requirements must be adjusted in accordance with individual activity levels. With unusual and strenuous physical activity, the body uses more glucose for energy. The insulin-dependent diabetic should either reduce insulin and/or increase carbohydrate intake during exercise to avoid hypoglycemia.

35.   In America, the major cause of death for diabetics is coronary disease, which occurs two to three times more frequently than in the nondiabetic.

36.   Neuropathy is an additional complication that can occur in those with uncontrolled diabetes, or in later years in the moderately well-controlled patient.

37.   For the hospitalized diabetic, unpredictable food intake is undesirable; small frequent feedings can prevent hypoglycemia and ketosis. It may also be desirable to revise the diet plan to lighter, more digestible foods emphasizing greater amounts of simple carbohydrates and lesser quantities of complex carbohydrates, protein, and fats. Caloric intake may need to be reduced temporarily and, with certain cases of extreme illness, the "diabetic diet" order may also need to be temporarily discontinued. The special replacement diet should be explained to the patient.

38.   Upon obtaining the necessary information from the nutrition and medical personnel, the diabetic is ultimately responsible for self-treatment. Self-monitoring includes blood sugar measuring (at mealtime and bedtime) with reagent strip packets—urine testing is less reliable—and record keeping of test results, dietary intake, insulin use, and activity levels.

Exercise on Juvenile-Onset Diabetes Counseling

Keeping in mind the preceding Juvenile-Onset Facts List, which provides some of the most current diet-related information to include in counseling individuals with insulin-dependent diabetes, prepare a simplified version for use as a patient handout. You may include graphics and/or prepare in a poster format, if desired; see the Sample Handout. Show your handout in rough draft form to classmates or co-workers for constructive criticism on the overall design, content, and potential effectiveness for use in pertinent diet counseling situations. Then prepare a final version for your own future use as a practicing dietetic technician.

Sample Handout

There is no known cure for diabetes mellitus, but the disease can be adequately controlled with close medical supervision and adherence to desirable lifestyle patterns, including proper diet.

○ *Symptoms:* Polyuria—excessive urination
Polydipsia—excessive thirst
Polyphagia—excessive hunger
Weight loss
Weakness, fatigue

○ *Acidosis (hyperglycemia) vs. insulin reaction (hypoglycemia):* See Table 11.3.

Table 11.3   Diabetic Acidosis vs. Insulin Reaction

	Diabetic acidosis (hyperglycemia)	Insulin reaction (hypoglycemia)
Onset	Slow (days)	Sudden (minutes–hours)
Causes	Inadequate insulin, overeating, anesthesia, pregnancy, infection or disease, vomiting or diarrhea, emotional stress, inadequate exercise	Insulin overdose, oral hypoglycemic agents, omission or delay of meals, excessive exercise, termination of pregnancy
Symptoms	Thirst, headache, nausea, vomiting, warm flushed skin, polyuria, drowsiness, difficult breathing, rapid pulse, fruity breath, unconsciousness	Hunger, cold sweat, anxiety, trembling, weakness, headache followed by dizziness, staggering, blurred vision, stupor, pallor, shallow respirations, numbness, unconsciousness
Blood glucose	>250 mg/100 ml	60 mg/100 ml or less
Plasma bicarbonate	Reduced	Normal
Urine glucose	Positive	Usually negative
Urine ketones	Positive	Negative
Treatment	Admission to hospital for insulin and intravenous (I.V.) fluids	Upon onset 10 g carbohydrate (such as $2\frac{1}{2}$ tsp sugar, 2–3 jelly beans or hard candies, $\frac{1}{2}$ cup soft drink) and 20 g 10 minutes later; if unconscious, a **glucagon** "shot" is given

glucagon: Hormone secreted by the pancreas (or prepared commercially) which increases blood glucose levels.

STEP 3: MATURITY-ONSET DIABETES

In most developed Western societies, 70 to 90% of all diabetics contract the disorder late in life. This mild to moderately severe form of the disease is termed *maturity-onset* diabetes, and most sufferers are overweight. For individuals with this type of diabetes, diet will not only control the disease, but can reverse it. For many of these individuals, weight loss can serve to eradicate the disorder, and proper diet with maintenance of a reasonable weight will prevent reoccurrences. The following Maturity-Onset Facts List provides some of the most current diet-related information to include in counseling individuals with noninsulin dependent diabetes.

Maturity-Onset Facts List

1. Diabetes is a hereditary metabolic disorder characterized by an inadequate supply of effective insulin which renders victims unable to regulate blood glucose levels within the normal ranges.

2. Maturity-onset diabetes is characterized by slow or ineffective insulin response and is also termed *noninsulin dependent.*

3.   Maturity-onset diabetes often appears after the age of thirty-five, and may be due to a delayed response to glucose or a decreased secretion of insulin; oral hypoglycemic agents may be prescribed.

4.   Maturity-onset diabetes appears gradually, often without symptoms other than fatigue or ill-defined complaints. Usually, there are not rapid changes in the blood glucose levels, and diet therapy with loss of excess body weight may be all that is required for treatment.

5.   If blood glucose levels rise to exceedingly high levels in those with maturity-onset diabetes, they will remain elevated for abnormally long periods of time and the kidneys will allow some of the glucose to spill out into the urine. Therefore, it is important to maintain a constant, steady, moderate flow of glucose into the bloodstream so that the pancreas is not overwhelmed. Also, concentrated forms of sugar are best avoided, with an emphasis on complex carbohydrates as part of the same well-balanced diet which is prescribed for normal, healthy, nondiabetic individuals.

6.   The two most common factors contributing to the development of maturity-onset diabetes are *genetic makeup* and *obesity;* appropriate diet modifications with weight loss have been shown to have the greatest potential for prevention and control of the disorder and some of the associated complications.

7.   Weight gain often precipitates the onset of diabetes, whereas weight reduction will normalize a number of the metabolic abnormalities in the maturity-onset diabetic, including insulin resistance and elevated levels of blood glucose and fats.

8.   In the United States, the average proportion of calories consumed as carbohydrate is 45%. This proportion, or higher, is usually acceptable for the diabetic because the limiting dietary factor is not carbohydrate but total caloric intake. Also, complex carbohydrates may enhance the efficiency of insulin usage, and by liberalizing dietary carbohydrate, fat intake can be reduced. This may lead to lower serum lipid levels, and thereby help to delay and/or minimize atherosclerosis.

9.   Arteriosclerosis advances at a faster rate in the diabetic, and even more rapidly in the uncontrolled diabetic. Arteriosclerosis is usually more extensive in the arteries of the lower extremities, so the diabetic must pay particular attention to proper foot care.

10.   Small hemorrhages and waxy deposits may develop in the retina of the diabetic. If extensive, blindness may result. The diabetic should have opthalmological examinations at least once each year.

11.   Alcohol may be restricted by the diabetic's physician because improper use can contribute to weight gain and may cause hypoglycemia. Since various drugs can affect blood glucose levels, physician approval should be obtained prior to use.

12.   It is important to determine the portion sizes and caloric contents of foods accurately, so that proper amounts can be included in the diet plan.

13.   A good understanding of the caloric contents of foods, Exchanges (see Table 11.4), and proper use of food labels will enable accuracy in caloric estimation, recipe modification, menu planning, and menu selection appropriate to individual diet requirements.

Table 11.4   Standard Food Exchanges

Exchange list	Carbohydrate (grams)	Protein (grams)	Fat (grams)	Calories
Starch/Bread	15	3	trace	80
Meat				
Lean	—	7	3	55
Medium-fat	—	7	5	75
High-fat	—	7	8	100
Vegetable	5	2	—	25
Fruit	15	—	—	60
Milk				
Skim	12	8	trace	90
Lowfat	12	8	5	120
Whole	12	8	8	150
Fat	—	—	5	45

14. Planning of meals in advance aids in adherence to the diet plan.

15. In the well-controlled diabetic, a minimum of 20 minutes of sustained daily activity is important to overall well-being.

16. In the past, diabetic diets have been lower in carbohydrate than diets for the nondiabetic. Recent studies show that the ratio of carbohydrate and fat to total calories does not affect diabetic control (as measured by plasma glucose levels) or the course of the disease and its complications. These observations appear to be true both in noninsulin dependent and in insulin-dependant patients. There no longer appears to be a need to restrict carbohydrate intake disproportionately in the diets of most diabetic patients.

17. Current studies indicate that high-fiber foods may be of some benefit for the diabetic patient; glucose tolerance may be improved, postprandial blood sugar may not rise as sharply, and insulin demands may be lessened following meals containing generous amounts of whole grains, legumes, vegetables, and fruits. Slowly absorbed (complex) carbohydrates such as starches are preferable to rapidly absorbed (simple) carbohydrates such as sugars. For example, whole grain cereal is preferable to fruit juice as a bedtime snack.

18. The composition of carbohydrates (i.e., whole grain vs. processed) and of meals (i.e., mixed with protein and/or fat) will affect blood glucose levels. Foods rich in "soluble" fibers (e.g., oat bran and legumes) may help to improve carbohydrate metabolism.

19. The theory that large intakes of sucrose will cause diabetes by overstraining the pancreas has not been supported by research. However, diabetes can be induced in animals fed diets high in fat, protein, or sugar, and the incidence can be diminished with a decrease in total food intake.

20. The advantages of using fructose as a replacement for sucrose in the diabetic diet have not been demonstrated to be as beneficial as some have claimed. Fructose is sweeter, but only by a small degree, so the amounts required for sweetening are not significantly less than for sucrose; also, most of the ingested fructose is converted to the insulin-requiring glucose form upon absorption. Caloric control must also be considered when the diet includes fructose-sweetened sweets and desserts.

21. A deficiency in the mineral-nutrient chromium is believed to cause a form of diabetes: chromium works closely with insulin, facilitating both the uptake of glucose by cells and the breakdown of glucose to release energy; if chromium is lacking, there is a decrease in the effectiveness of insulin.

22. With aging, the amount of chromium concentrated in human tissues appears to lessen; the incidence of abnormal carbohydrate tolerance also increases with age, making the results of tests administered for diabetes less accurate than during the younger years.

23. There is no documented need for the use of self-prescribed nutrition supplements, including chromium, by the diabetic. Unless a deficiency is diagnosed by the diabetic's physician, use of unnecessary supplements is unwise and may prove detrimental to health.

24. Large doses of vitamin C can interfere with the urine test used to diagnose diabetes and to indicate poor diabetic control. The use of vitamin supplementation should be confirmed prior to analysis of such tests.

25. During pregnancy, diabetes is a high-risk condition. At this time, it is essential for the mother with this disorder to maintain meticulous control of the diabetes in order to lessen risk for fetal and maternal morbidity and mortality. Pregnancy is *not* a time for weight reduction. Protein requirements increase by about 30 grams per day (to 1.3 g/kg for women, 1.5 g/kg for adolescent girls, 1.7 g/kg for younger girls). Carbohydrate intake should be increased by about 50 grams per day, with a bedtime snack containing at least 25 grams of complex carbohydrate. Frequent snacks need to be planned during the day. Special attention to calcium, iron, and folic acid in the diet is also important for the pregnant diabetic.

26. Diabetes can result in a more difficult pregnancy; the symptoms of diabetes may first appear during pregnancy, making it a wise idea to have a diabetes screening near the end of the second trimester. The pregnant woman with diabetes has an increased chance of developing toxemia.

27. Exercise is an important aspect of the treatment program for diabetes, but it is essential to balance caloric intake with expenditure (and with use of medication, if taking oral hypoglycemic agents or insulin).

28. Control of maturity-onset diabetes is successful if diet adherence is maintained

and a regular exercise program is adopted so that insulin levels are normalized and weight is controlled. Continued use of drug therapy in this country illustrates the difficulties of making the required long-term lifestyle changes (i.e., proper diet, weight loss, regular exercise).

Exercise on Maturity-Onset Diabetes Counseling

Keeping in mind the preceding Maturity-Onset Facts List, which provides some of the most current diet-related information to include in counseling individuals with noninsulin dependent diabetes, prepare a simplified version for use as a patient handout. You may include graphics and/or prepare in a poster format, if desired; see the Sample Handout. Show your handout in rough draft form to classmates or co-workers for constructive criticism on the overall design, content, and potential effectiveness for use in pertinent counseling situations. Then prepare a final version for your own future use as a practicing dietetic technician.

Sample Handout

Tip Sheet

1. Plan ahead:
   Plan menus using appropriate references.
   Make a shopping list and adhere to it.
   Choose and modify recipes carefully.
2. Employ learned nutrition concepts while shopping:
   Read labels carefully to check for ingredients, serving size, caloric and nutrient content—especially carbohydrate, protein, and fat. (See Table 11.4.)
   Be wary of "dietetic" foods, as labels may be misleading.
   Buy those foods allowed in unrestricted amounts to keep on hand for snacking.
3. Incorporate appropriate cooking methods:
   Weigh and measure portions until adept at judging serving sizes.
   Remove all visible fat, including skin, before cooking meat and poultry.
   Broil, boil, bake, and roast meat/fish/poultry without added fat.
   Use a rack when roasting meat/poultry/fish.
   Steam or simmer rather than frying, or use nonstick cooking utensils.
   Avoid nibbling during meal preparation.
   Use seasonings, vinegar, and lemon in cooking.
4. Consider the following additional tips if insulin dependent:
   Do not skip or delay meals; the interval between meals/snacks should not exceed 5 hours. Eat a small snack (include a combination of carbohydrate, protein, and fat) at bedtime or if a meal must be postponed.
   With unusual or continuous physical activity, such as backpacking or an extended bike trip, plan for more frequent meals with increased carbohydrate intake.
   Be especially careful to avoid a hypoglycemic reaction when swimming. Never swim alone.
   When ill, adhere to diet plan if possible; if unable to tolerate solid foods, include light foods at frequent intervals such as sweetened soft drinks, sweetened gelatin, light soups, fruits, and fruit juices.
   Keep sources of concentrated sugar (such as soft drinks, fruit, fruit juices, sugar cubes, Lifesavers, or candy) on hand in case of hypoglycemic reaction.

STEP 4: HYPOGLYCEMIA FACTS

Hypoglycemia may be defined as an abnormally low level of sugar in the blood—resulting either from an excessive rate of removal or a decreased rate of secretion. It is due to overproduction of insulin (or an overdosage of exogenous insulin), or to a depleted supply of liver glycogen. Mild bouts of symptomless hypoglycemia are tolerated by most people, but symptoms can be expected after extended periods of time without food, excessive alcohol intake, crash diets, and other common but undesirable lifestyle patterns. The vague symptomology of hypoglycemia resulted in its surge in popularity as the ready diagnosis for individuals with nebulous complaints. The following Hypoglycemia Facts List and the subsequent Suggested Readings provide some of the most current diet-related information on this topic.

Hypoglycemia Facts List

1. Carbohydrates are classified as complex (starches) or simple (sugars), normally serving as the body's chief source of energy to be utilized by the cells as glucose. Under normal circumstances, blood glucose levels are maintained within a narrow range. Hypoglycemia refers to a low concentration of glucose in the blood. Many people experience the symptoms of hypoglycemia when meals are skipped or delayed. Genuine hypoglycemia, however, is relatively rare.

2. Common symptoms of hypoglycemia include profuse sweating, nervousness, headache, weakness, faintness, and heart palpitations. Since these symptoms are often due to conditions other than hypoglycemia, a change in diet should not be initiated without proper medical diagnosis by a competent physician.

3. Hypoglycemia is classified as "reactive" or "organic." Reactive hypoglycemia (food stimulated, occurring 2–4 hours after a meal/snack) may be alimentary (post-**gastrectomy** or post-**gastroenterostomy**), functional (possible prediabetes), or early diabetes, and is usually a result of excessive insulin response to an ingested carbohydrate load. Crash dieting, frequent meal skipping, inadequate sleep, strenuous exercise, certain medications, and/or stimulants such as caffeine, nicotine, and alcohol may also trigger a reaction. Organic hypoglycemia can result from liver, pituitary, and adrenal disorders, or from tumors of the brain, abdomen, or pancreas.

gastrectomy: Total or partial removal of the stomach.

gastroenterostomy: Surgical connection of the stomach to the intestine.

4. Reactive hypoglycemia can occur when blood glucose levels drop, glycogen reserves are exhausted, and lack of food intake results in ketosis; muscle protein breakdown provides glucose to the brain, and body fat breakdown supplies other cells with energy. Prior to this body adjustment, the blood glucose level may fall too rapidly or too low, causing the symptoms of glucose deprivation of the brain (anxiety, hunger, dizziness) as well as muscle weakness, shakiness and trembling, and **tachycardia.** Most everyone experiences the reactive form of hypoglycemia at one time or another.

tachycardia: Abnormally rapid heart beat.

5. Organic hypoglycemia is an extremely rare condition in which the pancreas habitually oversecretes insulin, causing the level of blood glucose to drop and remain below normal. Treatment consists of an individualized diet plan which is relatively high in protein, with frequent feedings and the exclusion of simple sugars.

6. A normal blood sugar range is maintained by drawing on liver glycogen stores when the level is too low, and by siphoning off any excess into stored liver and muscle glycogen.

7. When the blood sugar level drops, the intake of a meal or snack will cause re-elevation; intake of complex carbohydrate is usually preferable to most simple sugars (which cause rapid increases in blood sugar and an immediate drop), and should be combined with protein and/or fat.

8. An excessive intake of carbohydrate-rich foodstuffs, especially the rapidly absorbed simple sugars, causes the blood glucose level to rise to an undesirably high level; the pancreas overreacts by secreting an excessive amount of insulin, which draws the

glucose into the cells and out of the bloodstream, causing the glucose level to fall too low and/or too rapidly.

9.   Treatment of hypoglycemia includes a nutritionally balanced diet with reduction in simple carbohydrates and such stimulants as caffeine, nicotine, and alcohol which might cause an exaggerated release of insulin into the bloodstream. Complex sources of carbohydrate, such as whole-grain products and legumes, influence insulin release to a lesser degree so are included in the diet plan.

10.   Six small feedings help to maintain an even level of glucose in the blood.

11.   A ready source of glucose should be carried in the event of hypoglycemic symptoms.

12.   Proper use of food labels will aid in the identification of those foods that can be included in the diet. Many "dietetic" foods contain **hexitols** (xylitol, sorbitol, and mannitol) that are metabolized as carbohydrate so should be used sparingly, as should those foods which contain **hexoses** (sucrose, glucose, maltose, dextrose, lactose, fructose, levulose).

13.   Self-diagnosis for hypoglycemia is unwise because the vague symptoms may be due to a number of other conditions, or can be psychologically induced or stress related.

14.   Maintenance of an even blood glucose level for most individuals merely requires a well-balanced dietary intake and adherence to a healthy lifestyle.

hexitol: Sugar alcohol derived from fruit or produced from dextrose.

hexose: Type of monosaccharide, such as dextrose and levulose.

Suggested Readings on Hypoglycemia

AMERICAN MEDICAL ASSOCIATION. 1973. Statement on hypoglycemia. J. Am. Med. Assoc. *223,* Feb. 5, 682.

ANDREANI, D., MARKS, V., and LEFEBRE, P. 1987. Hypoglycemia. New York: Raven Press.

BENNION, L. 1983. Hypoglycemia: Fact or Fad? New York: Crown.

BOHANNON, J., KARAM, H., and FORSHAM, P. 1980. Endocrine responses to sugar ingestion in man. J. Am. Dietet. Assoc. *77,* Jun., 555.

DANOWSKI, T., NOLAN, S., and STEPHAN, T. 1975. Hypoglycemia. World Rev. Nutr. Dietet., *22,* 288.

EDITOR. 1979. Hypoglycemia: Fact or fiction? Harvard Medical School Health Letter, Nov., 1.

HOFELDT, F. 1983. Preventing Reactive Hypoglycemia: The Great Medical Dilemma. St. Louis: Warren H. Green.

HUDNALL, M. 1981. Hypoglycemia: Myths and realities. American Council on Science and Health News and Views, Nov./Dec., 2.

MARKS, V., and ROSE, F. 1981. Hypoglycemia. Oxford, England: Blackwell Scientific Publications.

ROTWEIN, P., GIDDINGS, S., and PERMUTT, M. Diagnosis and management of hypoglycemic disorders in adults. In Special Topics on Endocrinology and Metabolism, M. Cohen and P. Foa (Editors), Vol. 3. New York: Alan R. Liss, Inc.

SERVICE, R. (Editor). 1983. Hypoglycemic Disorders: Pathogenesis, Diagnosis, and Treatment. Boston: G. K. Hall Medical Publishers.

YETIV, J. 1986. Hypoglycemia. In Popular Nutritional Practices: A Scientific Appraisal, pp. 150–154. Toledo, OH: Popular Medicine Press.

Exercise on Hypoglycemia Counseling

Keeping in mind the preceding Hypoglycemia Facts List and Suggested Readings, which provide some of the most current diet-related information on this popular topic, prepare a handout to use with individuals who believe that they are suffering from this condition. You may include graphics and/or prepare in a poster format, if desired; see the Sample Handout. Show your handout in rough draft form to classmates or co-workers for constructive criticism on the overall design, content, and potential effectiveness for use in pertinent diet counseling situations. Then prepare a final version for your own future use as a practicing dietetic technician. Also, begin to scan the media—television, magazines, newspapers, billboards, books, leaflets, etc.—for misleading advertisements for "hypoglycemia cures." You might want to develop a file on diet claims for use in counseling those seeking to cure vague symptoms attributed to hypoglycemia.

Sample Handout

Hypoglycemic Reaction Symptoms Record

Instructions: Use this chart to record all hypoglycemic symptoms. Be sure to describe any activity engaged in prior to onset of symptoms (e.g., eating candy, jogging, arguing with spouse). Estimate total number of minutes from onset to disappearance of symptoms.

Date	Time	Symptoms	Associated activities	Duration (min)

Table 11.5 lists foods that may elicit a hypoglycemic reaction in susceptible individuals.

Table 11.5   Foods That Can Trigger Hypoglycemic Reactions

Beverages	Desserts	Miscellaneous sweets
Alcohol	Candy	Cereals, presweetened
Chocolate drinks	Cookies, cakes, pies	Condensed milk
Coffee, tea	Doughnuts, pastries	Gum, breath fresheners
Soft drinks	Fruits, sweetened	Jams, jellies, preserves
Sweetened drinks	Gelatin (unless unsweetened)	Marshmallow
	Ice cream, ice milk, sherbet	Sugar—table, raw
	Puddings	Syrups, molasses, honey

STEP 5: DIABETES GUIDELINES

Eating Well While Eating Right[1]

Let's face it. Food is one of life's basic necessities, and eating is one of our greatest pleasures.

Throughout history we have had a tendency to overindulge in the kinds of foods that can eventually be harmful to us. In many countries, a campaign is underway to emphasize the importance of good nutrition.

When we hear the word "nutrition" we often think of "diet," and this word often has negative overtones. "Diet" can imply a set of rigid rules for eating dull, monotonous food. We tend to be conditioned to think that "good" foods must always be dull while "bad" foods are always tastier. Unfortunately, this attitude can carry on throughout life.

Developing the right attitude about food habits is the first, most important step in the right direction toward good health. Each of us, whether we are eating poorly or well, is on a diet. We are what we eat. While we often must compromise between the kinds and amounts of food we prefer and what is best for keeping us in good health, in most cases we can still have fun while eating, and still enjoy tasty, tempting dishes.

Of course, many people are eating well-balanced meals and only require a few simple changes in their diet. However, if a number of changes are necessary, the Exchange Lists offer a wide selection of foods for individual meal planning, for people with diabetes and others concerned about weight control, good health, and prevention of disease.

[1]Adapted from American Diabetes Association and American Dietetic Association (1976).

In order to be able to advise diabetics on the adoption of desirable dietary patterns, it is essential to have access to all of the hands-on material required for effective counseling sessions. It is also important to be able to record all of the pertinent information regarding each diet counseling session in the patient's medical charts. The following Suggested Readings and Counseling Guidelines should help to improve your confidence—and skills—regarding your counseling abilities.

This step includes suggested counseling strategies for use with diabetic patients. The following references may prove helpful.

Suggested Readings on Diet in Diabetes

AMERICAN DIABETES ASSOCIATION. 1978. Supplement to Exchange Lists for Meal Planning: Jewish Cookery. Alexandria, VA: ADA.

AMERICAN DIABETES ASSOCIATION. 1979. Supplement to Exchange Lists for Meal Planning: Vegetarian Cookery. Alexandria, VA: ADA.

AMERICAN DIABETES ASSOCIATION. 1981. Guidelines for Diabetes Care. Alexandria, VA: ADA.

AMERICAN DIABETES ASSOCIATION. 1982. Diabetes in the Family. Bowie, MD: Robert J. Brady Co.

AMERICAN DIABETES ASSOCIATION. 1984. Policy Statement: Glycemic effect of carbohydrates. Diabetes Care 7, Nov./Dec., 607.

AMERICAN DIABETES ASSOCIATION. 1986. Nutritional recommendations and principles for individuals with diabetes mellitus. Nutrition Today 21, Jan./Feb., 29.

AMERICAN DIABETES ASSOCIATION and AMERICAN DIETETIC ASSOCIATION. 1986. Exchange Lists for Meal Planning. Chicago, IL and Alexandria, VA: ADA.

AMERICAN DIABETES ASSOCIATION and AMERICAN DIETETIC ASSOCIATION. 1987. Family Cookbook, Volumes I, II, III. Englewood Cliffs, NJ: Prentice-Hall.

AMERICAN DIABETES ASSOCIATION and AMERICAN DIETETIC ASSOCIATION. 1988a. Meal Planning Approaches in the Nutrition Management of the Person with Diabetes. Chicago, IL and Alexandria, VA: ADA.

AMERICAN DIABETES ASSOCIATION and AMERICAN DIETETIC ASSOCIATION. 1988b. Nutrition Guide for Professionals: Diabetes Education and Meal Planning. Chicago, IL and Alexandria, VA: ADA.

AMERICAN DIETETIC ASSOCIATION. 1981. Handbook of Clinical Dietetics. New Haven, CT: Yale University Press.

AMERICAN DIETETIC ASSOCIATION. 1987. Ethnic Food Exchange Lists. Chicago: ADA.

AMERICAN DIETETIC ASSOCIATION. 1987. Position of The American Dietetic Association: Appropriate use of nutritive and non-nutritive sweeteners. J. Am. Dietet. Assoc. 87, Dec., 1689.

AMERICAN DIETETIC ASSOCIATION and AMERICAN DIABETES ASSOCIATION. 1987. A Nutrition Guide for Professionals: The Effective Application of Exchange Lists for Meal Planning. Chicago: ADA.

ANDERSON, J. 1981. Diabetes: A Practical Guide to Healthy Eating. New York: Simon & Schuster.

ANDERSON, J. 1984a. Dr. Anderson's HCF Diet. Lexington, KY: HCF Diabetes Foundation.

ANDERSON, J. 1984b. HCF Exchanges: A Sensible Plan for Healthy Eating. Lexington, KY: HCF Diabetes Foundation.

ANDERSON, J. 1984c. User's Guide to HCF Diets. Lexington, KY: HCF Diabetes Foundation.

ANDERSON, J. 1988. Nutrition Management of Metabolic Conditions: Professional Guide to HCF Diets. Lexington, KY: HCF Diabetes Foundation.

ANDERSON, J., et al. 1987. Dietary fiber and diabetes: A comprehensive review and practical application. J. Am. Dietet. Assoc. 87, Sept., 1189.

BARRETT, A. 1984. The Diabetic's Brand Name Food Exchange Handbook. Philadelphia: Running Press.

BERG, K. 1986. Diabetic's Guide to Health and Fitness: An Authoritative Approach to Leading an Active Life. Champaign, IL: Human Kinetics Publishers.

BIERMAN, J., and TOOHEY, B. 1980. The Diabetic's Total Health Book. Los Angeles: J. P. Tarcher.

BIRK, R. 1984. Emotional Adjustment to Diabetes. Wayzata, MN: Diabetes Center, Inc.

CHEW, I., et al. 1988. Application of glycemic index to mixed meals. Amer. J. Clin. Nutr. 47, Jan., 53.

CRAPO, P. 1986. Carbohydrate in the diabetic diet. J. Amer. Coll. Nutr. 5, 1, 31.

CRAPO, P., and VINIK, A. 1987. Nutrition controversies in diabetes management. J. Am. Dietet. Assoc. 87, Jan., 25.

DAVIDSON, J. 1986. Clinical Diabetes Mellitus: A Problem-Oriented Approach. New York: Thieme Medical Pubs., Inc.

ETZWILER, D., FRANZ, M., and HOLLANDER, P. (Editors). 1985. Learning to Live Well with Diabetes. Wayzata, MN: Diabetes Center, Inc.

FRANZ, M. 1987a. Exchanges for All Occasions. Wayzata, MN: Diabetes Center, Inc.

FRANZ, M. 1987b. Fast Food Facts. Wayzata, MN: Diabetes Center, Inc.

FRANZ, M., et al. 1986. Goals for Diabetes Educators. Alexandria, VA: American Diabetes Association.

FRANZ, M., et al. 1987. Exchange Lists: Revised, 1986. J. Am. Dietet. Assoc. *87,* Jan., 28.

HOLLERORTH, J. 1986. Diabetes Teaching Guide. Boston: Joselin Diabetes Center.

JENKINS, D., and JENKINS, A. 1987. The glycemic index, fiber, and dietary treatment. J. Amer. Coll. Nutr. *6,* 1, 11.

MARYNIUK, M. 1982. Practical aspects of nutrition in the management of diabetes mellitus. Primary Care *9,* Sept., 557.

MONK, A., and FRANZ, M. 1987. Convenience Food Facts. Wayzata, MN: Diabetes Center, Inc.

NUTTALL, F. 1987. Diet and diabetes: A brief overview. J. Amer. Coll. Nutr. *6,* 1, 5.

POWERS, M. 1987. Handbook of Diabetes Nutritional Management. Rockville, MD: Aspen Publishers.

SIMINERIO, L., and BETSCHART, J. 1986. Children with Diabetes. Alexandria, VA: American Diabetes Association.

TOMA, E. 1988. Food fiber choices for diabetic diets. Amer. J. Clin. Nutr. *47,* Feb., 243.

WHEELER, M. (Editor). 1983. Diabetes Mellitus and Glycemic Responses to Different Foods: A Summary and Annotated Bibliography. Chicago: Diabetes Care and Education Practice Group, ADA.

WHEELER, M., DELAHANTY, L., and WYLIE-ROSETT, J. 1987. Diet and exercise in noninsulin-dependent diabetes mellitus: Implications from the NIH Consensus Conference. J. Am. Dietet. Assoc. *87,* Apr., 480.

U.S. DEPARTMENT OF HEALTH AND HUMAN SERVICES. 1987. Noninsulin-dependent Diabetes, Publication No. 87-241. Bethesda, MD: National Diabetes Information Clearinghouse.

VINICK, A. 1988. Report of the American Diabetes Association's Task Force on Nutrition. Diabetes Care *11,* Feb., 127.

For journal subscriptions:

Diabetes. American Diabetes Association, 1660 Duke Street, Alexandria, VA 22314.

Diabetes Care. American Diabetes Association, 1660 Duke Street, Alexandria, VA 22314.

Diabetes '90. American Diabetes Association, 1660 Duke Street, Alexandria, VA 22314.

Diabetes Forecast. American Diabetes Association, 1660 Duke Street, Alexandria, VA 22314.

Diabetes Update. Greater Boston Diabetes Society, 1330 Beacon Street, Brookline, MA 02146.

The Diabetes Educator. American Association of Diabetes Educators, 500 North Michigan Avenue, Suite 1400, Chicago, IL 60611.

For further information:

American Association of Diabetes Educators, 500 North Michigan Drive, Suite 1400, Chicago, IL 60611.

American Diabetes Association, 1660 Duke Street, Alexandria, VA 22314.

American Dietetic Association, 216 West Jackson Boulevard, Chicago, IL 60606.

Diabetes Center, Inc., PO Box 739, Wayzata, MN 55391.

HCF Diabetes Foundation, PO Box 22124, Lexington, KY 40522.

Joselin Diabetes Association, Inc., One Joselin Place, Boston, MA 02215.

Juvenile Diabetes Foundation, 432 Park Avenue South, New York, NY 10016.

National Diabetes Information Clearinghouse, PO Box NDIC, Bethesda, MD 20892.

For audiovisuals:

Eating Healthy Foods. American Dietetic Association, 216 West Jackson Boulevard, Chicago, IL 60606 (picture version of Exchange Lists).

Gestational Diabetes. Media Medicine, Inc., Heritage Harbor, Building 200D, Monterey, CA 93940.

Learning to Live with Diabetes: Diet and Nutrition. Texas Department of Health, Division of Public Health Promotion, 110 West 49th Street, Austin, TX 78756.

The Diabetic Diet. Milner, Fenwick, Inc., 2125 Greenspring Drive, Timonium, MD 21093.

The Diabetes Picture Manual. Kettering Medical Center, 3535 Southern Boulevard, Kettering, OH 45429.

The 1986 Exchanges. Diabetes Center, Inc., PO Box 739, Wayzata, MN 55391 (video/slide set).

Table 11.6 General Outline for Diabetes Counseling

I. Initial Session
  A. General Guidelines
  B. Patient Records
    1. Medical History Form
    2. Weight Chart
    3. 24-Hour Recall Form
  C. Assignments
    1. Food Intake Record
    2. Insulin/Urine Record
    3. Activity Record
    4. Diet History
  D. Technician's Notes
II. Follow-up Session(s)
  A. General Guidelines
  B. Handouts
    1. Exchange Lists for Meal Planning
    2. Nonrestricted Foods
    3. Food Substitutions during Illness
    4. Baby Food Exchanges
    5. Learning Assessment Quiz
  C. Technician's Notes

Counseling Guidelines—Diabetes

Table 11.6 outlines the steps for diet counseling. The following material gives the details of each step.

I.   Initial Session

I.   A.   General Guidelines

1.   Use Medical History Form to assess patient's nutritional status.

2.   Weigh patient and record on Weight Chart. The chart is a helpful tool for visualization of weight status.

3.   Assist patient in recording 24-hour recall of food intake using 24-Hour Recall Form. This will aid patient in keeping an accurate Food Intake Record.

4.   Instruct patient to keep daily Food Intake Record so that typical food intake patterns can be evaluated. Advise patient not to deviate from normal eating pattern. Stress the importance of recording food intake immediately after eating.

5.   Instruct insulin-dependent patient to keep Insulin/Urine Record until next session so that insulin and diet can be evaluated. Knowledge of the patient's **renal threshold** is required before urine glucose and blood glucose can be correlated. Good control is usually indicated if about 75% of the test results are in the negative or trace range, with the remaining results positive but not occurring at the same time each day. Stress the importance of immediate recording of both insulin dosage and urine test values.

6.   Instruct patient to keep Activity Record in order to provide comparison of patient's conception of own activity with actual activity level. Advise patient not to deviate from normal activity pattern. This form can be utilized continually to emphasize the importance of regular physical activity.

7.   Instruct patient to complete Diet History. This provides for a basic evaluation of food intake patterns. (Use Pre-test from Chapter 2.)

8.   Record assessment and recommendation(s) using the SOAP method in Technician's Notes. This form can be kept in your files with a copy in the patient's medical records.

renal threshold: Individualized level above which the kidney can no longer process the constituent(s).

I.   B.   Patient Records

1. Medical History Form

Date _____ Referred by _____

Name _____ Date of birth _____

Address _____ Phone no. _____

Occupation _____ Hours per work week ____ Work phone no. _____

Educational background _____ Religious/ethnic background _____

Sex ____ Marital status ____

Household composition: Live alone _____ Spouse _____ Children/No. _____

Other: _____

General health status:

Physician _____ Address _____

Phone no. _____ Date of last visit _____

Ambulatory care required? ____ If so, describe: _____

Neuromuscular problems? ____ If so, how is eating affected? _____

Visual/auditory problems? ____ If so, describe: _____

Chewing difficulties? ____ If so, describe: _____

Appetite typically good? _____ fair? _____ poor? _____

Digestion/elimination difficulties? ____ If so, describe: _____

Food intolerances? ____ If so, describe: _____

Overweight? ____ If so, describe: _____

Hypertension? ____ If so, describe: _____

Hyperlipidemia? ____ If so, describe: _____

Gout? ____ If so, describe: _____

Other: _____

Height _____ Weight _____ Frame _____

Triceps skinfold thickness _____ Mid-arm circumference _____

Mid-arm muscle circumference _____

Weight changes/problems? ____ If so, describe: _____

Stage of diabetes _____ Age of onset _____
Blood glucose stable? _____ Mod. labile? _____ Severe labile? _____
Diabetes in family? ____ If so, describe: _____
History of use of insulin/oral hypoglycemic agents? ____ If so, describe: _____
History of symptoms/reactions? ____ If so, describe: _____

Clinical signs of nutritional status:

Skin _____ Mouth _____
Hair _____ Eyes _____
Teeth _____ Other: _____

Lab data:

Blood pressure _____
Fasting glucose _____ CTT _____ CGTT _____
Post-prandial glucose _____
Cholesterol _____ Triglycerides _____ Lipoprotein profile _____
CBC _____
Urine glucose _____ Urine acetone _____ Urine protein _____
Other: _____

Medications taken regularly: _____
Prescribed by: _____
Date(s) prescribed: _____
Nutrition supplements taken regularly: _____
Prescribed by: _____
Date(s) prescribed: _____
Special diet prescription: _____
Prescribed by: _____ Date of prescription: _____
How closely is diet followed? Always adhered to __ Sometimes __ Rarely __ Never __

Type of housing: Room _____ Apartment _____ Home _____ Institution _____
Prepare own meals? _____ Dine out? Often (more than once a day) _____ Rarely _____
Food shopping done independently? _____ If not, describe required assistance: _____
_____

Eligible for food stamps? ____ If so, are they currently being used? _____
Cigarette smoker? ____ If so, how much: _____
Exercise regularly? ____ If so, describe: _____
    No. times per week ____ No. minutes per session _____

Comments: _____

2. Weight Chart

Starting weight _____   Reasonable weight _____

Date	No. weeks on diet	Weight	Comments

3. 24-Hour Recall Form

Date	Time	Food and amount

I.   C.   Assignments

1. Food Intake Record

Date	Time	Food/Amount	Where[a]	With whom	Associated activity[b]

[a]Such as work, restaurant, kitchen, living room.
[b]For example, watching television, reading, socializing, driving, talking on the phone, cooking.

2. Insulin/Urine Record

Instructions: Record date and time, type of insulin and dosage, and test results in the designated columns. Test results should be recorded as 0 (negative); t (trace); 1, 2, 3, or 4 (degree of glycosuria). If test is not made, leave appropriate space blank. Note any variations in diet, exercise, emotions, etc. in Comments column. Do not make any changes in diet/insulin without physician approval.

Insulin		Urine test before:				Comments
Date/time	Type/amount	Breakfast	Lunch	Supper	Bedtime	

3. Activity Record

Instructions: Record those physical activities which were sustained for at least 20 minutes.

Date and time	Type of activity	Duration

4. Diet History

Use the Pre-test from Chapter 2 (p. 30) to provide a record of typical foods eaten.

I. D. Technician's Notes

Patient: _____   Date: _____

S   (Subjective data—how patient feels):
O   (Objective data—physical measurements including diet/nutritional status):
A   (Assessment—acceptability of dietary progress/nutritional status):
P   (Plan—diet prescription and instruction):
Comments:

II. Follow-up Session(s)

II. A. General Guidelines

1.   Weigh patient and record on Weight Chart.
2.   Review assignments and discuss.
3.   Aid patient in determining desired weight by using insurance company actuarial tables, skinfold thickness, and/or the following formulas: For women of medium build, use 100 lb for first 5 ft of height plus 5 lb for each additional inch; for men of medium build, use 106 lb for the first 5 ft of height plus 6 lb for each additional inch; for patients with small builds, subtract 10%, and for those with large builds add 10%.
4.   Using Activity Record, determine if patient's activity level is sedentary, moderate, or strenuous.
5.   Determine desired daily caloric level by using the following formulas: If activity level is sedentary, multiply desired weight by 13; if moderate, multiply by 15; if strenuous, multiply by 20. Estimate caloric level that would achieve or maintain desired body weight. (Note: 3500 calories = 1 lb.)
6.   Individualize the diet plan using Exchange Lists (Tables 11.7–11.12) for Meal Planning and instruct patient in their use. (Note that for the insulin-dependent diabetic, consistency in the timing of meals and in the ratios of carbohydrate, protein, and fat for each meal/snack is important.)
7.   Use other handouts depending on individual needs to enhance patient's understanding of the diet plan.
8.   Assign Learning Assessment Quiz to evaluate counseling process and to determine if additional counseling is needed.
9.   Instruct patient to continue to maintain daily Food Intake Record, Insulin/Urine Record, and Activity Record for next session and/or for self-review.
10.   Record assessment and recommendation(s) using the SOAP method in Technician's Notes. This form can be kept in your files with a copy in the patient's medical records.

Table 11.7 Starch/Bread Exchange List,[a] **Amounts Given for One Bread Exchange**

Kind	Amount	Kind	Amount
Cereals/grains/pasta		*Bread*	
Bran cereals, concentrated[b]	$\frac{1}{3}$ cup	Bagel	$\frac{1}{2}$ (1 oz)
(such as Bran Buds, All Bran)		Bread sticks, crisp, 4 in. long × $\frac{1}{2}$ in.	2 ($\frac{2}{3}$ oz)
Bran cereals, flaked[b]	$\frac{1}{2}$ cup	Croutons, low-fat	1 cup
Bulgur (cooked)	$\frac{1}{2}$ cup	English muffin	$\frac{1}{2}$
Cooked cereals	$\frac{1}{2}$ cup	Frankfurter or hamburger bun	$\frac{1}{2}$ (1 oz)
Cornmeal (dry)	$2\frac{1}{2}$ Tbsp	Pita, 6 in. across	$\frac{1}{2}$
Grapenuts	3 Tbsp	Plain roll, small	1 (1 oz)
Grits (cooked)	$\frac{1}{2}$ cup	Raisin, unfrosted	1 slice
Other ready-to-eat unsweetened	$\frac{3}{4}$ cup		(1 oz)
cereals		Rye, pumpernickel[b]	1 slice
Pasta (cooked)	$\frac{1}{2}$ cup		(1 oz)
Puffed cereal	$1\frac{1}{2}$ cups	Tortilla, 6 in. across	1
Rice, white or brown (cooked)	$\frac{1}{3}$ cup	White (including French, Italian)	1 slice
Shredded wheat	$\frac{1}{2}$ cup		(1 oz)
Wheat germ[b]	3 Tbsp	Whole wheat	1 slice
			(1 oz)
Dried beans/peas/lentils			
Beans and peas (cooked)[b]	$\frac{1}{3}$ cup	*Crackers/snacks*	
Lentils (cooked)[b]	$\frac{1}{3}$ cup	Animal crackers	8
Baked beans[b]	$\frac{1}{4}$ cup	Graham crackers, $2\frac{1}{2}$ in. square	3
		Matzoth	$\frac{3}{4}$ oz
Starchy vegetables		Melba toast	5
Corn[b]	$\frac{1}{2}$ cup	Oyster crackers	24
Corn on the cob, 6 in. long[b]	1	Popcorn (popped, no fat added)	3 cups
Lima beans[b]	$\frac{1}{2}$ cup	Pretzels	$\frac{3}{4}$ oz
Peas, green (canned or frozen)[b]	$\frac{1}{2}$ cup	Rye crisp, 2 in. × $3\frac{1}{2}$ in.	4
Plantain[b]	$\frac{1}{2}$ cup	Saltine-type crackers	6
Potato, baked	1 small	Whole wheat crackers, no fat added	2–4 ($\frac{3}{4}$ oz)
	(3 oz)	(such as crisp breads)	
Potato, mashed	$\frac{1}{2}$ cup		
Squash, winter (acorn, butternut)	$\frac{3}{4}$ cup		
Yam, sweet potato, plain	$\frac{1}{3}$ cup		
Starch foods prepared with fat			
(count as 1 starch/bread serving,			
plus 1 fat serving)			
Biscuit, $2\frac{1}{2}$ in. across	1	Muffin, plain, small	1
Chow mein noodles	$\frac{1}{2}$ cup	Pancake, 4 in. across	2
Corn bread, 2-in. cube	1 (2 oz)	Stuffing, bread (prepared)	$\frac{1}{4}$ cup
Cracker, round butter-type	6	Taco shell, 6 in. across	2
French-fried potatoes, 2 in. to	10 ($1\frac{1}{2}$ oz)	Waffle, $4\frac{1}{2}$ in. square	1
$3\frac{1}{2}$ in. long		Whole wheat crackers, fat added	4–6 (1 oz)

[a]One Exchange of Starch/Bread contains 15 grams of carbohydrate, 3 grams of protein, a trace of fat, and 80 calories.
[b]Contain 3 or more grams of fiber per serving.

Table 11.8   Meat Exchanges and Substitutes

	Kind	Amount
Lean meat and substitutes[a]		
Beef:	USDA Good or Choice grades of lean beef, such as round, sirloin, and flank steak; tenderloin; and chipped beef	1 oz
Pork:	Lean pork, such as fresh ham; canned, cured or boiled ham; Canadian bacon, tenderloin	1 oz
Veal:	All cuts are lean except for veal cutlets (ground or cubed); examples of lean veal are chops and roasts	1 oz
Poultry:	Chicken, turkey, Cornish hen (without skin)	1 oz
Fish:	All fresh and frozen fish	1 oz
	Crab, lobster, scallops, shrimp, clams (fresh or canned in water)	2 oz
	Oysters	6 medium
	Tuna (canned in water)	$\frac{1}{4}$ cup
	Herring (uncreamed or smoked)	1 oz
	Sardines (canned)	2 medium
Wild Game:	Venison, rabbit, squirrel	1 oz
	Pheasant, duck, goose (without skin)	1 oz
Cheese:	Any cottage cheese	$\frac{1}{4}$ cup
	Grated Parmesan	2 Tbsp
	Low-fat cheeses (with less than 55 calories per ounce)	1 oz
Other:	95% fat-free luncheon meat	1 oz
	Egg whites	3 whites
	Egg substitutes (with less than 55 calories per $\frac{1}{4}$ cup)	$\frac{1}{4}$ cup
Medium-fat meat and substitutes[b]		
Beef:	Most beef products fall into this category; examples are ground beef, roast (rib, chuck, rump), steak (cubed, Porterhouse, T-bone), and meatloaf	1 oz
Pork:	Most pork products fall into this category; examples are chops, loin roast, Boston butt, cutlets	1 oz
Lamb:	Most lamb products fall into this category; examples are chops, leg, and roast	1 oz
Veal:	Cutlet (ground or cubed, unbreaded)	1 oz
Poultry:	Chicken (with skin), domestic duck or goose (well-drained of fat), ground turkey	1 oz
Fish:	Tuna (canned in oil and drained)	$\frac{1}{4}$ cup
	Salmon (canned)	$\frac{1}{4}$ cup
Cheese:	Skim or part-skim milk cheeses, such as:	
	Ricotta	$\frac{1}{4}$ cup
	Mozzarella	1 oz
	Diet cheeses (with 55–80 calories per ounce)	1 oz
Other:	85% fat-free luncheon meat	1 oz
	Egg (high in cholesterol, limit to 3 per week)	1
	Egg substitutes with 55–80 calories per $\frac{1}{4}$ cup	$\frac{1}{4}$ cup
	Tofu ($2\frac{1}{2}$ in. × $2\frac{3}{4}$ in. × 1 in.)	4 oz
	Liver, heart, kidney, sweetbreads (high in cholesterol)	1 oz
High-fat meat and substitutes[c]		
Beef:	Most USDA Prime cuts of beef, such as ribs, corned beef	1 oz
Pork:	Spareribs, ground pork, pork sausage (patty or link)	1 oz
Lamb:	Patties (ground lamb)	1 oz
Fish:	Any fried fish product	1 oz

continued

Table 11.8 *(Continued)*

	Kind	Amount
Cheese:	All regular cheeses, such as American, blue, cheddar, Monterey, Swiss	1 oz
Other:	Luncheon meat, such as bologna, salami, pimento loaf	1 oz
	Sausage, such as Polish, Italian	1 oz
	Knockwurst, smoked	1 oz
	Bratwurst	1 oz
	Frankfurter (turkey or chicken)	1 frank (10/lb)
	Frankfurter (beef, pork, or combination) (count as one high-fat meat plus one fat exchange)	1 frank (10/lb)
	Peanut butter (contains unsaturated fat)	1 Tbsp

[a]One Exchange of Lean Meat or Substitute contains 7 grams of protein, 3 grams of fat, and 55 calories.
[b]One Exchange of Medium-Fat Meat or Substitute contains 7 grams of protein, 5 grams of fat, and 75 calories.
[c]One Exchange of High-Fat Meat or Substitute contains 7 grams of protein, 8 grams of fat, and 100 calories. These items are high in saturated fat, cholesterol, and calories, and should be limited to three servings per week.

Table 11.9   Vegetable Exchange List[a,b]

Artichoke ($\frac{1}{2}$ medium)	Mushrooms, cooked
Asparagus	Okra
Beans (green, wax, Italian)	Onions
Bean sprouts	Pea pods
Beets	Peppers (green)
Broccoli	Rutabaga
Brussels sprouts	Sauerkraut
Cabbage, cooked	Spinach, cooked
Carrots	Summer squash (crookneck)
Cauliflower	Tomato (one large)
Eggplant	Tomato/vegetable juice
Greens (collard, mustard, turnip)	Turnips
Kohlrabi	Water chestnuts
Leeks	Zucchini, cooked

[a]One Exchange of Vegetables contains about 5 grams of carbohydrate, 2 grams of protein, and 25 calories. One Exchange equals $\frac{1}{2}$ cup cooked vegetables or juice, or 1 cup raw unless otherwise noted.
[b]Starchy vegetables such as corn, peas, and potatoes are found on the Starch/Bread List.

Table 11.10 Fruit Exchange List,[a] Amounts Given for One Fruit Exchange

Kind	Amount	Kind	Amount
Fresh, frozen, and unsweetened canned fruit			
Apple (raw, 2 in. across)	1 apple	Mandarin oranges	$\frac{3}{4}$ cup
Applesauce (unsweetened)	$\frac{1}{2}$ cup	Mango (small)	$\frac{1}{2}$ mango
Apricots (medium, raw)	4 apricots	Nectarine ($1\frac{1}{2}$ in. across)[b]	1 nectarine
Apricots (canned)	$\frac{1}{2}$ cup, or 4 halves	Orange ($2\frac{1}{2}$ in. across)	1 orange
Banana (9 in. long)	$\frac{1}{2}$ banana	Papaya	1 cup
Blackberries (raw)[b]	$\frac{3}{4}$ cup	Peach ($2\frac{3}{4}$ in. across)	1 peach, or $\frac{3}{4}$ cup
Blueberries (raw)[b]	$\frac{3}{4}$ cup	Peaches (canned)	$\frac{1}{2}$ cup, or 2 halves
Cantaloupe (5 in. across) (cubes)	$\frac{1}{3}$ melon 1 cup	Pear	$\frac{1}{2}$ large, or 1 small
Cherries (large, raw)	12 cherries	Pears (canned)	$\frac{1}{2}$ cup, or 2 halves
Cherries (canned)	$\frac{1}{2}$ cup	Persimmon (medium, native)	2 persimmons
Figs (raw, 2 in. across)	2 figs	Pineapple (raw)	$\frac{3}{4}$ cup
Fruit cocktail (canned)	$\frac{1}{2}$ cup	Pineapple (canned)	$\frac{1}{3}$ cup
Grapefruit (medium)	$\frac{1}{2}$ grapefruit	Plum (raw, 2 in. across)	2 plums
Grapefruit (segments)	$\frac{3}{4}$ cup	Pomegranate[b]	$\frac{1}{2}$ pomegranate
Grapes (small)	15 grapes	Raspberries (raw)[b]	1 cup
Honeydew melon (medium) (cubes)	$\frac{1}{8}$ melon 1 cup	Strawberries (raw, whole)[b]	$1\frac{1}{4}$ cups
Kiwi (large)	1 kiwi	Tangerine ($2\frac{1}{2}$ in. across)	2 tangerines
		Watermelon (cubes)	$1\frac{1}{4}$ cups

Kind	Amount	Kind	Amount
Dried fruit		*Fruit juice*	
Apples[b]	4 rings	Apple juice/cider	$\frac{1}{2}$ cup
Apricots[b]	7 halves	Cranberry juice cocktail	$\frac{1}{3}$ cup
Dates	$2\frac{1}{2}$ medium	Grapefruit juice	$\frac{1}{2}$ cup
Figs[b]	$1\frac{1}{2}$	Grape juice	$\frac{1}{3}$ cup
Prunes[b]	3 medium	Orange juice	$\frac{1}{2}$ cup
Raisins	2 Tbsp	Pineapple juice	$\frac{1}{2}$ cup
		Prune juice	$\frac{1}{3}$ cup

[a]One Exchange of Fruit contains 15 grams of carbohydrate and 60 calories.
[b]Contains 3 or more grams of fiber per serving.

Table 11.11 Milk Exchange List,[a] Amounts Given for One Milk Exchange

Kind	Amount
Skim and very lowfat milk	
Skim milk	1 cup
$\frac{1}{2}$% milk	1 cup
1% milk	1 cup
Lowfat buttermilk	1 cup
Evaporated skim milk	$\frac{1}{2}$ cup
Dry nonfat milk	$\frac{1}{3}$ cup
Plain nonfat yogurt	8 oz
Lowfat milk	
2% milk	1 cup
Plain lowfat yogurt (with added nonfat milk solids)	8 oz
Whole milk[b]	
Whole milk	1 cup
Evaporated whole milk	$\frac{1}{2}$ cup
Whole plain yogurt	8 oz

[a]One Exchange of Milk contains 12 grams of carbohydrate and 8 grams of protein. Skim and very lowfat milk contain a trace of fat, lowfat milk contains 5 grams of fat, and whole milk contains 8 grams of fat.

[b]Try to limit choices from this high-fat group as much as possible.

Table 11.12 Fat Exchange List,[a]
Amounts Given for One Fat Exchange

Kind	Amount
Unsaturated fats	
Avocado	$\frac{1}{8}$ medium
Margarine	1 tsp
Margarine, diet	1 Tbsp
Mayonnaise	1 tsp
Mayonnaise, reduced-calorie	1 Tbsp
Nuts and Seeds:	
Almonds, dry roasted	6 whole
Cashews, dry roasted	1 Tbsp
Pecans	2 whole
Peanuts	20 small or 10 large
Walnuts	2 whole
Other nuts	1 Tbsp
Seeds, pine nuts, sunflower (without shells)	1 Tbsp
Pumpkin seeds	2 tsp
Oil (corn, cottonseed, safflower, soybean, sunflower, olive, peanut)	1 tsp
Olives	10 small or 5 large
Salad dressing, mayonnaise-type	2 tsp
Salad dressing, mayonnaise-type, reduced-calorie	1 Tbsp
Salad dressing (all varieties)	1 Tbsp
Salad dressing, reduced-calorie	2 Tbsp
Saturated fats	
Butter	1 tsp
Bacon	1 slice
Chitterlings	$\frac{1}{2}$ ounce
Coconut, shredded	2 Tbsp
Coffee whitener, liquid	2 Tbsp
Coffee whitener, powder	4 tsp
Cream (light, coffee, table)	2 Tbsp
Cream, sour	2 Tbsp
Cream (heavy, whipping)	1 Tbsp
Cream cheese	1 Tbsp
Salt pork	$\frac{1}{4}$ ounce

[a]One Exchange of Fat contains 5 grams fat and 45 calories.

II. B. Handouts

1. Exchange Lists for Meal Planning[1]

Your meal plan in Exchanges must be planned with the assistance of your Diet Counselor. The Exchange Lists are the basis of a meal planning system designed by a committee of the American Diabetes Association and the American Dietetic Association. While designed primarily for people with diabetes and others who must follow special diets, the Exchange Lists are based on principles of good nutrition that apply to everyone.

[1]Reprinted with permission from American Diabetes Association, Inc., American Dietetic Association, 1986.

Meal plan for (Name) _____

Carbohydrate _____ Protein _____ Fat _____ Calories _____

               grams   grams   grams

	Starch/Bread (See Table 11.7.)	Meat (See Table 11.8.)	Vegetable (See Table 11.9.)	Fruit (See Table 11.10.)	Milk (See Table 11.11.)	Fat (See Table 11.12.)
Breakfast time _____						
Snack time _____						
Lunch or dinner time _____						
Snack time _____						
Dinner or supper time _____						
Bedtime snack time _____						

2. Nonrestricted Foods

The foods listed in Table 11.13 can be used without restriction.

Table 11.13 Nonrestricted Foods

Artificial sweeteners	Dill	Mint	Salad greens (endive,
Broth, bouillon, or	Extracts (vanilla,	Mineral water	escarole, lettuce,
clear consommé[a]	etc.)	Mushrooms, raw	spinach)
Cabbage, raw	Garlic	Mustard[a]	Soft drinks, sugar-free
Carbonated water	Garlic powder	Onion, raw	Soy sauce[a]
Celery	Gelatin, unflavored/	Paprika	Spices
Celery seed	unsweetened or	Parsley	Tea
Chives	artificially flavored	Pepper, hot peppers	Vinegar
Club soda	Herbs	Pickles, sour or dill[a]	Worcestershire sauce[a]
Coffee	Horseradish	Pimento	Zucchini, raw
Cucumbers	Lemon/lime juice	Radishes	

[a]May have considerable sodium content.

3. Food Substitutions during Illness

Table 11.14 lists food substitutions that can be made during illness.

Table 11.14 Food Substitutions during Illness

Starch/Bread Exchange (15 grams carbohydrate)
    $\frac{1}{4}$ cup sherbet
    $\frac{1}{3}$ cup sweetened gelatin
    1 cup noodle/vegetable soup
    $\frac{3}{4}$ cup cream-style soup (water added, not milk)
    $\frac{1}{2}$ cup pudding
    1 cup custard
Milk Exchange (12 grams carbohydrate)
    5 oz carbonated beverage
    1 Tbsp sugar
Vegetable Exchange (5 grams carbohydrate)
    $\frac{1}{2}$ Fruit Exchange
Fruit Exchange (15 grams carbohydrate)
    $\frac{1}{2}$ cup carbonated beverage
    $\frac{1}{2}$ popsicle
    $\frac{1}{4}$ cup sweetened gelatin

4. Baby Food Exchanges

Table 11.15 lists the Baby Food Exchanges.

Table 11.15 Baby Food Exchanges[a]

	Protein/gram	Carbohydrate/gram	Fat/gram
Milk/Formula Exchanges—1 8-oz cup = 160 calories			
Whole milk[b]	8	12	10
Similac	3.6	17.0	8.8
Enfamil	3.6	16.8	8.8
SMA	3.6	17.3	8.6
Prosobee	6.0	16.3	8.4
Isomil	4.8	16.3	8.6

Kind	Amount	Kind	Amount
Bread Exchanges—each item is 1 Bread Exchange (80 calories)			
Dry baby rice cereal	5 Tbsp	Strained creamed corn	1 jar
Dry baby oatmeal cereal	5 Tbsp	Strained mixed vegetables	1 jar
Dry high protein cereal	9 Tbsp	Strained sweet potatoes	1 jar
"Strained" jar = 4.75 oz (135 g)		"Junior" jar = 7.75 oz (220 g)	
Strained baby rice cereal with mixed fruit (also count 1 fruit exchange)	1 jar	Junior rice with mixed fruit	½ jar
Strained baby oatmeal cereal with applesauce and banana	1 jar	Junior oatmeal with applesauce and banana	½ jar
Strained high protein cereal with applesauce and banana	1 jar	Junior creamed corn	½ jar
		Teething biscuits, arrowroot cookies, animal cookies, and pretzels	3
Meat Exchanges—each item is 1 Medium-fat Meat Exchange (75 calories)			
1 jar = 3.33 oz (94 g)		1 jar = 3.5 oz (99 g)	
Strained egg yolk	1 jar	Junior chicken	½ jar
Strained chicken	½ jar	ham	½ jar
ham	½ jar	lamb	½ jar
lamb	½ jar	beef	½ jar
beef	½ jar	pork	½ jar
pork	½ jar	meat sticks	½ jar
(above also must count 1 Fat Exchange)			
Fruit Exchanges—each item is 1 Fruit Exchange (60 calories)			
"Baby" can = 4.2 oz		Strained cherry vanilla pudding	½ jar
Baby apple juice	¾ can (3 oz)	chocolate custard	⅓ jar
Baby mixed fruit juice	½ can (2 oz)	dutch apple dessert	⅓ jar
Baby prune-orange juice	⅓ can (1½ oz)	"Junior" jar = 7.75 oz (220 g)	
"Strained" jar = 4.75 oz (135 g)		Junior applesauce	⅓ jar
Strained applesauce	½ jar	bananas	¼ jar
bananas	⅓ jar	peaches	⅓ jar
peaches	⅓ jar	pears	⅓ jar
plums	¼ jar	plums	⅓ jar
prunes	⅓ jar	prunes	⅓ jar
Vegetable Exchanges—each item is 1 Vegetable Exchange (25 calories)			
"Strained" jar = 4.5 oz (128 g)		"Junior" jar = 7.5 oz (213 g)	
Strained carrots	1 jar	Junior carrots	½ jar
beets	½ jar	creamed spinach	½ jar
creamed spinach	1 jar	green beans	½ jar
green beans	1 jar	squash	½ jar
squash	1 jar		
peas	1 jar		
Multiple Exchanges			
"Strained" jar = 4.5 oz (128 g)		"Junior" jar = 7.5 oz (213 g)	
Strained beef with egg noodles and vegetables	1 jar = ½ bread ½ meat	Junior beef with egg noodles	1 jar = 1 bread ½ meat
cereal and egg yolk	1 jar = ½ bread ½ meat	cereal and egg yolk	1 jar = 1 bread 1 fat
chicken and noodles	1 jar = ½ bread ½ meat	chicken and noodles	1 jar = 1 bread ½ meat
vegetables and chicken	1 jar = ½ bread ½ meat	vegetables and chicken	1 jar = 1 bread ½ meat
macaroni and cheese	1 jar = 1 bread ½ meat	macaroni and cheese	1 jar = 1 bread ½ meat
high meat dinners	1 jar = 1 meat ½ bread		

[a]Reprinted with permission from Benz and Kohler (1980).
[b]Not recommended under 1 year of age.

5. Learning Assessment Quiz

Answer true (T) or false (F) to the following statements:

____ 1. Diabetes is a very old disease, yet the exact cause is still unknown.
____ 2. Elevated glucose levels may frequently be related to overweight.
____ 3. The diabetic diet usually includes honey or molasses as desired.
____ 4. Normal blood glucose is 10 mg/100 ml.
____ 5. Hypoglycemia occurs when there is too much glucose in the blood.
____ 6. Those factors which increase the chances of developing diabetes include heredity, age, sex, and overweight.
____ 7. Insulin aids in the utilization and storage of glucose.
____ 8. If a hypoglycemic reaction occurs, the diabetic should inject insulin immediately.
____ 9. It is best for the diabetic to fast when exercising heavily.
____ 10. The three important factors to balance in diabetes are diet, exercise, and insulin.
____ 11. In uncontrolled diabetes, much of the carbohydrate from food cannot be used for energy.
____ 12. Excessive exercise can lead to insulin reaction.
____ 13. Insulin is produced by the beta (β) cells of the islets of Langerhans which are located in the liver.
____ 14. Alcohol is metabolized by the body in a manner similar to fats.
____ 15. Carbohydrates should be minimized and insulin intake curtailed during illness.
____ 16. Ketosis results from the breakdown of body fat when glucose is unable to be utilized for energy.
____ 17. In case of insulin reaction, diabetics should always carry a source of simple carbohydrate, such as jellybeans, hard candy, or sugar cubes.

Select the best answer to the following statements:

____ 18. Symptoms which may occur with diabetic acidosis include
(a) headache. (b) thirst. (c) warm flushed skin. (d) fruity breath. (e) rapid pulse. (f) polyuria. (g) all of these.
____ 19. Sign(s) of diabetes include
(a) excessive thirst. (b) excessive hunger. (c) excessive urination. (d) loss of weight. (e) weakness, fatigue. (f) all of these.

II. C. Technician's Notes

Patient: _____   Date: _____

S   (Subjective data—how patient feels):
O   (Objective data—physical measurements including diet/nutritional status):
A   (Assessment—acceptability of dietary progress/nutritional status):
P   (Plan—diet prescription and instruction):
Comments:

Diabetes Counseling Role Playing

Keeping in mind the preceding Suggested Readings and Counseling Guidelines, participate in the following role play situations; use the sample menu (Fig. 11.1) as a teaching aid. Select different partners for each situation, either classmates or co-workers, and elaborate on each role play situation to develop a patient/audience profile. You may want to use your handout from Steps 2, 3, or 4. Use the SOAP method to record in each patient's medical chart.

Name _____ Room _____
Diet **Calorie controlled** _____

Breakfast Please circle your selections below

Fruits and juices	**Cereals**	**Entrees**	**Breads**	**Miscellaneous**
Orange juice	Cream of wheat	Bacon	Bran muffin	Salt
Grapefruit juice	Grits	Sausage	Corn muffin	Pepper
Prune juice ¼ cup	Oatmeal	Scrambled egg	Plain muffin	Sugar substitute
Apple juice ⅓ cup	Cornflakes	Poached egg	English muffin	Butter
Cranberry juice LC	Rice Krispies	Egg substitute	White toast	Margarine
Grapefruit sections LC	Special K	Pancakes	Wheat toast	Lemon
Stewed prunes LC	Puffed rice	French toast	Rye toast	Dietetic jelly
Banana ½	Puffed wheat	Omelet of the Day		Dietetic syrup
	Shredded wheat			
	All Bran			
	Bran Flakes			

Beverages

Coffee

Tea   Cream

Decaffeinated coffee   Nondairy creamer

Whole milk

4 oz. whole milk

Skim milk

4 oz. skim milk

LC = Low Calorie

Name _____ Room _____
Diet **Calorie controlled** _____

Luncheon Please circle your selections below

Appetizers
Apple juice
Cranberry juice LC
Tomato juice
Fruit cup LC
Consomme/chicken/beef
Chicken noodle soup
Vegetable soup
Cream of tomato soup
Cream of chicken soup
Soup du jour

Entrees
Tomato with:
  Chicken salad, ½ cup
  Tuna salad, ½ cup
  Cottage cheese, ½ cup
  Egg salad, ½ cup
Chef's bowl/meat & cheese
Cottage cheese & fruit
Roast beef sandwich
Sliced turkey sandwich
Tuna salad sandwich
Chicken salad sandwich
Egg salad sandwich
Tuna noodle casserole
Turkey/gravy/dressing
Roast beef au jus
Macaroni and cheese
Scrod
Ham/plain
Steak/mushrooms
Chicken/cranberry LC
Grilled cheese/dill pickle
Veal/gravy
Pork chop/plain
Shell macaroni
Beefburger or cheeseburger
  (dill pickles)
Salisbury/gravy
Chef's special if allowed

Breads
White   Dinner Roll
Wheat   Crackers
Rye

Beverages
Coffee
Tea
Decaffeinated coffee
Cream
Nondairy creamer
Whole milk
4 oz. whole milk
Skim milk
4 oz. skim milk

Vegetables
Whipped potato
Baked potato
Noodles
Rice
Broccoli
Corn
Spinach
Carrots
Green beans
Beets
Peas
Squash

Salads and dressings
Lettuce/tomato
Tossed greens
Lettuce wedge
Cole slaw
Salad special
Mayonnaise
French LC
Italian LC
Oil & vinegar
Lemon and vinegar
Sour cream

Desserts
Unsweetened peaches
Unsweetened fruit cocktail
Unsweetened baked apple
Unsweetened pears
Unsweetened apricots
Unsweetened applesauce
Fresh fruit
Sunshine cup
Ice cream
Orange sherbet
Raspberry sherbet
Gelatin LC
Custard LC
Angel cake

Miscellaneous
Salt
Pepper
Sugar substitute
Butter
Margarine
Lemon
Dietetic jelly
Mustard
Catsup LC
Relish LC

LC = Low Calorie

Name _____ Room _____
Diet **Calorie controlled** _____

Dinner Please circle your selections below

Appetizers
Apple juice
Cranberry juice LC
Tomato juice
Fruit cup LC
Consomme/chicken/beef
Chicken noodle soup
Vegetable soup
Cream of tomato soup
Cream of chicken soup
Soup du jour

Entrees
Tomato with:
  Chicken salad, ½ cup
  Tuna salad, ½ cup
  Cottage cheese, ½ cup
  Egg salad, ½ cup
Chef's bowl/meat & cheese
Cottage cheese & fruit
Roast beef sandwich
Sliced turkey sandwich
Tuna salad sandwich
Chicken salad sandwich
Egg salad sandwich
Tuna noodle casserole
Turkey/gravy/dressing
Roast beef au jus
Macaroni and cheese
Scrod
Ham/plain
Steak/mushrooms
Chicken/cranberry LC
Grilled cheese/dill pickle
Veal/gravy
Pork chop/plain
Shell macaroni
Beefburger or cheeseburger
  (dill pickles)
Salisbury/gravy
Chef's special if allowed

Breads
White   Dinner Roll
Wheat   Crackers
Rye

Beverages
Coffee
Tea
Decaffeinated coffee
Cream
Nondairy creamer
Whole milk
4 oz. whole milk
Skim milk
4 oz. skim milk

Vegetables
Whipped potato
Baked potato
Noodles
Rice
Broccoli
Corn
Spinach
Carrots
Green beans
Beets
Peas
Squash

Salads and dressings
Lettuce/tomato
Tossed greens
Lettuce wedge
Cole slaw
Salad special
Mayonnaise
French LC
Italian LC
Oil & vinegar
Lemon and vinegar
Sour cream

Desserts
Unsweetened peaches
Unsweetened fruit cocktail
Unsweetened baked apple
Unsweetened pears
Unsweetened apricots
Unsweetened applesauce
Fresh fruit
Sunshine cup
Ice cream
Orange sherbet
Raspberry sherbet
Gelatin LC
Custard LC
Angel cake

Miscellaneous
Salt
Pepper
Sugar substitute
Butter
Margarine
Lemon
Dietetic jelly
Mustard
Catsup LC
Relish LC

LC = Low Calorie

Fig. 11.1 Controlled-calorie menu.
© *The Seiler Corporation. Reprinted by permission.*

As a dietetic technician in nutrition care, do you consider yourself capable of conducting effective counseling sessions with diabetics (juvenile-onset, maturity-onset, or pre-diabetic/hypoglycemic)? Would you be able to assess your patient's dietary compliance and revise diet plans when necessary? Would you or your family be able to adhere to your nutrition guidelines in order to control the undesirable symptoms of diabetes—including hypoglycemia—and prevent or delay the various complications?

Role Play Situation 1. You are working as a dietetic technician on the pediatric ward of a teaching hospital where a 12-year-old juvenile diabetic is referred to you for a discharge diet. Follow the guidelines to complete the charts and provide the patient with an individualized diet plan. Prepare a SOAP note that could be recorded in the patient's medical chart. Note: The boy has only recently been diagnosed and is slightly underweight.

Role Play Situation 2. In the obstetrics-gynecology clinic where you are employed as a dietetic technician, a young mother-to-be is referred to you by her obstetrician for a diabetic diet. Follow the guidelines to complete the charts and provide the patient with an individualized diet plan. Prepare a SOAP note for the patient's medical chart to be kept in the departmental files with a copy to be sent to the referring physician.

Role Play Situation 3. As an out-patient dietetic technician, you are participating in an ongoing Diabetes Club. Briefly outline and present a 15-minute talk on "Eating Enjoyment for Diabetics." Complete a written summary on the presentation for insertion in the clinic files.

Role Play Situation 4. Devise a number of different situations in order to practice calculating various diet plans using the Exchange Lists.

STEP 6: POST-TEST ON DIABETES

In order to evaluate your understanding of diabetes and the current diet therapy, complete the Post-test below. Section I is the Learning Assessment Quiz for Diabetics. (If the diet counselor is unable to complete the test successfully, how can the patient be expected to?) Section II incorporates much of the material from this chapter. Answers are given in the Answer Key. Will your diabetic patients be able to control the condition successfully using your nutrition guidelines to follow their individualized diet plans? Will they be able to avoid swings in blood glucose, and can those with the vague symptoms of "hypoglycemia" learn to balance their diets as well?

Section I: Complete the Learning Assessment Quiz (p. 279). Check your answers with the Answer Key.

Section II: Indicate whether you think the following statements are true (T) or false (F). Check your answers with the Answer Key.

_____ 1. Juvenile-onset diabetes appears gradually, often asymptomatically.
_____ 2. The juvenile-onset diabetic is usually insulin dependent.
_____ 3. Ketosis occurs when the body utilizes stored carbohydrate for energy.
_____ 4. Diet therapy should take into consideration insulin dose/timing and exercise degree/timing.
_____ 5. Insulin requirements tend to increase after puberty.
_____ 6. The basic nutritional requirements for diabetics differ markedly from those of their nondiabetic counterparts.
_____ 7. Drug therapy can readily compensate for dietary errors and excess body weight.
_____ 8. In overt diabetes, fasting blood glucose levels are elevated.
_____ 9. One symptom of insulin reaction is fruity breath due to ketosis.
_____ 10. PZI and ultra-lente are short-acting types of insulin.
_____ 11. The maturity-onset diabetic usually has little or no endogenous insulin.
_____ 12. One of the two most common contributing factors to the development of maturity-onset diabetes is excess body fat.

____ 13.   Carbohydrate intake should be minimized in the treatment of diabetes to 15–20% of total caloric intake.

____ 14.   Alcoholic beverages are to be excluded, even on liberal diabetic diets.

____ 15.   Fructose has little advantage over other simple carbohydrates in the diabetic diet.

____ 16.   Pregnancy can stimulate the progress of subclinical diabetes.

____ 17.   Individuals with diabetes are also at greater risk for heart disease.

____ 18.   Anyone noting the occurrence of the symptoms of hypoglycemia should immediately adopt a low-carbohydrate diet.

____ 19.   Reactive hypoglycemia is a serious and debilitating disorder.

____ 20.   For a majority of individuals, the maintenance of normal blood glucose levels requires adherence to a low-carbohydrate diet plan.

Select the answer that best completes the following statements and check your answers with the Answer Key.

____ 21.   For one Milk Exchange, use
(a) 1 cup lowfat milk. (b) 1 cup plain yogurt, lowfat. (c) either of these.

____ 22.   One Vegetable Exchange provides approximately
(a) 5 grams of carbohydrate. (b) 2 grams of protein. (c) negligible fat. (d) 25 calories. (e) a and d only. (f) all of these.

____ 23.   For one Fruit Exchange, use
(a) $\frac{1}{2}$ cup juice, any kind. (b) $\frac{1}{2}$ cup berries, any kind. (c) 1 large banana. (d) 1 large apple. (e) 1 small orange. (f) all of these. (g) none of these.

____ 24.   For one Starch/Bread Exchange, use
(a) $\frac{1}{2}$ frankfurter roll. (b) 1 tortilla (6-in. diameter). (c) 1 slice most breads. (d) $\frac{1}{2}$ cup cooked cereal. (e) 1 small corn-on-the-cob. (f) a and c only. (g) all of these.

____ 25.   For one lean Meat Exchange, use
(a) 1 egg. (b) 2 Tbsp peanut butter. (c) $\frac{1}{4}$ cup tuna. (d) 1 oz ground beef. (e) $\frac{1}{2}$ cup cottage cheese (regular, large curd). (f) all of these.

____ 26.   One Fat Exchange provides approximately
(a) 4 grams of fat. (b) 5 grams of fat. (c) 45 calories. (d) 100 calories. (e) b and c only.

REFERENCES

AMERICAN DIABETES ASSOCIATION and AMERICAN DIETETIC ASSOCIATION. 1976. Exchange Lists for Meal Planning. Chicago, IL and Alexandria, VA: ADA.

AMERICAN DIABETES ASSOCIATION and AMERICAN DIETETIC ASSOCIATION. 1986. Exchange Lists for Meal Planning. Chicago, IL and Alexandria, VA: ADA.

BENZ, M., and KOHLER, E. 1980. Baby Food Exchanges. Milwaukee, WI: Milwaukee Children's Hospital.

SCHUTT, C., and ARONSON, V. 1980. Diabetes Club at Union Hospital. J. Am. Dietet. Assoc. 77, Nov., 584.

Chapter Twelve

Cardiovascular Disease

CHAPTER BLUEPRINT

Step 1: Take the Pre-test on Cardiovascular Disease and participate in the assigned group discussion.
Step 2: Examine the Dietary Fat Facts List and prepare the assigned handout.
Step 3: Examine the Cholesterol Facts List and prepare the assigned handout.
Step 4: Examine the Sodium Facts List and prepare the assigned handout.
Step 5: Examine the CVD Guidelines and complete the role play assignment.
Step 6: Take the Post-test on Cardiovascular Disease to evaluate what you have learned from the information and activities provided in this chapter.

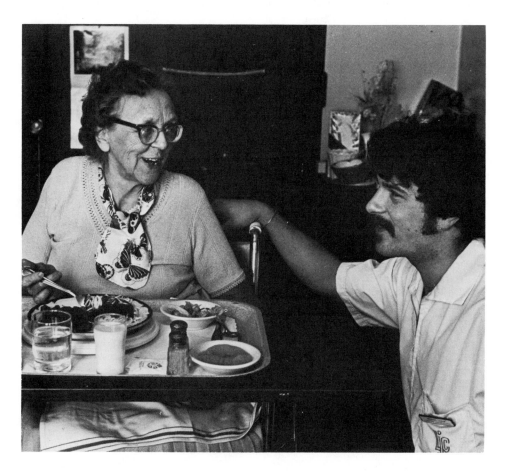

STEP 1: PRE-TEST ON CARDIOVASCULAR DISEASE

More than half of the deaths that occur in our society each year can be attributed to heart disease. Yet, the rate of death from cardiovascular disease (CVD) has actually declined from the late 1960s, and the drop is significant: over 200,000 fewer deaths from heart disease occurred during the 1970s than during the previous decade, and the number continued to drop in the '80s. To what do we owe this positive shift? Research is still underway, but several of the new trends in American lifestyle may prove to be the determining factors in our current "change of heart." In the late 1960s, 55% of American males smoked cigarettes, half of the existing cases of hypertension were undetected while half of those cases which had been discovered remained untreated, and the average (male) blood cholesterol was 240. A dozen years later, only 35% of this same population smoked cigarettes, more hypertensives were receiving adequate treatment, and the average cholesterol level for the middle-aged American (male) was 210.

Since evidence is still incomplete, there exists a great deal of controversy in the area of lifestyle influences on CVD. Except for cigarette smoking as a risk factor in CVD, a consensus has not been reached on the roles played by other lifestyle factors including fat, cholesterol, sodium, and total caloric intakes; the effects of other dietary components such as fiber (notably oat bran and legumes) and omega fatty acids; potassium, calcium, magnesium, and other minerals; alcohol; exercise; stress; and overall environmental influences.

Investigate the current professional opinions on the role of diet in the development and treatment of cardiovascular disease using some of the following Suggested Readings. Then complete the CVD and Diet Questionnaire, and discuss your answers with classmates or co-workers. As a dietetic technician in nutrition care, it is important for you to develop your own stand regarding the role of diet in CVD, and to have a working knowledge of the scientific facts as we now know them. Keep in mind the fact that nutrition is a relatively new science, and current theories will be altered as new evidence is uncovered.

Suggested Readings

AMERICAN HEART ASSOCIATION. 1982. Rationale of the Diet-Heart Statement of the AHA: Report of the Nutrition Committee. Dallas: AHA.

ANAKAWA, K. 1988. Nonpharmacological treatment of hypertension. Seminars in Nephrology *18,* Jun., 169.

ANDERSON, J., et al. 1984. Hypocholesterolemic effects of oat bran or bean intake. Amer. J. Clin. Nutr. *40,* Dec., 1146.

ATSCHUL, A., and GROMMET, J. 1980. Sodium intake and sodium sensitivity. Nutrition Rev. *38,* Dec., 393.

BRECKENRIDGE, A. 1988. Current controversies in the treatment of hypertension. Amer. J. Med. *84,* Jan. 29, 36.

BULPITT, C. 1982. Is there a new member in the high blood pressure mafia? Nutrition Today *17,* Mar./Apr., 6.

CASTELLI, W. 1979. How many drinks a day? J. Am. Med. Assoc. *242,* Nov. 2, 2000.

CHANDRA, R. 1988. There is more to fish than fish oils. Nutrition Res. *8,* Jan., 1.

EDITOR. 1988. Fish oil. Lancet *1,* Mar. 19, 624.

EVANS, D., WILLET, W., and HENNEKENS, C. 1980. Alcohol and coronary heart disease. Amer. Heart J. *100,* Oct., 584.

FALKNER, B. 1988. Sodium sensitivity: A determinant of essential hypertension. J. Amer. Coll. Nutr. *7,* Feb., 35.

FELDMAN, E., and KUSKE, T. 1987. Why, what, and how to implement reduction of cardiovascular risk factors by diet. J. Amer. Coll. Nutr. *6,* Dec., 475.

GLOMSET, J. 1985. Fish, fatty acids, and human health. New Engl. J. Med. *313,* May 9, 1253.

GRUNDY, S. 1986. Comparison of monounsaturated fatty acids and carbohydrates for lowering plasma cholesterol. New Engl. J. Med. *314,* Mar. 20, 745.

HENNEKENS, C., et al. 1979. Effects of beer, wine, and liquor in coronary deaths. J. Am. Med. Assoc. *242,* Nov. 2, 1979.

JAMES, T. 1981. Sure cures, quick fixes, and easy answers. Nutrition Today *16,* May/Jun., 19.

KAPLAN, N. 1985. Non-drug treatment of hypertension. Ann. Internal Med. *102,* Mar., 359.

KROMHOUT, D., BOSSCHIETER, E., and COULANDER, C. 1985. The inverse relation between fish consumption and 20-year mortality from coronary heart disease. New Engl. J. Med. *312,* May 9, 1205.

KURTZ, T., AL-BENDER, H., and MORRIS, C. 1987. "Salt-sensitive" essential hypertension in men: Is sodium alone important? New Eng. J. Med. *317,* Oct. 22, 1043.

MENSINK, R., and KATAN, M. 1987. Effect of monounsaturated fatty acids on HDLs in healthy men and women. Lancet *1,* Jan. 17, 22.

NATIONAL DAIRY COUNCIL. 1986. Nutrition controversies related to infants and children. Dairy Counc. Dig. *57,* Jul./Aug., 21.

NATIONAL DAIRY COUNCIL. 1987. The controversy regarding dietary cholesterol. Dairy Coun. Dig. *58,* Sept./Oct., 25.

NUBE, M., et al. 1987. Scoring of prudent dietary habits and its relation to 25-year survival. J. Am. Dietet. Assoc. *87,* Feb., 171.

OLSON, R. (Editor). 1988. Role of sodium vs. sodium chloride in hypertension. Nutrition Rev. *46,* May, 187.

ROBERTSON, J. 1988. Salt and hypertension—a dangerous myth? Public Health *102,* Nov., 513.

SHATERNIKOV, V. 1981. A Russian point of view. Nutrition Today *16,* Jan./Feb., 24.

SIMOPOULOS, A., KIFER, R., and MARTIN, R. 1986. Health Effects of Polyunsaturated Fatty Acids in Seafoods. Orlando, FL: Academic Press.

TOBIAN, L. 1988. Potassium and hypertension. Nutrition Rev. *46,* Aug., 273.

WASSERTHEIL, S., et al. 1985. Effective dietary intervention in hypertensives: Sodium restriction and weight reduction. J. Am. Dietet. Assoc. *85,* Apr., 423.

WEINSIER, R. 1985. Recent developments in the etiology and treatment of hypertension: Dietary calcium, fat, and magnesium. Amer. J. Clin. Nutr. *42,* Dec., 1331.

WHITE, P., and CROCCO, S. 1980. Hypertension: A Sodium-related Problem? Chicago: American Medical Association.

WILBER, J. 1982. The role of diet in the treatment of high blood pressure. J. Am. Dietet. Assoc. *80,* Jan., 25.

CVD and Diet Questionnaire

1. List the possible pros and cons for following a low-fat/modified fat diet plan.

    Pros   *Cons*
    1.   1.
    2.   2.
    3.   3.
    4.   4.
    5.   5.
    6.   6.
    7.   7.
    8.   8.
    .   .
    .   .
    .   .

2. List the possible pros and cons for following a low-cholesterol diet plan.

3. List the possible pros and cons for following a low/modified sodium diet plan.

4. List the possible pros and cons for following a high-fiber diet plan.

5. List the possible pros and cons for including fish in the diet several times each week.

6. List the possible pros and cons for taking fish oil supplements.

7. List the possible pros and cons for taking mineral supplements.

8. As a dietetic technician in nutrition care, summarize your viewpoint on reasonable, practical dietary guidelines for the prevention and control of cardiovascular disease.

STEP 2: DIETARY FAT FACTS

It is an accepted fact that diet affects blood lipid levels. The degree of influence of specific dietary factors is still a matter of debate. However, nutritionists advise the concerned public to eat a varied and well-balanced diet that meets the following criteria:

1. Maintenance of a reasonable body weight
2. Emphasis on starchy and fibrous foods
3. Limited intake of total fat
4. Emphasis on unsaturated fats
5. Limited intake of cholesterol
6. Moderate intake of sodium

The following Dietary Fat Facts List provides some of the most current diet-related information for counseling individuals who need a reduction in dietary fat intake.

Dietary Fat Facts List

1. Cardiovascular disease (CVD) is the leading cause of death in the United States.
2. The heart and blood vessels comprise the cardiovascular system responsible for establishing and maintaining circulation. The primary functions of the cardiovascular system are to deliver oxygen from the lungs to other organs and to return carbon dioxide back to the lungs.
3. Diseases of the cardiovascular system affect the heart and blood vessels, primarily the arteries. Coronary artery disease occurs with a deprivation of the blood supply to the heart, inducing atherosclerosis, **angina pectoris,** and **myocardial infarction.** Other cardiovascular disorders include **congenital heart disease, rheumatic heart disease,** and **congestive heart failure.**
4. The main goals of dietary care in CVD include (a) maximum rest for the heart, (b) prevention or elimination of edema, (c) maintenance of optimal nutritional status, and (d) diet tolerance/satisfaction for the individual patient.
5. The general diet plan for the patient with CVD is based on the following guidelines: (a) Attain and maintain a reasonable weight. (b) Avoid overeating (which puts extra strain on the heart, as well as extra fat on the body). (c) Include foods that are easy to eat and digest. (d) Restrict stimulants such as caffeine and nicotine. (e) Limit sodium, especially with hypertension and edema. (f) Divide food intake into several small meals instead of two or three larger ones. (g) Make mealtimes pleasant and unhurried.
6. It is important for the patient with CVD to attain and maintain a reasonable weight; with excess poundage, the heart is forced to work harder. Also, fat deposits in the **myocardium** decrease the overall efficiency of the heart, while abdominal fat interferes with the diaphragm and the pumping of the heart.
7. The incidence of CVD increases with age, but atherosclerosis has been reported in young individuals, and in the very young with inborn errors of metabolism. Uncommon in young women, CVD occurs more frequently after menopause.
8. Atherosclerosis is a degenerative disease of the arteries in which the inner layer is thickened by plaques consisting of lipid (primarily cholesterol) and fibrous tissue; as the plaques increase in size, blood flow is inhibited, leading to hypertension and CVD. The mechanisms by which plaque proliferates are still being researched. Atherosclerosis is characterized by a narrowing of the **lumen** of the blood vessels with loss of elasticity in arterial walls; a high level of fat in the blood is found in a majority of those with atherosclerosis, and a high dietary intake of saturated fat tends to elevate these levels further.
9. No one is totally free of atherosclerotic plaques, but it is possible to limit development through control of the CVD "risk factors," the predictors of future cardiovascular health.
10. The major predictors for CVD are cigarette smoking, high blood pressure, and elevated blood cholesterol levels; the recent decline in CVD may be correlated to the decrease in cigarette smoking, improved control of blood pressure, and a decrease in the average blood cholesterol level. Increased participation in physical activities probably influenced this decline as well.

angina pectoris: Chest pain radiating down the left side, due to insufficient supply of blood/oxygen to the heart.

myocardial infarction (MI): Heart attack.

congenital heart disease: Disorders of the heart that begin or exist at birth.

rheumatic heart disease: Serious pathological conditions of the heart that may occur following rheumatic fever, an inflammatory infectious disease characterized by fever and joint pain.

congestive heart failure (CHF): Condition in which the heart is unable to pump sufficiently, resulting in shortness of breath and edema.

myocardium: Cardiac muscle which forms the middle layer of the heart wall.

lumen: Cavity within a tube.

11.   The incidence of CVD can be correlated with the pressures of contemporary society, such as fast-moving urban lifestyles, career stress, alienation from family and peers, separation and divorce.

12.   The risk factors for CVD have multiple causes, and each plays an interrelated role in the predisposition to and development of the disease. Those factors which can be altered include hyperlipidemia, hypertension, and obesity (which are diet related), as well as smoking and physical activity; those factors which are more difficult but still possible to alter include underlying diseases, stress, and personality characteristics; and it is not possible to change heredity, the aging process, and sexual status.

13.   Lipid is a general term for fats that includes those naturally occurring substances insoluble in water but dissolvable in solvents: 95% of the lipids found in foods and the body are triglycerides; the other types of lipids are phospholipids (lecithin) and sterols (cholesterol).

14.   Blood lipid levels have been shown to be related to the incidence of myocardial infarction, cerebrovascular accident (CVA), and hypertension—or, in lay terms, heart attack, stroke, and high blood pressure.

15.   The blood lipid profile is a lab test used to determine the amounts of different lipids in the blood in order to assess the risk or presence of CVD.

16.   Primary hyperlipoproteinemia is an inherited disorder and/or associated with dietary constituents including fat. Secondary hyperlipoproteinemia is caused by other disorders including hypothyroidism, **dysproteinemia, nephrotic syndrome,** obstructive liver disease, and uncontrolled diabetes.

dysproteinemia: Abnormal amount of protein in the blood.

nephrotic syndrome: Nephrosis; kidney disease, most common in children, which is characterized by massive edema, loss of protein, and degenerative lesions in certain areas of the kidney.

17.   Hyperlipidemia or hyperlipoproteinemia is characterized by an elevated level of serum cholesterol, triglycerides, or both. Cholesterol and triglycerides are carried in the blood bound to specific proteins; these lipoproteins vary as to the amount of protein and fat they contain, and are identified according to their densities (Table 12.1).

18.   The four major categories of lipoproteins are (a) chylomicrons—mostly triglyceride, (b) pre-beta or very low density (VLDL)—containing mostly lipid and little protein, (c) beta or low density (LDL)—similar to VLDL but containing even more cholesterol, and (d) alpha or high density (HDL)—containing more protein and less lipid.

19.   There appears to be an inverse relationship for the level of HDL and the incidence of CVD; women tend to have higher levels, but alterations in both sexes can occur with changes in exercise, diet or alcohol intake, and use of certain medications.

20.   Food fats include the visible fats and oils (found in butter, oils, marbled meats, lard, etc.) and the hidden fats found in nuts, milk and milk products, avocados, and fried and processed foods (see Chapter 3, Step 6).

21.   In 1900, Americans consumed a daily average of 125 grams of fat, but by 1972, the intake had increased to around 159 grams. In 1980, the average fat intake was 168 grams, which is over 40% of the total caloric intake. There has been a shift from animal to vegetable sources of fat; especially notable is the increased use of vegetable oils by food processors and fast food chains.

22.   It is advisable for everyone over the age of 2 to modify fat intake; for those at high risk for CVD, regular screenings and dietary advice may be warranted.

Table 12.1   Lipoprotein Levels for Types of Hyperlipoproteinemias

Type	Triglycerides	Cholesterol	Chylomicrons	LDL[a]	VLDL[b]
I	↑	↑	↑	Normal	Normal
IIa	Normal	↑	—	↑	Normal
IIb	↑	↑	—	↑	↑
III	↑	↑	—	↑	↑
IV	↑	Normal or ↑	—	Normal or ↑	↑
V	↑	↑	↑	Normal or ↑	↑

[a]LDL is low density (or beta) lipoprotein.
[b]VLDL is very low density (or pre-beta) lipoprotein.

23.   Dietary treatment for hyperlipoproteinemia includes altered intake of some or all of the following: cholesterol, fat (saturated, polyunsaturated), carbohydrate, and alcohol (see Table 12.2).

24.   Plasma cholesterol levels tend to increase with immoderate intakes of saturated fats, whereas the substitution of polyunsaturated fats tends to have a lowering effect.

25.   Monounsaturated fats (found in olive oil, peanut oil, and avocado) are believed to help to reduce plasma cholesterol levels. The omega-3 fatty acids found in fatty fish may also play a role in the regulation of blood lipids.

26.   Individuals desiring to moderate fat intake should deemphasize meat in the diet (and substitute fish), replace high-fat dairy foods with low-fat milk products, avoid fried and greasy foods, and rely on grains, fruits, and vegetables for the bulk of daily calories.

27.   Carbohydrate intake can elevate serum levels of very low density lipoprotein (VLDL, composed of glucose and free fatty acids), and simple sugars can aggravate an existing hyperlipoproteinemia with elevated triglyceride levels; alcohol intake can also affect triglyceride levels and may require restriction.

28.   Diets for hyperlipoproteinemia may be low in vitamin A and iron, so the low-fat food sources of these nutrients should be emphasized.

29.   Research has indicated that soluble dietary fibers (found in oat bran and legumes) may help to decrease the reabsorption of bile salts and increase fecal excretion to help diminish hyperlipidemia.

30.   Diet is one of the cornerstones of treatment for hyperlipoproteinemia, and adherence to restrictions can improve the effects of drug treatment. The popular trend for dietary self-prescription, however, should be avoided. Infants, children, pregnant women, and those who are ill should not follow strict low-fat diets unless prescribed by a physician.

Exercise on Dietary Fat Counseling

Keeping in mind the preceding Dietary Fat Facts List, which provides some of the most current diet-related information for counseling individuals who need a reduction in dietary fat intake, prepare a simplified version for use as a patient handout. You may include graphics and/or prepare in a poster format, if desired; see the Sample Handout. Show your handout

Table 12.2   Treatment for Hyperlipoproteinemias[a]

	Type I	Type IIa	Type IIb and Type III	Type IV	Type V
Diet prescription	Low fat (25–30 g)	Low cholesterol; polyunsaturated fat increased	Low cholesterol; calories approx. 20% from protein, 40% from fat	Controlled carbohydrate—approx. 45% of calories; moderate cholesterol restriction	Restricted fat—30% of calories; controlled carbohydrate—50% of calories; moderate cholesterol restriction
Calories	Not restricted	Not restricted	Achieve and maintain a reasonable weight; reduction diet if necessary	Achieve and maintain a reasonable weight; reduction diet if necessary	Achieve and maintain a reasonable weight; reduction diet if necessary
Protein	Total protein intake not limited	Total protein intake not limited	High protein intake	Not limited other than control of patient's weight	High protein intake
Fat	Restricted to 25–30 g; type of fat not important	Saturated fat intake limited; polyunsaturated fat increased	Controlled to 40% of calories (polyunsaturated fats recommended over saturated fats)	Not limited other than control of patient's weight (polyunsaturated fats recommended over saturated fats)	Restricted to 30% of calories (polyunsaturated fats recommended over saturated fats)
Cholesterol	Not restricted	Low as possible	Less than 300 mg	Moderate restriction (300–500 mg)	Moderate restriction (300–500 mg)
Carbohydrate	Not limited	Not limited	Controlled; concentrated sweets restricted	Controlled; concentrated sweets restricted	Controlled; concentrated sweets restricted
Alcohol	Not recommended	May be used with discretion	No more than 2 servings	No more than 2 servings	Not recommended

[a]Adapted from Fredrickson et al. (1973).

in rough draft form to classmates or co-workers for constructive criticism on the overall design, content, and potential effectiveness for use in pertinent diet counseling situations. Then prepare a final version for your own future use as a practicing dietetic technician.

Sample Handout

CVD Risk Factors

Ask yourself the following questions to determine *your* risk for developing heart disease:

Heredity. Do you have any relatives who have had heart disease at a relatively young age?

Health. Do you have hypertension? hyperlipidemia? diabetes? Do these disorders affect close family members?

Age. Are you middle aged? older?

Sex. Are you a male? a post-menopausal female?

Smoking. Do you smoke cigarettes? How many packs per day? For how many years?

Exercise. Do you exercise daily? less than daily? occasionally? never?

Stress. Are you often uptight, anxious, or nervous? How often?

Weight. Are you overweight? by how many pounds?

Diet. Is your daily diet moderate in fat (30% of total caloric intake or less)? cholesterol (300 mg or less)? sodium (2 g or so)? Is it well balanced?

Table 12.3 Basic Terms Used in Dietary Control of CVD

Term	Definition
Lipid	A general term for fats, including triglycerides, cholesterol, phospholipids, and dietary fats.
Fatty acids	The building blocks of fats.
Triglycerides	The most common form of lipid in the diet, and the usual storage form of fats in the body. These fats are rapidly absorbed from food and can be synthesized by the body from sugar and alcohol. Excessive blood levels have been implicated in heart disease.
Cholesterol	A waxy fatlike substance found in every animal cell which is manufactured by the liver, and is present in all foods of animal origin. The amount of cholesterol in the diet may affect blood levels, and lead to a buildup of fatty deposits in the arteries (atherosclerosis). Egg yolks and organ meats are rich in cholesterol; fatty meats, shrimp, butter, cream, whole milk, and whole milk cheeses also contain considerable amounts.
Lecithin	A phospholipid (fat containing phosphorus) with emulsification properties involved in the transport and utilization of fats. It is found in many animal tissues and is used as a food additive. Synthesized by the body and abundant in egg yolk, meat, milk, soybeans, and corn, lecithin has *not* been shown to be effective in the dissolution of fatty accumulations in the blood, nor as an antidote to elevated cholesterol levels.
Saturated fats	Fats that are usually hard at room temperature and are found primarily in animal products (meat, eggs, lard, butter, cream, whole milk, and whole milk cheeses). These fats are also abundant in solid and hydrogenated vegetable fats and in coconut oil, palm oil, some margarines, and shortening. Since the body can convert saturated fats to cholesterol, it is believed that they have an elevating effect on blood cholesterol levels.
Polyunsaturated fats	Fats and oils that are usually liquid at room temperature are abundant in plant seed oils (safflower, sunflower, corn, soybean, cottonseed, sesame, walnut) and may be effective in lowering blood cholesterol levels.

continued

Table 12.3 *(Continued)*

Term	Definition
Monounsaturated fats	Liquid at room temperature, found primarily in olive and peanut oil, and believed to lower blood cholesterol levels.
Omega-3 fatty acids	Polyunsaturated fats abundant in cold water fish (such as salmon, mackerel, and tuna); intake can help lower blood lipids and reduce the risk for CVD and certain other diseases.
Hydrogenation	The chemical process used to convert unsaturated fats from liquid to semi-solid form in order to make the product more saturated and increase shelf life.

STEP 3: CHOLESTEROL FACTS

sterol: Type of steroid that includes alcohol and has lipidlike properties (e.g., cholesterol).

Cholesterol is a waxy, fatlike **sterol** found in all animal cells and present in foods of animal origin. Mainly manufactured by the liver, cholesterol plays an essential role in the body as a precursor for adrenal steroid hormones, male and female sex hormones, and bile acids. An elevated level of cholesterol in the blood, however, is undesirable and can be indicative of atherosclerosis.

The following Cholesterol Facts List provides some of the most current diet-related information to include in counseling individuals who need to reduce dietary cholesterol.

Cholesterol Facts List

1. Cardiovascular disease—those disorders which affect the heart or blood vessels—is the number one health problem in the United States today.

2. Studies conducted over a number of years indicate that preventive action can be undertaken through control over a number of risk factors now associated with cardiovascular disease. These include high blood pressure, smoking, stress, lack of exercise, elevated blood fat levels, obesity, diabetes, and family history of heart disease.

3. During the first decade of life, fatty streaks develop in the blood vessels, some of which develop into plaques—fibrous-covered fatty deposits prone to hemorrhage, ulceration, thrombosis, and calcification—which may narrow coronary blood vessels to cause angina pectoris, myocardial infarction, and death (or cerebral blockage to cause stroke).

4. Plaque formation is gradual and pernicious, sometimes without accompanying symptoms.

5. The three major risk factors associated with premature atherosclerosis are (a) cigarette smoking, (b) high blood pressure, and (c) hypercholesterolemia, but there exists no evidence to indicate that cholesterol intake alone causes coronary artery disease. Animal experiments, however, indicate that a high-cholesterol diet can produce atherosclerosis in those susceptible to the disease, and analysis of plaques reveals large amounts of cholesterol.

6. Cholesterol forms an essential lipid component of brain and nerve cell structure, and is both manufactured by the body and obtained through the diet.

7. Typical dietary cholesterol intake in this country approximates 250 mg/1000 calories, but nutritionists suggest a total daily intake of less than 300 mg. As serum cholesterol levels increase over 200 mg/dl, the incidence of coronary artery disease progressively rises.

8. To lower blood cholesterol levels, it is important to first attain and maintain a reasonable body weight; total fat intake should be lowered, with emphasis on unsaturated fats and minimal consumption of saturated fats. Less important is a restricted intake of dietary cholesterol.

9.   Diet plays a role in the control of blood lipids and should incorporate the following goals: (a) maintenance of a reasonable weight; (b) reduction of total fat intake; (c) reduction of saturated fat intake; (d) reduction of cholesterol intake.

10.   Other dietary considerations include the following:

○   Reduction of sodium intake when high blood pressure is evident.

○   Reduction of alcohol and refined sugar intake when blood triglyceride levels are elevated.

○   Increase in fiber intake.

11.   A basic understanding of the following terms is important in proper dietary control: lipid, fatty acids, triglycerides, cholesterol, lecithin, saturated fats, polyunsaturated fats, monounsaturated fats, omega-3 fatty acids, and hydrogenation. See Table 12.3 for definitions.

12.   About half of the average dietary intake of cholesterol is absorbed. Lipoproteins account for around 10% of total body cholesterol.

13.   The diet used to lower serum cholesterol is low in both cholesterol and saturated fat, minimizing the intake of: egg yolks; organ meats; fatty meats, luncheon meats, frankfurters, bacon, sausage, poultry skin, duck, and caviar; whole milk, cream, ice cream, sour cream, whole milk cheese and yogurt; butter, lard, gravies, and hydrogenated vegetable shortening; coconut, palm oil, and coconut oil; potato chips and other fried snacks; and commercially prepared baked goods made with the preceding foods.

14.   Soluble fiber (found in oat bran and legumes) may demonstrate a hypocholesterolemic effect by binding to bile acids to be excreted, reducing the body's cholesterol pool and lowering blood levels.

15.   Controversy exists as to the effect of dietary cholesterol on serum cholesterol levels: certain populations have a large cholesterol intake without experiencing hypercholesterolemia, whereas others report only a slight decrease in severity of the disorder upon lowering cholesterol intake.

16.   Despite advertising claims to the contrary, lecithin supplementation has not been shown to decrease serum cholesterol; widespread in foods, lecithin is also manufactured in the body in abundant amounts. Self-prescribed niacin supplementation is also undesirable, ineffective in safe doses and risky in megadoses.

17.   The low-cholesterol diet has become a popular self-prescription, but should only be undertaken upon a physician's recommendation.

18.   Control of risk factors through means other than diet should be undertaken as well. Stress reduction and regular exercise can help to reduce and control blood cholesterol levels.

Exercise on Cholesterol Counseling

Keeping in mind the preceding Cholesterol Fact List, which provides some of the most current diet-related information to include in counseling individuals who need to reduce dietary cholesterol, prepare a simplified version for use as a patient handout. You may include graphics and/or prepare in a poster format, if desired; see the Sample Handout. Show your handout in rough draft form to classmates or co-workers for constructive criticism on the overall design, content, and potential effectiveness for use in pertinent diet counseling situations. Then prepare a final version for your own future use as a practicing dietetic technician.

Sample Handout

The foods shown in Table 12.4 are high in total fat, saturated fat, and/or cholesterol.

Table 12.4   Foods High in Total Fat, Saturated Fat, and/or Cholesterol

Meats and alternates

Beef (unless lean)	Salt pork	Canned meats	Fish roe (including
Lamb (unless lean)	Spareribs	Organ meats	caviar)
Pork (unless lean)	Frankfurters, sausages,	Duck	Turkey or chicken skin
Bacon	cold cuts, luncheon	Goose	Eggs
	meats		Nuts, peanut butter

Milk and cheeses

Whole milk	Sour cream	Whole milk cheeses	
Cream, powdered	Whole milk yogurt	Ice cream	
creamer			

Fats and oils

Butter	Solid shortenings	Coconut oil	Cocoa butter
Stick margarines	Lard	Palm oil	Mayonnaise

Grains—bakery goods

Commercial biscuits	Doughnuts	Coffee cakes	
Croissants	Cookies	Pies	
Pastries	Cakes	Sweet rolls	

Desserts

Puddings	Custards	Rich sweets	Chocolate

Others

Sauces, gravies	Frozen dishes	Coconut	Fast Foods
Fried foods	Creamed dishes		

STEP 4: SODIUM FACTS

Diseases of the heart and blood vessels can lead to congestive heart failure and reduction in the blood pumping ability of the heart. Decreased blood flow results in an accumulation of fluids in surrounding tissues (edema), and a diminished ability of the kidney to excrete excess sodium (Na). Thus, sodium-restricted diets are often used in the management of congestive heart failure and edema, as well as to control hypertension (despite the fact that the exact relationship is unknown, as yet) and certain other conditions.

The following Sodium Facts List provides some of the most current diet-related information to include in counseling individuals requiring a reduction in dietary sodium intake.

Sodium Facts List

1.   The force of blood against the inside walls of the arteries is called blood pressure, and is controlled by the pumping action of the heart. Pressure increases with each heart contraction (systole), stretching artery walls. Pressure decreases during the rest between contractions (diastole), allowing relaxation of artery walls. The relation between the beating (systolic) and resting (diastolic) pressure is measured with a sphygmomanometer (blood pressure cuff) and expressed as systole/diastole (e.g., 120/80). Blood pressure varies, rising with excitement, stress, or anxiety, and dropping with relaxation. When blood pressure remains elevated the heart must work harder, blood vessels are stressed, and the risk of coronary disease, stroke, and organ damage is increased.

2.   Hypertension can be defined as a sustained increase in arterial blood pressure, either diastolic, systolic, or both.

3.   The upper limit of normal blood pressure is 140/90. The primary aim of hypertension therapy is to reduce diastolic pressure to below 90. In the hypertensive state, blood flows through the vessels under an increased pressure. Hypertension is sometimes secondary (the manifestation of an underlying disease such as kidney disease, adrenal tumor, or blood vessel defect), but more often is primary ("essential"), in which the cause is unknown.

4.   The symptoms of hypertension may go undetected for many years; millions of hypertensive Americans are unaware that they are victims of this dangerous disease. In fact, nearly one-sixth of the current population is hypertensive, yet only 50% are aware of their condition, and a mere 10–25% are currently receiving effective treatment.

5.   Primary or "essential" hypertension accounts for over 85% of the cases in the United States; secondary hypertension can be caused by renal disease, tumors of the adrenal gland, peripheral vascular disease, toxemia of pregnancy, and certain other disorders.

6.   Family history of hypertension suggests a genetic influence on the development of hypertension, but other factors such as obesity, stress, cigarette smoking, and sedentary lifestyle contribute to the disorder as well.

7.   Hypertension is a major risk factor in cardiovascular, cerebrovascular, and renal disease, but treatment to control blood pressure can decrease the associated morbidity and mortality.

8.   If untreated, hypertension can damage the heart, eyes, and kidneys; control of blood pressure can delay organ deterioration.

9.   Blood pressure tends to increase with age, with the upper limits of normal set as shown in Table 12.5.

10.   In addition to age, other factors influencing blood pressure include sex and race: more males than females suffer from hypertension (until menopause, when the incidence in females surpasses that for males), and hypertensive women tend to have a better prognosis; the incidence of hypertension in the black population in this country is twice that for whites; associated death rates are significantly higher.

11.   Controllable factors that can contribute to hypertension include lack of exercise, overweight, smoking, stress, diabetes, hyperlipidemia, family history of high blood pressure, and diet, including sodium intake for some.

12.   An excessive intake of sodium is believed to contribute to hypertension in susceptible individuals who are sodium sensitive, and sodium restriction can help to control high blood pressure. The restriction of sodium decreases arterial pressure by causing a negative sodium–water balance to prevent excessive retention.

13.   The Kempner diet, once used to reduce elevated blood pressure, allowed the consumption of only rice, fruit, and sugar; the Karell diet allowed only 800 cc (cubic centimeters) of milk given in four feedings for up to a week. It was these restrictive dietary measures that led to the trend away from the hard-to-follow low-sodium diets and toward the use of drug treatment for hypertension.

14.   The three common levels of sodium restriction are as follows: (a) mild (1–2 g)— no salt in cooking or at the table and avoidance of highly salted items; (b) moderate (1000

Table 12.5 Blood Pressure Norms: Upper Limits of Normal

Age (years)	Blood pressure (mmHg)
Infants	90/60
3–6	110/70
7–10	120/80
11–17	130/80
18–44	140/90
45–64	150/95
65 and older	160/95

mg)—minimal intake of sodium-rich foods and meat, milk, high-sodium vegetables; and (c) strict (250–500 mg)—requires use of low-sodium milk and other special foods, and may require hospitalization.

15.   Salt is composed of 40% sodium and 60% chloride, and is used as a flavor enhancer, preservative, color developer (in processed meats), binding agent (in smoked meats), texture aid (in cheeses, processed meats, and breads), and control agent to regulate the rate of fermentation (in pickles, sauerkraut, sausage, cheeses, and bread dough).

16.   Of the current sodium intake, approximately 20–40% is from the salt added during cooking or at the table, 40–60% is in commercially prepared foodstuffs, and 20–30% occurs naturally in our foods. Simply by eliminating use of the salt shaker, consumers can reduce sodium intake significantly.

17.   In the current American diet, commercially prepared grain products are a major contributor of sodium (breads, rolls, crackers, ready-to-eat cereals and biscuits), with mixed protein dishes (casseroles, chili, pizza, etc.), milk and milk products, soups, and meats contributing significant amounts. By reading ingredient lists one can determine if processed foods are relatively high in the following sodium-rich compounds: sodium bicarbonate (baking soda), sodium pyrophosphate (baking powder), sodium propionate (preservative), sodium carbonate (buffer), sodium nitrite (preservative), monosodium glutamate (flavor enhancer), sodium saccharin (nonnutritive sweetener), sodium benzoate (preservative), sodium alginate (emulsifier), and sodium sulfite (preservative).

18.   Animal foods have sodium contents that vary with the amount of protein: items high in protein tend to be high in sodium as well, so leaner meats and skim milk are richer in sodium than their fattier counterparts.

19.   The average daily intake of sodium in this country is 2–7 grams; the Food and Nutrition Board of the National Academy of Sciences recommends a sodium intake of 1100 to 3300 mg per day as a safe and adequate level for the healthy adult.

20.   A single teaspoon of salt contains over 2000 mg of sodium.

21.   Salt substitutes should only be used if prescribed by a physician, as some contain sodium (but in lowered amounts), others contain ammonium chloride which should be avoided by those with liver disease, and certain brands contain potassium chloride which is undesirable for those with certain renal disorders.

22.   Water softeners increase the sodium content of the water supply, so should only be attached to the hot water tap. Water with a sodium content of more than 5 mg per cup should be avoided by hypertensives, as should soft drinks and beers derived from high-sodium water supplies.

23.   The sodium contents of medications should be considered by hypertensives; even some dentifrices have a significant quantity of sodium.

24.   Products vary considerably in sodium contents. It is important to understand that the charts depicting the sodium contents of foodstuffs only provide representative values.

25.   Diuretics are medications which assist the kidney in the elimination of excess sodium and fluids. Certain diuretics increase dietary potassium (K) needs by causing potassium loss. The increased needs may be met by inclusion in the diet of foods high in potassium. Symptoms of hypokalemia (low level of potassium in the bloodstream) include weakness, muscle cramps, heart palpitations and arrythmias.

26.   Other dietary factors that may affect blood pressure include potassium, calcium, magnesium, caffeine, and alcohol.

27.   An increased dietary intake of potassium may prove to be beneficial in the treatment and prevention of hypertension; a ratio of less than one for Na : K (sodium/potassium) can be attained simply by including ample amounts of fruits and vegetables in the diet. In rats, an increased calcium intake tends to decrease elevated blood pressure, even with a high sodium intake. Inadequate magnesium intakes may also be linked to hypertension.

28.   Caffeine can elevate blood pressure, as can alcohol. Immoderate intakes of alcoholic beverages, along with popular snack foods rich in sodium, can replace more nutritious potassium-rich foods in the diet, and hypertension may develop.

29.   Licorice, ginseng, certain herbs, and some medications can elevate blood pressure; identification and elimination of the offending substance can reduce the elevation.

30.   It is well established that overweight hypertensives who successfully reduce body weight will concurrently decrease elevated blood pressure. Hypertensive individuals

should be encouraged to attain and maintain a reasonable weight, and to exercise regularly and adhere to individualized diet/drug therapy.

31.   Nutritionists, the National High Blood Pressure Education Committee, and many researchers recommend dietary alterations for control of hypertension, with use of drugs only if such measures prove unsuccessful.

32.   The popular tendency to self-prescribe low-sodium diets should be discouraged, as hypotension can be detrimental, even dangerous. Limited intakes of salty foods and curtailed addition of table salt is the more sensible approach to blood pressure control.

Exercise on Sodium Diet Counseling

Keeping in mind the preceding Sodium Facts List, which provides some of the most current diet-related information for counseling individuals requiring a reduction in dietary sodium intake, prepare a simplified version for use as a patient handout. You may include graphics and/or prepare in a poster format, if desired; see the Sample Handout. Show your handout in rough draft form to classmates or co-workers for constructive criticism on the overall design, content, and potential effectiveness for use in pertinent diet counseling situations. Then prepare a final version for your own future use as a practicing dietetic technician.

Sample Handout

You can utilize the following suggestions to assist in decreasing your daily sodium intake to a moderate (healthy) level:

○   Remove the salt shaker from the table.
○   Halt use of salt and sodium-rich seasonings in cooking.
○   Choose fresh foods over the processed items high in added sodium.
○   Read labels carefully for various forms of added sodium.
○   Be careful in purchasing costly, low-sodium, "dietetic" foods—oftentimes, the non-dietetic item is not excessively high in sodium.
○   Note that salt substitutes may lead to nutrient imbalances, and should only be used if prescribed by a physician.
○   Recognize foods, seasonings, and medicinals with high sodium content (see Table 12.6).

Table 12.6   High-Sodium Foods, Seasonings, and Medicinals

High sodium foods

Anchovies	Caviar	Fish (canned, dried, or
Bacon	Cheese food or spread	smoked)
Baking powder	Chips	Frankfurters
Beans, lima, frozen	Cocoa, instant	Frozen dinners and potpies
Beef, corned or dried	Cold cuts	Herring
Beets, pickled	Cornbread	Kosher meats
Biscuits	Crabmeat	Luncheon meats
Bouillon	Crackers (unless unsalted)	Meat (canned, dried, pickled, or
Bread sticks (unless	Danish pastry	smoked)
unsalted)	Dips	Mixed vegetables, frozen
Bread stuffing	Doughnuts	Nuts (unless unsalted)
Cake, from mixes	Egg substitutes	Olives
Canned fish or meat		Paté de foie gras

continued

Table 12.6   *(Continued)*

High sodium foods (continued)

Peanut butter (unless unsalted)	Pretzels	Sauerkraut
Peas, frozen	Relishes	Sausage
Pickles	Roe	Seeds (unless unsalted)
Pies	Salad dressings	Soups
Pizza	Salmon, canned or smoked	Stews, canned
Popcorn, commercial	Salt pork	Tomato juice
Potatoes, hash brown or scalloped	Sardines	Tongue, smoked
		Vegetable juice cocktail

High sodium seasonings

Catsup	Meat extracts	Mustard, peppered
Cooking wines	Meat marinades	Salts—celery, garlic, Kosher, onion, sea
Horseradish	Meat tenderizers	
Instant gravy mixes	Monosodium glutamate	Sauces (barbecue, chili, soy, Worcestershire)
Instant sauce mixes		

Medicinals high in sodium

Antacids	Cough medicines	Sodium bicarbonate (baking soda)
Antibiotics	Laxatives	
Buffered headache remedies	Sedatives	Also certain toothpastes and mouthwashes

STEP 5: CVD GUIDELINES

Certain individuals in the medical, scientific, and nutrition communities, as well as some health organizations (including the American Heart Association) now believe that most Americans should make some significant dietary alterations. Because of epidemiological evidence and the results of recent research, such groups have recommended overall reductions in the intake of total calories, fats (especially saturated fat), cholesterol, and sodium, with increased intakes of starchy, fibrous foods and fish. Advocates of immediate dietary change maintain that, although direct correlations between diet and CVD have not yet been established, this will soon occur and, in the meantime, the potential for adverse side effects from moderate diet modifications are negligible.

The ADA supports the proposed dietary modifications, but has acknowledged the importance of individualized diet planning. It is essential to tailor any CVD diet—preventive or therapeutic—to individual needs and desires. Certain individuals may not require severe dietary restrictions, whereas the overall health of other individuals (such as pregnant women or infants) may actually be threatened by major dietary changes. Thus, individualized diet counseling is essential.

In order to be able to advise individuals seeking to modify fat/cholesterol/sodium intake, it is essential to have all of the hands-on material required for effective counseling sessions. It is also important to be able to record all of the pertinent information regarding each diet counseling session in the patient's medical charts. The information provided below should help to improve your confidence—and skills—regarding your counseling abilities.

This step includes suggested strategies to use in counseling patients on the heart-healthy "prudent diet." The following references may prove helpful.

Suggested Readings for a "Prudent" Diet

AMERICAN ACADEMY OF PEDIATRICS. 1986. Prudent life-style for children: Dietary fat and cholesterol. Pediatrics *78*, Sept., 521.
AMERICAN DIETETIC ASSOCIATION. 1981. Handbook of Clinical Dietetics. New Haven, CT: Yale University Press.

AMERICAN HEART ASSOCIATION. 1980. American Heart Association Handbook: A Guide to Prevention and Treatment of Cardiovascular Disease. New York: E. P. Dutton.

AMERICAN HEART ASSOCIATION, 1981. An Older Person's Guide to Cardiovascular Health. Dallas: AHA.

AMERICAN HEART ASSOCIATION. 1983. Diet in the healthy child. Circulation 67, Jun., 1411-A.

AMERICAN HEART ASSOCIATION. 1984. Recommendations for treatment of hyperlipidemia in adults. Arteriosclerosis 4, Jul./Aug., 443A.

AMERICAN HEART ASSOCIATION. 1985. The American Heart Association Diet: An Eating Plan for Healthy Americans. Dallas: AHA.

AMERICAN HEART ASSOCIATION. 1988. Counseling the Patient with Hyperlipidemia. Dallas: AHA.

AMERICAN HEART ASSOCIATION. 1988. Dietary Guidelines for Healthy American Adults: A Statement for Physicians and Health Professionals. Dallas: AHA.

AMERICAN HEART ASSOCIATION. 1988. Eating for a Healthy Heart: Dietary Treatment of Hyperlipidemia. Dallas: AHA.

BENNETT, I., and SIMON, M. 1973. The Prudent Diet. New York: David White, Inc.

BRESLOW, J. 1987. Pediatric aspects of hyperlipidemia. Pediatrics 62, Oct., 510.

BURSZTYN, P. 1987. Nutrition and Blood Pressure. London, England: John Libbey & Co.

CONNOR, S., and CONNOR, W. 1986. The New American Diet. New York: Simon & Schuster.

COOPER, K. 1988. Controlling Cholesterol. New York: Bantam.

DEBAKEY, M., et al. 1984. The Living Heart Diet. New York: Simon & Schuster.

FELDMAN, E. (Editor). 1983. Nutrition and Heart Disease. New York: Churchill Livingstone.

FREDRICKSON, D., et al. 1973. The Dietary Management of Hyperlipoproteinemia: A Handbook for Physicians and Dietitians. Washington, DC: Government Printing Office.

GOOR, R., and GOOR, N. 1987. Eater's Choice: A Food Lover's Guide to Lower Cholesterol. Boston: Houghton Mifflin.

HALLGREN, B. (Editor). 1986. Diet and Prevention of Coronary Heart Disease and Cancer. New York: Raven Press.

HEPBURN, F., EXLER, J., and WEIHRAUCH, J. 1986. Provisional tables on the content of omega-3 fatty acids and other fat components of selected foods. J. Am. Dietet. Assoc. 86, Jun., 788.

HOEG, J., and BREWER, B. 1987. Definition and management of hyperlipoproteinemia. J. Amer. Coll. Nutr. 6, Apr., 157.

MAYES, K. 1984. The Sodium-Watchers Guide. Santa Barbara, CA: Pennant Books.

NATIONAL CHOLESTEROL EDUCATION PROGRAM. 1987. Report of the Expert Panel on Detection, Evaluation, and Treatment of High Blood Cholesterol in Adults. Bethesda, MD: National Institutes of Health.

NATIONAL DAIRY COUNCIL. 1988. Nutritional and health effects of unsaturated fatty acids. Dairy Coun. Dig. 59, Jan./Feb., 1.

NATIONAL HEART, LUNG, and BLOOD INSTITUTE. 1978. Dietary Management of Hyperlipoproteinemia (Types I, II, III, IV). Bethesda, MD: National Institutes of Health.

NATIONAL HEART, LUNG, and BLOOD INSTITUTE. 1984. The 1984 Report of the Joint National Committee on Detection, Evaluation, and Treatment of High Blood Pressure. Washington, DC: Government Printing Office.

NATIONAL INSTITUTES OF HEALTH. 1985. Consensus conference: Lowering blood cholesterol to prevent heart disease. J. Am. Med. Assoc. 253, Apr. 12, 2080.

NETTLETON, J. 1987. Seafood and Health. Huntington, NY: Osprey Books.

OREGON HEALTH SCIENCES UNIVERSITY. 1983. The Best from the Family Heart Kitchens: A Guide to Low-Fat, Low-Salt Cookery. Portland, OR: Oregon Health Sciences University.

PISCATELLA, J. 1983. Don't Eat Your Heart Out Cookbook. New York: Workman.

PISCATELLA, J. 1987. Choices for a Healthy Heart. New York: Workman.

RAAB, C., and TILLOTSON, J. (Editors). 1983. Heart to Heart: Nutrition Counseling for the Reduction of Cardiovascular Risk Factors, Publication No. HHS 83-1528. Washington, DC: Government Printing Office.

READER, D., and FRANZ, M. 1988. Pass the Pepper Please! Wayzata, MN: Diabetes Center, Inc.

REES, M. 1988. The Complete Guide to Living with High Blood Pressure. Englewood Cliffs, NJ: Prentice-Hall.

VAN HORN, L. 1988. Meeting the demands of the National Cholesterol Education Program. J. Am. Dietet. Assoc. 88, Feb., 161.

U.S. DEPARTMENT OF AGRICULTURE. 1980. Sodium Content of Your Food, USDA Home and Garden Bulletin No. 223. Washington, DC: Government Printing Office.

For audiovisuals:

Culinary Hearts Kitchen Course. New York Heart Association, 205 East 42nd Street, New York, NY 10017.

Dietary Management (Low Cholesterol). Milner-Fenwick, Inc., 2125 Greenspring Drive, Timonium, MD 21093.

Eat Right to Your Heart's Delight. American Heart Association Film Library, 8615 Directors Row, Dallas, TX 75231.

Mild Salt-Restricted Diet. Milner-Fenwick, Inc., 2125 Greenspring Drive, Timonium, MD 21093.

Potassium/Sodium Comparison Charts. Nutrition Graphics, PO Box 1527, Corvallis, OR 97339.

Salt and Hypertension. American Dietetic Association, 216 West Jackson Boulevard, Chicago, IL 60606.

Shake the Salt Habit! The Polished Apple, 3742 Seahorn Drive, Malibu, CA 90265.

Your Coronary Care Diet. The Polished Apple, 3742 Seahorn Drive, Malibu, CA 90265.

Your Hypertension Diet. The Polished Apple, 3742 Seahorn Drive, Malibu, CA 90265.

For further information:

American Heart Association, 7320 Greenville Avenue, Dallas, TX 75231.

Heart Information, National Heart, Lung, and Blood Institute, Building 31, Room 6A03, National Institutes of Health, Bethesda, MD 20892.

National Cholesterol Education Program, National Heart, Lung, and Blood Institute, C-200, National Institutes of Health, Bethesda, MD 20892.

National High Blood Pressure Information Center, 120/80, National Institutes of Health, Bethesda, MD 20892.

New York Heart Association, 205 East 42nd Street, New York, NY 10017.

Sports and Cardiovascular Nutritionists Council on Practice, American Dietetic Association, 216 West Jackson Boulevard, Chicago, IL 60606.

Counseling Guidelines—CVD

Table 12.7 General Outline for CVD Counseling

I. Initial Session
   A. General Guidelines
   B. Patient Records
      1. Medical History Form
      2. Weight Chart
      3. 24-Hour Recall Form
   C. Assignments
      1. Food Intake Record
      2. Diet History
   D. Technician's Notes
II. Follow-up Session(s)
   A. General Guidelines
   B. Handouts
      1. "Prudent" Diet Plan
      2. Learning Assessment Quizzes
   C. Technician's Notes

Table 12.7 outlines the steps for diet counseling with cardiovascular disease patients. The following material gives the details of each step.

I. Initial Session

I. A. General Guidelines

1. Use Medical History Form to assess patient's nutritional status.
2. Weigh patient and record on Weight Chart. The chart is a helpful tool for visualizing progress.
3. Assist patient in recording 24-hour recall of food intake using 24-Hour Recall Form. This will aid patient in keeping an accurate Food Intake Record.
4. Instruct patient to keep daily Food Intake Record so that typical food intake patterns can be evaluated. Advise patient not to deviate from normal eating pattern. Stress the importance of recording food intake immediately after eating.
5. Instruct patient to complete Diet History. This provides for a basic evaluation of food intake patterns. (Use Pre-test from Chapter 2.)
6. Record assessment and recommendation(s) using the SOAP method in Technician's Notes. This form can be kept in your files with a copy in the patient's medical records.

I. B. Patient Records

1. Medical History Form

Date _____ Referred by _____

Name _____ Date of birth _____

Address _____ Phone no. _____

Occupation _____ Hours per work week ____ Work phone no. _____

Educational background _____ Religious/ethnic background _____

Sex _____ Marital status _____

Household composition: Live alone _____ Spouse _____ Children/No. _____

Other: _____

General health status:

Physician _____ Address _____

Phone no. _____ Date of last visit _____

Ambulatory care required? _____ If so, describe: _____

Neuromuscular problems? _____ If so, how is eating affected? _____

Visual/auditory problems? _____ If so, describe: _____

Chewing difficulties? _____ If so, describe: _____

Appetite typically good? _____ fair? _____ poor? _____

Digestion/elimination difficulties? _____ If so, describe: _____

Food intolerances? _____ If so, describe: _____

Diabetes? _____ If so, describe: _____

Heart attack or stroke? _____ If so, describe: _____

Gout? _____ If so, describe: _____

Other: _____

Height _____ Weight _____ Frame _____

Triceps skinfold thickness _____ Mid-arm circumference _____

Mid-arm muscle circumference _____

Weight changes/problems? _____ If so, describe: _____

Clinical signs of nutritional status:

Skin _____ Mouth _____

Hair _____ Eyes _____

Teeth _____ Other: _____

Lab data:

Blood pressure _____ EKG _____ Exercise stress test _____

Cholesterol _____ Triglycerides _____ Lipoprotein profile _____

Fasting blood glucose _____

CBC _____

Serum albumin _____

Other: _____

Medications taken regularly: _____

Prescribed by: _____ Date(s) prescribed: _____

Nutrition supplements taken regularly: _____

Prescribed by: _____ Date(s) prescribed: _____

Special diet prescription: _____

Prescribed by: _____ Date of prescription: _____

How closely is diet followed? Always adhered to ___ Sometimes ___ Rarely ___ Never ___

Type of housing: Room _____ Apartment _____ Home _____ Institution _____

Prepare own meals? _____ Dine out? Often (more than once a day) _____ Rarely _____

Food shopping done independently? _____ If not, describe required assistance: _____
_____

Eligible for food stamps? _____ If so, are they currently being used? _____

Cigarette smoker? _____ If so, how much: _____

Exercise regularly? _____ If so, describe: _____

   No. times per week _____ No. minutes per session _____

Comments: _____

2. Weight Chart

Starting weight _____   Reasonable weight _____

Date	No. weeks on diet	Weight	Comments

3. 24-Hour Recall Form

Date	Time	Food and amount

I. C. Assignments

1. Food Intake Record

Date and time	Duration of meal (min)	Food and amount	Where[a]	With whom	Associated activity[b]	Associated emotions[c]

[a]Such as school, restaurant, kitchen, living room.
[b]For example, watching television, reading, talking.
[c]Attitude: bored, anxious, frustrated, depressed, happy, angry, tense, etc.

2. Diet History

Use the Pre-test from Chapter 2 (p. 30) to provide a record of typical foods eaten.

I. D. Technician's Notes

Patient: _____   Date: _____

S (Subjective data—how patient feels):
O (Objective data—physical measurements including diet/nutritional status):
A (Assessment—acceptability of dietary progress/nutritional status):
P (Plan—diet prescription and instruction):
Comments:

II. Follow-up Session(s)

II. A. General Guidelines
1. Weigh patient and record on Weight Chart.
2. Review assignments and discuss.
3. Individualize "Prudent" Diet Plan and instruct patient in its use.
4. Assign Learning Assessment Quizzes to evaluate counseling process and to determine if additional counseling is needed.
5. Record assessment and recommendation(s) using the SOAP method in Technician's Notes. This form can be kept in your files with a copy in the patient's medical records.

II. B. Handouts

1. "Prudent" Diet Plan

Name _____

How to use diet plan:

1. Select a variety of foods from each of the Basic Food Groups.
2. Include the recommended number of servings from each Food Group.
3. Limit foods high in fat (especially saturated fat), cholesterol, and sodium, such as those included in the Foods to Avoid List (Table 12.8).
4. Include generous amounts of High-Fiber Foods (Table 12.9), especially good sources of soluble fiber.

Note: If hyperlipoproteinemia is diagnosed, follow special diet plan (Type I, IIa, IIb, III, IV, or V) as prescribed.

Table 12.8 Foods to Avoid List

Food group	Foods to avoid
Fruits and vegetables	Vegetable juices (unless low-sodium)
	Pickled or brined vegetables, sauerkraut, pickles
	Frozen lima beans/mixed vegetables/peas
	Canned vegetables (unless low-sodium)
	Coconut
	Cream or butter sauces
	Seasoned preparations
Breads and cereals	Instant cereals
	Commercial baked goods and mixes
	Biscuits
	Egg noodles
	Crackers (unless unsalted)
	Chips, pretzels, and snack foods (unless unsalted)
	Any with significant amounts of added butter, saturated fats, or salt
Milk and cheeses	Whole milk
	Whole milk yogurt
	Whole milk cheeses (limit to low-fat types)

continued

Table 12.8 *(Continued)*

Food group	Foods to avoid
Meats and alternates	Ice cream
	Drinks made with whole milk, chocolate, ice cream, and/or egg yolk
	Organ meats
	Fatty meats
	Luncheon meats, frankfurters, sausage
	Fried/dried/smoked meat, poultry, or fish
	Duck, goose, or poultry skin
	Fish roe
	Eggs, fried or scrambled (limit yolks to 3 per week, boiled or poached)
	Baked beans prepared in pork fat
	Salted nuts, salted seeds
Others	Soups (unless low-sodium)
	Sweets prepared with chocolate/coconut/saturated fats
	Butter, shortening, hydrogenated oils
	Stick margarines
	Cream, sour cream, cream substitutes
	Bacon, salt pork
	Salad dressing (unless low-fat/low-sodium)
	Coconut oil, palm oil
	Condiments high in sodium (e.g., catsup, mustard, relishes)

Table 12.9   High-Fiber Foods

Fruits	(especially those eaten with seeds and/or skins)
Vegetables	(especially those eaten with seeds and/or skins)
Legumes[a]	
Whole grain	breads, cereals, muffins, pasta, crackers (especially bran products and oat bran[a]); popcorn

[a]Good source of soluble fiber.

2. Learning Assessment Quizzes

Hyperlipidemia. Answer true (T) or false (F) to the following statements:

____ 1. Hyperlipidemia is an excess of fatty materials in the blood.

____ 2. With increased blood triglyceride levels, the dietary intake of refined sugar and alcohol should be modified.

____ 3. Hydrogenation is the process by which hydrogen is added to saturated (solid) fat to produce unsaturated (liquid) fat.

____ 4. Saturated fats are usually hard at room temperature.

____ 5. Cholesterol occurs in varying amounts in all foods.

____ 6. Low grades of beef are less heavily marbled and contain less saturated fat than the higher grades.

____ 7. Food sources of soluble fiber include oat bran, lentils, and baked beans.

____ 8. Cholesterol performs a number of vital functions in the body.

____ 9. Lecithin supplementation has been proven to be an effective method for blood cholesterol clearance.

Select the best answer to the following statements:

____ 10. Some foods high in cholesterol include
(a) butter. (b) egg yolk. (c) liver. (d) margarine. (e) egg white. (f) a, b, and c. (g) all of these.

_____ 11. Some foods high in saturated fat include
(a) butter. (b) corn oil. (c) palm oil. (d) walnut oil. (e) a and c. (f) all of these.
_____ 12. Risk factors associated with CVD include
(a) overweight. (b) inadequate physical activity. (c) high blood pressure. (d) diabetes. (e) all of these.

Hypertension. Answer true (T) or false (F) to the following statements:

_____ 1. The upper limit of normal blood pressure for adults under age 45 is 140/90.
_____ 2. Secondary hypertension is a manifestation of another underlying disease.
_____ 3. Average sodium intake in the U.S. is about 500 mg per day.
_____ 4. Fresh fruits and vegetables are usually high in sodium.
_____ 5. Sodium is present in table salt, food additives, and as a natural component of most foods.
_____ 6. Water may contain an undesirably high level of sodium, depending on the source.
_____ 7. Certain laxatives may be high in sodium content and should be avoided unless prescribed by a physician.
_____ 8. Salt substitutes may be used by anyone on a sodium restricted diet.
_____ 9. Symptoms such as weakness, muscle cramps, and faintness may be indicative of a potassium depletion.
_____ 10. Certain diuretic medications can lead to excessive potassium losses.
_____ 11. For sodium restricted diets, bouillon and cooking wines should be used in place of table salt.
_____ 12. Unless symptoms of high blood pressure such as dizziness and headache are present, drug and/or diet therapy are unnecessary.
_____ 13. Table salt contains approximately 40% sodium.
_____ 14. Limiting sodium intake may help to prevent excess fluid accumulation in the body.
_____ 15. The kidneys normally excrete excess dietary sodium.
_____ 16. Sodium is an essential mineral, important for good health.
_____ 17. Blood pressure is the amount of pressure exerted by blood on the inside walls of the arteries.
_____ 18. Diastolic pressure is the amount of pressure exerted by blood on the inside walls of the arteries when the heart is contracting.

II. C. Technician's Notes
Patient: _____   Date: _____

S (Subjective data—how patient feels):
O (Objective data—physical measurements including diet/nutritional status):
A (Assessment—acceptability of dietary progress/nutritional status):
P (Plan—diet prescription and instruction):
Comments:

Cardiovascular Disease Counseling Role Playing

Keeping in mind the preceding Suggested Readings and Counseling Guidelines, participate in the following role play situations; use the sample menus (Figs. 12.1 and 12.2) as teaching aids. Select different partners for each situation, either classmates or co-workers, and elaborate on each role play situation to develop a patient/audience profile. You may want to use your handouts from Step 2, Step 3, and Step 4. Use the SOAP method to record in each patient's medical chart.

As a dietetic technician in nutrition care, do you consider yourself capable of conducting effective diet counseling sessions with patients who have cardiovascular disease? How about with those seeking to modify fat, cholesterol, and/or sodium intakes? Would you or your family be able to adhere to your nutrition guidelines in order to make such dietary alterations?

Role Play Situation 1. As a dietetic technician in a large teaching hospital, you are asked

Name _____ Room _____
Diet **Fat controlled** _____

Breakfast   Please circle your selections below

Fruits and juices
Orange juice
Grapefruit juice
Prune juice
Apple juice
Cranberry juice
Grapefruit sections
Stewed prunes
Banana

Cereals
Cream of wheat
Grits
Oatmeal
Cornflakes
Rice Krispies
Special K
Puffed rice
Puffed wheat
Shredded wheat
Raisin bran
All bran
Bran flakes

Entrees
Bacon
Scrambled egg
Poached egg
Egg substitute
Pancakes
French toast

Breads
Apple muffin
Blueberry muffin
Bran muffin
Corn muffin
Plain muffin
English muffin
White toast
Wheat toast
Rye toast

Miscellaneous ·
Salt
Pepper
Sugar
Sugar substitute
Butter
Margarine
Lemon
Jelly
Pancake syrup

Beverages
Coffee
Tea   Cream   Skim milk
Decaffeinated coffee   Nondairy creamer   4 oz. skim milk

Name _____ Room _____
Diet **Fat controlled** _____

Luncheon   Please circle your selections below

Appetizers
Apple juice
Cranberry juice
Tomato juice
Fruit cup
Consomme/chicken/beef
Chicken noodle soup
Vegetable soup
Cream of tomato soup
Cream of chicken soup
Soup du jour

Entrees
Tomato with:
  Chicken salad, $\frac{1}{2}$ cup
  Tuna salad, $\frac{1}{2}$ cup
  Cottage cheese, $\frac{1}{2}$ cup
Fruit and cottage cheese
Roast beef sandwich
Sliced turkey sandwich
Tuna salad sandwich
Chicken salad sandwich
Sandwich special (if allowed)
Tuna noodle casserole
Turkey/dressing/gravy
Roast beef au jus
Scrod
Ham/pineapple
Steak/mushrooms
Chicken/cranberry
Veal/gravy
Pork chop/applesauce
Shell macaroni
Beefburger
Salisbury/gravy
Chef's special (if allowed)

Breads
White   Dinner Roll
Wheat   Crackers
Rye

Beverages
Coffee
Tea
Decaffeinated coffee
Cream
Nondairy creamer
Skim milk
4 oz. skim milk

Vegetables
Whipped potato
Baked potato
Noodles
Rice
Broccoli
Corn
Spinach
Carrots
Green beans
Beets
Peas
Squash

Salads and dressings
Lettuce/tomato
Tossed greens
Lettuce wedge
Cole slaw
Salad special
Mayonnaise
French dressing
Italian dressing
Oil & vinegar
Lemon and vinegar
Sour cream

Desserts
Peaches
Fruit cocktail
Baked apple
Pears
Apricots
Applesauce
Fresh fruit
Sunshine cup
Orange sherbet
Raspberry sherbet
Gelatin
Low fat custard
Angel cake

Miscellaneous
Salt
Pepper
Sugar
Sugar substitute
Butter
Margarine
Lemon
Jelly
Mustard
Catsup
Relish

Name _____ Room _____
Diet **Fat controlled** _____

Dinner   Please circle your selections below

Appetizers
Apple juice
Cranberry juice
Tomato juice
Fruit cup
Consomme/chicken/beef
Chicken noodle soup
Vegetable soup
Cream of tomato soup
Cream of chicken soup
Soup du jour

Entrees
Tomato with:
  Chicken salad, $\frac{1}{2}$ cup
  Tuna salad, $\frac{1}{2}$ cup
  Cottage cheese, $\frac{1}{2}$ cup
Fruit and cottage cheese
Roast beef sandwich
Sliced turkey sandwich
Tuna salad sandwich
Chicken salad sandwich
Sandwich special (if allowed)
Tuna noodle casserole
Turkey/dressing/gravy
Roast beef au jus
Scrod
Ham/pineapple
Steak/mushrooms
Chicken/cranberry
Veal/gravy
Pork chop/applesauce
Shell macaroni
Beefburger
Salisbury/gravy
Chef's special (if allowed)

Breads
White   Dinner Roll
Wheat   Crackers
Rye

Beverages
Coffee
Tea
Decaffeinated coffee
Cream
Nondairy creamer
Skim milk
4 oz. skim milk

Vegetables
Whipped potato
Baked potato
Noodles
Rice
Broccoli
Corn
Spinach
Carrots
Green beans
Beets
Peas
Squash

Salads and dressings
Lettuce/tomato
Tossed greens
Lettuce wedge
Cole slaw
Salad special
Mayonnaise
French dressing
Italian dressing
Oil & vinegar
Lemon and vinegar
Sour cream

Desserts
Peaches
Fruit cocktail
Baked apple
Pears
Apricots
Applesauce
Fresh fruit
Sunshine cup
Orange sherbet
Raspberry sherbet
Gelatin
Low fat custard
Angel cake

Miscellaneous
Salt
Pepper
Sugar
Sugar substitute
Butter
Margarine
Lemon
Jelly
Mustard
Catsup
Relish

Fig. 12.1   Fat-controlled menu.
© *The Seiler Corporation. Reprinted by permission.*

Name _____ Room _____
Diet **Sodium controlled**

Breakfast   Please circle your selections below

Fruits and juices
Orange juice
Grapefruit juice
Prune juice
Apple juice
Cranberry juice
Grapefruit sections
Stewed prunes
Banana

Cereals
Cream of wheat LS
Grits LS
Oatmeal LS
Cornflakes LS
Puffed rice
Puffed wheat
Shredded wheat

Entrees
Scrambled egg LS
Poached egg
Egg substitute
Pancakes
French toast

Breads
Apple muffin
Blueberry muffin
Bran muffin
Corn muffin
Plain muffin
Danish pastry
English muffin
White toast
Wheat toast
Rye toast
LS toast

Miscellaneous
Pepper
Sugar
Sugar substitute
Butter
LS butter
Margarine
LS margarine
Lemon
Jelly
Pancake syrup

Beverages
Coffee
Tea
Decaffeinated coffee
Cocoa

Cream
Nondairy creamer

Whole milk
4 oz. whole milk
Skim milk
4 oz. skim milk

LS = Low Sodium

Name _____ Room _____
Diet **Sodium controlled**

Luncheon   Please circle your selections below

Appetizers
Apple juice
Cranberry juice
Tomato juice LS
Fruit cup
Consomme LS/chicken/beef
Chicken noodle soup LS
Vegetable soup LS
Cream of tomato soup LS
Cream of chicken soup LS

Entrees
Tomato with:
  Chicken salad LS
  Tuna salad LS
  Cottage cheese
  Egg salad LS
Fruit and cottage cheese
Roast beef sandwich
Sliced turkey sandwich
Tuna salad sandwich LS
Chicken salad sandwich LS
Egg salad sandwich LS
Tuna noodle casserole LS
Turkey/gravy LS
Roast beef au jus
Macaroni and cheese LS
Scrod
Steak/mushrooms
Chicken/cranberry
Grilled cheese LS
Veal/gravy
Pork chop/applesauce
Shell macaroni LS
Beefburger/cheeseburger LS
  (no pickles)
Salisbury steak/gravy LS

Breads
White   LS white
Wheat   Dinner roll
Rye   LS crackers

Beverages
Coffee
Tea
Decaffeinated coffee
Cocoa
Cream
Nondairy creamer
Whole milk
4 oz. whole milk
Skim milk
4 oz. skim milk

Vegetables
Whipped potato LS
Baked potato
Noodles LS
Rice LS
Broccoli LS
Corn LS
Spinach LS
Carrots LS
Green beans LS
Beets LS
Peas LS
Squash LS

Salads and dressings
Lettuce/tomato
Tossed greens
Lettuce wedge
Cole slaw LS
Mayonnaise LS
French LS
Italian LS
Oil & vinegar
Lemon and vinegar
Sour cream

Desserts
Peaches
Fruit cocktail
Baked apple
Pears
Apricots
Applesauce
Fresh fruit
Sugar cookies
Oatmeal cookies
Cupcake
Apple pie
Sunshine cup
Ice cream
Orange sherbet
Raspberry sherbet
Gelatin
Custard
Angel cake

Miscellaneous
Pepper
Sugar
Sugar substitute
Butter
LS butter
Margarine
LS margarine
Lemon
Jelly
LS Catsup

LS = Low Sodium

Name _____ Room _____
Diet **Sodium controlled**

Dinner   Please circle your selections below

Appetizers
Apple juice
Cranberry juice
Tomato juice LS
Fruit cup
Consomme LS/chicken/beef
Chicken noodle soup LS
Vegetable soup LS
Cream of tomato soup LS
Cream of chicken soup LS

Entrees
Tomato with:
  Chicken salad LS
  Tuna salad LS
  Cottage cheese
  Egg salad LS
Fruit and cottage cheese
Roast beef sandwich
Sliced turkey sandwich
Tuna salad sandwich LS
Chicken salad sandwich LS
Egg salad sandwich LS
Tuna noodle casserole LS
Turkey/gravy LS
Roast beef au jus
Macaroni and cheese LS
Scrod
Steak/mushrooms
Chicken/cranberry
Grilled cheese LS
Veal/gravy
Pork chop/applesauce
Shell macaroni LS
Beefburger/cheeseburger LS
  (no pickles)
Salisbury steak/gravy LS

Breads
White   LS white
Wheat   Dinner roll
Rye   LS crackers

Beverages
Coffee
Tea
Decaffeinated coffee
Cocoa
Cream
Nondairy creamer
Whole milk
4 oz. whole milk
Skim milk
4 oz. skim milk

Vegetables
Whipped potato LS
Baked potato
Noodles LS
Rice LS
Broccoli LS
Corn LS
Spinach LS
Carrots LS
Green beans LS
Beets LS
Peas LS
Squash LS

Salads and dressings
Lettuce/tomato
Tossed greens
Lettuce wedge
Cole slaw LS
Mayonnaise LS
French LS
Italian LS
Oil & vinegar
Lemon and vinegar
Sour cream

Desserts
Peaches
Fruit cocktail
Baked apple
Pears
Apricots
Applesauce
Fresh fruit
Sugar cookies
Oatmeal cookies
Cupcake
Apple pie
Sunshine cup
Ice cream
Orange sherbet
Raspberry sherbet
Gelatin
Custard
Angel cake

Miscellaneous
Pepper
Sugar
Sugar substitute
Butter
LS butter
Margarine
LS margarine
Lemon
Jelly
LS Catsup

LS = Low Sodium

Fig. 12.2   Sodium-controlled menu.
© *The Seiler Corporation. Reprinted by permission.*

to provide a discharge diet for a moderately overweight 40-year-old female patient; the diet prescription is for Type IV hyperlipoproteinemia. Follow the guidelines to complete the charts and provide the patient with an individualized diet plan. Prepare a SOAP note which could be recorded in the patient's medical chart.

Role Play Situation 2.   As an outpatient dietetic technician in a community clinic, you are asked to provide diet instruction for a slightly overweight middle-aged male whose lab tests show an elevated serum cholesterol level. Follow the guidelines to complete the charts and provide the patient with an individualized diet plan. Prepare a SOAP note for insertion in departmental files with a copy to be sent to the referring physician.

Role Play Situation 3.   A young female—a cigarette smoker who is on oral contraceptive medication—is referred to the out-patient nutrition clinic for a weight loss diet plan; her blood pressure is elevated and she has a family history of hypertension. As the assigned dietetic technician, follow the guidelines to complete the charts and provide the patient with an individualized diet plan. Prepare a SOAP note for insertion in departmental files with a copy to be sent to the referring physician.

Role Play Situation 4.   An elderly male with a history of atherosclerosis and hypertension is recovering from a CVA (stroke) and requires a discharge diet. As the assigned dietetic technician, follow the guidelines to complete the charts and provide the patient with an individualized diet plan. Prepare a SOAP note that could be recorded in the patient's medical chart.

Role Play Situation 5.   As a dietetic technician in a large, private nursing home, you have several elderly patients who are on restricted sodium diets to control hypertension. Prepare a brief outline and conduct a short class on diet therapy for hypertension (keeping in mind the individual learning capabilities of the patients) which includes the most current nutrition information on the "prudent" diet. Prepare a report on the class for insertion in departmental files.

STEP 6: POST-TEST ON CARDIOVASCULAR DISEASE

In order to evaluate your understanding of the role of diet in cardiovascular disease, complete the Post-test below. Sections I and II are the Learning Assessment Quizzes for hyperlipidemia and hypertension. (If the diet counselor is unable to complete the tests successfully, how can patients be expected to?) Section III incorporates much of the material from this chapter. Answers are given in the Answer Key. Will patients seeking to reduce dietary fat intake be able to use your nutrition guidelines in order to do so successfully? How about those desiring to lower dietary cholesterol intake? Or the amount of sodium in their diets? Can your patients acquire from you the guidance required to adopt prudent, individualized, health-promoting diet plans?

Sections I and II: Complete the Learning Assessment Quizzes on Hyperlipidemia and Hypertension given in Step 5. Check your answers with the Answer Key.

Section III: Indicate whether you think the following statements are true (T) or false (F). Check your answers with the Answer Key.

_____ 1. Cardiovascular disease is currently the leading cause of death in America.
_____ 2. Fats are transported through the bloodstream bound to proteins.
_____ 3. Chylomicrons are composed primarily of triglycerides.
_____ 4. High density lipoproteins (HDLs) have more fat than LDLs.
_____ 5. The diet prescribed for treatment of Type IV hyperlipoproteinemia is controlled in both carbohydrate and cholesterol content.
_____ 6. The appearance of fatty streaks in the arteries of Americans usually occurs early in life.
_____ 7. Cholesterol is both an essential body component and a major contributor to atherosclerotic plaque formation.

_____ 8. The diet recommended for lowering elevated blood cholesterol levels eliminates meat, cheese, milk, and eggs.

_____ 9. Niacin megadoses can be used to lower blood cholesterol levels safely.

_____ 10. Lecithin supplements have been shown to lower elevated cholesterol levels significantly.

_____ 11. Hypertension is rarely asymptomatic.

_____ 12. The upper limit for normal blood pressure for individuals over age 65 is set at 160/95.

_____ 13. Strict dietary sodium restrictions are required in mild hypertension therapy.

_____ 14. Mild sodium restrictions limit sodium intake to 500 mg per day.

_____ 15. The majority of sodium in the typical American diet is from that naturally present in foods.

_____ 16. An increased intake of potassium-rich foods may play a preventive role in hypertension.

Select the answer which best completes the following statements and check your answers with the Answer Key.

_____ 17. The "prudent" diet (see Table 12.8) advises followers to avoid
(a) sour cream. (b) more than three egg yolks per week. (c) coconut. (d) biscuits. (e) a and b. (f) all of these.

_____ 18. The "prudent" diet (see Tables 12.8 and 12.9) advises followers to include low-fat, low-cholesterol, low-sodium, high-fiber foods such as
(a) lentils. (b) lean roast beef. (c) fresh fruits. (d) low-fat yogurt. (e) oat bran cereal. (f) none of these. (g) all of these.

REFERENCE

FREDRICKSON, D., et al. 1973. Dietary Management of Hyperlipoproteinemia. Washington, DC: Government Printing Office.

Chapter Thirteen

Gastrointestinal Disorders

CHAPTER BLUEPRINT

Step 1: Take the Pre-test on Gastrointestinal Disorders and participate in the assigned group discussion.

Step 2: Examine the Ulcer Facts List and prepare the assigned handout.

Step 3: Examine the High-Fiber Facts List and prepare the assigned handout.

Step 4: Examine the Low-Residue Facts List and prepare the assigned handout.

Step 5: Examine the Low-Lactose Facts List and prepare the assigned handout.

Step 6: Examine the Diet as Tolerated (D.A.T.) Guidelines and complete the role play assignment.

Step 7: Examine the High-Fiber Diet Guidelines and complete the role play assignment.

Step 8: Take the Post-test on Gastrointestinal Disorders to evaluate what you have learned from the information and activities provided in this chapter.

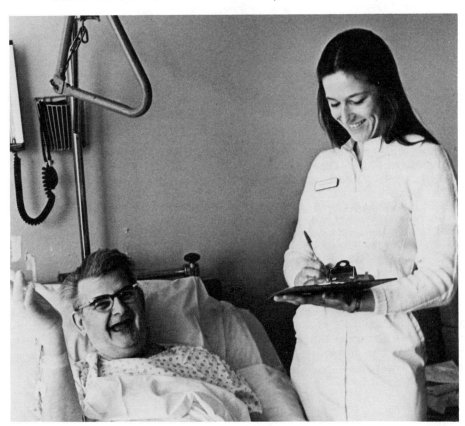

STEP 1: PRE-TEST ON GASTROINTESTINAL DISORDERS

Stress—anxiety, tension, nervous upset—is currently a topic of much public concern. Newspapers, magazines, and medical journals often deal with the subject, and numerous methods of stress control are practiced. Supposedly, stress has surpassed the common cold as the most prevalent health problem in America, and stress-related conditions that lead to the loss of industrial productivity are costing our society billions of dollars. In the early 1980s, around 100,000 physicians were asked to participate in a long-range national educational program on recognizing and managing stress.

Obviously, stress plays an important role in determining the overall physical and emotional health of America today. Although the term is relatively new, the associated health conditions have only recently been recognized, and methods for prevention and treatment are still being researched, the impact of stress cannot be overlooked by health educators, medical personnel, and the general public.

Suggested Readings on Stress

AMERICAN RUNNING AND FITNESS ASSOCIATION. 1985. Rate your susceptibility to stress. Running and FitNews, Jul., 1.

ARONSON, S., and MASCIA, M. 1981. The Stress Management Workbook: An Action Plan for Taking Control of Your Life and Health. East Norwalk, CT: Appleton & Lange.

BAMMER, K., and NEWBERRY, B. (Editors). 1981. Stress and Cancer. Toronto, Ont.: Hogrefe.

BENSON, H. 1975. The Relaxation Response. New York: Avon.

BIELIAUSKAS, L. 1982. Stress and Its Relationship to Health and Illness. Boulder, CO: Westview Press.

BLOOM, B. 1985. Stressful Life Event Theory and Research: Implications for Primary Prevention. Washington, DC: Government Printing Office.

COOPER, E. 1984. Stress, Immunity, and Aging. New York: M. Dekker.

DAVIS, M., ESHELMAN, E., and MCKAY, M. 1985. The Relaxation and Stress Reduction Workbook, 2nd Edition. Oakland, CA: New Harbinger Publications.

DOBSON, C. 1982. Stress: The Hidden Adversary. Ridgewood, NJ: Bogden.

DOHRENWEND, B. S., and DOHRENWEND, B. 1984. Stressful Life Events and their Contexts. New Brunswick, NJ: Rutgers University Press.

ELIOT, R. 1984. Is It Worth Dying For? New York: Bantam.

ELLIS, A., and HARPER, R. 1975. A New Guide to Rational Living. North Hollywood, CA: Wilshire Book Co.

FREUDENBERGER, H. 1980. Burnout: How to Beat the High Cost of Success. New York: Bantam.

HANSON, P. 1985. The Joy of Stress. Kansas City, MO: Andrews and McMeel.

HILL, J. 1987. Exercise prescription. Primary Care, 14, Dec., 817.

LAZARUS, R. 1984. Stress, Appraisal, and Coping. New York: Springer Publishing Co.

MCLAUGHLIN, W. 1987. The Relaxation Principle. Santa Fe, NM: Joy Publishing Co.

MEICHENBAUM, D. 1983. Coping with Stress. New York: Facts on File, Inc.

NATIONAL DAIRY COUNCIL. 1980. Nutritional demands imposed by stress. Dairy Coun. Dig. 51, Nov./Dec., 31.

PHILLIPS, E. 1982. Stress, Health, and Psychological Problems in the Major Professions. Washington, DC: University Press of America.

ROTH, R. 1987. Transcendental Meditation. New York: Donald I. Fine, Inc.

SELYE, H. 1976. The Stress of Life. New York: McGraw-Hill.

ZALES, M. (Editor). 1984. Stress in Health and Disease. Greenbelt, MD: American College of Psychiatrists.

Keeping in mind the preceding Suggested Readings and any other references on stress that you might have read recently, complete the questionnaire and discuss your answers with classmates or co-workers. As a dietetic technician in nutrition care, it is important for you to understand the psychological factors involved in certain diseases of the gastrointestinal tract, and to develop a working knowledge of the associated physical factors and dietary implications.

Questionnaire on Stress

1. List some lifestyle patterns and environmental factors which can contribute to stress:
    1.
    2.
    3.
    4.
    5.
    6.
    7.
    8.

2. Circle those factors which may be contributing to your current level of stress. Total no: _____

3. List some of the methods currently used to alleviate stress:

4. List the methods you use to relieve your own daily tensions:

5. List some of the possible side effects, both physiological and psychological, of continued stress:

STEP 2: ULCER FACTS

An ulcer is a lesion of the gastrointestinal **mucosa.** *Gastric* ulcers occur in the stomach, *duodenal* in the small intestine (duodenum), and *peptic* in either location. The diet therapies used in the treatment of peptic ulcer disease have varied considerably over the years, causing much confusion for both health care practitioners and their ulcer-prone patients.

The following Ulcer Facts List provides current diet-related information to include in counseling individuals with ulcers.

mucosa: Mucous membrane lining body passages and cavities that are reached by air.

Ulcer Facts List

1. The gastrointestinal tract is subject to a wide variety of disorders and diseases, appearing initially as digestive complaints, typically triggered by stressful situations. It is important to acknowledge the psychological aspects of gastrointestinal disturbances, as well as the physical symptoms of **dysphagia,** nausea, vomiting, abdominal pain, cramping, diarrhea, and constipation.

dysphagia: Difficulty in swallowing.

2. An ulcer is the erosion of a portion of the mucosal lining of the digestive tract that is in constant contact with the acidic gastric juices.

3. Ulcers can occur at many sites along the gastrointestinal tract: the esophagus, stomach (*gastric ulcer*), duodenum (*duodenal ulcer*), or jejunum (after a gastroje-junostomy); with a gastric ulcer, hypersecretion of gastric acid by the parietal cells is seen, whereas the duodenal ulcer victim displays weakened mucosal resistance to the hydro-chloric acid-containing gastric juices.

4. The primary goals for the medical treatment of peptic ulcers include the control of hyperacidity of the stomach, alleviation of tension and stress, and avoidance of stimulation of the gastrointestinal system.

5. The typical victim of gastric ulcers is the over-forty male, whereas duodenal ulcers occur more often in females.

6. Symptoms of a peptic ulcer include (a) burning pain when stomach is empty, often accompanied by hunger; (b) gastric hyperacidity; (c) melena (bloody, tarry stools); (d) nausea, vomiting; and (e) a general feeling of weakness.

7. Although the determining cause is not certain, peptic ulcer formation is believed to be influenced by the following factors: (a) tension and stress; (b) poor dietary habits; (c) cigarette smoking; (d) alcohol overindulgence; (e) impaired circulation; and (f) heredity. Ulcer pain can be relieved by consuming certain foods or antacids, or by vomiting.

8. Since the foods that aggravate the symptoms of peptic ulcer disease vary from person to person, individualized diet planning is essential.

9. Each ulcer victim is the best judge as to individual food tolerances and intolerances; most sufferers find that the following gastric stimulants are irritating: black and red pepper, chili powder, caffeine, alcohol, chocolate and cocoa, and decaffeinated coffee.

10. Alcohol, caffeine, and nicotine stimulate increased gastric acid production, making users of these substances more susceptible to ulcer development; even decaffeinated coffee and cola drinks can stimulate acidity. Omission of alcohol, caffeine, and nicotine helps to decrease gastric acidity. If included in the diet, beverages containing alcohol or caffeine should only be consumed with meals. Cold remedies, "diet pills," and stimulants may also contain caffeine.

11. Irregular meal patterns can contribute to gastrointestinal dysfunction. Small, frequent meals may be helpful in neutralizing gastric acidity.

12. Milk and cream were once prescribed for soothing ulcer pain (the "sippy" diet). Since protein can stimulate gastric acid secretion, milk is no longer the preferred buffer; all fats can serve as buffers, not just cream.

13. *Bland* foods can be defined as those items with a particularly flat, insipid taste and texture, but a diet of bland foods has not been shown to aid ulcer victims; thus, the current diet therapy is "diet as tolerated" (D.A.T.). This diet prescription is also utilized with gastritis, **esophagitis,** hiatus hernia, and gastrointestinal cancers.

esophagitis: Inflammation of the esophagus.

14. The same food item can cause different gastrointestinal responses depending on the circumstances of ingestion and the severity of existing stresses.

15. It is important to avoid rigid dietary guidelines in treating ulcer patients since the diet itself must not serve as an additional stress. Overweight individuals, however, should attempt to attain and maintain a reasonable weight.

16. The rationale behind the restrictive diets (e.g., bland, "sippy," milk and cream) used over the years had little scientific basis, and such practices can be attributed to folklore.

17. Peptic ulcer formation has been noted with megadoses of niacin; certain drugs, such as aspirin, may prove to be ulcerogenic.

18. Control of gastric acidity is the major emphasis of drug (anticholinergic, antacid, and antispasmodic) therapy. Antacids should be taken as prescribed by a physician; excessive usage leads to such side effects as **hypercalcemia, alkalosis,** phosphate deficiency, constipation, and diarrhea.

hypercalcemia: Excessive level of calcium in the blood.

alkalosis: Excessive alkalinity (baseness) of body fluids due to accumulated alkaline/basic compounds or reduced acids.

19. Bleeding ulcers cause a constant low-grade blood loss which can eventually lead to iron-deficiency anemia; antacids can do so also, as they tend to reduce iron absorption.

20. Bed rest can encourage the healing of peptic ulcers, but regularity in meal consumption and a relaxed lifestyle can prove to be the most effective therapy.

21. If medical intervention is ineffective, surgery may be required; surgery is usually required with a hemorrhage or perforation.

22. Following ulcer surgery, some patients experience the "dumping syndrome" after eating due to a reduced stomach capacity: food passes rapidly into the small intestine causing nausea, dizziness, sweating, tachycardia, stomach cramps, feeling of weakness, hypotension, hypoglycemia, and diarrhea; the best treatment includes frequent small feedings that are relatively high in protein and low in carbohydrate, restriction of liquids to between meals, and the avoidance of simple sugars.

23. *Hyperchlorhydria* is an excessive amount of hydrochloric acid in the gastric juice, which can irritate the stomach lining; *hypochlorhydria* is a deficiency of this acid, which can cause nutrient malabsorption and may be indicative of pernicious anemia.

24. Inflammation of the stomach mucosa is known as *gastritis. Chronic gastritis* may occur with ulcers—or with gastric carcinoma, pernicious anemia, endocrine disorders, or the use of certain drugs. But *acute* gastritis is due to overeating/drinking, or the consumption of highly seasoned foods, items of individual intolerance, or contaminated foodstuffs, and causes nausea, vomiting, and intestinal cramping. Treatment includes **NPO** until the acute symptoms subside, followed by diet as tolerated with the elimination of alcohol, caffeine, and aspirin.

NPO: Non per os (Latin); nothing by mouth.

25. Gastric hypersecretion can occur with **hyperparathyroidism,** chronic **pulmonary** disease, diabetes, central nervous system disorders, or collagen vascular disease; a reduced mucosal tissue resistance can arise from diminished production of mucus due to intake of salicylates, corticosteroids, or certain other drugs.

26. It is important to encourage persons with gastrointestinal disorders to show self-responsibility in dietary and other lifestyle pattern behaviors.

hyperparathyroidism: Condition resulting from increased parathyroid gland activity which causes calcium losses and bone damage.

pulmonary: Involving the lungs.

Exercise on Diet Counseling for Ulcer Patients

Keeping in mind the preceding Ulcer Facts List, which provides current diet-related information to include in counseling individuals afflicted with ulcers, prepare a simplified version for use as a patient handout. You may include graphics and/or prepare in a poster format, if desired; see the Sample Handout. Show your handout in rough draft form to classmates or co-workers for constructive criticism on the overall design, content, and potential effectiveness for use in pertinent diet counseling situations. Then prepare a final version for your own future use as a practicing dietetic technician.

Sample Handout

Instructions: Use the following chart to record any eating-related gastric upsets and to identify foods that are not well tolerated. Be sure to describe any activity (e.g., working, driving, arguing with spouse) engaged in prior to the onset of symptoms. Then complete the accompanying individualized diet plan.

Activities Associated with Gastric Upsets

Date	Time	Symptoms	Food eaten	Associated activities

Diet Plan

Foods to avoid	Foods not well tolerated under stress

STEP 3: HIGH-FIBER DIET FACTS

A diet with increased fiber content is currently believed to prevent or help to control the following disorders: constipation, hemorrhoids, colitis, diverticulosis, appendicitis, hiatus hernia, cancer of the colon, atherosclerosis, diabetes, and obesity. Although all the evidence is not yet in, a moderate intake of high-fiber foods appears to be beneficial for most individuals—including those with certain gastrointestinal disorders.

The following High-Fiber Facts List provides some of the most current diet-related information to include in counseling individuals with certain disorders of the gastrointestinal tract.

High-Fiber Facts List

1.   *Dietary fiber* is plant material consisting mainly of nondigestible carbohydrates, which cannot be completely broken down by the human digestive tract. *Crude fiber* estimates provided in nutrient values tables are representative of only a fraction of total dietary fiber content.

2.   Dietary fiber increases stool bulk, accelerates intestinal transit time, and leads to the passage of larger, softer stools. This allows for reduced proliferation of bacteria, decreased intralumenal pressure, and increased excretion of bile acids, sterols, and fats. Fiber aids in the relief of constipation, and may play a role in the prevention of colon cancer, large bowel disease, atherosclerosis, and other ills.

3.   *Insoluble* fibers (found in wheat bran, fruits and vegetables) are more important to digestive health than the *soluble* fiber of oat bran and legumes.

4.   Cereal grain is made up of three main components. Refining or milling of cereal grains removes the *bran* (fiber-rich outer husk) and *germ* (seed), leaving only the fiberless *endosperm.* Enriched flour restores only some of the lost nutrients and none of the fiber.

5.   The refining and processing of fruits, vegetables, and grains reduces the dietary fiber contents, so fresh fruits, fresh vegetables, and whole grains are usually the more fibrous choices; storage and cooking time should be minimized. Note that many "whole" flours and brown breads are not whole-meal. With true whole-meal flours, labeling should indicate 100% extraction (i.e., all the ground grain present). Thus, to ensure adequate dietary fiber, a variety of whole grain products, fruits, and vegetables should be included in the diet, and intake of refined products should be minimized.

6.   Excessive intake of dietary fiber can result in the loss of important nutrients, and may damage the large intestine.

7.   Adequate fluid intake helps to stimulate elimination.

8.   Natural laxative action occurs with the intake of dried fruits and their juices, particularly prunes.

9.   Constipation is a colonic disorder characterized by infrequent or difficult evacuation of feces with hard, dry stools. Preventive measures include proper hygiene, regularity in eating and bowel habits, and stability in emotional status.

10.   Chronic constipation can cause dull headache, lethargy, lassitude, anorexia, and low-back pain.

11.   *Atonic constipation* occurs with the loss of colonic muscle tone and is common in elderly persons, pregnant women, obese individuals, and following surgery. Treatment includes adherence to a well-balanced diet with adequate fiber and fluid intake.

12.   *Spastic constipation* can be caused by overstimulation of the peristaltic waves of the digestive tract, and is characterized by ineffectual movements and the inability to propel the undigested contents along through and out of the gastrointestinal tract; some of the known causes include the excessive use of **cathartics,** intake of spicy foods, cigarette smoking, and high intakes of caffeine or alcohol. Treatment measures parallel those for atonic constipation.

cathartic: Purgative which produces bowel movements.

13.   *Hemorrhoids* are varicose veins of the rectum. Constipation with straining during defecation and increased abdominal pressure may result in the development of hemorrhoids, and proper diet with adequate dietary fiber may help in prevention.

14.   The ruptured blood vessels around the anus which occur with hemorrhoids may be painful or asymptomatic. Avoiding constipation, especially during times of high susceptibility (such as pregnancy or immobilization), is important, so adequate fiber and fluid intake are essential. If hemorrhoids are inflamed, dietary treatment is aimed at symptom relief and may need to be nonirritating in nature; a high-fluid, low-fiber diet with stewed fruits to prevent constipation may be prescribed until inflammation subsides.

15.   *Colitis*—also known as spastic colon, irritable colon, mucous colitis—is characterized by irritation of the colon, causing alternating constipation and diarrhea due to abnormal, irregular colon contractions. Typically occurring in tense individuals with irregular eating habits and/or a history of laxative abuse, colitis is treated by restricting cigarette smoking and alcohol use, and by establishing regular patterns of eating, exercise, and rest. Individual food intolerances may also need to be pinpointed. After acute stages, a high-fiber diet may help to control symptoms.

16. *Diverticula* are small sacs which protrude through weakened areas along the colon due to high intralumenal pressure; irritation can occur with stress and/or individual food intolerances. Symptoms of diverticular disease include pain in the lower abdomen, abdominal distention, spasms, fever, and constipation. Diverticulitis in acute stages may require strict diet prescriptions (NPO to liquid to diet as tolerated), but diverticulosis is best controlled with a high-fiber diet because the bulk distends the walls of the colon to relieve the increased intralumenal pressure (*Note:* Acute attacks require immediate medical attention).

17. Diverticula can become infected with accumulated fecal matter, resulting in the ulcerations or perforations characteristic of acute diverticulitis; increased dietary fiber causes an increased diameter of the intestinal lumen and a decreased **viscosity** of the intestinal contents, leading to a more rapid fecal transit time, decreased intralumenal pressure, and possible prevention of acute diverticular attacks in individuals with diverticulosis.

viscosity: Thick, gummy, sticky quality; immovable property of a fluid.

18. *Appendicitis*—inflammation of the appendix—can be caused by a blockage of the lumen of the appendix, with increased intralumenal pressure due to fecalith formation or irregular muscle contractions. Diets high in fiber content can decrease the pressure, so are believed to alleviate the symptoms and possibly prevent the onset of appendicitis. (*Note:* Acute attacks require immediate medical attention.)

19. *Hiatus hernia* occurs when the stomach passes through the esophageal hiatus of the diaphragm into the thoracic cavity due to a herniation of the diaphragm; pressure on the abdomen from coughing, lifting, bending, and overeating causes slippage and results in reflux of the stomach contents. Symptoms of hiatus hernia include heartburn, dysphagia, **odynophagia,** and occasionally gastrointestinal bleeding. Antacids are prescribed (to be taken both after and between meals), and alcohol use, caffeine intake, and cigarette smoking should be curtailed in order to control gastric acidity.

odynophagia: Pain in swallowing.

20. Dietary treatment of hiatus hernia includes avoidance of large meals, with food intake divided into smaller, more frequent feedings. Liquids should not be consumed with meals, and a reasonable weight should be attained and maintained. It is often helpful to avoid lying down for several hours following food intake, as the stomach contents can exert pressure on the diaphragm and cause irritation of the hiatus hernia. Diet as tolerated is usually prescribed, but foods that irritate the gastric mucosa for most individuals should be avoided. These foods include black and red pepper, chili powder, caffeine, alcohol, chocolate and cocoa, and decaffeinated coffee.

21. With the presence of hiatus hernia, those foods that decrease esophageal pressure should be avoided (i.e., coffee, peppermint, chocolate) along with items that irritate the esophageal mucosa (i.e., citrus juices, alcoholic beverages, tomatoes and tomato juice); cigarette smoking should be curtailed. Fat may need to be modified, since a high-fat intake is believed to decrease esophageal sphincter pressure. Swallowing air can aggravate the hernia, so food should be properly chewed rather than gulped; carbonated beverages and chewing gum may also need to be restricted.

22. Although the etiology of hiatal hernias is uncertain, contributing factors include a congenital weakness of the diaphragmatic muscle, trauma, the aging process, and conditions that increase abdominal pressure such as obesity, pregnancy, **ascites,** tight-fitting clothing, and possibly a diet which is low in fiber. Thus, although a high-fiber diet is not usually prescribed as treatment, it may prove to be an essential component of the prevention of hiatus hernia.

ascites: Accumulation of fluid in the area surrounding the abdominal cavity.

Exercise on High-Fiber Diet Counseling

Keeping in mind the preceding High-Fiber Facts List, which provides some of the most current diet-related information to include in counseling individuals with certain disorders of the gastrointestinal tract, prepare a simplified version for use as a patient handout. You may include graphics and/or prepare in a poster format, if desired; see the Sample Handout. Show your handout in rough draft form to classmates or co-workers for constructive criticism on the overall design, content, and potential effectiveness for use in pertinent diet counseling situations. Then prepare a final version for your own future use as a practicing dietetic technician.

Sample Handout

Table 13.1 gives the fiber content of some high-fiber foods.

Table 13.1   Fiber Contents of Certain Foods[a]

Food	Total dietary fiber (g/100 g)	Food	Total dietary fiber (g/100 g)	Food	Total dietary fiber (g/100 g)
Flour		*Leafy vegetables*		*Fruits*	
White, bread-making	3.15	Broccoli tops (boiled)	4.10	Apples, flesh only	1.42
				peel only	3.71
Brown	7.87	Brussels sprouts (boiled)	2.86	Bananas	1.75
Whole-meal	9.51			Cherries (flesh and skin)	1.24
Bran	44.0	Cabbage (boiled)	2.83		
		Cauliflower (boiled)	1.80	Grapefruit (canned)	0.44
Breads					
White	2.72	Lettuce (raw)	1.53	Guavas (canned)	3.64
Brown	5.11	Onions (raw)	2.10	Mandarin oranges (canned)	0.29
Hovis	4.54	*Legumes*			
Whole-meal	8.50	Beans, baked (canned)	7.27	Mangoes (canned)	1.00
Cereals		Beans, runner (boiled)	3.35	Peaches (flesh and skin)	2.28
All-Bran	26.7				
Cornflakes	11.0	Peas, frozen (raw)	7.75	Pears, flesh only	2.44
Grapenuts	7.00	garden (canned)	6.28	peel only	8.59
Readibrek	7.60			Plums (flesh and skin)	1.52
Rice Krispies	4.47	processed (canned)	7.85		
Puffed Wheat	15.41			Rhubarb (raw)	1.78
Sugar Puffs	6.08	*Root vegetables*		Strawberries, raw	2.12
Shredded Wheat	12.26	Carrots, young (boiled)	3.70	canned	1.00
Swiss breakfast (mixed brands)	7.41	Parsnips (raw)	4.90	Sultanas	4.40
Weetabix	12.72	Swedes (raw)	2.40	*Nuts*	
		Turnips (raw)	2.20	Brazils	7.73
Biscuits		*Potatoes*		Peanuts	9.30
Chocolate digestive (half-coated)	3.50	Main crop (raw)	3.51	Peanut butter	7.55
		Chips (fried)	3.20		
Chocolate (fully coated)	3.09	Crisps	11.9		
		Canned, drained	2.51		
Crispbread, rye	11.73	*Peppers (cooked)*	0.93		
Crispbread, wheat	4.83				
Ginger biscuits	1.99	*Other vegetables*			
Matzo	3.85	Peppers (cooked)	0.93		
Oatcakes	4.00				
Semisweet	2.31	Tomatoes, fresh	1.40		
Short-sweet	1.60	canned, drained	0.85		
Wafers (filled)	1.62	Sweet corn, cooked	4.74		
		canned, drained	5.69		

[a]Reprinted by permission from NUTRITION—CONCEPTS AND CONTROVERSIES by E. Hamilton and E. Whitney © 1982 by West Publishing Company. All rights reserved. Reprinted with permission of the author, David Southgate © 1976.

STEP 4: LOW-RESIDUE DIET FACTS

Fecal material is 75% water, and of the remaining solids, less than half is composed of foodstuffs. Roughage and fat are the main dietary components of fecal residue, so a low-fiber/low-fat diet appears to be appropriate for those requiring a low-residue regime. Individual food intolerances should also be taken into account (e.g., lactose, caffeine, and gas-producing items) in diet planning.

The following Low-Residue Facts List provides some of the most current diet-related information to include in counseling individuals with certain gastrointestinal disorders.

Low-Residue Facts List

1. *Residue* is not equivalent to fiber, but is defined as the material which remains solid upon reaching the colon; this includes most fibers and milk curds. Thus, the low-residue diet includes restriction in the intake of fibrous foods and milk.

2. Diarrhea is characterized by frequent passage of liquidy stools, and is a symptom rather than a disease. Fluids and nutrients are lost, and food restriction during acute stages can compromise nutritional status. Causes include overeating, food intolerances, ingestion of spoiled foodstuffs, alcohol or caffeine, and emotional upset.

3. In *chronic diarrhea,* stools contain water, sodium, potassium, and undigested food particles. The etiology should be determined before treatment is initiated, but it is important to rapidly replace lost fluids and correct electrolyte imbalances.

4. *Acute diarrhea* may be caused by mucosal irritants (such as spices, drugs, and certain foods), overeating, nervous irritability, carbohydrate fermentation in the gut, bacterial overgrowth, or food poisoning. Treatment gradually advances to diet as tolerated with a low-residue intake.

5. Treatment of diarrhea—following NPO during the acute stages—includes the gradual addition of low-fiber, high-calorie, high-protein foods. High-fat foods may trigger bouts of diarrhea, as can caffeine, alcohol, and foods of individual intolerance.

6. *Steatorrhea*—fatty diarrhea—can lead to the decreased absorption of most nutrients and significant weight loss. A low-fat diet may be mandated in addition to a low-residue, nonirritating dietary intake.

7. Steatorrhea may be indicative of the presence of an organic disease; it is secondary to **celiac disease,** Crohn's disease, pancreatitis, and malabsorption disorders, and may occur after surgery.

celiac disease: Intestinal malabsorption syndrome characterized by diarrhea, flatulence, steatorrhea, and malnutrition; requires treatment which includes adherence to a gluten-free diet. (Also called nontropical sprue and gluten enteropathy.)

8. *Crohn's disease* (ileitis or nonspecific regional enteritis), a disorder of young adulthood, is characterized by cramps, diarrhea, fever, anorexia, and malabsorption symptoms due to an inflamed ileum. Vitamin B_{12} deficiency may develop, leading to the neurological damages of pernicious anemia. Weight loss is common.

9. The etiology of Crohn's disease is still uncertain, but it may be due to bacterial invasion or certain poisons. Although the disease is usually concentrated in the terminal ileum, occasionally the colon, duodenum, or other portions of the gastrointestinal tract are also affected.

10. The inflammation of Crohn's disease results in the shifting of fluids into the intestine with cramping, increased intestinal motility, diarrhea, and possibly steatorrhea.

11. Initial dietary treatment for Crohn's disease includes a high-protein, low-fat, low-residue diet with elimination of foods which tend to irritate the gastrointestinal tract.

12. Unlike simple colitis (spastic colon or irritable colon), *ulcerative colitis* is an organic inflammatory disease with lesions developing along the mucosal and submucosal linings of the large bowel. Colonic motility is greatly increased, with frequent diarrhea and stools which contain blood and mucous.

13. Although the etiology is unknown, ulcerative colitis may be inherited and/or caused by infection, stress, or protein deficiency. Symptoms include nausea, abdominal pain, anorexia, tachycardia, and anemia.

14. Occurring most frequently in women, especially the very young and those in their thirties, ulcerative colitis has periods of remission during which a high-fiber diet may prove beneficial. However, initial treatment generally includes a low-residue diet which is high in protein and calories to replace tissue losses and provide energy; with decreased stool frequency, diarrhea is controlled and bowel irritation diminished. Individual intolerances should be avoided, and a low-lactose diet is often required (see Step 5 of this chapter).

15. Vitamin supplementation may be required with severe cases of ulcerative colitis, iron supplements are needed with excessive blood losses, and calcium supplements may be necessary with milk/lactose restrictions.

Exercise on Low-Residue Diet Counseling

Keeping in mind the preceding Low-Residue Facts List, which provides some of the most current diet-related information to include in counseling individuals with certain gastrointestinal disorders, prepare a simplified version for use as a patient handout. You may include graphics and/or prepare in a poster format, if desired; see the Sample Handout. Show your handout in rough draft form to classmates or co-workers for constructive criticism on the overall design, content, and potential effectiveness for use in pertinent diet counseling situations. Then prepare a final version for your own future use as a practicing dietetic technician.

Sample Handout

Table 13.2 lists foods to avoid on a low-residue diet.

Table 13.2   Low-Residue Diet

Food Group[a]	Foods to avoid
Fruits and Vegetables	Fibrous produce eaten with seeds and/or skins such as artichokes, berries, celery, coconut, currants, dried fruits, dried peas and beans, guava, parsnips, peppers, and potato skins; prunes/prune juice; any prepared in rich sauces.
Breads and Cereals	Whole grain breads, cereals, flours, and pastas; brown rice; products containing fruit, nuts, or seeds; popcorn; fried snacks such as chips; rich products such as pastries.
Milk and Cheeses	Whole milk and whole milk products; cheese made with nuts, peppers, or seeds.
Meats and Alternates	Dried peas and beans, seeds, crunchy peanut butter, and nuts; fatty or fried meats, luncheon meats, sausage; poultry skin.
Others	Cream, cream cheese, avocado, bacon, chocolate, butter, lard, nuts and nut products, gravies, and rich sauces; desserts made with high-fiber or high-fat foods such as nuts, coconut, berries, dried fruits, seeds, chocolate; ice cream, rich cakes, pies, doughnuts, or cookies; milkshakes or eggnog; cream soups, chowders, and soups made with items listed above.

[a]Be sure to include the recommended number of servings from each of the Basic Food Groups every day.

STEP 5: LOW-LACTOSE DIET FACTS

Some individuals are unable to tolerate foods high in lactose content and, upon consumption, suffer from varying degrees of gastrointestinal upset including bloating, flatulence, diarrhea, nausea and vomiting. The disorder is due to an inadequate amount or total lack of lactase, the lactose-splitting enzyme, but can be controlled with proper dietary management.

The following Low-Lactose Facts List provides some of the most current diet-related information to include in counseling individuals with lactose intolerance.

Low-Lactose Facts List

congenital: Present at birth.

1.   Lactose intolerance may be the result of a **congenital** inborn error of metabolism, or may occur secondary to protein-calorie malnutrition, celiac disease, or infection, and may be caused by certain drugs.

2.   Lactose intolerance occurs more commonly in blacks, Orientals, and Jews, and affects nearly 80% of the world population.

3.   In children, the disorder is characterized by weakness, irritability, muscle wasting, chronic diarrhea and vomiting; in adults, lactose intolerance causes diarrhea, abdominal discomfort, **borborygmi,** flatulence, and nausea.

borborygmi: Intestinal rumbling noises caused by movement of gas through the intestine.

4.   Unabsorbed lactose remains in the intestinal lumen, increasing the osmotic load of the small intestine; as the normal intestinal bacteria act on the lactose, lactic acid wastes accumulate, fluids are drawn into the digestive tract, gas is produced, and diarrhea results.

5.   Increased peristalsis and diarrhea can cause malabsorption of nutrients and deficiencies may occur. Drug metabolism may also be impaired.

6.   Infants with lactose intolerance should be given lactose-free formulas until able to tolerate lactose.

7.   The majority of individuals who are lactose intolerant are able to ingest a small amount of milk (up to a cup, particularly when consumed with other foods and not all at once). Some individuals are able to tolerate fermented milk products, and chocolate milk is absorbed more slowly so may be better tolerated.

8.   Foods which are not lactose-rich may be allowed as desired, but individuals with a severe intolerance may need to restrict lactose intake rigorously. Labels need to be read carefully, and products containing whey—which contains lactose—may also have to be restricted. Certain medications contain lactose, so should be avoided by those requiring stringent restriction.

9.   Fermentation reduces the lactose in aged cheese, yogurt, and buttermilk, while processing removes the lactose-containing whey portion from cottage cheese. These products are tolerated by some individuals in moderate amounts.

10.   Individuals who are sensitive to lactose may try using lactose-hydrolyzed milk products such as Lact-Aid. These products are not always well-tolerated, however.

11.   Lactose enhances the absorption of calcium, so lactose restriction coupled with a decreased milk intake can cause calcium deficiency; alternative sources of calcium should be included in the diet in order to help prevent the onset of osteoporosis and other calcium-related disorders. Supplements may need to be prescribed.

12.   Once dietary intake is corrected, the symptoms of lactose intolerance disappear within several days. Individuals vary in their responses to lactose and to a low-lactose diet, so it is important to evaluate past food patterns and to monitor the diet carefully to determine the amount of lactose which can be tolerated. Calcium supplements may be required if dietary intake is inadequate. Iron absorption may also be impaired, so the inclusion of iron-rich foods is an essential aspect of the low-lactose diet. If diet restriction is severe, prescription of vitamin/mineral supplements may be required.

Exercise on Low-Lactose Diet Counseling

Keeping in mind the preceding Low-Lactose Facts List, which provides some of the most current diet-related information to include in counseling individuals with lactose intolerance, prepare a simplified version for use as a patient handout. You may include graphics and/or prepare in a poster format, if desired; see the Sample Handout. Show your handout in rough draft form to classmates or co-workers for constructive criticism on the overall design, content, and potential effectiveness for use in pertinent diet counseling situations. Then prepare a final version for your own future use as a practicing dietetic technician.

Sample Handout

Table 13.3 lists foods to avoid on a low-lactose diet.

Table 13.3   Low-Lactose Diet

Food Group[a]	Foods to avoid
Fruits and Vegetables	Any prepared in milk-based sauces[b]
Breads and Cereals	Any made with milk or whey
Milk and Cheese	Milk and milk substitutes over 1 cup per day; whey; ice cream; processed cheese foods/spreads
Meats and Alternates	Any made with milk-based gravies or sauces[b]
Others	Cream, creamed soups, cream pies, custard, puddings, milkshakes[b]

[a]Be sure to include the recommended number of servings from each of the Basic Food Groups every day. Divide milk intake into several small servings. Include yogurt, cheese, and fermented milk products as tolerated.

[b]Unless counted as part of daily cup of milk.

STEP 6: DIET AS TOLERATED (D.A.T.) GUIDELINES

For many years, individuals with gastrointestinal disorders were prescribed "bland" diets, which varied considerably in content depending on the attending physician and/or dietetics personnel. Within the past decade or so, evidence has indicated that these dietary restrictions are not only unnecessary, but may prove detrimental in the control of digestive diseases. Therefore, current diet therapy emphasizes a nonstressful, pleasant, appetizing diet—including all foods as tolerated by the individual patient.

In order to be able to advise individuals with peptic ulcer disease, gastritis, hiatus hernia, and acute diarrhea as to desirable dietary patterns, it is essential to have access to all of the hands-on material required for effective counseling sessions. It is also important to be able to record all of the pertinent information regarding each diet counseling session in the patients' medical charts. The information provided below should help to improve your counseling confidence and skills.

This step includes suggested strategies to use in counseling patients with peptic ulcer disease, lactose intolerance or other ailments for which *diet as tolerated* is prescribed. The following references may prove helpful.

Suggested Readings for Diet as Tolerated

AMERICAN DIETETIC ASSOCIATION. 1971. Position Paper on Bland Diet in the Treatment of Chronic Duodenal Ulcer. Chicago: ADA.

AMERICAN DIETETIC ASSOCIATION. 1985. Food sensitivity: Lactose Intolerance. Chicago: ADA.

BROSTOFF, J., and CHALLACOMBE, S. (Editors). 1987. Food Allergy and Intolerance. Philadelphia: W. B. Saunders Co.

CHERNOW, B., and CASTELL, D. 1979. Diet and Heartburn. J. Am. Med. Assoc. *241,* May 25, 2307.

FLOCH, M. 1981. Nutrition and Diet Therapy in Gastrointestinal Disease. New York: Plenum Press.

GROSSMAN, M. (Editor). 1981. Peptic Ulcer: A Guide by the Staff of the Center for Ulcer Research and Education (CURE). Chicago: Year Book Medical Publishers.

HALPERN, S. (Editor). 1987. Quick Reference to Clinical Nutrition, 2nd Edition. Philadelphia: J. B. Lippincott Co.

HORWITZ, C., and ROZEN, P. (Editors). 1988. Frontiers of Gastrointestinal Research: Progress in Diet and Nutrition. Basil, Switzerland: Karger.

JANOWITZ, H. 1985. Inflammatory Bowel Disease. Chicago: Year Book Medical Publishers.

JANOWITZ, H. 1987. Your Gut Feelings: A Complete Guide to Living Better with Intestinal Problems. New York: Oxford University Press.

KAPLAN, H. 1983. Peptic Ulcer. New Hyde Park, NY: Medical Examination Publishing Co.

KURTZ, R., YARBOROUGH, M., and CURRERI, P. (Editors). 1981. Nutrition in Gastrointestinal Disease. New York: Churchill Livingstone.

LESOFF, M. (Editor). 1984. Clinical Reactions to Food, Publication No. 84-2442. Washington, DC: Government Printing Office.

MCQUESTION, M. (Editor). 1983. Oral Rehydration Therapy: An Annotated Bibliography, 2nd Edition. Washington, DC: World Health Organization.

MIGLIOLI, M., et al. 1987. Optimal nutritional indexes in gastroenterology. J. Parenteral/Enteral Nutr. *11,* Sept./Oct., 1265-S.

MYLANDER, M. 1982. The Great American Stomach Book. New Haven, CT: Ticknor & Fields.

PAIGE, D., and BAYLESS, T. (Editors). 1981. Lactose Digestion: Clinical and Nutritional Implications. Baltimore: Johns Hopkins University Press.

READ, A., HARVEY, R., and NAISH, J. 1981. Basic Gastroenterology. Littleton, MA: Wright PSG.

READ, N. (Editor). 1985. Irritable Bowel Syndrome. Orlando, FL: Grune & Stratton.

ROBERSON, L., MCLAUGHLIN, A., and LUND, J. 1987. Promoting oral rehydration therapy for acute diarrhea. J. Am. Dietet. Assoc. *87,* Apr., 496.

RYDNING, A. 1987. Dietary fibre and peptic ulcer. Scandinavian J. Gastroenterol. *129,* Suppl., 232.

SKINNER, S., and MARTENS, R. 1985. The Milk Sugar Dilemma: Living with Lactose Intolerance. East Lansing, MI: Medi-Ed Press.

SLEISENGER, M., and FORDTRAN, J. 1983. Gastrointestinal Disease: Pathophysiology, Diagnosis, and Management, 3rd Edition. Philadelphia: W. B. Saunders Co.

STEIN, J., and GALLAGER-ALLRED, C. 1980. Dietary Management in Gastrointestinal Diseases. Columbus: Ohio State University College of Medicine.

TAYLOR, D., and ROCK, M. 1980. Gut Reactions: How to Handle Stress and Your Stomach. Philadelphia: W. B. Saunders Co.

ZUKIN, J. 1982. Milk-Free Cookbook: Cooking for the Lactose Intolerant. New York: Sterling Publishing Co.

For audiovisuals:

Gastrointestinal Reflux. Milner-Fenwick, Inc., 2125 Greenspring Drive, Timonium, MD 21903.
Irritable Bowel Syndrome. Milner-Fenwick, Inc., 2125 Greenspring Drive, Timonium, MD 21903.
Living with Stress. Milner-Fenwick, Inc., 2125 Greenspring Drive, Timonium, MD 21903.
Peptic Ulcer. Milner-Fenwick, Inc., 2125 Greenspring Drive, Timonium, MD 21903.
Your Ulcer Diet. The Polished Apple, 3742 Seahorn Drive, Malibu, CA 90265.

For further information:

American College of Gastroenterology, 299 Broadway, New York, NY 10017.
Center for Ulcer Research and Education (CURE), 11661 San Vincente Boulevard, Suite 304, Los Angeles, CA 90049.
National Digestive Diseases Education and Information Clearinghouse, 1555 Wilson Boulevard, Suite 600, Rosslyn, VA 22209.

Counseling Guidelines—D.A.T.

Table 13.4 outlines the steps for diet counseling when diet as tolerated is prescribed. The following material gives the details of each step.

I. Initial Session

I. A. General Guidelines

1. Use Medical History Form to assess patient's nutritional status.
2. Weigh patient and record on Weight Chart. The chart is a helpful tool for visualization of weight status.
3. Assist patient in recording 24-hour recall of food intake using 24-Hour Recall Form. This will aid patient in keeping an accurate Food Intake Record.
4. Instruct patient to keep daily Food Intake Record so that typical food intake patterns can be evaluated. Advise patient not to deviate from normal eating pattern. Stress the importance of recording food intake immediately after eating.
5. Instruct patient to complete Diet History. This provides for a basic evaluation of food intake patterns. (Use Pre-test from Chapter 2.)
6. Record assessment and recommendation using the SOAP method in Technician's Notes. This form can be kept in your files with a copy in the patient's medical records.

Table 13.4 General Outline for D.A.T. Counseling

I. Initial Session
  A. General Guidelines
  B. Patient Records
    1. Medical History Form
    2. Weight Chart
    3. 24-Hour Recall Form
  C. Assignments
    1. Food Intake Record
    2. Diet History
  D. Technician's Notes
II. Follow-up Session(s)
  A. General Guidelines
  B. Handouts
    1. Personal Diet Plan
    2. Learning Assessment Quiz
  C. Technician's Notes

I. B. Patient Records

1. Medical History Form

Date _____ Referred by _____
Name _____ Date of birth _____
Address _____ Phone no. _____
Occupation _____ Hours per work week ____ Work phone no. _____
Educational background _____ Religious/ethnic background _____
Sex _____ Marital status _____
Household composition: Live alone _____ Spouse _____ Children/No. _____
Other: _____

General health status:

Physician _____ Address _____
Phone no. _____ Date of last visit _____
Ambulatory care required? _____ If so, describe: _____
Neuromuscular problems? _____ If so, how is eating affected? _____
Visual/auditory problems? _____ If so, describe: _____
Chewing difficulties? _____ If so, describe: _____
Appetite typically good? _____ fair? _____ poor? _____
Digestion/elimination difficulties? _____ If so, describe: _____
Food intolerances? _____ If so, describe: _____

Diabetes? _____ If so, describe: _____
Heart attack or stroke? _____ If so, describe: _____
Gout? _____ If so, describe: _____
Other: _____

Height _____ Weight _____ Frame _____
Triceps skinfold thickness _____ Mid-arm circumference _____
Mid-arm muscle circumference _____
Weight changes/problems? _____ If so, describe: _____

Clinical signs of nutritional status:

Skin _____ Mouth _____
Hair _____ Eyes _____
Teeth _____ Other: _____

Lab data:

Blood pressure _____
CBC _____ Guaiac test _____
Serum albumin _____
Other: _____

Medications taken regularly: _____
Prescribed by: _____ Date(s) prescribed: _____
Nutrition supplements taken regularly: _____
Prescribed by: _____ Date(s) prescribed: _____
Special diet prescription: _____
Prescribed by: _____ Date of prescription: _____
How closely is diet followed? Always adhered to __ Sometimes __ Rarely __ Never __

Type of housing: Room _____ Apartment _____ Home _____ Institution _____
Prepare own meals? _____ Dine out? Often (more than once a day) _____ Rarely _____
Food shopping done independently? _____ If not, describe required assistance: _____
_____
Eligible for food stamps? _____ If so, are they currently being used? _____
Cigarette smoker? _____ If so, how much: _____
Exercise regularly? _____ If so, describe: _____
    No. times per week _____ No. minutes per session _____

Comments: _____

2. Weight Chart

Starting weight _____   Reasonable weight _____

Date	No. weeks on diet	Weight	Comments

3. 24-Hour Recall Form

Date	Time	Food and amount

I. C. Assignments

1. Food Intake Record

Date and time	Duration of meal (min)	Food and amount	Where[a]	With whom	Associated activity[b]	Associated emotions[c]

[a]Such as school, restaurant, kitchen, living room.
[b]For example, watching television, reading, talking.
[c]Attitude: bored, anxious, frustrated, depressed, happy, angry, tense, etc.

2. Diet History

Use the Pre-test from Chapter 2 (p. 30) to provide a record of typical foods eaten.

I. D. Technician's Notes

Patient: _____   Date: _____

S (Subjective data—how patient feels):
O (Objective data—physical measurements including diet/nutritional status):
A (Assessment—acceptability of dietary progress/nutritional status):
P (Plan—diet prescription and instruction):
Comments:

II. Follow-up Session(s)

II. A. General Guidelines
1. Weigh patient and record on Weight Chart.
2. Review assignments and discuss.

3. Individualize Personal Diet Plan and instruct patient in its use.
4. Assign Learning Assessment Quiz to evaluate the counseling process and to determine if additional counseling is needed.
5. Record assessment and recommendation(s) using the SOAP method in Technician's Notes. This form can be kept in your files with a copy in the patient's medical records.

II. B. Handouts

1. Personal Diet Plan

Name _____

How to use diet plan:

1. Select a variety of foods from each of the Basic Food Groups.
2. Include the recommended number of servings from each Food Group.
3. Divide daily food intake into small, frequent, regular meals.
4. Avoid stimulants such as alcohol and caffeine, especially between meals.
5. Avoid nicotine.
6. Omit Foods to Avoid (see Table 13.5) and those foods that produce symptoms of discomfort. List individual food intolerances:

Table 13.5 Foods to Avoid with Gastrointestinal Disorders

I. Ulcers or gastritis	II. Hiatus hernia	III. Acute diarrhea
Alcoholic beverages	List I. Plus	List I. Plus
Coffee, decaffeinated coffee	Peppermint	High-fiber foods
Tea	Citrus juices	High-fat foods
Chili powder	Tomato	Milk and milk products
Chocolate, cocoa	Tomato juice	(with lactose intolerance)
Cola drinks	High-fat foods	
Pepper, black and red		

2. Learning Assessment Quiz

Answer true (T) or false (F) to the following statements:

____ 1. Milk is highly effective in decreasing gastric acid secretions.
____ 2. Aspirin reduces gastric acidity.
____ 3. Gas-forming vegetables, such as cabbage and brussels sprouts, should be avoided by all individuals with peptic ulcer disease.
____ 4. Antacids are often prescribed to neutralize gastric acid.
____ 5. The establishment of regular meal times may be important for proper gastric function.
____ 6. Frequent, small meals may be effective in the control of gastric acidity.

Select the best answer to the following statements:

___ 7. To avoid excessive gastric secretion, omit foods such as
(a) coffee. (b) beer. (c) decaffeinated coffee. (d) a and b. (e) all of these.
___ 8. To help neutralize gastric secretions, include foods such as
(a) cream. (b) milk. (c) cream cheese. (d) a and c. (e) all of these.

II. C. Technician's Notes

Patient: _____   Date: _____

S (Subjective data—how patient feels):
O (Objective data—physical measurements including diet/nutritional status):
A (Assessment—acceptability of dietary progress/nutritional status):
P (Plan—diet prescription and instruction):
Comments:

D.A.T. Counseling Role Playing

Keeping in mind the preceding Suggested Readings and Counseling Guidelines, participate in the following role play situations; use the sample menus (Figs. 13.1 or 13.2) as a teaching aid. Select different partners for each situation, either classmates or co-workers, and elaborate on each role play situation to develop a patient/audience profile. You may want to use your handout from Steps 2, 4, or 5. Use the SOAP method to record in each patient's medical chart.

As a dietetic technician in nutrition care, do you consider yourself capable of conducting effective counseling sessions with individuals suffering from gastrointestinal disorders? Would you or your family be able to adhere to your nutrition guidelines in order to control or prevent the undesirable symptoms of gastrointestinal disorders?

Role Play Situation 1.   As a dietetic technician in a small, private hospital, you receive a memo from a physician: the patient has been complaining that the food served bothers his ulcer. A 45-year-old, overweight male, the patient has been on a house diet since admission. Follow the guidelines to complete the charts and provide the patient with an individualized diet plan. Prepare a SOAP note that could be recorded in the patient's medical chart. *Note:* Patient is hospitalized for upcoming disc surgery.

Role Play Situation 2.   A middle-aged overweight female is referred to the out-patient nutrition clinic with a diagnosis of hiatus hernia. As the assigned dietetic technician, follow the guidelines to complete the charts and provide the patient with an individualized diet plan. Prepare a SOAP note for insertion in department files with a copy to be sent to the referring physician.

Role Play Situation 3.   As a dietetic technician employed by a state public health agency, you are asked to help conduct a workshop on lactose intolerance. Prepare a brief outline and give a 15-minute talk on When You Can't Drink Milk. Prepare a report on the workshop for insertion in departmental files.

Name _____ Room _____
Diet **Clear or Full Liquid** _____

Breakfast Please √ check desired food items

☐ Orange juice   ☐ Cream of wheat cereal   ☐ Sparkle gelatin
☐ Apple juice   ☐ Chicken consomme   ☐ Plain yogurt
☐ Prune juice   ☐ Eggnog

☐ Coffee   ☐ Whole milk   ☐ Salt
☐ Tea   ☐ Skim milk   ☐ Sugar
☐ Decaffeinated coffee ☐ Teamilk   ☐ Sugar substitute
☐ Ginger ale   ☐ Cream   ☐ Lemon

Name _____ Room _____
Diet **Clear or Full Liquid** _____

Luncheon Please √ check desired food items

☐ Fruit juice
☐ Grape juice
☐ Eggnog
☐ Strained cream soup
☐ Beef consomme

☐ Orange gelatin
☐ Strawberry gelatin
☐ Butterscotch pudding
  ☐ Whipped topping
☐ Coffee ice cream
☐ Vanilla ice cream
☐ Custard
☐ Plain yogurt
☐ Water ice
☐ Popsicle
☐ Sherbet

☐ Coffee
☐ Tea
☐ Decaffeinated coffee
☐ Ginger ale
☐ Cream
☐ Whole milk
☐ Skim milk
☐ Teamilk

☐ Salt
☐ Sugar
☐ Sugar substitute
☐ Lemon

Name _____ Room _____
Diet **Clear or Full Liquid** _____

Dinner Please √ check desired food items

☐ Fruit juice
☐ Cranberry juice
☐ Eggnog
☐ Strained cream soup
☐ Chicken consomme

☐ Orange gelatin
☐ Strawberry gelatin
☐ Vanilla pudding
  ☐ Whipped topping
☐ Coffee ice cream
☐ Vanilla ice cream
☐ Custard
☐ Plain yogurt
☐ Water ice
☐ Popsicle
☐ Sherbet

☐ Coffee
☐ Tea
☐ Decaffeinated coffee
☐ Ginger ale
☐ Cream
☐ Whole milk
☐ Skim milk
☐ Teamilk

☐ Salt
☐ Sugar
☐ Sugar substitute
☐ Lemon

Fig. 13.1 Menu for clear or full liquid diets.
© *The Seiler Corporation. Reprinted by permission.*

STEP 7: HIGH-FIBER DIET GUIDELINES

The prevention and control of certain gastrointestinal disorders may be facilitated by a diet containing significant amounts of dietary fiber. Although epidemiological evidence suggests that the incidence of certain cancers, diabetes, and obesity are also reduced with high-fiber diets, research is still underway. It has been suggested that the typical American diet should include increased amounts of fiber-rich fruits, vegetables, and grains (see

Appendix III). Current therapy for individuals with constipation, colitis, and diverticulosis includes a high-fiber diet. *Note:* An excessive intake of high-fiber foods can lead to nutrient losses and dehydration.

In order to be able to advise individuals on increasing the fiber content of the diet, it is essential to have access to all of the hands-on material required for effective counseling sessions. It is also important to be able to record all of the pertinent information regarding each diet counseling session in the patient's medical charts. The information provided below should help to improve your counseling confidence and skills.

This step includes suggested counseling strategies to use with patients requiring an increase in fiber intake. A high-fiber diet may be contraindicated in patients with inflammatory bowel disease, threatened bowel obstruction, or renal disease. The following references may prove helpful.

Suggested Readings

AMERICAN DIETETIC ASSOCIATION. 1988. Position of The American Dietetic Association: Health implications of dietary fiber. J. Am. Dietet. Assoc. *88,* Feb., 216.

ANDERSON, J. 1984a. Dr. Anderson's HCF Diet. Lexington, KY: HCF Diabetes Foundation.

ANDERSON, J. 1984b. User's Guide to HCF Diets. Lexington, KY: HCF Diabetes Foundation.

ANDERSON, J. 1986. Plant Fiber in Foods. Lexington, KY: HCF Diabetes Foundation.

ANDERSON, J. 1988a. Fiber and health: An overview. Nutrition Today *21,* Nov./Dec., 22.

ANDERSON, J. 1988b. Nutrition Management of Metabolic Conditions: Professional Guide to HCF Diets. Lexington, KY: HCF Diabetes Foundation.

ANDERSON, J., and BRIDGES, S. 1988. Dietary fiber content of selected foods. Amer. J. Clin. Nutr. *47,* Mar., 440.

BURKITT, D. 1987. Dietary Fibre: Historical aspects. Scandinavian J. Gastroenterol. *129,* Supp., 1.

EASTWOOD, M., and PASSMORE, R. 1984. A new look at dietary fiber. Nutrition Today *19,* Sept./Oct., 6.

EGAN, J. 1987. Healthy High Fiber Cooking. Tucson, AZ: HP Books.

FLOCH, M., et al. 1988. Practical aspects of implementing increased dietary fiber intake. Nutrition Today *21,* Nov./Dec., 27.

HALPERN, S. (Editor). 1987. Quick Reference to Clinical Nutrition, 2nd Edition. Philadelphia: J. B. Lippincott Co.

IMES, S., PINCHBECK, B., and THOMSON, A. 1987. Diet counseling modifies nutrient intake of patients with Crohn's disease. J. Am. Dietet. Assoc. *87,* Apr., 457.

JENKINS, D., et al. 1986. Fiber and starchy foods: Gut function and implications in disease. Amer. J. Gastroenterol. *81,* Oct., 920.

KLURFELD, D. 1987. The role of dietary fiber in gastrointestinal disease. J. Am. Dietet. Assoc. *87,* Sept., 1172.

LIFE SCIENCES RESEARCH OFFICE. 1987. Physiological Effects and Health Consequences of Dietary Fiber. Bethesda, MD: Federation of American Societies for Experimental Biology Publications Office.

MADAR, Z. 1987. New sources of dietary fiber. Int. J. Obesity *11,* Supp., 57.

RATTAN, J., et al. 1981. A high-fiber diet does not cause mineral and nutrient deficiencies. J. Clin. Gastroenterol. *3,* Dec., 389.

SCHNEEMAN, B. 1987. Dietary fiber: Comments on interpreting recent research. J. Am. Dietet. Assoc. *87,* Sept., 1163.

SHARMA, S., et al. 1987. Role of dietary fiber in irritable bowel syndrome. Indian J. Med. Sci. *41,* Feb., 29.

SLAVIN, J. 1987. Dietary fiber: Classification, chemical analyses, and food sources. J. Am. Dietet. Assoc. *87,* Sept., 1164.

SOUTHGATE, D., and VAN SOEST, P. 1978. Dietary fiber: Analysis and food sources; fiber analysis tables. Amer. J. Clin. Nutr. *31,* Supp., 281.

TROWELL, H., BURKITT, D., and HEATON, K. (Editors). 1985. Dietary Fibre, Fibre Depleted Foods, and Disease. London: Academic Press.

VAHOUNY, G., and KRITCHEVSKY, D. 1982. Dietary Fiber in Health and Disease. New York: Plenum Press.

VAHOUNY, G., and KRITCHEVSKY, D. 1986. Dietary Fiber: Basic and Clinical Aspects. New York: Plenum Press.

For audiovisuals:

Constipation. Milner-Fenwick, Inc., 2125 Greenspring Drive, Timonium, MD 21093.

Crohn's Disease. Milner-Fenwick, Inc., 2125 Greenspring Drive, Timonium, MD 21093.

Diverticular Disease. Milner-Fenwick, Inc., 2125 Greenspring Drive, Timonium, MD 21093.
Fiber Charts. Nutrition Graphics, PO Box 1527, Corvallis, OR 97339.
Ulcerative Colitis. Milner-Fenwick, Inc., 2125 Greenspring Drive, Timonium, MD 21093.

Counseling Guidelines—High-Fiber Diet

Table 13.6 General Outline for High-Fiber Diet Counseling

I. Initial Session
   A. General Guidelines
   B. Patient Records
      1. Medical History Form
      2. Weight Chart
      3. 24-Hour Recall Form
   C. Assignments
      1. Food Intake Record
      2. Diet History
   D. Technician's Notes
II. Follow-up Session(s)
   A. General Guidelines
   B. Handouts
      1. Personal Diet Plan
      2. Learning Assessment Quiz
   C. Technician's Notes

Table 13.6 outlines the steps for high-fiber diet counseling. The following material gives the details of each step.

I. Initial Session

I. A. General Guidelines

1. Use Medical History Form to assess patient's nutritional status.
2. Weigh patient and record on Weight Chart. The chart is a helpful tool for visualization of weight status.
3. Assist patient in recording 24-hour recall of food intake using 24-Hour Recall Form. This will aid patient in keeping an accurate Food Intake Record.
4. Instruct patient to keep daily Food Intake Record so that typical food intake patterns can be evaluated. Advise patient not to deviate from normal eating pattern. Stress the importance of recording food intake immediately after eating.
5. Instruct patient to complete Diet History. This provides for a basic evaluation of food intake patterns. (Use Pre-test from Chapter 2.)
6. Record assessment and recommendation(s) using the SOAP method in Technician's Notes. This form can be kept in your files with a copy in the patient's medical records.

I. B. Patient Records

1. Medical History Form

Date _____ Referred by _____
Name _____ Date of birth _____
Address _____ Phone no. _____
Occupation _____ Hours per work week ____ Work phone no. _____
Educational background _____ Religious/ethnic background _____
Sex _____ Marital status _____
Household composition: Live alone _____ Spouse _____ Children/No. _____
Other: _____

General health status:

Physician _____ Address _____
Phone no. _____ Date of last visit _____
Ambulatory care required? _____ If so, describe: _____
Neuromuscular problems? _____ If so, how is eating affected? _____
Visual/auditory problems? _____ If so, describe: _____
Chewing difficulties? _____ If so, describe: _____
Appetite typically good? _____ fair? _____ poor? _____
Digestion/elimination difficulties? _____ If so, describe: _____
Food intolerances? _____ If so, describe: _____
Diabetes? _____ If so, describe: _____
Heart attack or stroke? _____ If so, describe: _____
Gout? _____ If so, describe: _____
Other: _____

Height _____ Weight _____ Frame _____
Triceps skinfold thickness _____ Mid-arm circumference _____
Mid-arm muscle circumference _____
Weight changes/problems? _____ If so, describe: _____

Clinical signs of nutritional status:

Skin _____ Mouth _____
Hair _____ Eyes _____
Teeth _____ Other: _____

Lab data:

Blood pressure _____

CBC _____ Guaiac test _____

Serum albumin _____

Other: _____

Medications taken regularly: _____

Prescribed by: _____ Date(s) prescribed: _____

Nutrition supplements taken regularly: _____

Prescribed by: _____ Date(s) prescribed: _____

Special diet prescription: _____

Prescribed by: _____ Date of prescription: _____

How closely is diet followed? Always adhered to __ Sometimes __ Rarely __ Never __

Type of housing: Room _____ Apartment _____ Home _____ Institution _____

Prepare own meals? _____ Dine out? Often (more than once a day) _____ Rarely _____

Food shopping done independently? _____ If not, describe required assistance: _____
_____

Eligible for food stamps? _____ If so, are they currently being used? _____

Cigarette smoker? _____ If so, how much: _____

Exercise regularly? _____ If so, describe: _____

   No. times per week _____ No. minutes per session _____

Comments: _____

2. Weight Chart

Starting weight _____   Reasonable weight _____

Date	No. weeks on diet	Weight	Comments

3. 24-Hour Recall Form

Date	Time	Food and amount

I. C. Assignments

1. Food Intake Record

Date and time	Duration of meal (min)	Food and amount	Where[a]	With whom	Associated activity[b]	Associated emotions[c]

[a]Such as school, restaurant, kitchen, living room.
[b]For example, watching television, reading, talking.
[c]Attitude: bored, anxious, frustrated, depressed, happy, angry, tense, etc.

2. Diet History

Use the Pre-test from Chapter 2 (p. 30) to provide a record of typical foods eaten.

I. D. Technician's Notes

Patient: _____   Date: _____

S (Subjective data—how patient feels):
O (Objective data—physical measurements including diet/nutritional status):
A (Assessment—acceptability of dietary progress/nutritional status):
P (Plan—diet prescription and instruction):
Comments:

II. Follow-up Session(s)

II. A. General Guidelines

1. Weigh patient and record on Weight Chart.
2. Review assignments and discuss.
3. Individualize Personal Diet Plan and instruct patient in its use.
4. Assign Learning Assessment Quiz to evaluate the counseling process and to determine if additional counseling is needed.
5. Record assessment and recommendation(s) using the SOAP method in Technician's Notes. This form can be kept in your files with a copy in the patient's medical records.

II. B. Handouts

1. Personal Diet Plan

Name _____

How to use diet plan:

1. Select a variety of foods from each of the Basic Food Groups.
2. Include the recommended number of servings from each Food Group.

3. Drink at least 8–10 cups of fluid daily.
4. Increase consumption of *high-fiber foods* (see Table 13.7).
5. Decrease consumption of highly refined (fiber-depleted) carbohydrate foods.

Table 13.7   High-Fiber Foods[a]

Vegetables[b]	Fruits[b]	Grains
Green leafy vegetables	Raw fruits (with skin	Breads, whole grain
Cabbage	and seeds)	Cereals, whole grain and bran-containing[c]
Tomato	Dried fruits	Crackers, whole grain and crispbreads
Carrots		Pasta, whole grain
Legumes		Popcorn, plain
Potato (with skin)		
Corn		
Peas		

[a]*Note:* Include one to two raw fruits and/or vegetable salads daily.
[b]Use all vegetables and fruits liberally; especially use those listed.
[c]Bran cereals contain more fiber per serving than other foods.

2. Learning Assessment Quiz

Answer true (T) or false (F) to the following statements:

_____ 1. Dietary fiber is that portion of plant material that cannot be fully digested.
_____ 2. Dietary fiber may play a role in the prevention of large bowel disease.
_____ 3. An adequate dietary fiber intake results in smaller, harder stools.
_____ 4. Dietary fiber increases the speed at which food moves through the digestive tract.
_____ 5. Reduction in fluid intake stimulates elimination.
_____ 6. Enriched breads and cereals are not always a good source of fiber.
_____ 7. Maintenance of proper muscle tone of the intestine may be enhanced by regular physical exercise.
_____ 8. Ingestion of excessive amounts of dietary fiber may lead to loss of important nutrients.
_____ 9. White flour is made from cereal grains from which the bran and germ have been removed.
_____ 10. Brown or dark breads are not always whole grain products.

II. C. Technician's Notes

Patient: _____   Date: _____

S   (Subjective data—how patient feels):
O   (Objective data—physical measurements including diet/nutritional status):
A   (Assessment—acceptability of dietary progress/nutritional status):
P   (Plan—diet prescription and instruction):
Comments:

High-Fiber Diet Counseling Role Playing

Keeping in mind the preceding Suggested Readings and Counseling Guidelines, participate in the following role play situations; use the sample menu (Fig. 13.2) as a teaching aid. Select different partners, either classmates or co-workers, for each situation and elaborate on each role play situation to develop a patient/audience profile. You may want to use your handout from Step 3. Use the SOAP method to record in each patient's medical chart.

As a dietetic technician in nutrition care, do you consider yourself capable of conducting effective counseling sessions with individuals suffering from certain gastrointestinal disorders? Would you or your family be able to adhere to your nutrition guidelines in order to control or prevent the undesirable symptoms of gastrointestinal disorders?

Name _____ Room _____
Diet **Regular plus Fiber** _____

Breakfast
Please circle your selections below

Fruits and juices	**Cereals**	**Entrees**	**Breads**	**Miscellaneous**
Orange juice	Cream of wheat	Bacon	Apple muffin	Salt
Grapefruit juice	Grits	Sausage	Blueberry muffin	Pepper
Prune juice	Oatmeal	Scrambled egg	Bran muffin	Sugar
Apple juice	Cornflakes	Poached egg	Corn muffin	Sugar substitute
Cranberry juice	Rice Krispies	Egg substitute	Plain muffin	Butter
Grapefruit sections	Special K	Pancakes	Danish pastry	Margarine
Stewed prunes	Puffed rice	French toast	Doughnut	Lemon
Banana	Puffed wheat	Omelet of the Day	English muffin	Jelly
	Shredded wheat		White toast	Pancake syrup
	Raisin bran		Wheat toast	
Beverages	All bran		Rye toast	
Coffee	Bran flakes	Whole milk		
Tea		4 oz. whole milk		
Decaffeinated coffee	Cream	Skim milk		
Cocoa	Nondairy creamer	4 oz. skim milk		

Luncheon
Please circle your selections below

Appetizers
Apple juice
Cranberry juice
Tomato juice
Fruit cup
Consomme/chicken/beef
Chicken noodle soup
Vegetable soup
Cream of tomato soup
Cream of chicken soup
Soup du jour

Entrees
Tomato with:
  Chicken salad
  Tuna salad
  Cottage cheese
  Egg salad
Chef's bowl/meat & cheese
Fruit and cottage cheese
Roast beef sandwich
Sliced turkey sandwich
Tuna salad sandwich
Chicken salad sandwich
Egg salad sandwich
Sandwich special
Peanut butter & jelly sandwich
Tuna noodle casserole
Turkey/gravy/dressing
Roast beef au jus
Chicken a la king/toast
Macaroni and cheese
Scrod
Ham/pineapple
Steak/mushrooms
Chicken/cranberry
Fish/chips
Veal parmesan
Grilled cheese/pickle
Veal/gravy
Pork chop/applesauce
Shell macaroni
Beefburger/cheeseburger
Salisbury/gravy
Chef's special

Breads
White Rye Dinner Roll
Wheat Crackers

Beverages
Coffee
Tea
Decaffeinated coffee
Cocoa
Cream
Nondairy creamer
Whole milk
4 oz. whole milk
Skim milk
4 oz. skim milk

Vegetables
Whipped potato
Baked potato
Steak-fried potato
Oven-browned potato
Noodles
Rice
Broccoli
Corn
Spinach
Carrots
Green beans
Beets
Peas
Squash

Salads and dressings
Lettuce/tomato
Tossed greens
Lettuce wedge
Cole slaw
Salad special
Mayonnaise
French dressing
Italian dressing
Thousand island dressing
Creamy Italian
Oil & vinegar
Lemon and vinegar
Sour cream

Desserts
Peaches
Fruit cocktail
Baked apple
Pears
Apricots
Applesauce
Fresh fruit
Dessert of the day
Sugar cookies
Oatmeal cookies
Cupcake
Apple pie
Cheesecake
Shortcake/topping
Chocolate pudding/topping
Butterscotch pudding/
  topping
Tapioca/topping
Sunshine cup
Ice cream
Orange sherbet
Raspberry sherbet
Gelatin
Custard
Eclair
Angel cake

Miscellaneous

Salt	Lemon
Pepper	Jelly
Sugar	Mustard
Sugar substitute	Catsup
Butter	Relish
Margarine	Bran

Dinner
Please circle your selections below

Appetizers
Apple juice
Cranberry juice
Tomato juice
Fruit cup
Consomme/chicken/beef
Chicken noodle soup
Vegetable soup
Cream of tomato soup
Cream of chicken soup
Soup du jour

Entrees
Tomato with:
  Chicken salad
  Tuna salad
  Cottage cheese
  Egg salad
Chef's bowl/meat & cheese
Fruit and cottage cheese
Roast beef sandwich
Sliced turkey sandwich
Tuna salad sandwich
Chicken salad sandwich
Egg salad sandwich
Sandwich special
Peanut butter & jelly sandwich
Tuna noodle casserole
Turkey/gravy/dressing
Roast beef au jus
Chicken a la king/toast
Macaroni and cheese
Scrod
Ham/pineapple
Steak/mushrooms
Chicken/cranberry
Fish/chips
Veal parmesan
Grilled cheese/pickle
Veal/gravy
Pork chop/applesauce
Shell macaroni
Beefburger/cheeseburger
Salisbury/gravy
Chef's special

Breads
White Rye Dinner Roll
Wheat Crackers

Beverages
Coffee
Tea
Decaffeinated coffee
Cocoa
Cream
Nondairy creamer
Whole milk
4 oz. whole milk
Skim milk
4 oz. skim milk

Vegetables
Whipped potato
Baked potato
Steak-fried potato
Oven-browned potato
Noodles
Rice
Broccoli
Corn
Spinach
Carrots
Green beans
Beets
Peas
Squash

Salads and dressings
Lettuce/tomato
Tossed greens
Lettuce wedge
Cole slaw
Salad special
Mayonnaise
French dressing
Italian dressing
Thousand island dressing
Creamy Italian
Oil & vinegar
Lemon and vinegar
Sour cream

Desserts
Peaches
Fruit cocktail
Baked apple
Pears
Apricots
Applesauce
Fresh fruit
Dessert of the day
Sugar cookies
Oatmeal cookies
Cupcake
Apple pie
Cheesecake
Shortcake/topping
Chocolate pudding/topping
Butterscotch pudding/
  topping
Tapioca/topping
Sunshine cup
Ice cream
Orange sherbet
Raspberry sherbet
Gelatin
Custard
Eclair
Angel cake

Miscellaneous

Salt	Lemon
Pepper	Jelly
Sugar	Mustard
Sugar substitute	Catsup
Butter	Relish
Margarine	Bran

Fig. 13.2 Menu for high-fiber diets.

Role Play Situation 1. As a dietetic technician in a large metropolitan hospital, you are asked by a physician to provide a discharge diet for a 52-year-old male with diverticulosis. Follow the guidelines to complete the charts and provide the patient with an individualized diet plan. Prepare a SOAP note which could be recorded in the patient's medical chart.

Role Play Situation 2. A 22-year-old new mother is referred to the out-patient nutrition clinic for dietary guidelines to control colitis and prevent recurrence of hemorrhoids. As the assigned dietetic technician, follow the guidelines to complete the charts and provide the patient with an individualized diet plan. Prepare a SOAP note for insertion in departmental files with a copy to be sent to the referring physician.

Role Play Situation 3. As a dietetic technician in a hospital which participates in an elderly congregate feeding program, you are asked to conduct a short postlunch talk on increasing dietary fiber. Prepare a brief outline and give a 10-minute talk on Let's Get Regular! Prepare a report on the talk for insertion in departmental files. *Note:* In a dining situation, detailed discussion of excretory functions is best kept to a minimum.

STEP 8: POST-TEST ON GASTROINTESTINAL DISORDERS

In order to evaluate your understanding of various common gastrointestinal disorders and the current diet therapies, complete the following Post-test. Sections I and II are the Learning Assessment Quizzes for peptic ulcer disease and high-fiber diets. (If the diet counselor is unable to complete the tests successfully, how can patients be expected to?) Section III incorporates much of the material from this chapter. Answers are given in the Answer Key. Will your patients with ulcers be able to use your nutrition guidelines in order to ease their pain and prevent further flare-ups? Will those requiring an increased fiber intake be able to adjust their diets successfully? How about those needing to restrict their dietary residue or lactose intake? Will your patients be able to learn how to optimize their own physical comfort and enhance overall health using your nutrition guidance?

Sections I and II. Complete the Quizzes for D.A.T. and High-Fiber Counseling in Steps 6 and 7. Check your answers with the Answer Key.

Section III. Indicate whether you think the following statements are true (T) or false (F). Check your answers with the Answer Key.

____ 1. Gastric ulcers occur most frequently in middle-aged males.
____ 2. Decaffeinated coffee is well tolerated by most ulcer patients.
____ 3. Milk is the preferred buffer in treating ulcers.
____ 4. Protein-rich foods do not stimulate gastric acid secretion.
____ 5. Once a poorly tolerated food item is identified, the ulcer patient should avoid it at all times.
____ 6. A high-fiber diet may prove to be effective in the prevention of certain cancers.
____ 7. Colitis commonly occurs in tense individuals with erratic lifestyle patterns and dietary habits.
____ 8. Diverticulitis is initially treated with a high-fiber diet.
____ 9. Treatment for inflamed hemorrhoids includes a high-fluid, low-fiber diet.
____ 10. With hiatus hernia, foods which increase esophageal pressure should be avoided.
____ 11. The terms residue and fiber are interchangeable.
____ 12. Lactose-intolerant individuals must eliminate milk and milk products from the diet.

Select the answer that best completes the following statements and check your answers with the Answer Key.

____ 13. Individuals suffering from peptic ulcers or gastritis may need to avoid
(a) black pepper. (b) red pepper. (c) decaffeinated coffee. (d) chocolate. (e) a and b. (f) all of these.

____ 14. Individuals suffering from hiatus hernia should avoid
(a) citrus juices. (b) large meals. (c) peppermint. (d) french fries. (e) alcoholic beverages. (f) b and e. (g) all of these.

____ 15. Individuals desiring an increase in dietary fiber should
(a) drink 6–8 cups of fluid daily. (b) read labels to ensure that bread and cereal products are 100% whole grain. (c) eat liberal amounts of fruits and vegetables. (d) avoid all refined foods. (e) eat a large amount of unprocessed bran every day. (f) a, b, and c. (g) all of these.

REFERENCE

HAMILTON, E., and WHITNEY, E. 1982. Nutrition—Concepts and Controversies. 2nd edition. St. Paul, MN: Nest Publishing Co.

Chapter Fourteen

Diseases of the Liver, Gallbladder, Pancreas, and Kidney

CHAPTER BLUEPRINT

Step 1: Take the Pre-test on Alcoholism and participate in the assigned group discussion.
Step 2: Examine the Liver Facts List and prepare the assigned handout.
Step 3: Examine the Gallbladder Facts List and prepare the assigned handout.
Step 4: Examine the Pancreas Facts List and prepare the assigned handout.
Step 5: Examine the Kidney Facts List and prepare the assigned handout.
Step 6: Examine the Alcoholism Guidelines and complete the role play assignment.
Step 7: Examine the Low-Fat Guidelines and complete the role play assignment.
Step 8: Examine the Renal Disease Guidelines and complete the role play assignment.
Step 9: Take the Post-test to evaluate what you have learned from the information and activities provided in this chapter.

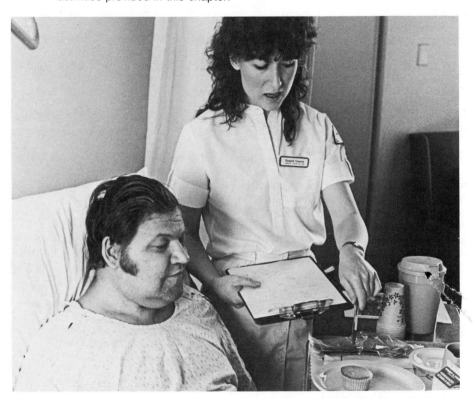

STEP 1: PRE-TEST ON ALCOHOLISM

During the past few decades, significant increases in both drug and alcohol abuse have occurred. There has been a concurrent growth in treatment facilities, therapeutic methodology, and trained substance-abuse counselors. Nutritional repletion measures have been adopted, and the importance of diet during rehabilitation has been recognized.

Use of alcohol for its intoxicating effects has been practiced for centuries. The medical, social, psychological, and nutritional consequences of alcohol abuse, however, have yet to be completely understood. Research has uncovered some important information regarding the psychological and physiological reasons for and side effects of alcohol ingestion—both desirable and undesirable—but much remains to be documented. Alcoholic beverages have been used throughout history, but the personal and social implications have changed.

Alcoholism Identification Signals

1. Frequent episodes of drunkenness (more than once a month).
2. Frequent hangovers or other physical side effects from overindulgence.
3. Interference with work/home/social life due to overindulgence.
4. Marked personality changes during drinking episodes (sometimes with small intakes).
5. Blackouts and/or memory lapses from drinking episodes.
6. Accidents during drinking episodes (car crashes, falling, cigarette burns).
7. "Out of character" behavior during drinking episodes.
8. Psychological dependence on alcohol for stress reduction, companionship, social confidence, or other purposes.
9. Psychological dependence on alcohol for accomplishment of everyday tasks.
10. Physical dependence on alcohol with recognized symptoms of withdrawal upon abstinence.

Suggested Readings on Alcoholism

AHLSTROM-LAAKSO, S. 1975. Drinking Habits Among Alcoholics. New Brunswick, NJ: Rutgers University Center for Alcohol Studies.

BISSELL, L. 1984. Alcoholism in the Professions. New York: Oxford University Press.

COOK, B., GARVEY, M., and SHUKLA, S. 1987. Alcoholism. Primary Care 14, Dec., 685.

DEUTSCH, C. 1982. Broken Bottles, Broken Dreams. New York: Columbia University Teachers College.

DONATELLE, R., DAVIS, L., and HOOVER, C. 1988. Access to Health, pp. 204–227. Englewood Cliffs, NJ: Prentice-Hall.

DUNCAN, D., and GOLD, R. 1982. Drugs and the Whole Person. New York: John Wiley & Sons.

EDWARDS, G., and GRANT, M. (Editors). 1980. Alcoholism Treatment in Transition. Baltimore: University Park Press.

ESTES, N., and HEINEMANN, M. (Editors). 1982. Alcoholism: Development, Consequences, and Interventions. St. Louis: C. V. Mosby Co.

FREE, J. 1977. Just One More. Palo Alto, CA: Bull Publishing Co.

GALLANT, D. 1987. Alcoholism. New York: W. W. Norton.

GOODWIN, D. 1981. Alcoholism: The Facts. New York: Oxford University Press.

GOODWIN, D. 1988. Is Alcoholism Hereditary? New York: Ballantine.

GROSS, L. 1983. How Much Is Too Much: The Effects of Social Drinking. New York: Random House.

HAZELDEN FOUNDATION. 1987. The 12 Steps of Alcoholics Anonymous. New York: Harper/Hazelden.

LUDWIG, A. 1988. Understanding the Alcoholic's Mind. New York: Oxford University Press.

MCCORMICK, R. 1982. Facing Alcoholism. San Diego, CA: Oak Tree Publications.

MILAN, J., and KETCHAM, K. 1981. Under the Influence: A Guide to Myths and Realities of Alcoholism. Seattle: Madrona Publishers.

NATIONAL INSTITUTE ON ALCOHOL ABUSE AND ALCOHOLISM. 1980. Facts About Alcohol and Alcoholism, Publication No. 81-1574. Washington, DC: Government Printing Office.

RIX, K. 1983. Alcohol Problems: A Guide for Nurses and other Health Professionals. Littleton, MA: Wright·PSG.

SCHLAADT, R., and SHANNON, P. 1986. Drugs of Choice, 2nd Edition. Englewood Cliffs, NJ: Prentice-Hall.

SHORE, R., and LUCE, J. 1976. To Your Health: The Pleasures, Problems, and Politics of Alcohol. New York: Seabury Press.

TARTER, R., and SUGARMAN, A. (Editors). 1976. Alcoholism: Interdisciplinary Approaches to an Enduring Problem. Reading, MA: Addison-Wesley.

WOITITZ, J. 1983. Adult Children of Alcoholics. Hollywood, FL: Health Communications, Inc.

ZIMBERG, S. 1982. Understanding Alcoholism. In The Clinical Management of Alcoholism, pp. 3–18. New York: Brunner/Mazel.

For further information:

Al-Anon Family Group Headquarters, PO Box 182, Madison Square Station, New York, NY 10159.

Alcoholics Anonymous, 468 Park Avenue South, New York, NY 10016.

American Council on Alcoholism, 3501 LaSalle Road, Suite 301, Towson, MD 21204.

National Council on Alcoholism, 12 West 21st Street, New York, NY 10017.

National Institute on Alcohol Abuse and Alcoholism, 1100 17th Street NW, Suite 710, Washington, DC 20036.

Keeping in mind the Alcoholism Identification Signals list and the preceding Suggested Readings, complete the Questionnaire on Alcoholism and discuss your answers with classmates or co-workers. As a dietetic technician in nutrition care, it is important for you to understand the psychological aspects underlining an alcohol addiction, and to develop a working knowledge of the physiological implications and related diet therapies.

Questionnaire on Alcoholism

1. List some of the physical and psychological indications and signs of alcoholism.

2. Briefly describe some of the theories about the physical cause(s) of alcoholism.

3. Briefly describe some of the theories about the psychological cause(s) of alcoholism.

4. Describe the role of the dietetics personnel in the treatment of alcoholics.

STEP 2: LIVER DISEASE FACTS

A majority of the cases of chronic liver disease require some specific dietary modifications, and most are influenced by alcohol intake. Nutrition therapy—in addition to abstinence from alcoholic beverages—is essential for complete recovery of health. Hepatitis and cirrhosis are two liver diseases which are treated with essentially the same dietary modifications; both disorders require vitamin and mineral supplementation, avoidance of alcohol, and a nutritionally adequate diet.

The following Liver Facts List provides current diet-related information to include in counseling individuals with alcohol-related liver disease.

Liver Facts List

1. The liver is the largest organ—actually a gland—in the body, and conducts a wide variety of functions (circulatory, metabolic, and **detoxification**) including the production of **bile.** Many of these functions affect nutritional status.

2. The liver is responsible for (a) carbohydrate metabolism—including glucose synthesis, glycogen storage, and blood glucose regulation; (b) protein metabolism—including plasma protein and **urea** formation; (c) fat metabolism—including lipoprotein synthesis and ketone formation; and (d) vitamin and mineral storage—including the fat-soluble vitamins, the B-complex, vitamin C, iron, and copper.

3. The bile produced by the liver is composed of (a) water; (b) bile salts (sodium and potassium); (c) bile pigments (bilirubin and biliverdin); (d) cholesterol, fatty acids, lecithin, fat; and (e) alkaline phosphatase (an enzyme).

4. In liver disease, laboratory tests will indicate the following parameters as elevated:

detoxification: Reduction of the toxic properties of a poison or drug.

bile: Fluid secreted by the liver, concentrated in the gallbladder, and excreted into the small intestine to help in the digestion of fats.

urea: Main nitrogenous compound of urine; the colorless, odorless end product of protein metabolism.

(a) bilirubin (serum, urine); (b) alkaline phosphatase; (c) cholesterol; (d) SGOT (serum glutamic oxalacetic transaminase, an enzyme); and (e) BSP (sulfobromophthalein in Bromsulphalein, a dye used in testing for liver disease).

5. In liver disease, laboratory tests will indicate reductions in the following parameters: (a) prothrombin time (due to decreased production of fibrinogen and prothrombin, the two proteins involved in clotting, also known as clotting factors I and II); and (b) albumin (serum) due to decreased protein synthesis.

6. *Hepatitis* is characterized by inflammation of the liver due to injury to liver cells from toxins or bacterial/viral infection; these cases are either (a) *viral/infectious* via the oral–fecal route—contaminated drinking water, food, or sewage; or (b) *serum* through the use of nonsterile medical instruments or contaminated blood transfusions. Both types of hepatitis have similar clinical manifestations and treatment modes.

7. The symptoms of hepatitis include anorexia, malaise, nausea and vomiting after eating, headache, fever, and after several days the increased circulating bilirubin can cause **jaundice** and darkened urine. The liver becomes enlarged (hepatomegaly), and the spleen may become distended (splenomegaly). The amazing regenerative powers of the liver lead to rapid recovery, usually in only 6–8 weeks.

8. Treatment of hepatitis focuses on bed rest. Diet therapy provides high-calorie, high-quality protein meals, with vitamin/mineral supplementation if required. Alcohol use is prohibited.

9. The diet is high enough in protein to allow for the regeneration of damaged tissue, yet not so high as to cause **hepatic coma,** and calories are increased to counteract catabolism, weight loss, and impaired metabolism. Carbohydrate intake is liberal, and fat should be consumed in moderate amounts. With ascites and edema, sodium intake is restricted.

10. *Cirrhosis* is end-stage liver injury, with **fibrosis** of the connective tissue gradually replacing the degenerating liver cells to cause loss of liver function. Most often found in chronic alcoholics, cirrhosis can also occur with malnutrition, **biliary** obstruction, infectious hepatitis, poisons, drugs, congestive heart failure, and atherosclerosis. Alcohol abuse first results in **steatosis;** the accompanying malnutrition can be due to nutrient malabsorption, decreased hepatic storage of nutrients, disturbances in nutrient metabolism, and poor dietary habits.

11. The symptoms of cirrhosis include anorexia, nausea, vomiting, abdominal pain and distention, and—if the biliary tract is involved—jaundice. Impairment of the circulation causes hypertension, **esophageal varices,** abdominal varicose veins, ascites, and edema. With esophageal varices, food intake may be limited, requiring tube feedings or a liquid diet advancing to small, frequent feedings and avoidance of irritating foods.

12. Nutritional assessment in cirrhosis is difficult: body weight is altered due to the presence of edema, while protein status is difficult to determine because plasma proteins are decreased but enzyme activity (of serum ribonuclease) is elevated.

13. Protein should be of high biological value, but intake is restricted in the presence of hepatic coma. Hepatic coma can develop with serious liver disease if the **ammonia** buildup enters the cerebral circulation; treatment includes medication to decrease ammonia production and temporary restriction in high-quality protein. Fat may need to be modified if biliary obstruction occurs. Hematocrit and hemoglobin may become depressed, and decreased nutrient absorption leads to low serum levels of folic acid, vitamin B_{12}, and pyridoxine, resulting in various anemias. Acute alcohol intake can actually increase iron absorption which, in combination with high-iron wines, can aggravate liver damage.

14. The most common form of cirrhosis is *Laennec's cirrhosis,* which is usually associated with alcohol abuse; a number of normal metabolic activities are disturbed which causes formation of scar tissue, accumulation of fat, portal hypertension, vitamin deficiencies (particularly of thiamin), and **delirium tremens,** as well as the usual cirrhotic symptoms of ascites, edema, esophageal varices, hepatomegaly, jaundice, etc.

15. It has been estimated that there are over ten million alcoholics in America today, and although the majority tend to consume inadequate diets, proper nutrition offers no protection against the **hepatotoxic** effects of alcohol excess.

16. For unknown reasons, only a small percentage of alcoholics develop cirrhosis, and significantly excessive quantities of alcohol must be consumed before any evidence of liver damage occurs.

---

jaundice: Condition characterized by yellowed skin from excess bilirubin in the blood.

hepatic coma: Condition in which impaired liver function causes accumulation of those products in the blood which are usually metabolized by the liver, resulting in impaired speech, stupor, and coma.

fibrosis: An abnormal formation of fibrous tissue.

biliary: Pertaining to bile.

steatosis: Fatty degeneration.

esophageal varices: Twisted enlarged veins in the esophagus.

ammonia: Gas formed by protein or amino acid breakdown.

delirium tremens: Disorder characterized by hallucinations; usually occurs during alcohol withdrawal.

hepatotoxin: Substance which is specifically poisonous for liver cells.

17. Alcohol is directly toxic to other tissues in addition to the liver, and the synergism of malnutrition and alcoholism is still under research.

18. Much of the liver toxicity from alcohol is due to the accumulation of **NADH,** acetate, and acetaldehyde, the poisonous by-products of alcohol metabolism.

NADH: Reduced form of the enzyme nicotinamide adenine dinucleotide.

19. Alcoholics are one of the few populations in this country in which multiple nutritional deficiencies are common—with the accompanying neurological manifestations of **polyneuropathy, Wernicke–Korsakoff syndrome,** nutritional **amblyopia, pellagra,** and other relatively rare ills. Alcohol abusers are especially prone to vitamin B deficiencies.

polyneuropathy: Disorder affecting the nerves caused by disease, nutritional deficiencies, and/or chronic alcoholism.

20. Chronic alcohol abuse can cause other diet-related disorders including loss of appetite, gastritis, decreased release of pancreatic enzymes, diminished fat absorption, and altered nutrient absorption; hyperuricemia, hypoglycemia, gout, and diabetes can occur.

Wernicke–Korsakoff syndrome: Condition characterized by loss of memory, disorientation, confabulation, and hallucinations; occurs secondary to alcoholism.

21. Alcoholics may have decreased plasma levels of zinc, calcium, magnesium, plus low stores of potassium, retention of sodium and water, and prolonged prothrombin time necessitating intramuscular injections of vitamin K. Abnormalities in the status of other nutrients are currently under investigation.

amblyopia: Dimmed vision.

22. Routine iron supplementation in alcoholics is inadvisable, as deficiencies are uncommon (possibly occurring with gastrointestinal bleeding or chronic infections); use of iron supplements can mask other, more common anemias, and may contribute to an undesirably high iron intake with the threat of **hematochromatosis.**

pellagra: Disease caused by niacin deficiency, characterized by diarrhea and rough, patchy skin, and resulting in death; often occurs secondary to alcoholism.

23. Small, frequent feedings may prove to be more acceptable to the individual recovering from alcoholism, and will be more efficiently digested and absorbed; meals should be as tasteful, and mealtimes as pleasant as possible in order to combat anorexia and loss of interest in eating a variety of foods.

hematochromatosis: Abnormal, excessive iron deposits in tissues from blood or dietary intakes.

24. Although moderate alcohol intake may have cardiovascular benefits, alcohol abuse can lead to elevated serum cholesterol and/or triglyceride levels, thereby unmasking subclinical hyperlipoproteinemias.

25. Fetal alcohol syndrome is currently emerging as the most prevalent cause of mental impairment in the Western world; the liver is not the only organ which can be seriously damaged by alcohol abuse, and the alcohol user is not the only organism to be adversely affected (see p. 100).

26. The success of dietary treatment for recovering alcoholics can be enhanced by familial involvement and support.

Exercise on Diet Counseling for Liver Disease

Keeping in mind the preceding Liver Facts List, which provides current diet-related information to include in counseling individuals with liver disease, prepare a simplified version for use as a patient handout. You may include graphics and/or prepare in a poster format, if desired; see the Sample Handout. Show your handout in rough draft form to classmates or co-workers for constructive criticism on the overall design, content, and potential effectiveness for use in pertinent diet counseling situations. Then prepare a final version for your own future use as a practicing dietetic technician.

Sample Handout

Hints to Help Your Recovery from Alcoholism

1. First, note that alcohol abuse can lead to significant changes in eating patterns and health including the following:

○ Strong preference for concentrated carbohydrates/sweets
○ Avoidance of meat
○ Reliance on large daily consumption of caffeine
○ Increase in weight without increase in food intake
○ Gastritis

2. Eat a well-balanced diet that includes a variety of foods chosen from the Basic Food Groups.

3. Eat regular meals and snacks. Avoid skipping meals, including breakfast.
4. Exercise regularly.
5. If you are overweight, it is best to reduce your intake of high-fat foods and rich sweets and to be moderate in portion size for other foods regularly eaten. Cravings for sweets can be quelled with fresh fruits and their juices, chocolate-flavored milk, and artificially sweetened soft drinks or mints.
6. If you need to gain weight, increase the portion sizes of foods from each of the Basic Food Groups. You may want to try commercial dietary supplements as high-calorie snacks.
7. Large quantities of caffeine can contribute to gastritis and nervousness. Decaffeinated coffee and tea can be substituted.
8. Avoid hidden sources of alcohol in "over-the-counter" medicinal products such as cough and cold remedies, mouthwashes, etc. Also, check with your physician before taking *any* medication.

STEP 3: GALLBLADDER DISEASE FACTS

cholecystitis: Inflammation of the gallbladder.

cholelithiasis: Presence of stones in the gallbladder or adjoining duct.

cholecystectomy: Removal of the gallbladder.

Because dietary fat stimulates the gallbladder to contract and secrete bile, disorders in this organ—such as **cholecystitis, cholelithiasis,** and immediate pre/post-**cholecystectomy**—require fat restriction in order to prevent postprandial irritation and pain. Food intolerances specific for those with gallbladder disease do not exist, but individual dietary intolerances need to be identified and controlled.

The following Gallbladder Facts List provides current diet-related information to include in counseling individuals with gallbladder disorders.

Gallbladder Facts List

1. The gallbladder stores and concentrates bile, and rests full and immobile between feedings.

2. Upon stimulation by the hormone cholecystokinin, which is secreted from the intestinal mucosa in the presence of food, the gallbladder contracts and releases bile into the common bile duct to enter the duodenum. The amount of bile that is released is appropriate for handling the quantity of fat present.

3. *Cholecystitis* is characterized by inflammation of the gallbladder due to infection or abnormalities in function, and is common during pregnancy and with obesity. Cholecystitis usually occurs due to the obstruction of the cystic duct with gallstones.

epigastric: Pertaining to the region over the pit of the stomach.

4. Symptoms of cholecystitis include **epigastric** pain, nausea, vomiting, flatulence, and indigestion, especially after consumption of large, high-fat meals. Control of symptoms includes a low-fat, nonirritating diet.

5. *Cholelithiasis* develops from an infection or with changes in the composition of bile, and may be influenced by heredity, sex (females are more prone), diet (including alcohol intake), and body weight (the obese are more susceptible); the stones are primarily composed of cholesterol, bilirubin, and calcium, with a small percentage composed of crystalline cholesterol.

6. Although gallstones can be present for years without major symptoms, the most common complication occurs when a stone leaves the gallbladder and lodges in the common bile duct to block bile flow; obstructive jaundice and liver damage can result, and biliary colic causes extreme pain. After severe symptoms reside, surgery can be performed.

7. Gallstones are more common in overweight women (often postpregnancy) and in those over age 35, so the symptom cluster is sometimes referred to as "the three Fs" (female, fat, and forty).

8. Treatment for cholelithiasis includes drugs, surgery, and individualized dietary regimens; diet as tolerated is advisable to uncover individual intolerances—many sufferers seem to react unfavorably to the intake of rich foods, fatty products, and chocolate. Since fat stimulates the gallbladder to contract, a low-fat diet is recommended prior to gallbladder surgery. For several months after cholecystectomy, a low-fat diet, with a gradual increase in fat content, is advised.

9. Feedings are best tolerated if divided into small, frequent meals and snacks.

10. Alcohol is usually restricted with cholecystitis and cholelithiasis.

11. Vitamin/mineral supplements should be individually prescribed; since bile salts are necessary for the absorption of fat-soluble vitamins, diet after cholecystectomy should include adequate amounts of these nutrients.

12. Overweight individuals should attain and maintain a reasonable weight.

Exercise on Diet Counseling for Gallbladder Disease

Keeping in mind the preceding Gallbladder Facts List, which provides some of the most current diet-related information to include in counseling individuals with gallbladder disorders, prepare a simplified version for use as a patient handout. You may include graphics and/or prepare in a poster format, if desired; see the Sample Handout. Show your handout in rough draft form to classmates or co-workers for constructive criticism on the overall design, content, and potential effectiveness for use in pertinent diet counseling situations. Then prepare a final version for your own future use as a practicing dietetic technician.

Sample Handout

Fat Restricted Diet

Foods to avoid:

Avocado; any fruits or vegetables in sauces with added fat or cream.

Any grains prepared with added cream sauces; corn chips or potato chips; fried breads or potatoes; commercial bakery goods or mixes.

Canned, dehydrated, or whole milk; milk drinks prepared with whole milk, chocolate, cream, ice cream, or egg yolk; whole milk yogurt; all cheeses except for low-fat varieties.

Fried or fatty meats, brisket, sausage, duck, goose, frankfurters, luncheon meats (canned or packaged); oil-packed fish; any meats or fish prepared with added fat, cream sauces, or gravies (unless fat free); eggs prepared with cream sauces or added fat; dried beans or peas in pork fat; commercial peanut butter with added fat.

Any sweets prepared with chocolate, coconut, nuts, or other foods listed above.

Other restrictions:

Beverages should not contain whole milk, cream, or alcohol.
Fats should be limited to 3 servings daily:

1 serving = 1 tsp: Margarine, shortening, oil, mayonnaise, butter
1 serving = 1 Tbsp: Salad dressing, cream (whipping, half and half, light),
                       cream cheese
1 serving = 2 Tbsp: Whipped topping, whipped cream, and sour cream

Note: Include the recommended number of daily servings from the Basic Food Groups. Food is better tolerated if eaten in small amounts several times daily. Try to plan menus to include five or six light meal/snacks each day. If you are overweight, it is advisable to reach and maintain a reasonable weight. See your dietitian/dietetic technician for an individualized diet plan.

STEP 4: PANCREATITIS FACTS

Inflammation of the pancreas (pancreatitis) requires an individualized diet that is low in fat, moderate in protein, and given in small, frequent feedings. All alcoholic beverages and any foods that stimulate pancreatic activity should be avoided. Oftentimes, recovery leads to increased dietary tolerance.

The following Pancreas Facts List provides current diet-related information to include in counseling individuals with pancreatitis.

Pancreas Facts List

exocrine: External secretion of a gland.

1.   The pancreas is a large gland which produces the hormone insulin and provides **exocrine** secretions to aid digestion in the small intestine; pancreatic enzymes aid in the digestion of carbohydrate, protein, and fat.

2.   Pancreatitis is characterized by inflammation of pancreatic tissue due to the presence of stones in the common bile duct or a backflow of pancreatic secretions and bile into the pancreas.

3.   Symptoms of chronic pancreatitis include bouts of pain in the upper abdomen, which range from moderate to severe and last for several hours or days; jaundice is common and, depending on severity, other symptoms may occur including weight loss, steatorrhea, malabsorption, diabetes, and pancreatic calcification. Chronic pancreatitis sometimes develops following diseases of the gallbladder.

hemorrhage: Bleeding due to injury.

4.   Acute pancreatitis occurs when chronic pancreatitis results in **hemorrhage** into the gland, and diet is usually NPO until pain subsides.

5.   Treatment for chronic pancreatitis includes restriction of fat intake and moderation in protein consumption, since the presence of these nutrients in the small intestine stimulates pancreatic secretions. Protein is gradually added to the diet as tolerated, with fat restriction continued until steatorrhea disappears.

6.   Feedings should be divided into small frequent meals and snacks.

7.   Stimulants such as caffeine and nicotine may need to be restricted.

8.   Pancreatic function can be altered by acute or chronic alcohol abuse, so treatment includes restricted alcohol intake. Glucose intolerance can occur, possibly due to a reduction in the number of glucose-responsive pancreatic cells caused by chronic intakes of alcohol.

9.   Pancreatic extracts are sometimes prescribed during treatment; the use of self-prescribed "health" food extracts should be avoided—by both healthy individuals and those with pancreatitis.

Exercise on Diet Counseling for Pancreatitis

Keeping in mind the preceding Pancreas Facts List, which provides some of the most current diet-related information to include in counseling individuals with pancreatitis, prepare a simplified version for use as a patient handout. You may include graphics and/or prepare in a poster format, if desired; see the Sample Handout. Show your handout in rough draft form to classmates or co-workers for constructive criticism on the overall design, content, and potential effectiveness for use in pertinent diet counseling sessions. Then prepare a final version for your own future use as a practicing dietetic technician.

Sample Handout

Fat Restricted Diet

Foods to avoid:

Avocado; any fruits or vegetables in sauces with added fat or cream.

Any grains prepared with added cream sauces; corn chips or potato chips; fried breads or potatoes; commercial bakery goods or mixes.

Canned, dehydrated, or whole milk; milk drinks prepared with whole milk, chocolate, cream, ice cream, or egg yolk; whole milk yogurt; all cheeses except for low-fat varieties.

Fried or fatty meats, brisket, sausage, duck, goose, frankfurters, luncheon meats (canned and packaged); oil-packed fish; any meats or fish prepared with added fat, cream sauces, or gravies (unless fat free); eggs prepared with cream sauces or added fat; dried beans or peas in pork fat; commercial peanut butter with added fat.

Any sweets prepared with chocolate, coconut, nuts, or other foods listed above.

Other restrictions:

Beverages should not contain whole milk, cream, or alcohol.
Fats should be limited to 3 servings daily:

1 serving = 1 tsp: Margarine, shortening, oil, mayonnaise, butter
1 serving = 1 Tbsp: Salad dressing, cream (whipping, half and half, light),
                        cream cheese
1 serving = 2 Tbsp: Whipped topping, whipped cream, and sour cream

Note: Include the recommended number of servings from the Basic Food Groups; minimize your servings from the Milk and Cheeses Group and the Meat and Alternates Group, with gradual increases as condition improves. Divide your daily food intake into five or six small meals or snacks. See your dietitian/dietetic technician for an individualized diet plan.

STEP 5: KIDNEY DISEASE FACTS

Serious kidney disorders, such as acute and chronic **renal** failure or acute **glomerulonephritis,** require careful dietary control. The diet must be individualized, flexible, and carefully regulated to meet specific nutrient needs—especially for protein, sodium, potassium, and fluid.

renal: Pertaining to the kidney.

glomerulonephritis: Inflammation of the blood vessels of the kidney; frequently occurs secondary to other infections.

The following Kidney Facts List provides current diet-related information to include in counseling individuals with renal disease.

Kidney Facts List

1. The kidney is the body's major excretory organ, capable of excreting all wastes except for carbon dioxide, and second only to the liver in diversity of function. Functions of the kidney include (a) removal of wastes from the bloodstream, such as metabolic end products (urea, uric acid, **creatinine,** ammonia), some toxic substances, and excess mineral salts (calcium, chloride, magnesium, phosphate, oxalate, potassium, sodium sulfate); (b) reabsorption of needed substances and excretion of those that are toxic or present in excess amounts; (c) maintenance of fluid balance and regulation of blood pressure; (d) maintenance of body pH; (e) stimulation of red blood cell production; and (f) conversion of inactive vitamin D to the active form.

creatinine: Nonproteinous constituent of blood and urine; a breakdown product of creatine.

2. The kidneys can effectively regulate the body's physiological state and handle all of the essential nutrients. With diminished renal function, the kidneys are no longer able to eliminate the multitude of wastes which result from an unrestricted diet.

3. Serum elevation of nitrogenous constituents such as urea and creatinine can indicate renal disease; serum urea nitrogen (SUN) measurements are used more often than the blood urea nitrogen (BUN) levels. **Proteinuria and hematuria** can also be indicative of renal dysfunction.

proteinuria: Albumin in the urine.

hematuria: Blood in the urine.

parenchyma: Functional part of an organ.

4. Renal diseases are either primary, involving **parenchymal** structures of the kidney, or secondary to other diseases such as **systemic lupus erythematosus,** diabetes, **Wilson's disease,** and **septic** shock.

systemic lupus erythematosus: Chronic inflammatory disease affecting the connective tissue (i.e., skin, joints, nerves, etc.) which occurs most commonly in young females; cause is unknown.

5. The primary dietary goal with kidney disease is to achieve optimal nutritional status by minimizing protein catabolism and maintaining fluid and electrolyte balance through altered intake of water (including the water found in foods), protein, calories, sodium, potassium, phosphorus and calcium; all of these nutrients need not be altered for each individual, so dietary individualization is important.

Wilson's disease: Hereditary disorder in which excessive amounts of copper are absorbed and accumulate in certain organs (brain, kidney, liver, eyes).

6. Renal dysfunction can appear as nephrotic syndrome, nephrosclerosis, acute or chronic glomerulonephritis, or acute or chronic renal failure.

septic: Pertaining to the presence of disease-causing bacteria in the blood stream.

7. *Nephrotic syndrome* is a group of symptoms that can occur secondary to other diseases such as glomerulonephritis, or in response to the ingestion of toxins, but frequently appears in children without any apparent cause. Symptoms include edema, **albuminuria, hypoalbuminemia,** hypercholesterolemia, hyperlipidemia, and hypertension, and can lead

albuminuria: Presence of protein in the urine.

hypoalbuminemia: Inadequate amount of protein in the blood.

dialysis: Process of removing toxic substances from blood when kidney function is impaired.

glomerular filtration rate (GFR): Specific speed at which the kidney is continuously filtering toxic wastes from the blood.

uremia: Retention in the blood of toxic wastes usually excreted by the kidney.

glomeruli: Clusters of blood vessels found in the kidney.

oliguria: Diminished urine formation.

azotemia: Excessive amount of urea in the blood.

anuria: Absence of urine.

hyperkalemia: Excessive amount of potassium in the blood.

nephron: Functional unit of the kidney.

pyuria: Presence of pus in the urine.

cylinduria: Presence of twisted casts in the urine.

retinopathy: Disorder of the retina of the eye.

purpura: Condition characterized by multiple hemorrhages in skin, internal organs, and other tissues.

pruritis: Itching.

to serious renal disease requiring **dialysis** or transplant. If the **glomerular filtration rate (GFR)** is normal, diet should be high in calories and protein, but with diminished GFR, protein should be restricted and of high quality; sodium and cholesterol restrictions may also be required.

8. *Nephrosclerosis* occurs most frequently in older persons due to arteriosclerosis and hypertension, and is also known as malignant hypertension; treatment focuses on decreasing elevated blood pressure and preventing the progressively fatal **uremia.**

9. *Acute glomerulonephritis* is characterized by inflammation of the **glomeruli,** usually due to infection. Symptoms include hematuria, albuminuria, **oliguria, azotemia,** edema, and hypertension. If SUN levels are elevated, protein intake is restricted and calories are derived mainly from carbohydrate; with edema and/or hypertension, sodium intake may be restricted, and fluid intake is carefully regulated if oliguria occurs.

10. *Chronic glomerulonephritis* can develop when acute glomerulonephritis fails to heal and becomes latent/subacute with fibrotic and hyalinized glomeruli; renal insufficiency leads to the symptoms of proteinuria, edema, hypertension, and nocturia, and renal failure may occur. Protein intake is restricted (severely if uremia occurs) and sodium intake is modified to reduce the kidney workload, edema, and hypertension.

11. *Acute renal failure* can result from glomerulonephritis, severe burns, injuries or infections, ingestion of toxic agents, shock, surgery, heart attack, and obstructions in either blood flow to the kidney or urine flow out of the kidney. During renal failure, the kidney loses all excretory capacity, resulting in oliguria or **anuria,** and the excretory products (urea, uric acid, creatinine) are retained in the bloodstream; sodium and water retention also occur. Treatment includes restrictions in the intakes of nitrogen/protein, potassium, phosphate, and sulfate by keeping dietary protein low, monitoring of sodium and fluid intakes, with gradual dietary liberalization based on SUN levels, and on serum creatinine, potassium, and sodium levels.

12. In acute renal failure, adequate energy is required to support basal metabolic needs, reduce protein breakdown, and prevent ketosis; protein intake should be restricted, fluid and electrolyte imbalance corrected, **hyperkalemia** controlled, and phosphate levels monitored.

13. *Chronic renal failure* may progress slowly and asymptomatically for years, with a gradual decline in the number of functioning **nephrons** and loss of the ability to excrete waste products and balance body fluids and electrolytes. This leads to a decrease in the GFR, with increased plasma levels of SUN, uric acid, and creatinine, as well as altered metabolism of sodium, phosphate, calcium, potassium, and glucose; the net result is acidosis and the terminal stage of uremia. Symptoms of chronic renal failure include proteinuria, **pyuria, cylinduria,** with urine of low specific gravity, anorexia, nausea, vomiting, constipation and diarrhea, as well as hypertension and anemia. Arteriosclerotic and hypertensive **retinopathy,** skin infections, **purpura,** and **pruritis** may also occur.

14. Dietary treatment of chronic renal failure includes restricted protein intake (limited to high-quality protein, with use of special low-protein breads), careful control of fluid, sodium, and potassium, plus adequate calories to prevent breakdown in body tissue. Chronic renal failure can be managed by such dietary manipulation and dialysis, or by renal transplant.

15. The primary dietary problem in renal failure is determining the ideal amount of protein for positive nitrogen balance. As renal function declines, protein intake must also be reduced; at least two thirds of the protein should be of high quality, served at each meal to enhance the quality of poorer proteins. Diets prescribed for chronic renal failure are highly restrictive, unappealing, and complex, which makes adherence difficult.

16. The Giordano–Giovanetti diet can produce significant reductions in both uremic symptoms and blood urea, but adequate amounts of calories as carbohydrate and fat are difficult to provide; the primary source of protein is a powdered amino acid mixture or egg, with the remainder of the caloric intake limited to sugar, honey, jelly, unsalted butter, vegetable oils, and special low-protein starches. Fortunately, less restrictive diets may elicit a similar amelioration of uremic symptoms in some individuals, with far better patient adherence.

17.   In chronic renal failure, the less serious stages require a low sodium intake (if hypertension is present), fluid control, and potassium monitoring; the onset of azotemia requires protein restriction, with sodium, potassium, phosphorus and fluid intakes dependent on individual needs. Terminal or end-stage uremia may require the use of a low-protein plan (e.g., Giordano–Giovannetti diet) with the intake of other nutrients limited to the amounts determined individually; multi-vitamin supplements are usually prescribed. Dialysis can help to liberalize the diet.

18.   Whenever the diet contains less than 40 grams of protein, vitamin/mineral supplementation may be required; supplementary vitamin A and magnesium are generally not recommended in renal disease.

19.   Long-term chronic renal failure can lead to renal **osteodystrophy,** a process which can be slowed with a high-calcium/low-phosphorus diet, calcium supplementation, and phosphorus-binding gels (aluminum gels interfere with phosphorus absorption by binding the nutrient in the gastrointestinal tract).

osteodystrophy: Abnormal bone formation.

20.   Hyperkalemia is an ever-present danger and a common cause of death in patients with chronic renal failure, but does not occur unless the GFR (see item 7) is severely compromised or sodium restriction is severe. However, unnecessarily large intakes of potassium-rich foods and the use of potassium-sparing diuretics or drugs high in potassium should be avoided.

21.   Patients with advanced renal disease appear to tolerate hyperkalemia better than healthy individuals, but if serum potassium rises too rapidly or reaches an extremely high level, potassium intoxication can occur, causing cardiac arrhythmias and ultimately cardiac arrest.

22.   Magnesium-containing laxatives or antacids should be avoided with renal insufficiency, as magnesium excretion is impaired and an excess can result in **hypermagnesemia;** symptoms include **hypotension** and respiratory paralysis.

hypermagnesemia: Excessive amount of magnesium in the blood.

hypotension: Below normal blood pressure.

23.   Even though glucose intolerance occurs frequently in renal disease, carbohydrate intake is usually not restricted and concentrated sweets may be well tolerated, even by diabetics.

24.   Hyperlipidemias and vascular disease are common complications of chronic renal failure, partially due to the high fat-calorie intake. Dehydration also occurs frequently with imbalances in fluids and electrolytes, as does overhydration; weight loss, lethargy, and oliguria can indicate a possible need for increased sodium or water, while hypertension, weight gain, and edema may be indicative of the need to reduce intake of these nutrients.

25.   During dialysis, nitrogenous compounds, some vitamins, and other water-soluble nutrients can be lost, and less iron is incorporated into red blood cells; with dietary restriction as well, nutritional status can become significantly impaired.

26.   Successful renal transplantation erases the need for dietary restrictions (except in patients who develop hypertriglyceridemia). But, despite the great advances in technology (including the development of dialysis, as well as kidney transplantation), nutrition support and diet therapy continue to serve as integral components of renal disease treatments.

27.   In renal diseases, the diet is not static and must change with the different stages of the individual disease.

28.   Renal **calculi**—a common ailment in the United States—can be found anywhere along the urinary tract, often asymptomatically; stones can damage the kidney by causing pressure **necrosis,** obstruction, or infection. Renal calculi appear as one of the following:

calculi: Stones.

necrosis: Destruction and death of body tissue.

○   Calcium stones.   The majority of renal stones contain calcium and are due to hyperparathyroidism, excessive vitamin D intakes, milk–alkali syndrome in peptic ulcer treatment, prolonged immobilization, or **ideopathic hypercalcuria;** these stones are composed of calcium oxalate, calcium phosphate, or a mixture of both. Calcium oxalate stones occur with an excessive intake of high-oxalate foods (such as vegetable greens, chocolate, and cocoa; see also Table 14.1) or due to congenital oxaluria. Treatment includes high fluid intake, sometimes a low-calcium diet, and an acid ash diet to render urine acidic in order to dissolve the calcium stones (which are insoluble in an alkaline pH).

ideopathic: Pertaining to disorders of unknown origin.

hypercalcuria: Excessive amount of calcium in the urine.

○   Uric acid stones.   A small percentage of renal stones are composed of uric acid, an end product of purine metabolism; drug treatment may be combined with a low-purine diet (see Table 14.1) and restricted alcohol consumption. Fluid intake should be generous.

○   **Cystine** stones.   A small percentage of renal stones are due to **cystinuria,** a genetically determined disorder, and can be treated with an alkaline ash diet which is low in methionine (see Table 14.1) to render urine alkaline in order to dissolve the cystine stones (which are insoluble in an acidic urine). Fluid intake should be generous.

Table 14.1   Foods to Avoid[a]

High in oxalates		High in purines	High in methionine
Rhubarb	Almonds	Organ meats	Milk and milk products
Spinach	Cashews	Anchovies	Cheeses
Swiss chard	Chocolate	Meat extracts	Eggs
Dandelion, beet, and	Cocoa	Gravies	Fish
collard greens		Sardines	Certain fruits and vege-
Asparagus			tables
Cranberries			

[a]See Appendix IV for recommended acid ash and alkaline ash diets.

29.   Renal calculi can be removed surgically, or may be passed spontaneously via medicinal use and/or dietary manipulations. There is no general agreement, however, as to the overall effectiveness of dietary treatment.

30.   A low-carbohydrate diet can lead to kidney problems from a buildup of nitrogen and overworked kidneys; crash diets may precipitate renal stones. Megadoses of vitamin C may aggravate gout and elevate uric acid levels to precipitate the condition in predisposed individuals; large doses of zinc can cause renal failure. Thus, a lifetime of sensible dietary habits is important in the maintenance of renal health.

Note: Protein is the only major food constituent containing nitrogen (1 g/6.25 g of protein); 80–90% is excreted in the urine as urea, 4–5% as creatinine, 3% as ammonia, and 1–2% as uric acid. When the kidneys fail, the nitrogenous end products are improperly excreted, necessitating protein restriction in accordance with monitoring of laboratory data and clinical conditions.

Exercise on Diet Counseling for Kidney Disease

Keeping in mind the preceding Kidney Facts List, which provides some of the most current diet-related information to include in counseling individuals with renal disease, prepare a simplified version for use as a patient handout. You may include graphics and/or prepare in a poster format, if desired; see the Sample Handout. Show your handout in rough draft form to classmates or co-workers for constructive criticism on the overall design, content, and potential effectiveness for use in pertinent diet counseling situations. Then prepare a final version for your own future use as a practicing dietetic technician.

Sample Handout

Table 14.2 lists good sources of potassium.

Table 14.2   Foods (A) High and (B) Relatively High in Potassium

A.	Fruits (and their juices)[a]		Vegetables (and their juices)[a]	
	Apricots	Melons—cantaloupe,	Artichokes	Mushrooms
	Bananas	casaba, honeydew	Carrots	Parsnips
	Berries—elderberries,	Nectarines	Celery	Potatoes
	raspberries, straw-	Oranges	Dark green, leafy vegeta-	Rhubarb
	berries	Papayas	bles—beet greens, chicory,	Squash, winter
	Currants	Peaches	collards, dandelion greens,	Tomatoes
	Dried fruits—apricots,		kale, mustard greens,	
	dates, figs, peaches,		parsley, spinach, Swiss	
	prunes, raisins		chard	

B.	Breads and Cereals[b]	Milk and Cheeses[b]	Meats and Alternates[b]		Others[b]
	Bran	Low-sodium milk	Dried beans and peas		Chocolate, cocoa
	Oatmeal		Peanuts, other nuts		Coconut
	Pumpernickel bread				Coffee
					Molasses
					Salt substitutes
					(containing potassium)

[a]Listed foods are high in potassium.
[b]Listed foods are higher in potassium than other foods in each of these Groups.

STEP 6: ALCOHOLISM GUIDELINES

Although the many different diseases and disorders resulting from alcoholism have specific nutritional implications and require varying dietary prescriptions, there are some general guidelines to follow in educating the recovering alcoholic. The primary emphasis is on a well-balanced and calorically adequate diet, with special attention to those nutrients commonly found in short supply when alcohol intake is excessive. Used in moderation, alcoholic beverages can enhance eating enjoyment, but if abused, alcohol can wreak nutritional havoc.

In order to be able to advise those individuals recovering from alcoholism on the adoption of desirable dietary patterns, it is essential to have access to all of the hands-on material required for effective counseling sessions. It is also important to be able to record all of the pertinent information regarding each diet counseling session in the patient's medical charts. The information provided below should help to improve your confidence—and skills—regarding your counseling abilities.

This step includes suggested strategies to use in counseling recovering alcoholics on improving nutritional status. The following references may prove helpful.

Suggested Readings on Alcoholism and Recovery Diets

AMERICAN DIETETIC ASSOCIATION. 1981. Handbook of Clinical Dietetics. New Haven, CT: Yale University Press.

BARNES, H., ARONSON, M., and DELBANCO, T. (Editors). 1987. Pathophysiology and medical complications. In Alcoholism: A Guide for the Primary Care Physician, pp. 111–158. New York: Springer-Verlag.

CASTELLI, W. 1979. How many drinks a day? J. Am. Med. Assoc. 242, Nov. 2, 2000.

CLARK, P., and KRICKA, L. 1980. Medical Consequences of Alcohol Abuse. New York: Halsted Press.

EISENSTEIN, A. 1982. Nutritional and metabolic effects of alcohol. J. Am. Dietet. Assoc. *81,* Sept., 247.

EVANS, D., WILLET, W., and HENNEKENS, C. 1980. Alcohol and coronary heart disease. Amer. Heart J. *100,* Oct., 584.

EVIAS, I. (Editor). 1988. The Liver: Biology and Pathobiology. New York: Raven Press.

HALL, P. (Editor). 1985. Alcoholic Liver Disease. New York: John Wiley & Sons.

HALPERN, S. 1987. Quick Reference to Clinical Nutrition, 2nd Edition. Philadelphia: J. B. Lippincott Co.

HENNEKENS, C., et al. 1979. Effects of beer, wine, and liquor in coronary deaths. J. Am. Med. Assoc. *242,* Nov. 2, 1979.

HODGES, R. 1980. Nutrition in Medical Practice. Philadelphia: W. B. Saunders Co.

HOLM, E., and KASPER, H. (Editors). 1984. Metabolism and Nutrition in Liver Disease. Hingham, MA: MTP Press.

HURLEY, R., and GALLAGER-ALLRED, C. 1980. Dietary Management for Alcoholic Patients. Columbus: Ohio State University College of Medicine.

LIEBER, C. 1982. Medical Disorders of Alcoholism. Philadelphia: W. B. Saunders Co.

LIEBER, C. 1988. The influence of alcohol on nutritional status. Nutrition Rev. *46,* Jul., 241.

MACDONALD, J. 1982. Moderate amounts of alcoholic beverages and clinical nutrition. J. Nutr. Educ. *14,* Jun., 58.

MAJCKVOWICZ, E., and NOBLE, E. (Editors). 1980. Biochemistry and Pharmacology of Ethanol. New York: Plenum Press.

MERLI, M., et al. 1987. Optimal nutritional indexes in chronic liver disease. J. Parenteral/Enteral Nutr. *11,* Sept./Oct., 130-S.

MEZEY, E. 1986. Alcohol abuse and digestive diseases. Alcohol Health/Res. World *10,* Winter, 6.

MEZEY, E., et al. 1988. Alcohol and dietary intake in the development of chronic pancreatic and liver disease in alcoholism. Amer. J. Clin. Nutr. *48,* Jul., 148.

NATIONAL INSTITUTE ON ALCOHOL ABUSE AND ALCOHOLISM. 1984. The fifth special report to Congress on alcohol and health. Alcohol Health/Res. World *9,* Fall, 20.

OLSON, R. (Editor). 1988. Nutritional management of cirrhosis. Nutrition Rev. *46,* Jul., 259.

ROE, D. 1985. Drug-induced Nutritional Deficiencies, 2nd Edition. Westport, CT: AVI Publishing Co.

SCHNEIDER, H., ANDERSON, D., and COURSIN, D. (Editors). 1983. Nutritional Support of Medical Practice, 2nd Edition. New York: Harper & Row.

TOFLER, O. 1985. The Heart of the Social Drinker. London, England: Lloyd-Luke Medical Books.

WORTHINGTON-ROBERTS, B. 1982. Alcoholism and malnutrition. In Alcoholism: Development, Consequences, and Interventions, N. Estes and M. Heinemann (Editors), pp. 109–135. St. Louis: C. V. Mosby Co.

VITALE, J., and COFFEY, J. 1971. Alcohol and vitamin metabolism. In The Biology of Alcoholism, B. Kissin and H. Bergleiter (Editors), Volume 1. New York: Plenum Press.

For journal subscriptions:

Alcohol and Health Notes. 1100 17th Street NW, Suite 710, Washington, DC 20036.

Alcohol Health and Research World. PO Box 2345, Rockville, MD 20852.

Alcoholism: Clinical and Experimental Research. Williams & Wilkins, 428 East Preston Street, Baltimore, MD 21202.

Journal of Studies on Alcohol. Center of Alcohol Studies, PO Box 969, Piscataway, NJ 08854.

For further information:

Center of Alcohol Studies, Rutgers University, New Brunswick, NY 08903.

Finnish Foundation for Alcohol Studies, Helsinki, Finland.

National Clearinghouse for Alcohol Information, PO Box 2345, Rockville, MD 20852.

Table 14.3   General Outline for Diet Counseling for Alcoholics

I. Initial Session
   A. General Guidelines
   B. Patient Records
      1. Medical History Form
      2. Weight Chart
      3. 24-Hour Recall Form
   C. Assignments
      1. Food Intake Record
      2. Diet History
   D. Technician's Notes
II. Follow-up Session(s)
   A. General Guidelines
   B. Handouts
      1. Personal Diet Plan
      2. Good Eating Checklist
   C. Technician's Notes

Counseling Guidelines—Recovering Alcoholics

Table 14.3 outlines the steps for diet counseling with recovering alcoholics. The following material gives the details of each step.

I.   Initial Session

I.   A.   General Guidelines

1. Use Medical History Form to assess patient's nutritional status.
2. Weigh patient and record on Weight Chart. The chart is a helpful tool for visualization of patient's weight status.

3. Assist patient in recording 24-hour recall of food intake using 24-Hour Recall Form. This will aid in keeping an accurate Food Intake Record.

4. Instruct patient to keep daily Food Intake Record so that typical food intake patterns can be evaluated. Advise patient not to deviate from normal eating pattern. Stress the importance of recording food intake immediately after eating.

5. Instruct patient to complete Diet History. This provides for a basic evaluation of food intake patterns. (Use Pre-test from Chapter 2.)

6. Record assessment and recommendation(s) using SOAP method in Technician's Notes. This form can be kept in your files with a copy in the patient's medical records.

I. B. Patient Records

1. Medical History Form

Date _____ Referred by _____

Name _____ Date of birth _____

Address _____ Phone no. _____

Occupation _____ Hours per work week ____ Work phone no. _____

Educational background _____ Religious/ethnic background _____

Sex ____ Marital status _____

Household composition: Live alone _____ Spouse _____ Children/No. _____ Other: _____

General health status:

Physician _____ Address _____

Phone no. _____ Date of last visit _____

Ambulatory care required? _____ If so, describe: _____

Neuromuscular problems? _____ If so, how is eating affected? _____

Visual/auditory problems? _____ If so, describe: _____

Chewing difficulties? _____ If so, describe: _____

Appetite typically good? _____ fair? _____ poor? _____

Digestion/elimination difficulties? _____ If so, describe: _____

Food intolerances? _____ If so, describe: _____

Gastritis? _____ If so, describe: _____

Diabetes? _____ If so, describe: _____

Hypertension? _____ If so, describe: _____

Ascites/edema? _____ If so, describe: _____

Hepatitis? _____ If so, describe: _____

Cirrhosis? _____ If so, describe: _____

Neurological manifestations? _____ If so, describe: _____

Other: _____

Height _____ Weight _____ Frame _____

Triceps skinfold thickness _____ Mid-arm circumference _____

Mid-arm muscle circumference _____

Weight changes/problems? _____ If so, describe: _____

Clinical signs of nutritional status:

Skin (jaundice?) _____ Mouth _____

Hair _____ Eyes _____

Teeth _____ Other: _____

Lab data:

Blood pressure _____

Cholesterol _____ Triglycerides _____ Lipoprotein profile _____

Fasting blood glucose _____

CBC _____

Bilirubin: serum _____ urine _____ Serum albumin _____

SGOT _____ BSP _____ Alkaline phosphatase _____

Prothrombin time _____ Hematocrit _____ Hemoglobin _____

Other: _____

Medications taken regularly: _____
Prescribed by: _____ Date(s) prescribed: _____
Nutrition supplements taken regularly: _____
Prescribed by: _____ Date(s) prescribed: _____
Special diet prescription: _____
Prescribed by: _____ Date of prescription: _____
How closely is diet followed? Always adhered to ___ Sometimes ___ Rarely ___ Never ___

Type of housing: Room _____ Apartment _____ Home _____ Institution _____
Prepare own meals? _____ Dine out? Often (more than once a day) _____ Rarely _____
Food shopping done independently? _____ If not, describe required assistance: _____
_____
Eligible for food stamps? _____ If so, are they currently being used? _____
Cigarette smoker? _____ If so, how much: _____
Exercise regularly? _____ If so, describe: _____
    No. times per week _____ No. minutes per session _____

Comments: _____

2. Weight Chart

Starting weight _____   Reasonable weight _____

Date	No. weeks on diet	Weight	Comments

3. 24-Hour Recall Form

Date	Time	Food and amount

I.   C.   Assignments

1. Food Intake Record

Date and time	Duration of meal (min)	Food and amount	Where^a	With whom	Associated activity^b	Associated emotions^c

^{a}Such as school, restaurant, kitchen, living room.
^{b}For example, watching television, reading, talking.
^{c}Attitude: bored, anxious, frustrated, depressed, happy, angry, tense, etc.

2. Diet History

Use the Pre-test from Chapter 2 (p. 30) to provide a record of typical foods eaten.

I.   D.   Technician's Notes

Patient: _____   Date: _____

S   (Subjective data—how patient feels):
O   (Objective data—physical measurements including diet/nutritional status):
A   (Assessment—acceptability of dietary progress/nutritional status):
P   (Plan—diet prescription and instruction):
Comments:

II.   Follow-up Session(s)

II.   A.   General Guidelines

1.   Weigh patient and record on Weight Chart.
2.   Review assignments and discuss.
3.   Individualize Personal Diet Plan and instruct patient in its use.
4.   Using Food Intake Record and Good Eating Checklist, assist patient in a general evaluation of nutrient intake.
5.   Instruct patient to self-evaluate adherence to Personal Diet Plan and development of new habits through continued use of Food Intake Record and Good Eating Checklist.
6.   Record assessment and recommendation(s) using the SOAP method in Technician's Notes. This form can be kept in your files with a copy in the patient's medical records.

II.   B.   Handouts

1. Personal Diet Plan

Name _____

How to use diet plan:

1.   Select a variety of foods from each of the Basic Food Groups.

2. Include the recommended number of servings from each Food Group.
3. Divide daily intake into small, frequent, regular meals.
4. Emphasize foods high in B vitamins (especially thiamin, niacin, and folic acid), magnesium, and zinc (see Table 14.4) to replenish depleted body stores.
5. Use nutrition supplements as prescribed for increased caloric/vitamin/mineral intake.

Table 14.4   Foods High in Needed Nutrients

Thiamin	Niacin	Folic Acid	Magnesium	Zinc
Pork, lean[a]	High-quality protein foods[b]	Organ meats[a]	Nuts	Oysters[a]
Liver and other organ meats[a]	Enriched breads and cereals[a]	Legumes[a]	Legumes[a]	Herring
Yeast	Legumes[a]	Bean sprouts	Whole grains	Milk
Legumes[a]	Nuts	Dark green leafy vegetables[a]	Dark green leafy vegetables[a]	Egg yolk
Dark green leafy vegetables[a]		Wheat germ	Seafood	Most animal foods
Whole grain and enriched breads and cereals[a]		Bran	Chocolate	
		Brewer's yeast	Cocoa	

[a]With hematochromatosis, iron intake should be minimal.
[b]Tryptophan is converted to niacin in the body.

2. Good Eating Checklist

Instructions: Using Food Intake Record, total the number of daily servings from each Food Group and transfer to this chart. Evaluate by comparison to Recommended Daily Servings (RDSs).

Day	No. of servings/Food Group					
	Fruits	Vegetables	Grains	Milk	Meats	Others
1						
2						
3						
4						
5						
RDSs	2	2	4	3	2	—

II. C. Technician's Notes

Patient: _____   Date: _____

S (Subjective data—how patient feels):
O (Objective data—physical measurements including diet/nutritional status):
A (Assessment—acceptability of dietary progress/nutritional status):
P (Plan—diet prescription and instruction):
Comments:

Alcoholism Diet Counseling Role Playing

Keeping in mind the preceding Suggested Readings and Counseling Guidelines, participate in the following role play situations; use the sample menu (Fig. 14.1) as a teaching

Name _____ Room _____
Diet **Special Restriction** _____

Breakfast   Please circle your selections below

Fruits and juices	**Cereals**	**Entrees**	**Breads**	**Miscellaneous**
Orange juice	Cream of wheat	Bacon	Apple muffin	Salt
Grapefruit juice	Oatmeal	Scrambled egg	Plain muffin	Sugar
Prune juice	Cornflakes	Poached egg	Danish pastry	Sugar substitute
Apple juice	Rice Krispies	Egg substitute	English muffin	Butter
Cranberry juice	Special K	Pancakes	White toast	Margarine
Grapefruit sections	Puffed rice	French toast	Wheat toast	Lemon
Banana	Puffed wheat	Omelet of the day	Rye toast	Jelly
				Pancake syrup

Beverages		Whole milk
Coffee		4 oz. whole milk
Tea	Cream	Skim milk
Decaffeinated coffee	Nondairy creamer	4 oz. skim milk
Cocoa		

Name _____ Room _____
Diet **Special Restriction** _____

Luncheon   Please circle your selections below

Appetizers	**Vegetables**
Apple juice	Whipped potato
Cranberry juice	Baked potato
Tomato juice	Noodles
Soft fruit cup	Rice
Consomme/chicken/beef	Broccoli buds
Chicken noodle soup	Spinach
Vegetable soup	Carrots
Cream of tomato soup	Green beans
Cream of chicken soup	Beets
Soup du jour	Peas
	Squash

Entrees	**Salads and dressings**
Soft fruit/cottage cheese	Mayonnaise
Roast beef sandwich	Sour cream
Sliced turkey sandwich	
Tuna salad sandwich plain	
Chicken salad sandwich plain	**Desserts**
Egg salad sandwich plain	Peaches
Peanut butter & jelly sandwich	Fruit cocktail
Tuna noodle casserole	Baked apple
Turkey/gravy	Pears
Roast beef au jus	Apricots
Chicken a la king/toast	Applesauce
Macaroni and cheese	Dessert of the day
Scrod	Sugar cookies
Ham/plain	Cupcake
Steak/mushrooms	Apple pie
Chicken/cranberry	Cheese cake
Grilled cheese	Chocolate pudding/topping
Veal/gravy	Butterscotch pudding/
Pork chop/applesauce	topping
Shell macaroni	Tapioca/topping
Beefburger plain	Sunshine cup
Cheeseburger plain	Ice cream
Plain salisbury/gravy	Orange sherbet
Chef's special (if allowed)	Raspberry sherbet
	Gelatin

Breads		Custard
White	Dinner Roll	Eclair
Wheat	Crackers	Angel cake
Rye		
		Miscellaneous
Beverages		Salt
Coffee		Sugar
Tea		Sugar substitute
Decaffeinated coffee		Butter
Cocoa		Margarine
Cream		Lemon
Nondairy creamer		Jelly
Whole milk		Mustard
4 oz. whole milk		Catsup
Skim milk		
4 oz. skim milk		

Name _____ Room _____
Diet **Special Restriction** _____

Dinner   Please circle your selections below

Appetizers	**Vegetables**
Apple juice	Whipped potato
Cranberry juice	Baked potato
Tomato juice	Noodles
Soft fruit cup	Rice
Consomme/chicken/beef	Broccoli buds
Chicken noodle soup	Spinach
Vegetable soup	Carrots
Cream of tomato soup	Green beans
Cream of chicken soup	Beets
Soup du jour	Peas
	Squash

Entrees	**Salads and dressings**
Soft fruit/cottage cheese	Mayonnaise
Roast beef sandwich	Sour cream
Sliced turkey sandwich	
Tuna salad sandwich plain	
Chicken salad sandwich plain	**Desserts**
Egg salad sandwich plain	Peaches
Peanut butter & jelly sandwich	Fruit cocktail
Tuna noodle casserole	Baked apple
Turkey/gravy	Pears
Roast beef au jus	Apricots
Chicken a la king/toast	Applesauce
Macaroni and cheese	Dessert of the day
Scrod	Sugar cookies
Ham/plain	Cupcake
Steak/mushrooms	Apple pie
Chicken/cranberry	Cheese cake
Grilled cheese	Chocolate pudding/topping
Veal/gravy	Butterscotch pudding/
Pork chop/applesauce	topping
Shell macaroni	Tapioca/topping
Beefburger plain	Sunshine cup
Cheeseburger plain	Ice cream
Plain salisbury/gravy	Orange sherbet
Chef's special (if allowed)	Raspberry sherbet
	Gelatin

Breads		Custard
White	Dinner Roll	Eclair
Wheat	Crackers	Angel cake
Rye		
		Miscellaneous
Beverages		Salt
Coffee		Sugar
Tea		Sugar substitute
Decaffeinated coffee		Butter
Cocoa		Margarine
Cream		Lemon
Nondairy creamer		Jelly
Whole milk		Mustard
4 oz. whole milk		Catsup
Skim milk		
4 oz. skim milk		

Fig. 14.1   Menu for special restriction diets.
© *The Seiler Corporation. Reprinted by permission.*

aid. Select different partners, either classmates or co-workers, for each situation and elaborate on each role play situation to develop a patient/audience profile. You may want to use your Handout from Step 2 in this chapter. Use the SOAP method to record in each patient's medical chart.

As a dietetic technician in nutrition care, do you consider yourself capable of conducting effective counseling sessions with individuals recovering from alcoholism or alcohol-related disorders? Would you or your family be able to adhere to your nutrition guidelines in order to ensure optimal nutritional status during a recovery phase?

Role Play Situation 1. You are a dietetic technician in a large metropolitan hospital; a 39-year-old female who is a recovering alcoholic is referred to you by her physician for a discharge diet. Follow the guidelines to complete the charts and provide the patient with an individualized diet plan. Prepare a SOAP note that could be recorded in the patient's medical chart. Note: The patient does not need any dietary restrictions, but is underweight and has some borderline nutritional deficiencies.

Role Play Situation 2. As a dietetic technician in a community public health agency, you are asked to assist in a high school program on alcohol abuse. Prepare an outline and present a 10-minute talk on "Nutrition and the Beer Facts," which includes the dietary implications of alcoholism. Complete a written summary of the presentation for insertion in the departmental files.

Role Play Situation 3. Derive your own role play situation requiring dietary guidance for a recovering alcoholic, and provide information on the dietary implications of alcoholism and alcohol-related disorders.

STEP 7: LOW-FAT GUIDELINES

Myths have long existed surrounding the best dietary treatment for disorders of the liver, gallbladder, and pancreas. Diet as tolerated appears to be the most effective nutrition therapy in most cases. However, during certain stages of some of the diseases which afflict these organs, fat intake should be limited. Successful nutrition therapy, however, requires a palatable, appetizing diet which does not result in further stress for the patient, nor lead to anorexia and poor nutritional status due to an unappetizing menu.

In order to be able to advise individuals requiring a low-fat intake—due to disorders of the liver, gallbladder, or pancreas—about desirable dietary patterns, it is essential to have access to all of the hands-on material required for effective counseling sessions. It is also important to be able to record all of the pertinent information regarding each diet counseling session in the patient's medical charts. The information provided below should help to improve your confidence—and skills—regarding your counseling abilities.

This step includes suggested counseling strategies for patients afflicted with certain diseases of the liver, gallbladder, or pancreas. The following references may prove helpful.

Suggested Readings for Low-Fat/Gallbladder Diet

AMERICAN DIETETIC ASSOCIATION. 1981. Handbook of Clinical Dietetics. New Haven, CT: Yale University Press.
BANKS, P. 1979. Pancreatitis. New York: Plenum Press.
BARBER, J., and TEASLEY, K. 1984. Nutritional support of patients with hepatic failure. Clin. Pharmacol. *3,* 245.
BOYAR, A., and LOUGHRIDGE, J. 1985. The Fat Portion Exchange List: A tool for teaching and evaluating low-fat diets. J. Am. Dietet. Assoc. *85,* May, 589.
ENLOE, C. (Editor). 1982. The pancreas. Nutrition Today *17,* Mar./Apr., 20.
FISHER, M. (Editor). 1979. Gallstones. New York: Plenum Press.
FITZGERALD, P., and MORRISON, A. 1980. The Pancreas. Baltimore: Williams & Wilkins.
FLOCH, M. 1981. Gallbladder disease. In Nutrition and Diet Therapy in Gastrointestinal Disease. New York: Plenum Press.
FOLEY, L. (Editor). 1985. Low Fat Cooking. Des Moines, IA: Meredith Corp.
GITNICK, G. (Editor). 1980. Current Hepatology. Boston: Houghton Mifflin.
HALPERN, S. (Editor). 1987. Quick Reference to Clinical Nutrition, 2nd Edition. Philadelphia: J. B. Lippincott Co.

HODGES, R. 1980. Nutrition in Medical Practice. Philadelphia: W. B. Saunders Co.

HURLEY, R. and MEKHJIAN, H. 1987. Dietary habits of patients with cholelithiasis. J. Am. Dietet. Assoc. *87*, Feb., 209.

MAKHLOUF, G. 1982. Function of the gallbladder. Nutrition Today *17*, Jan./Feb., 10.

MOGADAM, M., et al. 1984. Gallbladder dynamics in response to various meals. Amer. J. Gastroenterol. *79*, 745.

SCHEIN, C. 1972. Postcholecystectomy Syndromes. New York: Harper & Row.

WELDON, D. 1984. Pathology of the Gallbladder. New York: Masson Publishing.

Counseling Guidelines—Low Fat

Table 14.5 outlines the steps for low-fat diet counseling. The following material gives the details of each step.

I. Initial Session

I. A. General Guidelines

1. Use Medical History Form to assess patient's nutritional status.
2. Weigh patient and record on Weight Chart. The chart is a helpful tool for visualization of patient's weight status.
3. Assist patient in recording 24-hour recall of food intake using 24-Hour Recall Form. This will aid in keeping an accurate Food Intake Record.
4. Instruct patient to keep daily Food Intake Record so that typical food intake patterns can be evaluated. Advise patient not to deviate from normal eating pattern. Stress the importance of recording food intake immediately after eating.
5. Instruct patient to complete Diet History. This provides for a basic evaluation of food intake patterns. (Use Pre-test from Chapter 2.)
6. Record assessment and recommendation(s) using SOAP method in Technician's Notes. This form can be kept in your files with a copy in the patient's medical records.

Table 14.5 General Outline for Low-Fat Diet Counseling

I. Initial Session
  A. General Guidelines
  B. Patient Records
    1. Medical History Form
    2. Weight Chart
    3. 24-Hour Recall Form
  C. Assignments
    1. Food Intake Record
    2. Diet History
  D. Technician's Notes
II. Follow-up Session(s)
  A. General Guidelines
  B. Handouts
    1. Personal Diet Plan
    2. Good Eating Checklist
  C. Technician's Notes

I. B. Patient Records

1. Medical History Form

Date _____ Referred by _____

Name _____ Date of birth _____

Address _____ Phone no. _____

Occupation _____ Hours per work week _____ Work phone no. _____

Educational background _____ Religious/ethnic background _____

Sex _____ Marital status _____

Household composition: Live alone _____ Spouse _____ Children/No. _____ Other: _____

General health status:

Physician _____ Address _____

Phone no. _____ Date of last visit _____

Ambulatory care required? _____ If so, describe: _____

Neuromuscular problems? _____ If so, how is eating affected? _____

Visual/auditory problems? _____ If so, describe: _____

Chewing difficulties? _____ If so, describe: _____

Appetite typically good? _____ fair? _____ poor? _____

Digestion/elimination difficulties? _____ If so, describe: _____

Food intolerances? _____ If so, describe: _____

Gastritis? _____ If so, describe: _____

Diabetes? _____ If so, describe: _____

Hypertension? _____ If so, describe: _____

Ascites/edema? _____ If so, describe: _____

Hepatitis? _____ If so, describe: _____

Cirrhosis? _____ If so, describe: _____

Neurological manifestations? _____ If so, describe: _____

Other: _____

Height _____ Weight _____ Frame _____
Triceps skinfold thickness _____ Mid-arm circumference _____
Mid-arm muscle circumference _____
Weight changes/problems? _____ If so, describe: _____

Clinical signs of nutritional status:

Skin (jaundice?) _____ Mouth _____
Hair _____ Eyes _____
Teeth _____ Other: _____

Lab data:

Blood pressure _____
Cholesterol _____ Triglycerides _____ Lipoprotein profile _____
Fasting blood glucose _____
CBC _____
Bilirubin: serum _____ urine _____ Serum albumin _____
SGOT _____ BSP _____ Alkaline phosphatase _____
Prothrombin time _____ Hematocrit _____ Hemoglobin _____
Other: _____

Medications taken regularly: _____
Prescribed by: _____ Date(s) prescribed: _____
Nutrition supplements taken regularly: _____
Prescribed by: _____ Date(s) prescribed: _____
Special diet prescription: _____
Prescribed by: _____ Date of prescription: _____
How closely is diet followed? Always adhered to __ Sometimes __ Rarely __ Never __

Type of housing: Room __ Apartment __ Home __ Institution __
Prepare own meals? __ Dine out? Often (more than once a day) __ Rarely __
Food shopping done independently? _____ If not, describe required assistance: _____
_____
Eligible for food stamps? _____ If so, are they currently being used? _____
Cigarette smoker? _____ If so, how much: _____
Exercise regularly? _____ If so, describe: _____
     No. times per week _____ No. minutes per session _____

Comments: _____

2. Weight Chart

Starting weight _____   Reasonable weight _____

Date	No. weeks on diet	Weight	Comments

3. 24-Hour Recall Form

Date	Time	Food and amount

I. C. Assignments

1. Food Intake Record

Date and time	Duration of meal (min)	Food and amount	Where[a]	With whom	Associated activity[b]	Associated emotions[c]

[a]Such as school, restaurant, kitchen, living room.
[b]For example, watching television, reading, talking.
[c]Attitude: bored, anxious, frustrated, depressed, happy, angry, tense, etc.

2. Diet History

Use the Pre-test from Chapter 2 (p. 30) to provide a record of typical foods eaten.

I. D. Technician's Notes

Patient: _____   Date: _____

S (Subjective data—how patient feels):
O (Objective data—physical measurements including diet/nutritional status):
A (Assessment—acceptability of dietary progress/nutritional status):
P (Plan—diet prescription and instruction):
Comments:

II. Follow-up Session(s)

II. A. General Guidelines

1. Weigh patient and record on Weight Chart.
2. Review assignments and discuss.
3. Individualize Personal Diet Plan and instruct patient in its use.
4. Using Food Intake Record and Good Eating Checklist, assist patient in a general evaluation of nutrient intake.

5.   Instruct patient to self-evaluate adherence to Personal Diet Plan and development of new habits through continued use of Food Intake Record and Good Eating Checklist.

6.   Record assessment and recommendation(s) using the SOAP method in Technician's Notes. This form can be kept in your files with a copy in the patient's medical records.

II.   B.   Handouts

1. Personal Diet Plan

Name _____

How to use diet plan:

1.   Select a variety of foods from each of the Basic Food Groups.
2.   Include the recommended number of servings from each Food Group.
3.   Divide daily food intake into small, frequent, regular meals.
4.   Avoid stimulants such as alcohol and caffeine, especially between meals.
5.   Avoid nicotine.
6.   Avoid high-fat foods (see Table 14.6); limit fats to three daily servings.
7.   Omit foods which produce symptoms of discomfort. Make a list of individual intolerances:

Table 14.6   High-Fat Foods

Fruits and Vegetables

Any prepared with added fat, cream, or cheese sauce

Milk and Cheeses

Whole milk, chocolate milk, milkshakes
Cheeses (except for low-fat varieties)
Whole milk yogurt

Breads and Cereals

Any prepared with added fat
Fried products including potatoes, chips, breaded items
Commercial baked goods
Packaged mixes with added fat

Meats and Alternates

Fried meat, poultry, fish, eggs; refried beans
High-fat meats including brisket, ground beef, cold cuts, frankfurters,
    sausage, spareribs; capon, duck, goose; poultry skin; oil-packed fish
Any prepared with added fat, gravy, or cream sauce
Dried beans or peas in pork fat
Commercial peanut butter with added fat

Others

Avocado; bacon; chocolate; coconut; desserts, rich[a]; lard; nuts; olives;
    salt pork; tartar sauce

Fats

One serving = 1 tsp:	Butter, margarine, mayonnaise, oil, shortening
One serving = 1 Tbsp:	Cream, cream cheese, salad dressing
One serving = 2 Tbsp:	Sour cream
One serving = 3 Tbsp:	Nondairy creamer

[a]Cakes, cookies, doughnuts, ice cream, pastries, pie, etc.

2. Good Eating Checklist

Instructions: Using the Food Intake Record, total the number of daily servings from each Food Group and transfer to this chart. Evaluate by comparison to Recommended Daily Servings (RDSs).

Day	No. of servings/Food Group					
	Fruits	Vegetables	Grains	Milk	Meats	Others
1						
2						
3						
4						
5						
RDSs	2	2	4	3	2	—

II. C. Technician's Notes

Patient: _____   Date: _____

S (Subjective data—how patient feels):
O (Objective data—physical measurements including diet/nutritional status):
A (Assessment—acceptability of dietary progress/nutritional status):
P (Plan—diet prescription and instruction):
Comments:

Low-Fat Diet Counseling Role Playing

Keeping in mind the preceding Suggested Readings and Counseling Guidelines, participate in the following role play situations; use the sample menu (Fig. 14.2) as a teaching aid. Select different partners, either classmates or co-workers, for each situation and elaborate on each role play situation to develop a patient profile. You may want to use your Handouts from Steps 3 and 4. Use the SOAP method to record in each patient's medical chart.

As a dietetic technician in nutrition care, do you consider yourself capable of conducting effective counseling sessions with individuals suffering from liver, gallbladder, or pancreatic disorders? Would you or your family be able to adhere to your nutrition guidelines in order to ensure optimal nutritional status despite liver, gallbladder, or pancreatic disease?

Role Play Situation 1. As a dietetic technician in a large teaching hospital, you are assigned to a 40-year-old female who needs instructions on a post-cholecystectomy discharge diet. Follow the guidelines to complete the charts and provide the patient with an individualized diet plan. Prepare a SOAP note that could be recorded in the patient's medical chart.

Role Play Situation 2. As a dietetic technician in a rural hospital/clinic, you are assigned to a 55-year-old male with pancreatitis who needs a low-fat discharge diet. Follow the guidelines to complete the charts and provide the patient with an individualized diet plan. Prepare a SOAP note that could be recorded in the patient's medical chart.

Role Play Situation 3. Derive your own role play situation requiring dietary guidance on a low-fat diet for treatment of liver, gallbladder, or pancreatic disorder(s).

Name _____ Room _____
Diet **Fat controlled** _____

Breakfast   Please circle your selections below

Fruits and juices	**Cereals**	**Entrees**	**Breads**	**Miscellaneous**
Orange juice	Cream of wheat	Bacon	Apple muffin	Salt
Grapefruit juice	Grits	Scrambled egg	Blueberry muffin	Pepper
Prune juice	Oatmeal	Poached egg	Bran muffin	Sugar
Apple juice	Cornflakes	Egg substitute	Corn muffin	Sugar substitute
Cranberry juice	Rice Krispies	Pancakes	Plain muffin	Butter
Grapefruit sections	Special K	French toast	English muffin	Margarine
Stewed prunes	Puffed rice		White toast	Lemon
Banana	Puffed wheat		Wheat toast	Jelly
	Shredded wheat		Rye toast	Pancake syrup
	Raisin bran			
	All bran			
	Bran flakes			

Beverages
Coffee
Tea   Cream   Skim milk
Decaffeinated coffee   Nondairy creamer   4 oz. skim milk

Name _____ Room _____
Diet **Fat controlled** _____

Luncheon   Please circle your selections below

Appetizers	**Vegetables**
Apple juice	Whipped potato
Cranberry juice	Baked potato
Tomato juice	Noodles
Fruit cup	Rice
Consomme/chicken/beef	Broccoli
Chicken noodle soup	Corn
Vegetable soup	Spinach
Cream of tomato soup	Carrots
Cream of chicken soup	Green beans
Soup du jour	Beets
	Peas
	Squash

Entrees
Tomato with:
   Chicken salad, ½ cup
   Tuna salad, ½ cup
   Cottage cheese, ½ cup
Fruit and cottage cheese
Roast beef sandwich
Sliced turkey sandwich
Tuna salad sandwich
Chicken salad sandwich
Sandwich special (if allowed)
Tuna noodle casserole
Turkey/dressing/gravy
Roast beef au jus
Scrod
Ham/pineapple
Steak/mushrooms
Chicken/cranberry
Veal/gravy
Pork chop/applesauce
Shell macaroni
Beefburger
Salisbury/gravy
Chef's special (if allowed)

Salads and dressings
Lettuce/tomato
Tossed greens
Lettuce wedge
Cole slaw
Salad special
Mayonnaise
French dressing
Italian dressing
Oil & vinegar
Lemon and vinegar
Sour cream

Desserts
Peaches
Fruit cocktail
Baked apple
Pears
Apricots
Applesauce
Fresh fruit
Sunshine cup
Orange sherbet
Raspberry sherbet
Gelatin
Low fat custard
Angel cake

Breads
White   Dinner Roll
Wheat   Crackers
Rye

Beverages
Coffee
Tea
Decaffeinated coffee
Cream
Nondairy creamer
Skim milk
4 oz. skim milk

Miscellaneous
Salt
Pepper
Sugar
Sugar substitute
Butter
Margarine
Lemon
Jelly
Mustard
Catsup
Relish

Name _____ Room _____
Diet **Fat controlled** _____

Dinner   Please circle your selections below

Appetizers	**Vegetables**
Apple juice	Whipped potato
Cranberry juice	Baked potato
Tomato juice	Noodles
Fruit cup	Rice
Consomme/chicken/beef	Broccoli
Chicken noodle soup	Corn
Vegetable soup	Spinach
Cream of tomato soup	Carrots
Cream of chicken soup	Green beans
Soup du jour	Beets
	Peas
	Squash

Entrees
Tomato with:
   Chicken salad, ½ cup
   Tuna salad, ½ cup
   Cottage cheese, ½ cup
Fruit and cottage cheese
Roast beef sandwich
Sliced turkey sandwich
Tuna salad sandwich
Chicken salad sandwich
Sandwich special (if allowed)
Tuna noodle casserole
Turkey/dressing/gravy
Roast beef au jus
Scrod
Ham/pineapple
Steak/mushrooms
Chicken/cranberry
Veal/gravy
Pork chop/applesauce
Shell macaroni
Beefburger
Salisbury/gravy
Chef's special (if allowed)

Salads and dressings
Lettuce/tomato
Tossed greens
Lettuce wedge
Cole slaw
Salad special
Mayonnaise
French dressing
Italian dressing
Oil & vinegar
Lemon and vinegar
Sour cream

Desserts
Peaches
Fruit cocktail
Baked apple
Pears
Apricots
Applesauce
Fresh fruit
Sunshine cup
Orange sherbet
Raspberry sherbet
Gelatin
Low fat custard
Angel cake

Breads
White   Dinner Roll
Wheat   Crackers
Rye

Beverages
Coffee
Tea
Decaffeinated coffee
Cream
Nondairy creamer
Skim milk
4 oz. skim milk

Miscellaneous
Salt
Pepper
Sugar
Sugar substitute
Butter
Margarine
Lemon
Jelly
Mustard
Catsup
Relish

Fig. 14.2   Menu for fat-controlled diets.
© The Seiler Corporation. Reprinted by permission.

STEP 8: RENAL DISEASE GUIDELINES

The prognosis for patients with renal disease has improved significantly during the past few decades. Due to the increased possibility for rehabilitation and longevity, maintenance of optimal nutritional status has become an integral component of renal disease therapy; what used to be a means for the temporary postponement of death has become a way to improve the quality of life, sometimes a relatively long life. Somewhat restrictive and complex, successful diet therapy for the renal patient requires understanding, acceptance, and adherence.

In order to be able to advise individuals with renal disease on the adoption of desirable dietary patterns, it is essential to have access to all of the hands-on material required for effective counseling sessions. It is also important to be able to record all of the pertinent information regarding each diet counseling session in the patient's medical charts. The information provided below should help to improve your confidence—and skills—regarding your counseling abilities.

This step includes suggested counseling strategies to use with renal patients. The following references may prove helpful.

Suggested Readings

ALFREY, A. 1988. Effect of dietary phosphate reduction on renal function and deterioration. Amer. J. Clin. Nutr. *47,* Jan., 153.

AMERICAN DIETETIC ASSOCIATION. 1981. Handbook of Clinical Dietetics. New Haven, CT: Yale University Press.

AMERICAN DIETETIC ASSOCIATION. 1987. A Clinical Guide to Nutrition Care in End-stage Renal Disease. Chicago: ADA.

BRENNER, B., and RECTOR, F. (Editors). 1981. The Kidney, 2nd Edition. Philadelphia: W. B. Saunders Co.

BRENNER, B., and STERN, J. (Editors). 1981. Contemporary Issues in Nephrology. New York: Churchill Livingstone.

CASS-RYAN, T., and RIGGIN, K. 1988. Teaching tools for the young renal patient. J. Nutr. Educ. *20,* Jul./Aug., 190-D.

CUMMINGS, N., and KLAHR, S. 1985. Chronic Renal Disease: Causes, Complications, Treatment. New York: Plenum Press.

GIORDANO, C., et al. 1980. Modulated nitrogen intake for patients on low-protein diets. Amer. J. Clin. Nutr. *33,* Jul., 1638.

HALPERN, S. (Editor). 1987. Quick Reference to Clinical Nutrition, 2nd Edition. Philadelphia: J. B. Lippincott Co.

HODGES, R. 1980. Nutrition in Medical Practice. Philadelphia: W. B. Saunders Co.

KEANE, W., KASISKE, B., and O'DONNELL, M. 1988. Hyperlipidemia and the progression of renal disease. Amer. J. Clin. Nutr. *47,* Jan., 157.

KINCAID-SMITH, P., and WHITWORTH, J. 1988. Pathogenesis of hypertension in chronic renal disease. Seminars in Nephrology *8,* Jun., 155.

KLAHR, S., and PURKESON, M. 1988. Effects of dietary protein on renal function and the progression of renal disease. Amer. J. Clin. Nutr. *47,* Jan., 146.

MARTINEZ-MALDONADO, M. (Editor). 1983. Manual of Renal Therapeutics. New York: Plenum Press.

MIRTALLO, J., KUDSK, K., and EBBERT, M. 1984. Nutritional support of patients with renal disease. Clin. Pharmacol. *3,* 253.

MITCH, W., and KLAHR, S. (Editors). 1988. Nutrition and the Kidney. Boston: Little, Brown & Co.

MITCH, W., and STEINMAN, T. 1983. Can the course of renal disease be altered by diet? Kidney *16,* 31.

NATIONAL DAIRY COUNCIL. 1983. Diet and urolithiasis. Dairy Counc. Dig. *54,* Sept./Oct., 25.

PATEL, C., and DENNY, M. 1988. Cultural Foods and Renal Diets. Concord, CA: Council on Renal Nutrition, Northern California/Northern Nevada.

PIPER, C. 1985. Very-low-protein diets in chronic renal failure: Nutrient contents and guidelines for supplementation. J. Am. Dietet. Assoc. *85,* Oct., 1344.

RICHARD, C. (Editor). 1986. Comprehensive Nephrology Nursing. Boston: Little, Brown & Co.

RUDMAN, D. 1988. Kidney senescence: A model for aging. Nutrition Rev. *46,* Jun., 209.

SCHNEIDER, H., ANDERSON, C., and COURSIN, D. (Editors). 1983. Nutritional Support of Medical Practice, 2nd Edition. New York: Harper & Row.

SPRITZER, M., DICKINSON, B., and RODGERS, P. 1976. A Renal Failure Diet Manual Utilizing the Food Exchange System. Springfield, IL: Charles C. Thomas.

WALSER, M. 1980. Does diet therapy have a role in the pre-dialysis patient? Amer. J. Clin. Nutr. *33,* Jul., 1629.

For journal subscription:

Seminars in Nephrology. Grune & Stratton, Inc., The Curtis Center, Independence Square West, Philadelphia, PA 19106.

For audiovisuals:

Sodium and Potassium Comparison Charts. Nutrition Graphics, PO Box 1527, Corvallis, OR 97339. Your Renal Diet. The Polished Apple, 3742 Seahorn Drive, Malibu, CA 90265.

For further information:

Council on Renal Nutrition, National Kidney Foundation, Two Park Avenue, New York, NY 10003.

Counseling Guidelines—Renal Disease

Table 14.7 General Outline for Renal Disease Counseling

Table 14.7 outlines the steps for diet counseling with renal disease patients. The following material gives the details of each step.

I. Initial Session

I. A. General Guidelines

1. Use the Medical History Form to assess patient's nutritional status.
2. Weigh patient and record on Weight Chart. The chart is a helpful tool for visualization of patient's weight status.
3. Assist patient in recording 24-hour recall of food intake using 24-Hour Recall Form. This will aid in keeping an accurate Food Intake Record.
4. Instruct patient to keep daily Food Intake Record so that typical food intake patterns can be evaluated. Advise patient not to deviate from normal eating pattern. Stress the importance of recording food intake immediately after eating.
5. Instruct patient to complete Diet History. This provides for a basic evaluation of food intake patterns. (Use Pre-test from Chapter 2.)
6. Record assessment and recommendation(s) using SOAP method in Technician's Notes. This form can be kept in your files with a copy in the patient's medical records.

I. B. Patient Records

1. Medical History Form

Date _____ Referred by _____

Name _____ Date of birth _____

Address _____ Phone no. _____

Occupation _____ Hours per work week ____ Work phone no. _____

Educational background _____ Religious/ethnic background _____

Sex ____ Marital status _____

Household composition: Live alone _____ Spouse _____ Children/No. _____ Other: _____

General health status:

Physician _____ Address _____

Phone no. _____ Date of last visit _____

Ambulatory care required? _____ If so, describe: _____

Neuromuscular problems? _____ If so, how is eating affected? _____

Visual/auditory problems? _____ If so, describe: _____

Chewing difficulties? _____ If so, describe: _____

Appetite typically good? _____ fair? _____ poor? _____

Digestion/elimination difficulties? _____ If so, describe: _____

Food intolerances? _____ If so, describe: _____

Diabetes? _____ If so, describe: _____

Hypertension? _____ If so, describe: _____

Heart attack or stroke? _____ If so, describe: _____

Kidney stones? _____ If so, describe: _____

Systemic lupus erythematosus? _____ If so, describe: _____

Wilson's disease? _____ If so, describe: _____
Nephrotic syndrome? _____ If so, describe: _____
Nephrosclerosis? _____ If so, describe: _____
Acute/chronic glomerulonephritis? _____ If so, describe: _____
Acute/chronic renal failure? _____ If so, describe: _____
Other: _____

Height _____ Weight _____ Frame _____
Triceps skinfold thickness _____ Mid-arm circumference _____
Mid-arm muscle circumference _____
Weight changes/problems? _____ If so, describe: _____

Clinical signs of nutritional status:

Skin _____ Mouth _____
Hair _____ Eyes _____
Teeth _____ Other: _____

Lab data:

Blood pressure _____
Cholesterol _____ Triglycerides _____ Lipid profile _____
SUN _____ BUN _____ GFR _____
Serum: Urea ___ Uric acid ___ Creatinine ___ Ammonia ___ Albumin ___ Electrolytes ___
Urine: Albumin _____ Pyuria _____ Cylinduria _____ Specific gravity _____
Blood gases _____ Fluid intake/output: _____
CBC _____
Other: _____

Medications taken regularly: _____
Prescribed by: _____ Date(s) prescribed: _____
Nutrition supplements taken regularly: _____
Prescribed by: _____ Date(s) prescribed: _____
Special diet prescription: _____
Prescribed by: _____ Date of prescription: _____
How closely is diet followed? Always adhered to ___ Sometimes ___ Rarely ___ Never ___

Type of housing: Room ___ Apartment ___ Home ___ Institution ___
Prepare own meals? ___ Dine out? Often (more than once a day) ___ Rarely ___
Food shopping done independently? _____ If not, describe required assistance: _____
_____

Eligible for food stamps? _____ If so, are they currently being used? _____
Cigarette smoker? _____ If so, how much: _____
Exercise regularly? _____ If so, describe: _____
   No. times per week _____ No. minutes per session _____

Comments: _____

2. Weight Chart

Starting weight _____   Reasonable weight _____

Date	No. weeks on diet	Weight	Comments

3. 24-Hour Recall Form

Date	Time	Food and amount

I. C. Assignments

1. Food Intake Record

Date and time	Duration of meal (min)	Food and amount	Where[a]	With whom	Associated activity[b]	Associated emotions[c]

[a]Such as school, restaurant, kitchen, living room.
[b]For example, watching television, reading, talking.
[c]Attitude: bored, anxious, frustrated, depressed, happy, angry, tense, etc.

2. Diet History

Use the Pre-test from Chapter 2 (p. 30) to provide a record of typical foods eaten.

I. D. Technician's Notes

Patient: _____   Date: _____

S (Subjective data—how patient feels):
O (Objective data—physical measurements including diet/nutritional status):
A (Assessment—acceptability of dietary progress/nutritional status):
P (Plan—diet prescription and instruction):
Comments:

II. Follow-up Session(s)

II. A. General Guidelines

1. Weigh patient and record on Weight Chart.
2. Review assignments and discuss.
3. Individualize Personal Diet Plan and instruct patient in its use.
4. Provide patient with High-Sodium Foods List if required.
5. Provide patient with High-Potassium Foods List if required.
6. Provide patient with Approximate Water Content of Foods list if required.
7. Record assessment and recommendation(s) using the SOAP method in Technician's Notes. This form can be kept in your files with a copy in the patient's medical records.

II. B. Handouts

1. Personal Diet Plan

Name _____

How to use diet plan:

1. Select a variety of foods from each of the Basic Food Groups.
2. Include the recommended number of servings from each Food Group.
3. If required, restrict intake of foods high in sodium (see Table 14.8).
4. If required, restrict intake of foods high in potassium (see Table 14.9).
5. If required, restrict fluid intake (see Table 14.10).

2. High-Sodium Foods List

Table 14.8 lists foods high in sodium.

3. High-Potassium Foods List

Table 14.9 lists foods high in potassium.

4. Approximate Water Content of Foods

Table 14.10 gives the average fluid contents of foods.

II. C. Technician's Notes

Patient: _____   Date: _____

S (Subjective data—how patient feels):
O (Objective data—physical measurements including diet/nutritional status):
A (Assessment—acceptability of dietary progress/nutritional status):
P (Plan—diet prescription and instruction):
Comments:

Renal Disease Diet Counseling Role Playing

Keeping in mind the preceding Suggested Readings and Counseling Guidelines, participate in the following role play situations; use the sample menu (Fig. 14.3) as a teaching aid. Select different partners, either classmates or co-workers, for each situation and elaborate on each role play situation to develop a patient/audience profile. You may want to use your Handout from Step 5. Use the SOAP method to record in each patient's medical chart.

As a dietetic technician in nutrition care, do you consider yourself capable of conducting effective counseling sessions with individuals suffering from renal disease? Would you or your family be able to adhere to your nutrition guidelines in order to ensure optimal nutritional status despite renal disease?

Role Play Situation 1.   As a dietetic technician for the renal unit of a teaching hospital, you are assigned to a 69-year-old female with chronic renal failure who needs diet instructions. Her diet prescription requires restrictions in sodium, potassium, protein, and/or fluids. Follow the guidelines to complete the charts and provide the patient with an individualized diet

Table 14.8   High-Sodium Foods List

Fruits and Vegetables Group

Brined or highly salted items:

Lima beans, frozen	Sauerkraut
Mixed vegetables, frozen	Seasoned frozen vegetables
Peas, frozen	Tomato juice
Pickled beets	Vegetable juice cocktail
Pickled salad mix	

Breads and Cereals Group

Highly salted items:

Bread sticks, salted tops	Rolls, salted tops
Crackers, salted tops	Seasoned croutons
Popcorn, salted	Seasoned rice and pasta mixes
Pretzels	Seasoned stuffing mixes

Meats and Alternates Group

Smoked, dried, cured, or salty items:

Bologna	Meats, smoked	Fish, dried
Chipped beef	Pastrami	Fish, frozen fillets
Corned beef	Pickled meats	Fish, smoked
Frankfurters	Sausage	Herring
Ham	Smoked tongues	Sardines
Kosher meats	Stews, canned	Cheese spreads
Luncheon meats	Anchovies	Processed cheeses
Meats, canned	Caviar	Nuts, salted
Meats, dried	Fish, canned	Seeds, salted

Others

Highly salted items:

Bacon	Olives
Bacon bits	Salted snack foods—cheese curls, chips, pret-
Condiments—catsup, horseradish, mustard,	zels, etc.
pickles, relishes, salad dressings, and sauces	Salt pork
(barbecue, chili, soy, Worcestershire)	Soups
Dips	

Seasonings

High in sodium content:

Bouillon	Meat/vegetable extracts
Cooking wines	Monosodium glutamate
Instant gravy and sauce mixes	Salts—celery salt, garlic salt, Kosher salt, onion
Meat marinades	salt, sea salt, seasoned salts
Meat tenderizers	Salt, table

Medicinals high in sodium

Antacids	Laxatives
Antibiotics	Sedatives
Buffered headache remedies	Sodium bicarbonate (or baking soda)
Cough medicines	

Table 14.9   High-Potassium Foods List

Fruits and Vegetables Group:

Apricots	Currants	Parsnips
Artichokes	Dark green leafy vegetables	Peaches
Bananas	Dried fruits and juices—	Potatoes
Cantaloupe, casaba,	apricots, dates, figs,	Raspberries
honeydew melon	peaches, prunes, raisins	Rhubarb
Carrots	Elderberries	Squash, winter
Celery	Mushrooms	Strawberries
Citrus fruits and juices—	Nectarines	Tomatoes
grapefruit, orange	Papayas	Tomato juice (low-sodium)

Breads and Cereals Group:

Bran	Oatmeal	Pumpernickel bread

Milk and Cheeses Group:

Milk (low sodium)

Meats and Alternates Group:

Dried beans and peas	Peanuts

Others:

Chocolate, cocoa	Coffee	Molasses

Table 14.10   Approximate Water Content of Foods

Food group	Amount of water (in ml/100 g)
Fruits and Vegetables (all)	50–96
Breads and Cereals	
Cooked cereal	90
Cooked rice, pastas	80–90
Breads	30–40
Dry cereal	0–14
Crackers	0–14
Milk and Cheeses	
Cheese	30–40
Meats and Alternates	
Meat, fish, poultry, eggs	50–75
Others	
Butter, margarine	15–20
Oils	0–14
Sugars	0–14

plan. Prepare a SOAP note that could be recorded in the patient's medical chart. Then repeat the role play several times using varying levels in the dietary restrictions.

Role Play Situation 2.   As a dietetic technician for the renal unit of a large metropolitan hospital, you are required to assist the dialysis patients (see Step 5, items 14–27) in menu selection. Prepare a brief outline to delineate the importance of different dietary factors in the treatment and control of renal failure; present a 10-minute talk to the dialysis unit patients. Complete a written summary on the presentation for insertion in the departmental files.

Role Play Situation 3.   Derive your own role play situation requiring dietary guidance for a patient with renal disease.

STEP 9: POST-TEST ON NUTRITION FOR LIVER, GALLBLADDER, PANCREAS, AND KIDNEY DISEASES

In order to evaluate your understanding of the current diet therapies for diseases of the liver, gallbladder, pancreas, and kidney, complete the Post-test. Answers are given in the Answer Key. Will your patients with diseases affecting the liver (or gallbladder, or pancreas, or kidney) be able to use your nutrition guidelines in order to control the disorder and optimize nutritional status?

Indicate whether you think the following statements are true (T) or false (F). Check your answers with the Answer Key.

_____   1.   The kidney is the largest organ in the body.
_____   2.   The liver serves as a storage place for certain nutrients.
_____   3.   In liver disease, serum albumin is reduced.
_____   4.   In liver disease, SGOT is elevated.
_____   5.   With hepatitis, fat intake is severely restricted.
_____   6.   Cirrhotic edema makes measurements of body weight an unreliable parameter of nutritional status.
_____   7.   With hepatic coma, protein intake should be increased.

Name _____ Room _____
Diet **Special Restriction** _____

Breakfast
Please circle your selections below

Fruits and juices	Cereals	Entrees	Breads	Miscellaneous
Orange juice	Cream of wheat	Bacon	Apple muffin	Salt
Grapefruit juice	Oatmeal	Scrambled egg	Plain muffin	Sugar
Prune juice	Cornflakes	Poached egg	Danish pastry	Sugar substitute
Apple juice	Rice Krispies	Egg substitute	English muffin	Butter
Cranberry juice	Special K	Pancakes	White toast	Margarine
Grapefruit sections	Puffed rice	French toast	Wheat toast	Lemon
Banana	Puffed wheat	Omelet of the day	Rye toast	Jelly
				Pancake syrup

Beverages — Whole milk

Coffee		4 oz. whole milk
Tea	Cream	Skim milk
Decaffeinated coffee	Nondairy creamer	4 oz. skim milk
Cocoa		

Name _____ Room _____
Diet **Special Restriction** _____

Luncheon
Please circle your selections below

Appetizers

	Vegetables
Apple juice	Whipped potato
Cranberry juice	Baked potato
Tomato juice	Noodles
Soft fruit cup	Rice
Consomme/chicken/beef	Broccoli buds
Chicken noodle soup	Spinach
Vegetable soup	Carrots
Cream of tomato soup	Green beans
Cream of chicken soup	Beets
Soup du jour	Peas
	Squash

Entrees

	Salads and dressings
Soft fruit/cottage cheese	Mayonnaise
Roast beef sandwich	Sour cream
Sliced turkey sandwich	
Tuna salad sandwich plain	
Chicken salad sandwich plain	**Desserts**
Egg salad sandwich plain	Peaches
Peanut butter & jelly sandwich	Fruit cocktail
Tuna noodle casserole	Baked apple
Turkey/gravy	Pears
Roast beef au jus	Apricots
Chicken a la king/toast	Applesauce
Macaroni and cheese	Dessert of the day
Scrod	Sugar cookies
Ham/plain	Cupcake
Steak/mushrooms	Apple pie
Chicken/cranberry	Cheese cake
Grilled cheese	Chocolate pudding/topping
Veal/gravy	Butterscotch pudding/
Pork chop/applesauce	topping
Shell macaroni	Tapioca/topping
Beefburger plain	Sunshine cup
Cheeseburger plain	Ice cream
Plain salisbury/gravy	Orange sherbet
Chef's special (if allowed)	Raspberry sherbet
	Gelatin
Breads	Custard
White Dinner Roll	Eclair
Wheat Crackers	Angel cake
Rye	
	Miscellaneous
Beverages	Salt
Coffee	Sugar
Tea	Sugar substitute
Decaffeinated coffee	Butter
Cocoa	Margarine
Cream	Lemon
Nondairy creamer	Jelly
Whole milk	Mustard
4 oz. whole milk	Catsup
Skim milk	
4 oz. skim milk	

Name _____ Room _____
Diet **Special Restriction** _____

Dinner
Please circle your selections below

Appetizers

	Vegetables
Apple juice	Whipped potato
Cranberry juice	Baked potato
Tomato juice	Noodles
Soft fruit cup	Rice
Consomme/chicken/beef	Broccoli buds
Chicken noodle soup	Spinach
Vegetable soup	Carrots
Cream of tomato soup	Green beans
Cream of chicken soup	Beets
Soup du jour	Peas
	Squash

Entrees

	Salads and dressings
Soft fruit/cottage cheese	Mayonnaise
Roast beef sandwich	Sour cream
Sliced turkey sandwich	
Tuna salad sandwich plain	
Chicken salad sandwich plain	**Desserts**
Egg salad sandwich plain	Peaches
Peanut butter & jelly sandwich	Fruit cocktail
Tuna noodle casserole	Baked apple
Turkey/gravy	Pears
Roast beef au jus	Apricots
Chicken a la king/toast	Applesauce
Macaroni and cheese	Dessert of the day
Scrod	Sugar cookies
Ham/plain	Cupcake
Steak/mushrooms	Apple pie
Chicken/cranberry	Cheese cake
Grilled cheese	Chocolate pudding/topping
Veal/gravy	Butterscotch pudding/
Pork chop/applesauce	topping
Shell macaroni	Tapioca/topping
Beefburger plain	Sunshine cup
Cheeseburger plain	Ice cream
Plain salisbury/gravy	Orange sherbet
Chef's special (if allowed)	Raspberry sherbet
	Gelatin
Breads	Custard
White Dinner Roll	Eclair
Wheat Crackers	Angel cake
Rye	
	Miscellaneous
Beverages	Salt
Coffee	Sugar
Tea	Sugar substitute
Decaffeinated coffee	Butter
Cocoa	Margarine
Cream	Lemon
Nondairy creamer	Jelly
Whole milk	Mustard
4 oz. whole milk	Catsup
Skim milk	
4 oz. skim milk	

Fig. 14.3 Menu for special restriction diets.
© *The Seiler Corporation. Reprinted by permission.*

_____ 8. A large percentage of alcoholics eventually develop cirrhosis.

_____ 9. Alcoholics often develop deficiencies in B vitamins, zinc, magnesium, and other nutrients.

_____ 10. Between feedings, the gallbladder rests in an empty state.

_____ 11. Cholecystokinin is released from the gallbladder upon consumption of fat.

_____ 12. Males are more prone to cholelithiasis than are females.

_____ 13. After cholecystectomy, fat intake must remain restricted indefinitely.

_____ 14. Carbohydrate intake is severely restricted with pancreatitis.

_____ 15. Pancreatic extracts are helpful for those with minor digestive complaints.

_____ 16. Renal dysfunction causes an elevation in SUN and BUN levels.

_____ 17. Nephrosclerosis requires a sodium restriction.

_____ 18. Dietary protein intake is usually restricted in patients with renal failure.

_____ 19. A high-calcium diet may help to slow or prevent renal osteodystrophy after chronic renal failure.

_____ 20. Vitamin A supplements are usually recommended for patients with renal failure.

_____ 21. Successful renal transplantation can help to ease dietary restrictions.

_____ 22. Most renal stones contain calcium.

_____ 23. Cranberries are high in oxalates.

_____ 24. Anchovies are high in purines.

_____ 25. The water content of most fruits and vegetables is over 50%.

Select the answer which best completes the following statements and check your answers with the Answer Key.

_____ 26. A diet increased in thiamin content could include
(a) spinach. (b) baked beans. (c) lean pork chops. (d) whole wheat bread. (e) enriched wheat bread. (f) b, c, and d. (g) all of these.

_____ 27. A diet increased in magnesium content could include
(a) Swiss chard. (b) hot chocolate. (c) peanut butter. (d) whole wheat bread. (e) enriched wheat bread. (f) a, d. (g) a, b, c, d. (h) all of these.

_____ 28. A reduction in dietary fat would exclude
(a) olives. (b) commercial baked goods. (c) eggs Benedict. (d) canned beans 'n franks. (e) guacamole. (f) none of these. (g) all of these.

_____ 29. One serving of fat is equivalent to
(a) 1 Tbsp margarine. (b) 3 Tbsp nondairy creamer. (c) 2 Tbsp cream cheese. (d) 1 Tbsp Italian dressing. (e) 1 tsp butter. (f) b, d, e. (g) a, d. (h) all of these.

_____ 30. A reduction in dietary potassium would require moderation in the intake of
(a) potatoes. (b) oatmeal. (c) strawberries and raspberries. (d) citrus fruit. (e) c and d. (f) all of these.

Chapter Fifteen

Other Clinical Conditions[1]

CHAPTER BLUEPRINT

Step 1: Take the Pre-test on Hospital Malnutrition and participate in the assigned group discussion.

Step 2: Examine the Anemia Facts List and prepare the assigned handout.

Step 3: Examine the Parenteral/Enteral Facts List and complete the accompanying assignment.

Step 4: Examine the Trauma Facts List and complete the accompanying assignment.

Step 5: Examine the Cancer and AIDS Facts List and complete the accompanying assignment.

Step 6: Examine the Developmental Disabilities Facts List and prepare the assigned handout.

Step 7: Examine the Anemia Guidelines and complete the role play assignment.

Step 8: Examine the Extended Illness Guidelines and complete the role play assignment.

Step 9: Take the Post-test on Other Clinical Conditions to evaluate what you have learned from the information and activities provided in this chapter.

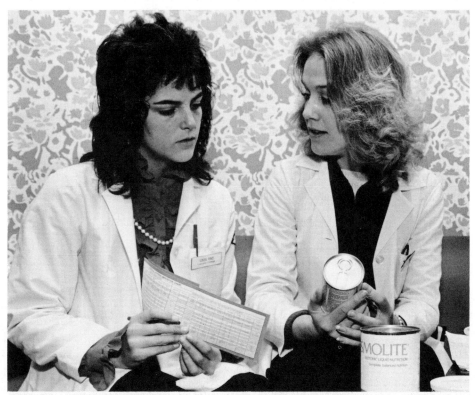

[1]*Note:* This chapter is appropriate for practicing dietetic technicians who are actively involved in clinical nutrition and who have achieved a high level of competency.

STEP 1: PRE-TEST ON HOSPITAL MALNUTRITION

With the rapid increases in hospital costs during the 1970s, attention finally focused on one of the major factors contributing to the national health expenditure: nutrition mis-management of patients caused by ignorance, neglect, and error on the part of medical staffs. Once one of the largest undiscovered malnourished populations in America, in-house hospital patients are overlooked less often now, their nutritional needs are identified and the proper nutrition therapies are prescribed.

iatrogenic: Physician induced.

However, the problem of **iatrogenic** malnutrition in hospitalized patients still exists, largely due to lack of nutrition education in medical schools. The situation also exists where dietetics departments fail to utilize and vocalize their nutrition skills and know-how. Thus, despite immense technological advances and ever-expanding knowledge about the role of nutrition in preventive and curative medicine, appropriate use of such information is not always made. Fortunately, in many hospitals and health care institutions, this is no longer the rule, but the exception.

Malnutrition can contribute to morbidity, mortality, and prolonged hospitalization. Yet, relatively minor alterations in hospital policy and staff practice can prevent the unnecessary development of nutritional deficiencies. The nutritional status of most hospitalized patients can be improved by establishing the following desirable daily practices: (a) monitoring of patient's daily food intake; (b) monitoring of patient's weight status; (c) proper nutritional assessment; (d) application of nutrition support as soon as the patient is in need; (e) proper administration of tube feedings; and (f) on-going communication between the dietetics department and other medical staff members.

Suggested Readings on Malnutrition

ANDERSON, C., et al. 1984. The sensitivity and specificity of nutrition-related variables in relationship to the duration of hospital stay and the role of complications. Mayo Clin. Proc. *59,* Jul., 477.

ASPEN. 1987. Proceedings of the First International Workshop on Nutrition and Metabolism in Hospital Malnutrition. J. Parenteral/Enteral Nutr. *11,* Sept./Oct., Supplement.

BISTRIAN, B., et al. 1976. Prevalence of malnutrition in general medical patients. J. Am. Med. Assoc. *235,* Apr. 12, 1567.

BROLLET, J., and OWENS, S. 1973. Evaluation of nutrition status of selected hospitalized patients. Amer. J. Clin. Nutr. *26,* Sept., 931.

BUTTERWORTH, C. 1974. The skeleton in the hospital closet. Nutrition Today *10,* Mar./Apr., 4.

BUTTERWORTH, C., and BLACKBURN, G. 1975. Hospital malnutrition. Nutrition Today *11,* Mar./Apr., 8.

HEDBERG, A., et al. 1988. Nutrition risk screening: Development of a standardized protocol using dietetic technicians. J. Am. Dietet. Assoc. *88,* Dec., 1553.

HILL, G., et al. 1977. Malnutrition in surgical patients: An unrecognized problem. Lancet *1,* Mar. 26, 689.

KAMATH, S., et al. 1986. Hospital malnutrition: A 33-hospital screening study. J. Am. Dietet. Assoc. *86,* Feb., 203.

LIPSCHITZ, D. 1982. Protein-calorie malnutrition in the hospitalized elderly. Primary Care *9,* Sept., 531.

LONG, J. 1982. Opening the closet door: The key is education. J. Parenteral/Enteral Nutr. *6,* Jul./Aug., 280.

OLSON, R. (Editor). 1988. Hospital malnutrition still abounds. Nutrition Rev. *46,* Sept., 315.

PARSONS, H., et al. 1980. The nutritional status of hospitalized children. Amer. J. Clin. Nutr. *33,* May, 1140.

PINCHOFSKY-DEVIN, G., and KAMENSKI, M. 1987. Incidence of protein-calorie malnutrition in the nursing home. J. Amer. Coll. Nutr. *6,* 2, 109.

ROUBENOFF, R., et al. 1987. Malnutrition among hospital patients: A problem of physician awareness. Arch. Internal Med. *147,* Aug., 1462.

STEFFE, W. 1980. Malnutrition in hospitalized patients. J. Am. Med. Assoc. *244,* Dec. 12, 2630.

SUSKIND, R. (Editor). 1977. Malnutrition and the Immune Response. New York: Raven Press.

WEINSIER, R., et al. 1979. Hospital malnutrition: A prospective evaluation of general medical patients during the course of hospitalization. Amer. J. Clin. Nutr. *32,* Feb., 418.

WEISSBERGER, L., SOWA, D., and WEDDLE, D. 1982. Clinical nutritional assessment: A two-month evaluation. J. Am. Dietet. Assoc. *81,* Jul., 58.

Keeping in mind the preceding Suggested Readings, complete the following questionnaire and discuss your answers with classmates or co-workers. As a dietetic technician in nutrition care, it is important for you to understand the importance of *adequate* nutrition in the treatment of degenerative diseases and diet-related disorders, and to develop a working knowledge of the pertinent physiological implications and accepted diet therapies. It is also your responsibility to help patients receive the *adequate* nutrition care that they deserve.

Questionnaire on Hospital Malnutrition

1. List some of the indications and signs of malnutrition:

2. List some of the common causes for hospital-induced malnutrition:

3. Briefly describe acceptable methods for the prevention of hospital-induced malnutrition:

4. Describe the role of the physician in the prevention of hospital-induced/iatrogenic malnutrition:

5. Describe the role of the dietetics department in the prevention of hospital-induced malnutrition:

STEP 2: ANEMIA FACTS

Anemia is a deficiency of the oxygen-carrying capacity of the blood which is caused by inadequate quantity and/or quality of red blood cells. The nutritional anemias are due to dietary lack or intestinal malabsorption of iron, folic acid, and/or vitamin B_{12}. Thus, appropriate nutrition guidelines are important in the prevention and control of these disorders.

The following Anemia Facts List provides current diet-related information for counseling individuals with nutritional anemias.

Anemia Facts List

1. Anemia is a decrease in total red cell mass due to fewer red blood cells (RBC) or smaller RBC containing less hemoglobin.
2. Anemia is the result of either increased loss or destruction of RBC or a decrease in RBC formation; **microcytic** anemias are usually due to iron deficiency, **macrocytic** to folic acid and/or vitamin B_{12} deficiencies, and **normocytic** to the inhibition of **marrow** formation from chronic disease, infection, uremia, malignancy, or marrow **aplasia.**
3. Many nutrients are involved in the formation of blood—iron, folic acid, vitamin B_{12}, pyridoxine, ascorbic acid, vitamin E—so nutritional anemias are common in individuals with nutritionally inadequate diets. Deficiencies of certain other nutrients can also play a role in the development of anemia, including niacin, thiamin, riboflavin, pantothenic acid, biotin, copper, and cobalt.
4. Anemia also occurs in individuals with diets that are deficient in protein; anemias are best treated with an adequate intake of high-quality protein.
5. Despite the many advances that have been made in the area of **hematology,** anemia is still prevalent all over the world.
6. The most common nutritional deficiency is an iron deficiency, which can be found in every age group, impairing the health and performance of millions of people.
7. *Iron deficiency anemia* is insidious in onset and can be difficult to diagnose until the condition is in the advanced stages.
8. Red blood cells contain hemoglobin, of which iron is an essential component. Hemoglobin is involved in the transport of oxygen from the lungs to the tissues, and of carbon dioxide from the tissues to the lungs. A deficiency in iron leads to tissue **hypoxia** with the resultant symptoms of anemia.

microcyte: Abnormally small red blood cell.

macrocyte: Abnormally large red blood cell.

normocyte: Red blood cell of normal size.

marrow: Soft tissue found inside the long bones.

aplasia: Failure of an organ or tissue to develop normally.

hematology: Science of blood and blood-forming tissues.

hypoxia: Oxygen deficiency.

9.   Iron-deficiency anemia results in RBC which are reduced in size and pale in color. The condition is most common in (a) pregnancy; (b) infancy (at birth, infant requires enough stored iron for 3–6 months; iron-fortified cereals should then be introduced); (c) growing children and teens (due to increased blood volumes); (d) women of child-bearing ages (due to monthly menstrual losses); and (e) the elderly (due to poor dietary intake).

10.   Although the average American diet contains 10–20 mg (milligrams) of iron per day, only around 10% is absorbed; absorption is enhanced with (a) simultaneous consumption of vitamin C-rich foods; (b) an increase in gastric secretions; or (c) a depletion in iron stores.

11.   Iron absorption may be improved by increasing either the amount of iron in the diet or the availability. There are two forms of dietary iron (heme and nonheme), each absorbed by different mechanisms. Absorption of heme iron is not affected by meal content, whereas nonheme iron absorption is influenced by the nature of the meal: phytates, phosphates, and oxalates interfere with the absorption of nonheme iron, while vitamin C enhances it; meals and snacks containing meat, fish, or poultry also improve the availability of nonheme iron.

tetracycline: An antibiotic.

12.   Iron absorption can be reduced with use of certain medications, including **tetracycline** and antacids.

13.   Approximately 40% of the total iron in meat, fish, and poultry is heme iron; the remaining 60% (and all other dietary iron) is nonheme iron. The total iron available per meal or snack can be calculated by adding together the amounts of heme iron and available nonheme iron. Daily iron intake can then be determined by totaling the values from each meal and snack. (See Table 15.1).

Table 15.1   Nonheme Iron Intake

Meal content	Absorption of nonheme iron (%)
Low	
<25 mg vitamin C <1 oz meat/fish/poultry	2
Medium	
25–75 mg vitamin C 1–3 oz meat/fish/poultry	5
High	
≥75 mg vitamin C ≥3 oz meat/fish/poultry	8

desquamation: Process of shedding an outer layer of the skin.

14.   The total iron content of the body is around 3–4 g; normal iron losses are mostly due to **desquamation** of iron-containing intestinal mucosal cells. Daily losses average around 1 mg/day, increasing to about 2 mg/day with menstruation, and 3 mg/day during pregnancy to provide for fetal iron needs.

15.   Due to diets typically low in iron-rich foods, many females fail to meet their iron requirements, and most average around 6 mg/1000 kcal. Thus, supplementation may need to be prescribed during the childbearing years, especially during pregnancy.

16.   Treatment of iron-deficiency anemia is simple and relatively inexpensive: in conjunction with a well-balanced diet, one of several forms of ferrous iron is given orally several times daily; plus, monthly evaluations are made to track dietary and hematologic progress to determine the cause(s) and prevent recurrence.

17.   Although ferrous sulfate is the form of iron best absorbed by the body, the other forms—ferrous gluconate, ferrous fumarate, and iron dextran for intravenous or intramuscular injection—are also absorbed enough for use in supplementation.

18.   Transferrin is a visceral protein which helps to combat infection (by preventing bacterial growth) and binds/transports iron in the plasma. If transferrin is depleted, iron supplementation before repletion can cause serum bacterial infestation.

19. *Megaloblastic anemia* results in RBC which are large and immature, and is due to deficiency in vitamin B_{12} (*pernicious anemia*) or folic acid.

20. A deficiency in folic acid leads to impaired synthesis of the **DNA** vital to cell growth and division, resulting in abnormally large red blood cells (megaloblasts) in the bone marrow and abnormally large red blood cells (macrocytes) in the peripheral blood.

DNA: Deoxyribonucleic acid; complex protein which carries genetic information.

21. Possibly the most common hypovitaminosis, *folic acid deficiency* can occur with (a) chronic alcoholism, (b) certain diseases, (c) long-term use of oral contraceptives, (d) constant adherence to poor diet, (e) reliance on overcooked foodstuffs (folic acid is heat labile, so prolonged cooking can cause inactivation), (f) inadequate absorption or utilization of the vitamin or increased requirements, (g) injury to skin from burns or certain illnesses, (h) intestinal damage from ailments such as **dysentery,** and (i) rapid destruction of RBC (as in chemolytic anemia). Inadequate intakes of vitamin C or B_{12} can impair the utilization of absorbed folate.

dysentery: Intestinal disorder caused by bacterial or viral infection, characterized by abdominal pain and diarrhea.

22. With megaloblastic anemia due to folic acid deficiency, an adequate intake of vitamin C is essential, as this vitamin is necessary for the conversion of folic acid to the metabolically active form. Recovery from iron deficiency anemia is also enhanced by adequate intake of vitamin C-rich foods, which will increase iron absorption.

23. Folacin is readily absorbed from the digestive tract, and is synthesized by the bacteria normally present in the intestines (although availability is speculative). Since cooking can destroy folacin, raw fruits and salad greens are better sources of this vitamin.

24. Since folacin is essential to proper RBC formation, supplementation can mask pernicious anemia by aiding normal cell development while the progressive nerve damage of a vitamin B_{12} deficiency continues unabated. Vegans (restrictive vegetarians) often consume large amounts of folacin-rich vegetables and fruits with an intake of little or no vitamin B_{12}.

25. Treatment of folic acid deficiency usually includes supplementation with 500 mg/day, but therapy should not begin until the cause or causes of the deficiency have been determined.

26. Folic acid is the only vitamin which cannot be sold over the counter in doses greater than the RDA because of the risk of a delayed diagnosis of pernicious anemia.

27. A deficiency in vitamin B_{12} leads to impaired synthesis of the DNA vital to cell growth and division. One result is abnormally large red blood cells (megaloblasts) in the bone marrow and abnormally large red blood cells (macrocytes) in the peripheral blood.

28. Since vitamin B_{12} aids in the preservation of the integrity of the central nervous system, clinical deficiency symptoms include **paresthesia,** forgetfulness, irritability, and other manifestations of nerve degeneration and neurologic change.

paresthesia: Numbness or tingling sensations.

29. In pernicious anemia, the "intrinsic factor" needed for transport of vitamin B_{12} across the intestinal mucosa is inadequate or missing. Vitamin B_{12} is known as the "extrinsic factor" (found in foods), and requires the "intrinsic factor" (of gastric secretions) for absorption. Lifelong **parenteral** injections are required so that the vitamin can bypass the intestine.

parenteral: Referring to any route other than oral (e.g., intravenous).

30. Vitamin B_{12} occurs naturally in foods of animal origin almost exclusively. Required in small amounts, this vitamin is rarely inadequate in the American diet (except for the strict vegan diet).

31. A deficiency in vitamin B_{12} develops quite gradually, as the liver stores quantities sufficient for as long as 3 years.

32. Symptoms of pernicious anemia include fatigue, weakness, glossitis, and intestinal injury. Symptoms of folacin-deficiency megaloblastic anemia are similar, but headache, irregular heartbeat, labored respiration, anorexia, weight loss, irritability, and forgetfulness can also occur.

33. Pernicious anemia begins insidiously, with gradual progression of symptoms and nerve damage. This anemia can occur with gastrectomy, **iliectomy, "blind loop" syndrome,** certain malabsorption syndromes, antibiotic therapy, and tapeworms. It appears frequently in individuals of Northern European descent, and is more common in older persons. The neurological abnormalities include degeneration of the spinal cord and peripheral neuritis, but recovery can be complete if the deficiency is treated before neurologic lesions are severe.

iliectomy: Surgical removal of part of the small intestine.

"blind loop" syndrome: Bacterial overgrowth in the intestine that causes malabsorption.

34. Anemic children often have multiple nutritional deficiencies, but iron deficiency is the most common problem.

35. The "physiologic anemia of infancy" is due to the fact that, in newborns, RBC values are usually 10–20% greater than normal, but fall below normal for the first 6 months of life.

dermatitis: Inflammation of the skin characterized by redness, itching, and skin lesions.

36.   *Milk anemia* is iron deficiency anemia due to an excessive milk intake, which displaces iron-rich foods in the diet.

37.   Anemia can serve as an early sign of lead poisoning. Pica is not uncommon in those with severely depleted iron stores, but the ingestion of clay or laundry starch will only hinder iron absorption.

38.   Vitamin B_6-deficiency anemia is usually mild and is accompanied by other signs of B_6 deficiency including **dermatitis** and neuropathy; simple treatment with oral supplementation is usually sufficient.

39.   Vitamin B_6-deficiency anemia which does not respond to oral supplementation is a more severe form requiring parenteral doses and seldom resulting in complete hematologic remission.

40.   Hemoglobin consists of heme (a pigmented compound containing iron) and globin (a protein), and carries oxygen from the lungs to the tissues; hematocrit is the normal value of packed RBC in 100 ml of blood, and is used as an aid in the diagnosis of iron deficiency and the classification of anemias.

41.   With anemia, the normal serum level of RBC (4.2–5.9 million/mm^3) is decreased, as is the normal hemoglobin level (13–16 g/dl for males, 12–15 g/dl for females); a low value for hematocrit, or the percentage volume of packed RBC (normally 42–50% for males, 40–48% for females) is indicative of inadequate dietary iron. Serum iron levels, normally 50–150 mg/dl, are increased with pernicious anemia and decreased with inadequate dietary iron.

42.   Iron is transported in the circulation bound to protein—globin—as transferrin or siderophilin. Iron-binding capacity, normally 350–400 mg/dl, is increased with low serum iron in iron-deficiency anemia and decreased with high serum iron in pernicious anemia.

Exercise on Anemia

Keeping in mind the preceding Anemia Fact List, which provides some of the most current diet-related information to include in counseling individuals with nutritional anemias, prepare a simplified version for use as a patient handout. You may include graphics and/or prepare in a poster format, if desired; see the Sample Handout. Show your handout in rough draft form to classmates or co-workers for constructive criticism on the overall design, content, and potential effectiveness for use in pertinent diet counseling situations. Then prepare a final version for your own future use as a practicing dietetic technician.

Sample Handout

Table 15.2 gives dietary information for treating nutritional anemias.

Table 15.2   Diet in Nutritional Anemias

Foods high in iron

Meat, especially organ meats	Dried fruits and their juices
Oysters, clams	Dark green leafy vegetables
Legumes	Potato, sweet potato
Whole grain and enriched breads and cereals	Foods prepared in iron cookware

Foods high in folic acid

Organ meats	Legumes, cooked
Dark green leafy vegetables	

Foods high in vitamin B_{12}

Animal foods	Soy milk fortified with B_{12}
Fortified yeasts	

Foods high in vitamin C

Citrus fruits and juices	Papaya
Broccoli	Mango
Strawberries	Tomato
Cantaloupe	Potato

STEP 3: PARENTERAL/ENTERAL FACTS

Until relatively recently, the medical community did not have access to parenteral support and **enteral** feeding. These essential nutrition support services now help to prolong lives by promoting tissue growth and repair, and assist in health recovery for neonates, infants, children, teens, adults, and the elderly suffering from a variety of clinical conditions. Different brands and combinations of the various feeding modes can be utilized in order to optimize nutritional status. With appropriate prescription and monitoring, parenteral/enteral nutrition can serve as life-saving therapy.

The following Parenteral/Enteral Fact List provides current information on these state-of-the-art methods for nutrition support.

enteral: Referring to the intestinal route.

Parenteral/Enteral Fact List

1. According to Stanley Dudrick, an early researcher in parenteral nutrition (Dudrick 1969), nutrition support is deemed necessary when an individual "cannot eat, should not eat, will not eat, or cannot eat enough."

2. It is important to understand the metabolic response to trauma and stress before designing the appropriate nutrition support plan; route of administration (enteral versus parenteral), required degree of nutrition repletion, and level of **hypermetabolism/hypercatabolism** will also need to be considered for each individual patient.

hypermetabolism: Abnormally increased metabolism.

hypercatabolism: Abnormally increased metabolic breakdown with excessive excretion of body substances.

3. Enteral feeding formulas generally fit into two basic types: (a) Defined formulas or nutrition supplements and (b) elemental diets. These products are used as oral or tube feedings for **anabolism,** or as dietary supplements. Most contain whole proteins or protein isolates, sugar (such as sucrose, lactose, corn syrup, glucose) and fat (as oil, animal fat, or glycerides), and may be vitamin/mineral fortified, low-sodium, low-lactose, and/or **isotonic.**

anabolism: A constructive metabolic process with building up of body substances.

isotonic: Having the same tone; with solutions, the concentration of electrolytes and/or nonelectrolytes exert an equivalent osmotic pressure.

4. Defined formulas or nutrition supplements can be (a) polymeric (averaging 1 kcal/cc with a balance of protein, carbohydrate, and fat), (b) high-caloric-density polymeric (with 1.5–6 kcal/cc for smaller volume feedings), or (c) modular, which supply specific nutrients to supplement other formulas (e.g., hydrolyzed protein, essential fatty acids, specific vitamins/minerals). Polymeric formulas have fixed nutrient compositions requiring specific volumes to supply adequate nutrition, so may be contraindicated in renal, liver, and cardiac patients. High-caloric-density polymeric formulas can provide as much as 4500–6000 calories per day, so are used in hypermetabolic states (such as with severe burns and in cancer patients) as well as with patients requiring volume restrictions.

5. Elemental diets are predigested (so do not require pancreatic enzymes for absorption), low in fat (to decrease the need for bile salts), and low residue (to rest the bowel). They usually contain easily absorbed protein (as crystalline amino acids or egg albumin), simple sugars requiring little amylase activity (such as maltose and glucose), essential fatty acids, vitamins and minerals; some products are high density (for fluid restriction) or low sodium–potassium–protein (for renal failure). These diets provide 1 cal/ml.

6. If the gastrointestinal tract is functioning, either a regular diet—with or without nutrition supplements—or an elemental diet is given, orally or as tube feedings. However, if the gastrointestinal tract is not functioning, use of parenteral nutrition is indicated. Also, since elemental diets are costly and often unpalatable, the alternative parenteral route may be considered even if tube feeding is acceptable.

7. Tube feedings can cause vomiting and/or diarrhea due to the following errors of administration: (a) excessive amounts are given at once, instead of starting at one quarter of the target level with gradually increasing quantities; (b) excessive concentrations with high osmolalities are used; (c) the presence of lactose, intolerable to some patients, is overlooked; and (d) bacterial contamination causes iatrogenic food poisoning. Tube feedings can be effective and well tolerated if they are started slowly, if overconcentration and hyperosmolality are avoided, and if feedings are administered in small quantities (enough for 3 hours) using sterile containers for each new portion.

8. Tube feedings for adults are generally started at 40–50 ml/hour, with a gradual increase over 7–10 days to a maximum of 100–200 ml every 2 hours. Large volumes administered rapidly can overstimulate gastric mucosa and cause hemorrhage.

9. Tube feedings must supply adequate nutrition that can be well tolerated and in a form modified so as to meet individual needs and dietary restrictions; feedings should be the

desired consistency and particle size and easily prepared from readily available materials at an affordable cost. They should also be reasonably palatable.

10. Tube feedings can be purchased as commercial liquids or dissolvable powders, and can be prepared from diluted solid foods or baby food.

11. Some of the advantages of tube feedings include the high nutritional value, consistent content, sterility, and ease of preparation.

12. Constipation can occur with long-term tube feeding, especially with inadequate fluid intake.

13. Patients who cannot be fed orally but have a functioning gastrointestinal tract can be tube fed through the nose, hypopharynx, or esophagus; during comas, a gastrostomy tube may be used, and with tumor obstruction of the stomach or total gastrectomy, a jejunostomy tube may be required.

14. With acute gastric ulceration and bleeding (e.g., as induced by major stress such as severe burns, multiple injuries, renal or respiratory failure), continuous nasogastric tube feeding is important to provide the necessary nutrition support without inducing further bleeding.

15. Enteral feeding is safer than parenteral therapy (with less of a risk for infection and fluid/electrolyte imbalances) and is less costly, requiring less equipment and staff time. There is no need to sterilize tubing, and feeding can be performed outside the hospital setting. Caloric intake is simple to assess, and the gastrointestinal (GI) system is stimulated by enteral feedings. However, if neither oral nor tube feeding is feasible, parenteral routes can provide the nutritional substrates required to support normal growth and development in the young and to maintain or improve nutritional status in adults.

16. Elemental diets are absorbed in the proximal small bowel, requiring little or no enzymatic digestion, so can be used when a functioning GI tract has digestive or absorptive dysfunctions (e.g., pancreatic insufficiencies or inflammatory bowel disease).

17. Elemental diets are contraindicated in infancy due to hyperosmolality; the offensive taste makes tube feeding advisable. The major drawbacks for adult use include the potential side effects of hyperglycemia, hypervitaminosis K, nasopharyngeal and mucosal irritation, fluid overload, cramping and diarrhea, hypertonic dehydration, hyperosmolar coma, and pulmonary **aspiration.**

aspiration: Process of sucking in or out by which foreign objects can be inspired into the nose, throat, or lungs.

18. The term *hyperalimentation* appeared in the 1960s and referred to the supplemental intravenous feeding of fat, but is now used extensively as a general term for total parenteral nutrition (TPN). Total parenteral nutrition is used to maintain optimal nutritional status for prolonged periods so that underlying diseases can be treated.

19. Total parenteral nutrition allows the delivery of large amounts of amino acids and calories (up to 200 g and 2000–5000 kcal every 24 hours) directly into the bloodstream in order to eliminate the need for absorption by the gastrointestinal tract; thus TPN allows for long-term maintenance or improvement of nutritional status solely by the intravenous infusion of nutrients.

20. The typical TPN solution provides around 1000 cal/L of solution, and the volume can be increased or decreased to meet individual caloric needs: glucose—250 g and 1000 kcal; protein—36 g (6 g nitrogen) and 120 kcal; sodium—30 **mEq (milliequivalent);** potassium—15 mEq; chloride—22 mEq; calcium—5 mEq; magnesium—4 mEq; phosphate—30 mEq; and multivitamin solution—10 ml. Fat soluble vitamins are administered once a week, and Intralipid or Liposyn is usually given several times each week.

milliequivalent (mEq): Concentration of electrolyte (e.g., sodium) in solution.

21. Some of the problems associated with TPN include the establishment of an individually adequate formulation, sterile preparation techniques, and safe administration procedures.

22. Calories provided by TPN should be sufficient to meet individual requirements, either enough to maintain weight or increased to promote weight gain. Essential amino acids should be included in the amounts required for adequate protein synthesis. Vitamins and minerals should be provided to meet individual requirements without excessive wastage or toxicity. Water should be provided in the volumes consistent with cardiovascular and renal needs, yet in amounts adequate to replace abnormal fluid losses.

hemolysis: Red cell destruction with the release of hemoglobin into the surrounding fluid.

23. The high osmolality of parenteral solutions necessitates administration into large veins in order to avoid **hemolysis** and **phlebitis.**

phlebitis: Inflammation of a vein.

24. Total parenteral nutrition is provided through a central vein, whereas short-term supplementary feeding can be given via a peripheral vein. Peripheral parenteral nutrition

(PPN) is limited in nutrient concentrations due to the small size of the veins into which solutions are infused.

25.   Peripheral parenteral nutrition consists of amino acids and dextrose, so can meet protein needs but not caloric requirements.

26.   Peripheral parenteral nutrition is often used for several days with patients who are in reasonably good health and who can soon return to oral intake routes; in the malnourished and those unable to utilize other feeding routes for longer than several days, TPN should be administered.

27.   If TPN is not introduced gradually and in stages, with careful monitoring of serum phosphate levels, hypophosphatemia can occur, leading to coma and death. Aluminum hydroxide antacids, which bind phosphates, should be avoided.

28.   If glucose intolerance (due to pancreatic dysfunction, shock, malnutrition, or other causes) prevents adequate caloric support, insulin can be added to TPN treatments.

29.   Hypertonic, hyperglycemic, nonketonic coma can occur with TPN (especially in the adult patient who is obese, inactive, and mildly diabetic) causing an increased need for fluid, sodium, and insulin.

30.   Preventable side effects associated with TPN use include metabolic acidosis; **cholestatic** jaundice; **hyperammonemia;** and essential fatty acid, zinc, and copper deficiencies; mechanical injury and infection can also be avoided. Involvement of a skilled TPN team is essential for the prevention or rapid control of potential side effects.

31.   The assessment of nutritional status is required prior to use of TPN, and continual reassessment includes daily measurements of body weight and intake/output.

32.   Parenteral preparations do not include vitamin K, which can be given intramuscularly on a weekly or biweekly basis; supplementary folic acid and vitamin B_{12} may also be required. If fluid is insufficient, separate intravenous (IV) solutions can be administered. With long-term TPN, a liter of lipid emulsion should be administered several times weekly to provide essential fatty acids, as deficiencies have been observed within the first month of parenteral nutrition use.

33.   Fat emulsions of castor oil and cottonseed oil were first used in hyperalimentation, but the undesirable side effects led to a ban on their use in 1964. Subsequent research showed that soybean oil and safflower oil emulsions had no significant side effects, so the soybean oil emulsion Intralipid and the safflower oil emulsion Liposyn were approved for parenteral use.

34.   Much research is still needed in order to document the specific requirements for trace elements during parenteral nutrition, as changes occur in these requirements with stress, malnutrition, and fluid loss. Eventually, improved laboratory measurements and recognition of toxic levels will lead to the development of products that can meet individual mineral needs of TPN patients; until that time, supplements must be individualized as carefully as possible.

35.   Despite extensive research, the changes in vitamin requirements with injury and disease are still unclear. Thus, intravenous requirements are uncertain, and elevations in catabolism and protein/caloric intakes can further complicate the situation.

36.   Elemental diets can provide nutrition in clear liquid form when minimal residue is required (e.g., Mead Johnson's Flexical, Doyle's Precision LR or Precision HN, Cutter's Vipep, Ross's Vital, Eaton's Vivonex or Vivonex HR).

37.   In parenteral feedings, caloric intake at a rate of 40–45 cal/kg/day with 1.5 g of protein per kilogram can achieve positive nitrogen balance, as will oral intakes of 35–40 cal/kg/day. Fat emulsions (e.g., Intralipid and Liposyn) are isotonic, providing 1.1 calorie/gram, and supplying essential fatty acids during long-term use of TPN (but should not constitute more than 60% of total calories).

38.   It is important not to make abrupt changes from one modality to another, so patients should gradually progress from

(parenteral → parenteral + enteral → enteral → enteral + food → food),

receiving adequate nutrition from the second feeding method before discontinuation of the first.

39.   It is important to recognize and assess catabolic losses, provide appropriate nutrition support, and avoid nutritional depletion as early as possible in the treatment program; anabolism becomes increasingly difficult to achieve during illness once malnutrition is

cholestasia: Halted excretion of bile.

hyperammonemia: Excessive amount of ammonia in the blood.

present. Vigorous nutrition support, however, can significantly reduce the morbidity and mortality associated with prolonged starvation.

40.   The nutrition support team (who prescribes and provides the parenteral and/or enteral feedings) usually includes specially trained physician(s) and nurse(s), a pharmacist, and a dietitian; the team may also involve physical therapists, social workers, dietetic technicians, laboratory technicians, and data processors/clerical workers.

Exercise on Parenteral/Enteral Feeding

Keeping in mind the preceding Parenteral/Enteral Facts List, which provides some of the most current information on the subject, prepare a sheet that lists the available products, major components, and features. A sample product list (Table 15.3) is given. Show your sheet in rough draft form to several members of a nutrition support team to determine whether it is both complete and accurate. Then prepare a final version for your own future use as a practicing dietetic technician. Note: Leave extra space to add in new products as they become available.

Sample Product Sheet

Table 15.3 lists available products and their major components.

Table 15.3   Nutrition Supplements: Sample Product List

Product	Source	Special features
Amin-Aid	McGaw Labs	High-calorie powder; low in protein but contains essential amino acids
Carnation Instant Breakfast	Carnation Company	Calorie/protein powder; mixed into milk
Compleat-B	Doyle Pharmaceutical Co.	Blenderized formula for tube feeding
Controlyte	Doyle Pharmaceutical Co.	Low-protein high-calorie supplement
Citroitein	Doyle Pharmaceutical Co.	Lactose-free powdered source of protein, vitamins, and minerals
Ensure	Ross Labs	Lactose-free liquid source of calories, protein, vitamins, and minerals
Ensure Plus	Ross Labs	Higher level of protein and calories than Ensure
Formula 2	Cutter Labs	Blenderized formula for tube feeding
Isocal	Mead Johnson and Co.	Lactose-free, elemental, low-residue formula
Isotein HN	Doyle Pharmaceutical Co.	Lactose-free, powdered source of calories, protein, vitamins, and minerals
Meritene	Doyle Pharmaceutical Co.	Calorie/protein supplement with vitamins and minerals
Nutrament	Dracket Products Co.	Calorie/protein milkshake-like liquid supplement
Nutri-Aid	McGaw Labs	Lactose-free formula for tube feeding
Osmolite	Ross Labs	Lactose-free liquid source of calories, protein, vitamins, and minerals
Polycose	Ross Labs	Tasteless calorie supplement to mix into foods and beverages
Precision LR	Doyle Pharmaceutical Co.	Lactose-free, low-residue, calorie/protein powdered supplement with vitamins and minerals
Sustacal	Mead Johnson and Co.	Calorie/protein lactose-free liquid supplement with vitamins and minerals
Susta Pudding	Mead Johnson and Co.	Milk-based calorie/protein ready-to-eat supplement
Trauma-Aid HN Drink	McGaw Labs	High-nitrogen, nutritionally complete liquid supplement

continued

Table 15.3 *(Continued)*

Product	Source	Special features
Trauma-Cal	Mead Johnson and Co.	Lactose-free, low-volume liquid source of calories and protein
Travasorb MCT	Travenol	Easily digestible fat source; lactose-free and high in calories, protein, vitamins, and minerals
Vital	Ross Labs	Lactose-free, low-residue calorie/protein powdered supplement with vitamins and minerals
Vivonex	Eaton Labs	Lactose-free elemental powdered calorie/protein formula with vitamins and minerals
Vivonex HN	Eaton Labs	High-nitrogen, low-residue liquid supplement
Other (Insert additional products in alphabetical order, using a footnote system to indicate where the products fit into the above list.):		

STEP 4: TRAUMA FACTS

The survival of a seriously injured individual, burn victim, or postsurgical patient depends on overall ability to handle physical stress, minimize weight loss, and meet increased nutritional needs. Catabolism is the usual response to such trauma, but the chances for developing the accompanying protein-caloric malnutrition, vitamin/mineral deficiencies, and potential complications can be minimized with optimal nutritional management.

The following Trauma Facts List provides current diet-related information to include in counseling individuals recovering from burns, surgery, or other physical trauma.

Trauma Facts List

1.   Wounds, fractures, and burns are some of the major reasons for hospitalization in this country. Adequate nutrition therapy can help to enhance recovery significantly, whereas poor nutrition will delay the return to good health.

2.   Illness imposes varying degrees of stress on the traumatized body, which leads to significant alterations in nutritional requirements. With the stress of surgery, high fever, or extensive burns, the body's need for protein may increase fivefold and vitamin/mineral requirements may increase even more, especially with certain drug therapies. Thus, individual nutrient needs may be altered significantly from the stress which accompanies surgery, fractures, severe burns, and serious illnesses.

3.   With aggressive nutrition support, anabolism can be established soon after trauma in order to diminish metabolic losses and shorten the recovery period.

4.   Stress can be defined as physical or emotional tension resulting in altered **homeostasis** with a definite physiological reaction.

5.   Stress causes nitrogen loss. Stress-related factors that increase metabolism include (a) hormones, (b) severely cold temperatures, (c) infection, and (d) tissue destruction.

6.   The *catabolic response* occurs when starvation is complicated by stress/trauma-induced metabolic changes, including increased oxygen consumption and urinary nitrogen

homeostasis: Internal state of balance maintained by the body's regulatory processes.

losses exceeding amounts from tissue injury. The administration of parenteral nutrition does not prevent the catabolic response, but can compensate for the negative nitrogen balance.

7.   Significant alterations in body metabolism develop secondary to the trauma of surgery, burns, injury, and infection with (a) an acute phase—certain hormones are released and hyperglycemia, reduced insulin levels, and anorexia occur, along with the mobilization of skeletal muscles and fat reserves; and (b) an adaptive phase—blood glucose is reduced, ketones are released, insulin levels are high, while nitrogen losses are elevated; substantial nutritional repletion is mandatory for recovery.

8.   The major nutritional goals of post-trauma treatment are to minimize catabolism during the acute phase and restore body mass during the adaptive phase.

9.   The post-trauma nutrition support plan should take into consideration the following factors: (a) type and extent of malnutrition, (b) degree of hypermetabolism, (c) protein/calorie requirements, (d) gastrointestinal function, (e) appetite, (f) delivery route for nutrition therapy, and (g) organ dysfunction that may require nutritional restrictions.

10.   The various options for post-trauma therapeutic nutrition include (a) oral, (b) nasogastric tube feedings, (c) gastrostomy feedings, (d) jejunostomy feedings, (e) elemental diets, and (f) intravenous hyperalimentation (IVH).

11.   In this age of modern nutrition support, the protein–calorie malnutrition associated with trauma should not develop but, if it does, treatment should be prompt and vigorous.

12.   Intravenous hyperalimentation (IVH) can be used as supplemental or total parenteral nutrition when the overall state of gastrointestinal function precludes oral intake or use of tube feedings, such as with the following conditions: (a) persistent diarrhea, (b) malabsorption syndromes, (c) loss or absence of pancreatic enzymes, (d) reduced biliary secretions, (e) chronic bowel obstruction, (f) radiation injury to the intestine, and (g) short bowel syndrome.

13.   With essential fatty acid deficiency, which can occur following long-term use of glucose/amino acid IVH, administration of linoleic acid may be required. A fat emulsion such as Intralipid can be used.

14.   Even with minor surgery, the ensuing catabolism can cause weight loss and protein–calorie malnutrition. The more prolonged and severe the stress, the greater the weight loss (as lean tissue, fat stores, and fluids); without adequate nutrition, the patient can die of malnutrition rather than from the illness or surgery.

15.   Individuals undergoing minor surgery lose around 5–8% of their preoperative body weight, and complicated surgery can lead to losses of 15–25%, making adequate body reserves essential. Surgery may be postponed if nutritional status is less than optimal, so that the chances for developing postoperative complications will be lessened and recovery can be completed more rapidly.

16.   Individuals with reasonable body weights should have adequate body fat stores to meet energy needs during postoperative stages, but underweight patients should gain and obese patients should lose weight prior to surgery in order to avoid complications and enhance recovery.

17.   Preoperative nutritional status can be optimized with the use (singly or in combination) of the following: (a) oral high-protein/high-calorie diet, (b) liquid supplements, (c) tube feedings, (d) intravenous therapy, (e) total parenteral nutrition (TPN), and (f) vitamin/mineral supplements.

18.   Surgical patients who may be especially susceptible to nutritional deficiencies include those with (a) obstruction of the GI tract, (b) bowel tumors, (c) diseases of the liver, gallbladder, or pancreas that affect digestion and/or absorption, (d) neurological disorders with impaired eating abilities and/or GI function, (e) renal or liver failure, and (f) increased metabolism due to cancer, major trauma, or hormonal disorders; neonates with congenital disorders are also at risk.

19.   The risk of postsurgical complications is increased with (a) pre-surgical malnutrition, (b) underweight of 20–30%, (c) obesity, (d) alcoholism, (e) certain gastrointestinal disorders that cause diarrhea, (f) increased metabolism from fever, trauma, burns, hyperthyroidism, pregnancy, or infancy, (g) fistulas or abscesses, and (h) inability to ingest adequate protein/calories after a week or more.

20.   Adequate glycogen stores in the liver can protect this organ from the toxic effects of anesthesia.

21.   After surgery, patients are in negative nitrogen balance with tissue catabolism so may require 100–200 g of protein daily and sufficient calories to spare protein. It is also important to monitor fluid intake to prevent dehydration—due to vomiting, hemorrhage, and diuresis—and electrolyte imbalance.

22.   After surgery (or with burns and other traumas), patients are often dehydrated with depleted intravascular fluid volumes. Thus, initial parenteral nutrition can cause fluid retention until fluid volume is replenished; solutions that reflect normal serum electrolyte concentration are preferable to hypotonic solutions, which can cause fluids to shift into extravascular spaces. Fluid requirements during stress may be increased 10% for each degree of body temperature elevation.

23.   With surgery or severe burns, blood and fluid losses cause water intoxication when water is replaced without the necessary sodium; symptoms include headache, muscular weakness, lack of concentration, poor memory, and anorexia, which will disappear upon replenishment of both sodium and water.

24.   Following gastric surgery, patients may have difficulty tolerating osmotic loads, and the **dumping syndrome** can occur; preventive measures include a diet limited in carbohydrate, fluids given 30 minutes prior to or following the ingestion of solids, and food intake divided into six small feedings. Milk may not be tolerated; supplements may need to be prescribed.

dumping syndrome: Disorder following food ingestion characterized by sweating and weakness, due to rapid emptying of stomach contents into the small intestine.

25.   Following intestinal surgery, a low-residue diet is best at first, gradually progressing to diet as tolerated; supplements may need to be prescribed.

26.   Following cholecystectomy, adherence to a low-fat diet for several months is required; supplements may need to be prescribed.

27.   Vitamin C supplements may be given (orally or parenterally) after surgery in amounts averaging 500–1500 mg/day; vitamin E supplementation is not prescribed postoperatively as it can cause repair tissue to form in a weakened state.

28.   In patients requiring immediate surgery, there is inadequate time for preoperative nutritional repletion; blood transfusions can elevate hemoglobin and hematocrit levels, and supplementation with vitamins C and K can enhance wound healing and help to prevent hemorrhage.

29.   Psychological support and sympathetic understanding are needed with postoperative feeding because patients often refuse to eat due to pain, remembered pain, and anorexia. Mealtimes should be as pleasurable as possible.

30.   During recovery from the trauma and stress of surgery, the requirements for protein can be five times greater and caloric needs far greater than normal. Once nitrogen losses have been replenished, fat alone is regained until body fat stores are back to normal. Since some of the weight gain may be due to water retention as well, weight gain is not always equivalent to gain in lean body mass.

31.   There have been major advances in surgical techniques and postoperative monitoring, yet nutrition therapy remains an integral component of life support systems, and has contributed to the improved morbidity and mortality rates.

32.   Severe burns can lead to greater increases in nutritional needs than any other trauma. Burns cause massive losses of fluids, electrolytes, and proteins from the burn site; the first concern is fluid replacement. Caloric intake should increase significantly, and protein needs are greater due to rapid body metabolism, protein losses, decreased protein synthesis, and breakdown of body tissue. Loss of weight is proportional to the extent of the burn, but high-protein/high-calorie intakes can lead to rapid healing.

33.   With severe burns, it is imperative that nutrition support is aggressive and include intravenous fluids, low-residue elemental diets, commercial supplements, and nutrient-rich foodstuffs; since a diet prescription for 3000–5000 calories with 150–200 grams of protein is not uncommon, all routes—oral, tube, TPN including fat emulsions—may need to be utilized. Care must be taken to avoid hemorrhage from overstimulation of the GI tract with large volumes of nutrient-rich material.

34.   Once the burn victim can handle an oral intake, an individualized high-calorie high-protein diet is prescribed, but usually requires between-meal supplementation with high-protein liquid preparations.

35.   Burns can be classified by the degree of severity as (a) small—less than 15–20% of the total body surface area (BSA) affected; (b) intermediate—20–40% BSA affected; and (c) severe—more than 40–50% BSA affected.

36. Burns can be classified by the depth of the injury as (a) partial-thickness—epithelium still present to spontaneously re-epithelialize; and (b) full-thickness—all epithelial remnants are destroyed mandating the use of grafts.

37. The primary goals for management of burn patients are (a) to support respiration and circulation until skin cover is restored and basal metabolic rate is normalized through the maintenance of normal fluid/electrolyte balance, blood volume, and nutritional status; and (b) the prevention of infection.

38. Patients with small burns or partial-thickness burns who were in good health at the time of trauma rarely develop nutritional problems.

39. Patients with extensive burns and those who were malnourished at the time of trauma require extensive nutrition support; survival ultimately depends on ability to withstand the stress. Weight loss with full-thickness burns may be as much as 30–40%, while protein, fat, and insensible water losses also contribute to increased caloric needs; elevated energy expenditures can be 30–300% above normal while grafting is underway.

40. Individualization of the post-burn diet is important, generally based upon the following:

$$\text{Calories} = 25 \times \text{body weight (kg)} + 40 \times \% \text{ BSA affected}$$
$$\text{Protein} = 2\text{–}4 \text{ g/kg (of body weight)/day}$$
$$\text{Supplements as required}$$

41. It is important to provide enough nonprotein calories so that protein can be utilized for tissue building and repair; protein should be of high quality and provide around 15% of total caloric intake.

42. The need for water-soluble vitamins, especially ascorbic acid, and zinc may be increased in burn victims.

43. Serum potassium should be monitored carefully following severe burns since hypokalemia can occur. During immobilization, high calcium intakes from the use of milk-based supplements can result in renal calculi.

44. Immediately following severe burns, gastrointestinal distress is common; intravenous feeding with gradual progression to oral intake plus nutrition supplements should be prescribed. Anorexia can occur due to pain, depression, and difficulty in moving the body.

45. Frequent weighings can aid in nutrition assessment while patients gradually return to pre-burn weight status, wound healing is completed, and metabolic rate normalizes.

46. Burns can result in permanent disability and disfigurement and may involve many weeks of constant pain. Thus, the psychological needs of the patient (as well as the financial strains) must be considered during treatment.

Exercise on Trauma and Nutrition

Keeping in mind the preceding Trauma Facts List, which provides current diet-related information to include in counseling individuals recovering from burns, surgery, or other physical trauma, prepare a sheet that lists available parenteral and/or enteral products and their major components and functions. A sample product list is given in Table 15.4. Show your sheet in rough draft form to several members of a nutrition support team to determine whether it is both complete and accurate. Then prepare a final version for your own future use as a practicing dietetic technician. Note: Leave extra space to add in new products as they become available.

Sample Product Sheet

Table 15.4 lists available products and their major components and functions.

Table 15.4   Nutrition Supplements and Meal Replacements: Sample Product List[a]

	cal/mL	mOsm/L	% cal protein	% cal carbohydrate	% cal fat	N:Cal	Protein source	Carbohydrate source	Fat source	mEq Na/L	Function
Supplements											
Citrotein	0.53		24.1	73.2	2.3	1:93	Egg white solids	Sucrose Dextrin maltose	Mono and diglycerides	23	Contains 50% RDA of protein, vitamins and minerals
Lanolac	0.66		21	30	49	1:81	Casein	Lactose	Coconut oil	1.1	Protein supplement for low-sodium diets
Lolactene vanilla	0.8	670 mOsm/kg	26	52.8	21	1:70	Low lactose non-fat milk	Corn syrup Sucrose	Vegetable oil	36.2	Protein supplement, minimal lactose content
Meritene (liquid) vanilla chocolate	1.0	640	24	46	30	1:79	Skim milk Casein	Sucrose Lactose Corn syrup solids	Vegetable oil	40.5	Protein supplement
Sustacal (liquid) vanilla chocolate	1.0	638, 616	24	41.3	20.7	1:79	Skim milk	Sucrose Lactose Corn syrup solids	Partially hydro-genated soy oil	47.1	Protein supplement, low lactose content
Meritene powder + skim milk	1.0		35.9	62.4	1.7	1:43	Skim milk	Lactose Corn syrup solids	Cow milk fat	39.1	Protein supplement utilizing skim milk
Meritene powder + whole milk	1.0		26.4	44.8	28.8	1:48	Milk	Lactose Corn syrup solids	Cow milk fat	39.1	Protein supplement utilizing whole milk
Sustagen powder (normal dilution) vanilla chocolate	1.8	721	24	68	8	1:79	Nonfat dry milk Powdered whole milk	Glucose Lactose Corn syrup solids	Cow milk fat	54.3	Protein supplement
Meal Replacements											
Compleat-B	1.0	468	16	48	36	1:131	Skim milk Beef	Lactose Sucrose	Corn oil Beef fat	59	Tube feeding—unflavored blenderized house diet for anabolism
Ensure vanilla black walnut	1.06	460	14	54.5	31.5	1:155	Casein Soy protein isolate	Sucrose Corn syrup solids	Corn oil	32	Tube or oral feeding, lactose-free for anabolism
Isocal	1.05	350	12.9	49.6	38.5	1:169	Soy protein isolate Casein	Glucose Corn syrup solids	MCT Soy oil	22.6	Tube feeding—unflavored iso-tonic for anabolism
Nutri-1000	1.06	400	13	40	47	1:167	Skim milk	Glucose Sucrose Lactose Dextrin maltose	Corn oil	23	Tube or oral feeding for anabolism
Portagen	1.0	354	16	44	40	1:160	Casein	Sucrose Corn syrup solids	MCT Safflower oil	27	Oral feeding for malabsorption of long chain fats for ana-bolism
Precision isotonic vanilla	1.0	300 mOsm/kg	12	60	28	1:183	Egg albumin	Glucose Oligosaccharides Sucrose	Vegetable oil	34	Tube or oral feeding Isotonic lactose-free
Precision moderate Nitrogen vanilla citrus	1.2	395 mOsm/kg	12	60	28	1:169	Egg albumin	Maltodextrin Sucrose	Vegetable oil	43.3	Easily absorbed protein source Moderate fat content, low osmolality
Other (Insert additional products in alphabet-ical order, using a footnote system to in-dicate where products fit into above list.):											

[a]Adapted from Schneider *et al.* (1977, p. 85).

STEP 5: CANCER AND AIDS FACTS

Degenerative diseases such as cancer and AIDS are frequently complicated by anorexia and the accompanying ill effects of malnutrition. Metabolic disorders as well as side effects from medications and therapies can also contribute to the depletion of nutrient stores and to poor nutritional status. Yet, morbidity and mortality can be reduced with optimization of nutritional status.

The following Cancer and AIDS Facts List provides current diet-related information to include in counseling individuals with various types of cancer and AIDS.

Cancer and AIDS Facts List

1.   Approximately one out of every four Americans will develop cancer during his/her lifetime. Although cancer is still one of the major health problems for Americans, significant progress has been made during the past several decades in research, treatment, and prevention.

2.   Almost half of all fatal cancers affect the lung, large intestine, or breast. Epidemiological studies have provided most of the information on the correlations between food, nutrition, and these and other cancers, so much remains to be documented.

3.   The term cancer can be used interchangeably with *neoplasm* and *malignant tumor,* and is defined as a growth disturbance with excessive and unnecessary cell proliferation. When nonspreading and localized, a cancer might not produce serious illness or invade other tissues; such increases in cell numbers are termed *benign.* If the cells multiply rapidly and invade other tissues (metastasize), the cancer is *malignant.*

4.   If discovered early, cancer may be controlled by use of proper treatment modes; if left untreated, cancer can spread, with significant metabolic side effects including elevated metabolism, disturbances in metabolic processes, and destruction of body tissues.

5.   It is important for cancer patients to avoid the onset of malnutrition since it is easier to prevent than overcome a debilitated state.

6.   There is no special diet or nutrient which has been proven to cure cancer, but a well-balanced nourishing diet can help to maintain the strength and resistance required to combat the disease and enhance the treatment.

7.   Inadequate nutrient intake may occur with cancer due to the following associated factors: (a) anorexia and weight loss; (b) alterations in taste and smell; (c) difficulty in chewing and swallowing; (d) early satiety; (e) rapid physical feelings of "fullness"; (f) severe pain; and (g) anxiety.

mucositis: Inflammation of the mucous membranes.

stomatitis: Inflammation of the mouth.

gingivitis: Inflammation of the gums (gingiva).

8.   Cancer treatments that can lead to poor nutrient intake include: (a) chemotherapy—nausea, vomiting, diarrhea, constipation, **mucositis, stomatitis, gingivitis,** glossitis, anorexia, malabsorption; (b) radiotherapy—dry mouth, loss of taste acuity, difficulty chewing and swallowing, esophagitis, nausea, vomiting, diarrhea, constipation, mucositis, anorexia, malabsorption; and (c) surgery—difficulty chewing and swallowing, diarrhea, malabsorption.

9.   Optimal nutritional status is required during the course of the disease and with treatment therapies; symptoms affecting nutrient intake should be treated individually. Aggressive nutrition therapy can mean the difference between life and death for cancer patients, as many patients actually die from the starvation associated with cancer rather than from the disease itself.

10.   The malnutrition that accompanies cancer results from: (a) reduced food intake; (b) impaired digestion and absorption; (c) loss of nutrients; (d) competition for nutrients by tumors; and (e) increased energy expenditure from illness.

11.   The effects of the malnutrition that accompanies cancer include (a) reduced tolerance to treatment procedures; (b) weight loss; (c) decrease in tissue repair; (d) impaired **immunocompetence;** and (e) altered drug metabolism.

immunocompetence: Ability to resist infection, disease.

12.   Nutrition management in cancer patients is highly individualized and depends on the type and degree of severity of the disease. It is important to realize that, for patients in advanced stages of untreatable cancer, food may be one of the few remaining pleasures of life, so may contribute as much to emotional health as to nutritional and physical status.

13.   Appetite may increase with successful pain control and the alleviation of depression; periodic evaluations of nutritional status are essential for proper care of cancer patients.

14.   Oftentimes, cancer patients experience an increased taste threshold for sweets and a decreased threshold for or aversion to certain other foods; this allows for the inclusion of high-calorie sugar-rich products, but often requires the use of meat substitutes as well as special care in meal preparation. Taste acuity and food preferences usually return to normal when cancer is responding to therapy.

15. Specific nutrition treatments are associated with each type of cancer therapy, including chemotherapy, radiotherapy, surgery, and immunotherapy:

○ *Chemotherapy.* Chemotherapy, the use of drugs to destroy cancerous cells, can serve as the sole treatment or an adjunct to other modes; the goal is to attain the maximum benefits without causing severe toxicity, since the drugs are toxic to normal cells as well as cancerous tissue. Usually a low-residue or elemental diet is prescribed on an individual basis.

○ *Radiotherapy.* Radiotherapy, the use of radiation selectively to destroy abnormal cells, can cause a number of nutrition problems depending on the site of the radiation.

○ *Surgery.* Surgery and the associated nutrition problems depend upon the site of the surgery, with the same preoperative and postoperative nutrition guidelines as for other surgical conditions.

○ *Immunotherapy.* Immunotherapy attempts to alter tumors or increase the patient's immune response and may be used as an adjunct to chemotherapy, radiotherapy, or surgery; side effects include anorexia, nausea, vomiting, diarrhea, constipation, malabsorption and altered taste, each of which requires the appropriate nutrition guidelines.

16. Radiation treatment in the head and neck area frequently causes dryness of the mouth, mucositis, stomatitis, changes in taste, pain with swallowing, burning sensations, anorexia and, if affecting the salivary glands, alterations in the composition and quantity of saliva. The diet should be modified to ease swallowing and minimize pain by avoiding (a) acidic foods such as citrus juices, (b) spicy foodstuffs, (c) foods served at temperature extremes, (d) dry foods (unless moistened with milk, gravies, etc.), and (e) large meals (small frequent feedings are preferable). Individualization of the diet is important (with use of supplements if required) to ensure adequate intake of calories, protein, and other nutrients.

17. Drug metabolism may be altered with malnutrition and cancer, due in part to the following: (a) malnutrition—decreased tissue uptake, altered gastrointestinal absorption, alterations in liver enzymes and body hydration status, changes in protein metabolism, hormonal changes, and cardiac or renal abnormality; and (b) cancer—catabolism, chemotherapy, radiotherapy, alcohol carcinogenesis, fluid overload, and certain types of tumors.

18. **Granulocytopenic** patients often receive antibiotics that destroy gastrointestinal bacteria and increase the susceptibility to infection from foodborne pathogenic microorganisms; patients with a reduced white blood cell count and a lowered resistance to infection may require a *Reduced Bacteria Diet,* which eliminates fresh fruits and vegetables, and allows only processed foods, cooked foods, and sterile water, all served in disposable dishware with disposable utensils.

granulocytopenia: Condition characterized by an abnormal reduction of certain white blood cells.

19. The ultimate success of diet therapy depends on the ability to meet individual physical and psychological needs. It is important to take into consideration the effect on appetite of anxiety, fear, hair loss and poor body image, loss of control over body functions, and depression.

20. Weight loss in cancer patients is due to the combination of decreased caloric intake, increased caloric utilization, and altered metabolism; when caloric deficits occur or physical disturbances interfere with oral intake, use of parenteral/enteral feedings should be considered.

21. Elemental diets can provide nutrition in clear liquid form when minimal residue is required (e.g., Mead Johnson's Flexical, Doyle's Precision LR or Precision HN, Cutter's Vipep, Ross's Vital, Eaton's Vivonex or Vivonex HR).

22. Parenteral and enteral support are required by patients with increased needs for energy and protein that cannot be met solely by oral intake. There is no universal formula for enteral feeding or parenteral nutrition that is applicable to all patients; product taste, osmolality, digestibility, and specific disease state must be taken into consideration.

23. In parenteral feedings caloric intake at a rate of 40–45 cal/kg/day with 1.5 grams of protein per kilogram can achieve positive nitrogen balance, as will oral intakes of 35–40 cal/kg/day. Fat emulsions (e.g., Intralipid and Liposyn) are isotonic, providing 1.1 calories/gram, and supplying essential fatty acids during long-term use of TPN (but should not constitute more than 60% of total calories).

24. Total parenteral nutrition may require the intake of vitamins K and B_{12}, folic acid, and iron via another route of administration. Deficiency syndromes, especially of the water-

soluble vitamins, may develop rapidly with parenteral nutrition use. Since a single solution providing the proper amounts of vitamins has yet to be developed, several different solutions need to be administered. To avoid possible side effects, only RDA levels for the fat-soluble vitamins should be given.

25.   It is important not to make abrupt changes from one modality to another, so patients should gradually progress from

$$(parenteral \rightarrow parenteral + enteral \rightarrow enteral \rightarrow enteral + food \rightarrow food),$$

receiving adequate nutrition from the second feeding method before discontinuation of the first.

26.   Better response to chemotherapy, radiotherapy, and cancer surgery has been observed in patients receiving total parenteral nutrition. Yet, the metabolism or growth of cancerous tumors can be stimulated by an increased intake of nutrients, so supplementation must be an adjunct to anti-tumor therapies.

27.   Numerous unproven claims blame the development of cancer on diet and offer nutrient megadoses and food fads as cures; adherence to such programs can result in nutritional toxicities and deficiencies, diminished nutritional status, and delay of important medical treatment (see Chapter 6). Attention to proper nutrition is important for cancer patients, but diet is only part of the overall treatment plan and should not be substituted for complete, effective therapy.

28.   During the decade following the identification of AIDS, the acquired immune deficiency syndrome has sharply increased in prevalence, and the rise in the associated mortality rate is alarming. Transmission of the virus that causes this fatal disease is by exchange of body fluids (e.g., blood and semen). Victims appear to acquire the disease through inoculation with contaminated blood, sexual contact with an AIDS carrier, or perinatal transmission from a maternal AIDS host. Casual contact does not appear to be involved in the transmission of the AIDS virus.

29.   So far, there is no known cure for AIDS. The drug zidovudine (AZT), which inhibits the replication of the virus, has been approved for treatment of AIDS patients. Various other drugs are used to treat the myriad illnesses that occur when the immune system is compromised. The side effects from drug therapy, in addition to the symptoms of the disease, can have nutrition implications.

30.   AIDS patients may suffer from anorexia, weight loss, malabsorption, diarrhea, fever, and depression. Nutrition support can help to treat the symptoms as they arise and is essential for the prevention of secondary malnutrition. Specific nutrition problems vary markedly from patient to patient, so diet therapy should be highly individualized.

31.   Debilitated AIDS patients may require enteral and/or parenteral support. Since AIDS is terminal, difficult ethical questions arise when patients are maintained for prolonged periods of time on total parenteral nutrition. Therapies should be tailored to suit the individual patient's needs and desires.

32.   Unproven claims for dietary cures may attract the victims of AIDS and can appeal to those fearful of contacting the disease. Good nutrition is essential to promote optimal health of the immune system, but adherence to unproven diet programs (e.g., vitamin/mineral megadoses, "immune power" diets, "detoxification" regimens) can result in nutritional toxicities and deficiencies, diminished nutritional status, and delay of important medical care (see Chapter 6). Attention to proper nutrition is important for AIDS patients, but diet is only part of the overall treatment and should not be substituted for complete therapy.

Exercise on Cancer, AIDS, and Nutrition

Keeping in mind the preceding Cancer and AIDS Facts List, which provides some of the most current diet-related information to include in counseling individuals with various types of cancer and AIDS, prepare a sheet which lists available parenteral and/or enteral products and their major components and functions. A sample product list is given in Table 15.5. Show your sheet in rough draft form to several members of a nutrition support team to determine whether it is both complete and accurate. Then prepare a final version for your own future use as a practicing dietetic technician. Note: Leave extra space to add in new products as they become available.

Sample Product Sheet

Table 15.5 lists available products and their major components and functions.

Table 15.5   Elemental Diets: Sample Product List[a]

Defined formula diets (DFD)	cal/mL	mOsm/L	% cal protein	% cal carbohydrate	% cal fat	% cal linoleic acid	N:cal	Protein source	Carbohydrate source	Fat source	mEq Na/L	Function (all DFD are low residue clear liquid diets)
For maintenance												
Flexical orange vanilla banana fruit punch	1.0	805	8.8	61.1	30.1	2.16	1:264	Hydrolyzed protein + Methionine, tyrosine, tryptophan	Sucrose Dextrooligo-saccharides	MCT Partially hydro-genated soy oil	15.2	30% cal from fat 60% cal from carbohydrate Protein source requires some digestion
Jejunal beef broth beverage, cherry pudding	.91	990 1200	9.1	90.0	0.82	0.56	1:252	Crystalline amino acids	Glucose Dextrins	Safflower oil	33.7	60:40 essential to non-essential amino acid Easily absorbed protein source of high biological value
Precision LR cherry lemon lime orange	1.08	600	8.8	90.8	0.65	0.48	1:258	Egg albumin	Maltose Dextrins	Safflower oil	27.4	Low osmolality Protein source requires some digestion
Vivonex vanilla beef broth orange grape tomato chocolate	1.0	550	8.1	90.3	1.3	1.04	1:286	Crystalline amino acids	Maltose Dextrins	Safflower oil	37.3	High osmolality when fla-vored Easily absorbed protein source of high biological value
W-T low residue beef bouillon	.98	649	8.6	90.7	0.7	0.56	1:304	Crystalline amino acids	Dextrins	Safflower oil	68.8	Easily absorbed protein source of high biological value
For anabolism												
Precision HN citrus fruit vanilla	1.0	580	16.6	82.9	0.42	0.33	1:125	Egg albumin	Maltose Dextrins	Safflower oil	40.5	Low osmolality Protein source requires some digestion
Vivonex HN beef broth orange grape strawberry	1.0	800	16.6	84.1	0.78	0.62	1:127	Crystalline amino acids	Glucose Maltose	Safflower oil	27.4	Easily absorbed protein source
Special DFD Aminade	2.02	1050	4	68	28	11	1:418	Essential amino acids	Sucrose Dextrins	Soybean oil	2	Provides high-calorie, low-protein diet of high bio-logical value (only es-sential amino acids) for use as Giordano-Giovan-etti diet in renal failure Contains no vitamins
Others (Insert addi-tional products using a footnote system to indicate where products fit into above list.):												

[a]Adapted from Schneider *et al.* (1977, p. 86).

STEP 6: DEVELOPMENTAL DISABILITIES FACTS

Until recently, little professional attention was devoted to the diets and feeding prac-tices of the developmentally disabled population. Widespread recognition of the need for vocational rehabilitation and a normalized lifestyle has led to the development of disability-specific dietary guidelines and improved feeding practices.

The following Developmental Disabilities Facts List provides some of the most current diet-related information to include in counseling individuals with feeding problems.

Developmental Disabilities Facts List

1.   The mentally retarded and/or developmentally disabled (MRDD) individual may have feeding difficulties. Problems differ for each person depending on his/her individual degree of mental and physical disability.

2.   MRDD individuals and their families usually need coordinated care provided by the health care team; effective services require cooperative efforts for early identification and assessment, development of individual care plans, and open communication between team members and care provisioners.

3.   Some MRDD individuals do not have feeding difficulties (and some nonhandicapped children do suffer from feeding problems). Unless feeding difficulties are recognized and managed, they can lead to more serious problems. Abnormal social and behavioral development in children can lead to mealtime tantrums, bizarre food habits, poor food acceptance and/or food rejection, and delayed acquisition of self-feedings skills. The associated nutritional problems include obesity, anorexia nervosa, pica, and **rumination.**

4.   Feeding problems can also be due to the physical defects that arise from deviations in normal growth or disorders of body organs, tissues, or systems. Proper nutrition is important for the maximization of genetic potential.

5.   The major nutrition-related deviations in the MRDD are linear growth delay, underweight, overweight, and anemia; the one preventable cause is inappropriate feeding due to a lack of understanding as to what, how, and how much to feed the MRDD individual.

6.   The nutrition assessment of the MRDD individual is important, but may prove difficult due to the lack of standard criteria; little data is available for the determination of individual dietary needs, and special growth charts are unavailable.

7.   Some of the feeding problems and nutritional side effects that affect MRDD individuals include (a) mechanical feeding problems; (b) delayed feeding skills; (c) inborn errors of metabolism; (d) anemia; (e) overweight; (f) underweight; (g) growth delay and/or delayed weaning; (h) anorexia; and (i) poor or bizarre food habits.

8.   Most feeding problems appear to fit into one or more of four distinct categories: (a) mechanical feeding difficulties; (b) feeding skill difficulties; (c) behavior problems; and (d) disorders requiring diet therapy.

8a.   Oral–motor problems interfere with the normal ingestion of foods (e.g., with profound retardation, severe neurological or physical defects, or both), leading to the inability to chew and swallow properly; the potential for overcoming such disabilities is limited. The main dietary goal is to ensure adequate food intake with modified consistency and to keep both the food and the feeding process as normal as possible. Frequent dietary analysis and body weight assessments are important to assure optimal growth and proper weight maintenance. If adequate energy and/or protein cannot be obtained, supplements should be used. Some individuals with neurological disorders may require tube feedings, or TPN if disorders of the digestive tract preclude oral food intake. Some oral–motor problems improve, while others do not. Delayed oral development can also cause abnormal tongue/mouth behaviors and drooling or choking. Persistence of primitive reflexive responses beyond infancy can interfere with desirable motor control and cause feeding problems. Improper reflexes and feeding implications common in the MRDD are included in Table 15.6.

8b.   Nutritional status can be affected when outside assistance with feeding is required. The goal of nutrition management is to devise diet plans based on foods which are easy to eat (e.g., finger foods, mashed foods, etc.) yet meet nutritional needs. Behavior

rumination: Practice of regurgitating and rechewing food which has already been swallowed.

Table 15.6   Common Feeding Difficulties of the MRDD

Reflex	Description	Implications
ATNR (asymmetrical tonic neck reflex)	As head is turned, arms have increased muscle tone, hand looked at is extended.	Interferes with ability to bring hands to mouth.
Moro	If let head drop, arms are flung.	Interferes with ability to hold bottle, eating utensils, or finger foods.
Tonic labyrinthine	When lying down, muscle tone is increased.	Choking occurs when fed while lying down.
STNR (symmetrical tonic neck reflex)	Moving the head causes arms and legs to flail.	Interferes with ability to pick up food or eating utensils and bring to the mouth.

management techniques and mini-meals are helpful. It is important to monitor food intake and height/weight status. Use of specially designed equipment and recipes can allow for self-feeding and self-preparation of foods; an excellent book which outlines basic nutrition, meal planning and food preparation, as well as providing over a hundred recipes—all written on a fourth to fifth grade reading level—is "Effective Meal Planning and Food Preparation for the MRDD" by Amary (see Suggested Readings in Step 8).

8c. Nutrition intervention is required with problems of food acceptance, mealtime behavior, pica, rumination, and anorexia nervosa. The goal of nutrition management is to improve the variety of the diet and eliminate undesirable behaviors at mealtime. Dietary intake should be monitored, as should height/weight status. Rumination often occurs in MRDD children who appear to eat great quantities of food but are not overweight, and the practice can lead to malnutrition. The MRDD can have (i) learning disabilities and poor eye/hand coordination resulting in difficulties with use of eating utensils, (ii) abnormal muscle tone which interferes with the ability to sit erectly, (iii) orthopedic problems which can impair the ability to sit properly, and (iv) bony deformities which can hamper self-feeding skills.

8d. Disorders requiring diet therapy which are common to the MRDD include overweight, underweight, anemia, and inborn errors of metabolism. The goals of nutrition intervention are weight management (to normalize in proportion to height) and proper treatment for anemia. The most common inborn errors of metabolism are (i) phenylketonurea (PKU), (ii) **galactosemia,** and (iii) **maple syrup urine disease (MSUD),** which require the provision of a nutritionally adequate diet while limiting the intake of the nutrient which is improperly metabolized: (i) phenylalanine in PKU, (ii) galactose in galactosemia; and (iii) leucine, isoleucine, and valine in MSUD; the amount of the problem nutrient provided in the diet must be sufficient for growth and development without exceeding the individual's ability to metabolize it. Dietary intake, height/weight, and laboratory parameters need to be carefully monitored.

9. It is important to assess typical dietary patterns and evaluate health/dietary records; anthropometric measurements to determine height, weight, and skinfold thickness may require segmental measures using flexible metal tape and sling balances for weighing. Assessment and reassessment should be a continuous procedure.

10. An individualized assessment chart to aid in developing a feeding plan for each MRDD individual is essential (see Table 15.7 for sample Developmental Feeding Tool).

galactosemia: Inborn error of metabolism with a lack of the enzyme responsible for converting galactose to glucose; characterized by anorexia, vomiting, and diarrhea after ingestion of foods containing galactose or lactose.

maple syrup urine disease (MSUD): Inborn error of metabolism with a deficiency in the enzyme responsible for the metabolism of certain proteins; characterized by mental and physical retardation, early death, and urine and sweat that smell like maple syrup.

Table 15.7 Developmental Feeding Tool (DFT)

Physical handicaps	Neuromotor/muscular handicaps	Oral/motor handicaps
Underweight _____	Body tonicity _____	Facial muscle tone _____
Overweight _____	Head control _____	Gag reflex _____
Short _____	Trunk control _____	Bite _____
Tall _____	Range of motion _____	Rooting _____
Abnormal body proportions _____	Dominance established _____	Suck/swallow _____
Microcephalic _____	Grasp _____	Respiration _____
Macrocephalic _____	Reflexes _____	Oral sensitivity _____
Anemic _____	**Scoliosis** _____	Tongue movements _____
Diabetic _____	**Lordosis** _____	Drools _____
Gastrointestinal disorder _____	**Kyphosis** _____	
Food allergies/intolerances _____	Other: _____	
Special diet: _____		
Medication(s): _____		
Other: _____		
Feeding patterns (describe): _____		

Current diet status		Comments: _____
Blenderized food _____	Finger feeds _____	_____
Limited texture _____	Uses spoon _____	_____
Chopped table food _____	Uses fork _____	_____
Table foods _____	Uses knife _____	_____
Fed under full aid _____	Drinks from cup _____	_____
Feeds with some aid _____	Drinks with straw _____	_____
Feeds unassisted _____	Slow eater _____	_____
	Normal eating rate _____	_____
	Fast eater _____	_____

microcephalic: Having an abnormally small head.

macrocephalic: Having an abnormally large head.

scoliosis: Lateral curvature of the spine.

lordosis: Abnormal spinal concavity.

kyphosis: Abnormal spinal convexity; hunchback.

11. The nutrition care plan for MRDD individuals needs to be practical and usable. Each diet plan needs to address the basic techniques for facilitation of eating with adaptive equipment, include behavioral management and positioning techniques, and outline the individualized diet and any potential diet/drug interactions.

12. Drugs are often used to help treat the MRDD. Those individuals using stimulants need to be monitored to ensure adequate caloric intake; use of anticonvulsants may require supplementation with folic acid and regular hematological profiles to monitor serum levels of folic acid and vitamin B_{12}.

13. Successful diet counseling with MRDD individuals must address other factors which can influence diet acceptance—such as mealtime environment, emotions, overall appearance of food, and family interactions—and emphasize the importance of individualization in order to suit both the patient and his/her family or caretaker(s).

14. It is important to encourage self-motivation, foster feelings of accomplishment, and prepare MRDD individuals to be able to deal with life as efficiently and enjoyably as possible.

Exercise on Diet and the Developmentally Disabled

Keeping in mind the preceding Developmental Disabilities Facts List, which provides some of the most current diet-related information to include in counseling individuals with feeding problems, prepare a simplified version for use as a patient handout. You may include graphics and/or prepare in a poster format, if desired; see the Sample Handout. Show your handout in rough draft form to classmates or co-workers for constructive criticism on the overall design, content, and potential effectiveness for use in pertinent diet counseling situations. Then prepare a final version for your own future use as a practicing dietetic technician.

Sample Handout

Table 15.8 lists some tips that can help simplify meals.

Table 15.8 Simplifying Meals—Tip Sheet

1. Prepare a shopping list in advance by designing complete weekly menus. Try to stick to the list when shopping.
2. Budget money for food shopping carefully so that there is always enough.
3. Choose recipes that meet your dietary needs, appear appetizing, and are easy to follow. Make sure that you have all of the ingredients and utensils required.
4. Invite friends to share meals. Be sure to prepare enough for everyone.
5. Cook carefully, prepare foods carefully, and enjoy your kitchen activities by being *careful*. Keep these practical hints in mind:

    ○ Make sure your hands are *dry* when you cook.
    ○ Cut with a knife facing away from you. Use a cutting board.
    ○ Wipe up spills immediately.
    ○ Always use pot holders for hot items.
    ○ Set hot dishes on special boards or pads.
    ○ Always set pans on the stove so that handles are not hanging out over the stove top.
    ○ Make sure your hands are dry when using a plug in an electrical outlet.
    ○ Do not remove a plug by pulling on the cord.
    ○ Keep matches in a safe place.
    ○ Check gas stoves daily to make sure that the pilot light is still on.

STEP 7: ANEMIA GUIDELINES

Poverty, ignorance, and indifference can lead to the development of nutritional anemia, as can certain metabolic states and diseases. Yet, appropriate dietary information can assist individuals in the prevention of this nutritional disorder. Foods contain the preventive nutrients, as well as substances that can inactivate or interfere with utilization and contribute to anemic states. The prescribed diet should be acceptable, practical, affordable, and compatible with lifestyle to be effective in the prevention and treatment of nutritional anemia.

In order to be able to advise individuals with nutritional anemias as to desirable dietary patterns, it is essential to have access to all of the hands-on material required for effective counseling sessions. It is also important to be able to record all of the pertinent information regarding each diet counseling session in the patient's medical charts. The information provided here should help to improve your confidence—and skills—regarding your counseling abilities.

This step includes suggested counseling strategies to use with patients who have nutritional anemias (i.e., iron, folic acid, and vitamin B_{12} deficiency anemias); although each nutritional anemia is discussed independently of the others, it is essential to consider the ramifications of cases with more than one complicating factor. The following references may prove helpful.

Suggested Readings on Nutritional Anemias

BAKER, S., and DEMAEYER, E. 1979. Nutritional anemia: Its understanding and control. Amer. J. Clin. Nutr. 32, Feb., 368.

BEARD, J. 1986. Yin, yang, and iron. Nutr. Today 21, Jul./Aug., 17.

BEUTLER, E. 1988. The common anemias: State of the art review. J. Am. Med. Assoc. 259, Apr. 22, 2433.

BEZKOROVAINY, A. 1980. Biochemistry of Non-Heme Iron. New York: Plenum Press.

CHANARIN, I. 1979. The Megaloblastic Anemias. New York: Blackwell Scientific Publications.

CROSBY, W. 1972. Iron: A Total Clinical Learning Experience. New York: MEDCOM, Inc.

DALLMAN, P., YIP, R., and JOHNSON, C. 1984. Prevalence and causes of anemia in the U.S. Amer. J. Clin. Nutr. 39, Mar., 437.

HALL, C. (Editor). 1983. The Cobalamins. New York: Churchill Livingstone.

HERBERT, V. 1959. The Megaloblastic Anemias. Philadelphia: Grune & Stratton.

KASS, L. 1976. Pernicious Anemia. Philadelphia: W. B. Saunders Co.

KELCHER, J. 1980. Anemia in infancy and childhood. Primary Care 7, Sept., 473.

PILCH, S., and SENLI, F. (Editors). 1984. Assessment of the Iron Nutrition Status of the U.S. Population, 1976–1980. Bethesda, MD: Federation of American Societies for Experimental Biology.

POLLITT, E., and LIEBEL, R. (Editors). 1982. Iron Deficiency. New York: Raven Press.

STEINBERG, D. 1982. Anemia. Philadelphia: W. B. Saunders Co.

STROBACH, R., et al. 1988. The value of the physical examination in the diagnosis of anemia. Arch. Internal Med. 148, Apr., 831.

WILLIAMS, W. (Editor). 1983. Hematology. New York: McGraw-Hill.

WINTROBE, W. (Editor). 1981. Clinical Hematology. Philadelphia: Lea & Febiger.

For journal subscriptions:

Blood. Grune and Stratton, 210 West Washington Square, Philadelphia, PA 19106.

British Journal of Hematology. Blackwell Scientific Publications, 527 Madison Avenue, Suite 1217, New York, NY 10022.

Seminars in Hematology. The Curtis Center, Independence Square West, Philadelphia, PA 19106.

For audiovisual:

Anemia. University of Kansas Medical Center, Hematology Department, Lawrence, KS 66045.

Counseling Guidelines—Anemia

Table 15.9 outlines the steps for diet counseling with an anemic patient. The following material gives the details of each step.

I.   Initial Session

I.   A.   General Guidelines

1.   Utilize the Differential Diagnoses, Morphologic Classification, and Comparative Anemias Charts to assist in the diagnosis/assessment.
2.   Use Medical History Form to assess patient's nutritional status.
3.   Weigh patient and record on Weight Chart. The chart is a helpful tool for visualization of progress.
4.   Assist patient in recording 24-hour recall of food intake using 24-Hour Recall Form. This will aid in home record keeping of food intake.
5.   Instruct patient to keep daily Food Intake Record so that typical food intake patterns can be evaluated. Advise patient not to deviate from normal eating pattern. Stress the importance of recording food intake immediately after eating.
6.   Instruct patient to complete Diet History. This provides for a basic evaluation of food intake patterns. (Use Pre-test from Chapter 2.)
7.   Record evaluation and recommendation(s) using the SOAP method in Technician's Notes. This form can be kept in your files with a copy in the patient's medical records.

I.   B.   Differential Diagnoses Chart

Table 15.10 may aid in the diagnosis of the type and severity of anemia. Only those laboratory tests used to identify *nutritional* anemias are included. Note that other diseases and conditions may cause these abnormal results as well.

I.   C.   Morphologic Classification Chart

Use the RBC indices given in Table 15.11 for morphologic classification.

I.   D.   Comparative Anemias Chart

Table 15.12 gives comparative information on nutritional anemias.

Table 15.10   Differential Diagnoses Chart

Laboratory test	Reason for test	Interpretation of results
Hematology:		
Hemoglobin	To evaluate hemoglobin status	Decreased levels occur in anemia.
Hematocrit	To evaluate red blood cell (RBC) status	Decreased levels occur in anemia.
RBC	To evaluate red blood cell (RBC) status	Decreased levels occur in anemia.
RBC indices	To estimate the size and hemoglobin content of red blood cells	MCV,[a] MCH,[b] and MCHC[c] values help indicate type of anemia.
Reticulocyte count	To measure bone marrow activity and the status of RBCs in circulation	Elevation indicates an increased number of new RBCs in circulation; depression indicates a decreased rate of RBC production.
WBC	To evaluate white blood cell (WBC) status	Decreased levels are common in megaloblastic anemias.
Platelets	To evaluate platelet production and survival	Decreased levels are indicative of an abnormality affecting hemopoiesis or platelet survival.

(continued)

Table 15.10   (Continued)

Laboratory test	Reason for test	Interpretation of results
Ferritin	To evaluate body iron stores	Decreased levels indicate iron deficiency.
Iron and total iron-binding capacity (TIBC)	To evaluate iron content of red blood cells	A decreased iron level with an elevated TIBC points to an iron deficiency; low iron and TIBC levels indicate a possible anemia of chronic disease.
Folic acid	To differentiate the megaloblastic anemias	A decreased level indicates folic acid deficiency anemia.
Vitamin B_{12}	To differentiate the megaloblastic anemias	A decreased level indicates pernicious or vitamin B_{12} deficiency anemia.
Blood smear	To identify red blood cell abnormalities that might be peculiar to a specific anemia	The presence of macrocytes and polymorphonuclear cells (PMNs) suggest megaloblastic anemia. The presence of pale microcytes indicates iron deficiency anemia.
Bone marrow analysis: Bone marrow aspirate	To observe the site of red blood cell production and to assess iron stores	The presence of megaloblasts indicates folic acid or vitamin B_{12} deficiency anemia. The absence or lack of hemosiderin indicates iron deficiency anemia.
Urinalysis: FIGlu Test	To aid in definitive diagnosis of folic acid deficiency anemia	An increased output of FIGlu indicates folic acid deficiency anemia.
Schilling test	To aid in definitive diagnosis of pernicious anemia	A decreased output of radioactive vitamin B_{12} occurs when the intrinsic factor is missing.
Methylmalonic acid test	To distinguish between vitamin B_{12} and folate deficiencies	An increased urinary excretion of methylmalonic acid indicates vitamin B_{12} deficiency.
Gastric analysis: Histidine load test	To aid in definitive diagnosis of pernicious anemia	Achlorhydria is common in pernicious anemia.
Other: Guaiac test	To aid in diagnosis of GI bleeding	A positive result indicates the presence of stool blood and possible iron deficiency.

[a,b,c]See Table 15.11.

Table 15.11   Morphologic Classification Chart

Type of anemia	MCV[a]	MCH[b]	MCHC[c]
Normocytic	82–92	27–31	32–36
Macrocytic	>94	>31	32–36
Microcytic	<80	<27	<32
Normal	82–92	27–31	32–36

[a]MCV (mean corpuscular volume)

$$= \frac{\text{Hematocrit}}{\text{RBC}} = \text{Average size of a RBC.}$$

[b]MCH (mean corpuscular hemoglobin)

$$= \frac{\text{Hemoglobin}}{\text{RBC}} = \text{Weight of hemoglobin in the average RBC.}$$

[c]MCHC (mean corpuscular hemoglobin concentration)

$$= \frac{\text{Hemoglobin}}{\text{Hematocrit}} = \text{Concentration of hemoglobin in the average RBC.}$$

Table 15.12   Comparative Anemias Chart[a]

	Iron deficiency	Folic acid deficiency	Vitamin B$_{12}$ deficiency
Hematology:			
Hemoglobin	Decreased[b]	Decreased	Decreased
Hematocrit	Decreased[b]	Decreased	Decreased
RBC	Normal or decreased	Decreased	Decreased
RBC indices:			
MCV	<80	>100	>100
MCH	<27	>32	>32
MCHC	<32.5	Normal	Normal
WBC	Decreased in pro-longed deficiency	Decreased	Decreased
Ferritin	Decreased	Normal	Normal
Platelets	Normal or elevated	Decreased	Decreased
Iron[c]	<50 mcg/dL	Normal or elevated	Normal or elevated
TIBC[c]	>400 mcg/dL	Normal	Normal or decreased
Folic acid	Normal	Decreased	Normal
Vitamin B$_{12}$	Normal	Normal	Decreased
Blood smear	Hypochromic micro-cytes	Hypersegmented PMNs, oval macro-cytes	Hypersegmented PMNs, oval macro-cytes
Bone marrow analysis:			
Bone marrow aspirate	Little or no hemo-siderin	Megaloblasts present	Megaloblasts present
Urinalysis:			
FIGlu test	Negative	Positive	Negative
Schilling test	Negative	Negative	Positive
Methylmalonic acid test	Negative	Negative	Positive
Gastric analysis:			
Histidine load test	Achlorhydria some-times present	Achlorhydria uncom-mon	Achlorhydria common
Other:			
Guaiac test	Sometimes positive	Negative	Negative
Additional clinical symptoms:	Pallor, dry and scanty hair; spoon nails and glossitis pres-ent in severe cases	Glossitis, weight loss, diarrhea	Glossitis, pale yellow complexion, neuro-logical symptoms such as paresthesia
Likely causes:[d]	1. Inadequate diet 2. Blood loss 3. Deficient iron utili-zation (i.e., infec-tion and renal fail-ure) 4. Malabsorption (i.e., partial gas-trectomy, achlor-hydria) 5. Increased need, as in pregnancy	1. Inadequate diet 2. Chronic alcohol-ism 3. Liver disease 4. Malabsorption syndromes (i.e., sprue, celiac dis-ease) 5. Folate antagonists such as anti-con-vulsant drugs and oral contracep-tives 6. Increased need, as in pregnancy	1. Inadequate diet (unlikely except among vegans) 2. Lack of intrinsic factor (i.e., perni-cious anemia, gastric resection) 3. Malabsorption syndromes (i.e., Crohn's disease, sprue, diverticulo-sis, "blind loop" syndrome)

[a]See Tables 15.10 and 15.11 for explanations of abbreviations.
[b]Not indicative of iron deficiency until the anemia is well advanced.
[c]A percentage of transferrin saturation [(Iron × 100)/TIBC] of less than 15 indicates impaired erythropoiesis as this is a reflection of the amount of iron available to the erythroid marrow. Serum iron does not fall until iron stores are exhausted.
[d]To treat any anemia, the underlying cause(s) must be determined and eliminated, if possible. With those anemias not caused by nutrient deficiencies, vitamin and/or iron therapy will be of no value. Usual laboratory measures may be inaccurate when blood volume is abnormal (e.g., dehydration, overhydra-tion).

I. E. Patient Records

1. Medical History Form

Date _____ Referred by _____

Name _____ Date of birth _____

Address _____ Phone no. _____

Occupation _____ Hours per work week ____ Work phone no. _____

Educational background _____ Religious/ethnic background _____

Sex ____ Marital status _____

Household composition: Live alone _____ Spouse _____ Children/No. _____ Other: _____

General health status:

Physician _____ Address _____

Phone no. _____ Date of last visit _____

Ambulatory care required? _____ If so, describe: _____

Neuromuscular problems? _____ If so, how is eating affected? _____

Visual/auditory problems? _____ If so, describe: _____

Chewing difficulties? _____ If so, describe: _____

Appetite typically good? _____ fair? _____ poor? _____

Digestion/elimination difficulties? _____ If so, describe: _____

Food intolerances? _____ If so, describe: _____

Pica? _____ If so, describe: _____

Liver disease? _____ If so, describe: _____

Renal disease? _____ If so, describe: _____

Other: _____

Height _____ Weight _____ Frame _____

Triceps skinfold thickness _____ Mid-arm circumference _____

Mid-arm muscle circumference _____

Weight changes/problems? _____ If so, describe: _____

Clinical signs of nutritional status:

Skin _____ Mouth _____

Hair _____ Eyes _____

Teeth _____ Other: _____

Lab data:

Hematocrit _____ Hemoglobin _____ RBC _____

MCV _____ MCH _____ MCHC _____

Serum Iron _____ TIBC _____

Blood smear _____

Serum albumin _____

Other: _____

Medications taken regularly: _____

Prescribed by: _____ Date(s) prescribed: _____

Nutrition supplements taken regularly: _____

Prescribed by: _____ Date(s) prescribed: _____

Special diet prescription: _____

Prescribed by: _____ Date of prescription: _____

How closely is diet followed? Always adhered to ___ Sometimes ___ Rarely ___ Never ___

Type of housing: Room ____ Apartment ____ Home ____ Institution ____

Prepare own meals? _____ Dine out? Often (more than once a day) _____ Rarely _____

Food shopping done independently? _____ If not, describe required assistance _____

Eligible for food stamps? _____ If so, are they currently being used? _____

Cigarette smoker? _____ If so, how much: _____

Exercise regularly? _____ If so, describe: _____

    No. times per week _____ No. minutes per session _____

Comments: _____

2. Weight Chart

Starting weight _____   Reasonable weight _____

Date	No. weeks on diet	Weight	Comments

3. 24-Hour Recall Form

Date	Time	Food and amount

I. F. Assignments

1. Food Intake Record

Date and time	Duration of meal (min)	Food and amount	Where[a]	With whom	Associated activity[b]	Associated emotions[c]

[a]Such as school, restaurant, kitchen, living room.
[b]For example, watching television, reading, talking.
[c]Attitude: bored, anxious, frustrated, depressed, happy, angry, tense, etc.

2. Diet History

Use the Pre-test from Chapter 2 (p. 30) to provide a record of typical foods eaten.

I. G. Technician's Notes

Patient: _____   Date: _____

S (Subjective data—how patient feels):
O (Objective data—physical measurements including diet/nutritional status):
A (Assessment—acceptability of dietary progress/nutritional status):
P (Plan—diet prescription and instruction):
Comments:

II. Follow-up Session(s)

II. A. General Guidelines

1. Weigh patient and record on Weight Chart.
2. Review assignments and discuss.
3. Individualize Personal Diet Plan and instruct patient in its use.
4. Instruct patient to self-evaluate adherence to Personal Diet Plan and development of good eating habits through continued use of Food Intake Record and Good Eating Checklist.
5. Record evaluation and recommendation(s) using the SOAP method in Technician's Notes. This form can be kept in your files with a copy in the patient's medical records.

II. B. Handouts

1. Personal Diet Plan

Name _____

How to use diet plan:

1. Select a variety of foods from each of the Basic Food Groups.
2. Include the recommended number of servings from each Food Group.
3. See Table 15.13.
   Iron deficiency anemia: Choose foods from Foods High in Iron list. Include beef, fowl, fish, and/or vitamin C-rich food with all meals or snacks to enhance absorption of iron. Avoid tea and foods containing metal chelates such as EDTA; also avoid the overconsumption of substances high in the iron-binding phytates and oxalates.
   Folic acid deficiency anemia: Choose foods from Foods High in Folic Acid list.
   Vitamin B_{12} deficiency anemia: Choose foods of animal origin and/or foods fortified with vitamin B_{12}.

2. Good Eating Checklist

Instructions: Using the Food Intake Record, total the number of daily servings from each Food Group and transfer to this chart. Evaluate by comparison to Recommended Daily Servings (RDSs).

Day	No. of servings/Food Group					
	Fruits	Vegetables	Grains	Milk	Meats	Others
1						
2						
3						
4						
5						
RDSs	2	2	4	3	2	—

Table 15.13   Diet in Nutritional Anemias

Foods high in iron

Meat, especially organ meats	Dried fruits and their juices
Oysters, clams	Dark green leafy vegetables
Legumes	Potato, sweet potato
Whole grain and enriched breads and cereals	Foods prepared in iron cookware

Foods high in vitamin C

Citrus fruits and juices	Papaya
Broccoli	Mango
Strawberries	Tomato
Cantaloupe	Potato

Foods commonly containing EDTA

Beer	Mayonnaise
Carbonated drinks	Sandwich spreads
Commercial salad dressings	Sauces

Foods high in phytates

Bran	Oatmeal
Whole grains	

Foods high in oxalates

Swiss chard and spinach	Rhubarb
Beet tops and greens	Collard and dandelion greens
Asparagus	Chocolate, cocoa
Almonds, cashews	Cranberries

Foods high in folic acid

Organ meats	Legumes, cooked
Dark green leafy vegetables	

II. C. Technician's Notes

Patient: _____   Date: _____

S   (Subjective data—how patient feels):
O   (Objective data—physical measurements including diet/nutritional status):
A   (Assessment—acceptability of dietary progress/nutritional status):
P   (Plan—diet prescription and instruction):
Comments:

Diet Counseling for Anemia Role Playing

Keeping in mind the preceding Suggested Readings and Counseling Guidelines, participate in the following role play situations; use the sample menu (Fig. 15.1) as a teaching aid. Select different partners for each situation, either classmates or co-workers, and elaborate on each role play situation to develop a patient profile. You may want to use your handout from Step 2. Use the SOAP method to record in each patient's medical chart.

As a dietetic technician in nutrition care, do you consider yourself capable of conducting effective counseling sessions with individuals suffering from nutritional anemias? Would you or your family be able to adhere to your nutrition guidelines in order to overcome anemia?

Role Play Situation 1.   As a dietetic technician in an outpatient clinic, you are often asked to counsel individuals on the dietary methods used in treating iron-deficiency anemia. An anemic pregnant 25-year-old woman and her anemic 2-year-old child are referred to you for nutrition counseling on increasing iron in the diet. Follow the guidelines to complete two sets of charts—one for the mother and one for her child—and provide the mother with indi-

Breakfast

Name _____ Room _____
Diet **Regular+** _____

Please circle your selections below

Fruits and juices	Cereals	Entrees	Breads	Miscellaneous
Orange juice	Cream of wheat	Bacon	Apple muffin	Salt
Grapefruit juice	Grits	Sausage	Blueberry muffin	Pepper
Prune juice	Oatmeal	Scrambled egg	Bran muffin	Sugar
Apple juice	Cornflakes	Poached egg	Corn muffin	Sugar substitute
Cranberry juice	Rice Krispies	Egg substitute	Plain muffin	Butter
Grapefruit sections	Special K	Pancakes	Danish pastry	Margarine
Stewed prunes	Puffed rice	French toast	Doughnut	Lemon
Banana	Puffed wheat	Omelet of the Day	English muffin	Jelly
	Shredded wheat		White toast	Pancake syrup
Beverages	All Bran		Wheat toast	
Coffee	Bran Flakes	Whole milk	Rye toast	
Tea		4 oz. whole milk		
Decaffeinated coffee	Cream	Skim milk		
Cocoa	Nondairy creamer	4 oz. skim milk		

Name _____ Room _____
Diet **Regular+** _____

Luncheon

Please circle your selections below

Appetizers
Apple juice
Cranberry juice
Tomato juice
Fruit cup
Consomme/chicken/beef
Chicken noodle soup
Vegetable soup
Cream of tomato soup
Cream of chicken soup
Soup du jour

Entrees
Tomato with:
  Chicken salad
  Tuna salad
  Cottage cheese
  Egg salad
Chef's bowl/meat & cheese
Fruit and cottage cheese
Roast beef sandwich
Sliced turkey sandwich
Tuna salad sandwich
Chicken salad sandwich
Egg salad sandwich
Sandwich special
Peanut butter & jelly sandwich
Tuna noodle casserole
Turkey/gravy/dressing
Roast beef au jus
Chicken a la king/toast
Macaroni and cheese
Scrod
Ham/pineapple
Steak/mushrooms
Chicken/cranberry
Fish/chips
Veal parmesan
Grilled cheese/pickle
Veal/gravy
Pork chop/applesauce
Shell macaroni
Beefburger/cheeseburger
Salisbury/gravy
Chef's special

Breads
White Rye Dinner Roll
Wheat   Crackers

Beverages
Coffee
Tea
Decaffeinated coffee
Cocoa
Cream
Nondairy creamer
Whole milk
4 oz. whole milk
Skim milk
4 oz. skim milk

Vegetables
Whipped potato
Baked potato
Steak-fried potato
Oven-browned potato
Noodles
Rice
Broccoli
Corn
Spinach
Carrots
Green beans
Beets
Peas
Squash

Salads and dressings
Lettuce/tomato
Tossed greens
Lettuce wedge
Cole slaw
Salad special
Mayonnaise
French dressing
Italian dressing
Thousand island dressing
Creamy Italian
Oil & vinegar
Lemon and vinegar
Sour cream

Desserts
Peaches
Fruit cocktail
Baked apple
Pears
Apricots
Applesauce
Fresh fruit
Dessert of the day
Sugar cookies
Oatmeal cookies
Cupcake
Apple pie
Cheesecake
Shortcake/topping
Chocolate pudding/topping
Butterscotch pudding/
  topping
Tapioca/topping
Sunshine cup
Ice cream
Orange sherbet
Raspberry sherbet
Gelatin
Custard
Eclair
Angel cake

Miscellaneous

Salt	Jelly
Pepper	Mustard
Sugar	Catsup
Sugar substitute	Relish
Butter	
Margarine	
Lemon	

Name _____ Room _____
Diet **Regular+** _____

Dinner

Please circle your selections below

Appetizers
Apple juice
Cranberry juice
Tomato juice
Fruit cup
Consomme/chicken/beef
Chicken noodle soup
Vegetable soup
Cream of tomato soup
Cream of chicken soup
Soup du jour

Entrees
Tomato with:
  Chicken salad
  Tuna salad
  Cottage cheese
  Egg salad
Chef's bowl/meat & cheese
Fruit and cottage cheese
Roast beef sandwich
Sliced turkey sandwich
Tuna salad sandwich
Chicken salad sandwich
Egg salad sandwich
Sandwich special
Peanut butter & jelly sandwich
Tuna noodle casserole
Turkey/gravy/dressing
Roast beef au jus
Chicken a la king/toast
Macaroni and cheese
Scrod
Ham/pineapple
Steak/mushrooms
Chicken/cranberry
Fish/chips
Veal parmesan
Grilled cheese/pickle
Veal/gravy
Pork chop/applesauce
Shell macaroni
Beefburger/cheeseburger
Salisbury/gravy
Chef's special

Breads
White Rye Dinner Roll
Wheat   Crackers

Beverages
Coffee
Tea
Decaffeinated coffee
Cocoa
Cream
Nondairy creamer
Whole milk
4 oz. whole milk
Skim milk
4 oz. skim milk

Vegetables
Whipped potato
Baked potato
Steak-fried potato
Oven-browned potato
Noodles
Rice
Broccoli
Corn
Spinach
Carrots
Green beans
Beets
Peas
Squash

Salads and dressings
Lettuce/tomato
Tossed greens
Lettuce wedge
Cole slaw
Salad special
Mayonnaise
French dressing
Italian dressing
Thousand island dressing
Creamy Italian
Oil & vinegar
Lemon and vinegar
Sour cream

Desserts
Peaches
Fruit cocktail
Baked apple
Pears
Apricots
Applesauce
Fresh fruit
Dessert of the day
Sugar cookies
Oatmeal cookies
Cupcake
Apple pie
Cheesecake
Shortcake/topping
Chocolate pudding/topping
Butterscotch pudding/
  topping
Tapioca/topping
Sunshine cup
Ice cream
Orange sherbet
Raspberry sherbet
Gelatin
Custard
Eclair
Angel cake

Miscellaneous

Salt	Jelly
Pepper	Mustard
Sugar	Catsup
Sugar substitute	Relish
Butter	
Margarine	
Lemon	

Fig. 15.1 Regular-plus menu.

vidualized diet plans for both herself and her child. Prepare a SOAP note for insertion in departmental files with a copy to be sent to the referring physician.

Role Play Situation 2.   As a dietetic technician in a community-based family planning clinic, you are often asked to counsel users of oral contraceptives who have folic acid deficiency anemia. Prepare a brief outline for counseling such clients on a folic acid-rich diet (see Table 15.13) by following the guidelines, and prepare a general handout for use in future individualized counseling sessions. Using your outline and handout, counsel an 18-year-old female with megaloblastic anemia due to folic acid deficiency. Prepare a SOAP note for insertion in departmental files with a copy to be sent to the referring physician.

Role Play Situation 3.   A physician refers a college coed to the university hospital outpatient clinic where you are employed. The student has been on and off a strict vegan diet for 4 years, and requires diet counseling to help treat the megaloblastic anemia that has developed. Follow the guidelines to complete the charts and provide the patient with an individualized diet plan. Prepare a SOAP note which could be recorded in departmental files with a copy to be sent to the referring physician.

STEP 8: EXTENDED ILLNESS GUIDELINES

Patients who are recovering from extended illnesses such as recent surgery, severe burns, or multiple injuries, patients with AIDS or cancer, and individuals who are MRDD all require individualized dietary planning and constant monitoring of nutritional status. Use of parenteral/enteral feeding may be required, and special consideration must be given to altered metabolic states and any corresponding changes in nutrient needs. The proper planning of adequate diets mandates input from a skilled nutrition support team, of which you may be an active or ancillary member.

This step includes suggested counseling strategies to use with patients who have extended illnesses due to surgery, burns, multiple injuries, AIDS or cancer, and the families or caretakers of individuals with developmental disabilities. The following references may prove helpful.

Suggested Readings on Nutrition in Extended Illnesses

AMARY, I. 1979. Effective Meal Planning and Food Preparation for the Mentally Retarded/Developmentally Disabled. Springfield, IL: Charles C. Thomas.

AMERICAN CANCER SOCIETY. 1986. Cancer Facts and Figures. New York: ACS.

AMERICAN DIETETIC ASSOCIATION. 1987. Position of The American Dietetic Association: Issues in feeding the terminally ill. J. Am. Dietet. Assoc. 87, Jan., 78.

AMERICAN DIETETIC ASSOCIATION. 1987. Position of The American Dietetic Association: Nutrition in comprehensive program planning for persons with developmental disabilities. J. Am. Dietet. Assoc. 87, Aug., 1068.

ASPEN. 1987. Proceedings of the First International Workshop on Nutrition and Metabolism in Hospital Malnutrition. J. Parenteral/Enteral Nutr. 11, Sept./Oct., Supplement.

BEACH, R. 1983. Nutrition and AIDS. Ann. Internal Med. 99, Oct., 565.

BEATLER, M., and STANISH, M. 1987. Nutrition support of the pediatric patient with AIDS. J. Am. Dietet. Assoc. 87, Apr., 488.

CARP, D., KRICK, J., and WEBSTER, C. 1981. Eating for Good Health: A Nutrition Handbook for Caretakers of the Handicapped Child. Baltimore: John F. Kennedy Institute for Handicapped Children.

CHANDRA, R. 1988. Nutrition, immunity, and outcome: Past, present, and future. Nutrition Res. 8, Mar., 225.

CHUMP, I. 1987. Nutrition and Feeding of the Handicapped Child. Boston: Little, Brown & Co.

CREASEY, W. 1985. Diet and Cancer. Philadelphia: Lea & Febiger.

DIETEL, M. (Editor). Nutrition in Clinical Surgery. Baltimore: Williams & Wilkins.

DRESSER, R., and BOISAUBIN, E. 1985. Ethics, law, and nutritional support. Arch. Internal Med. 145, Jan., 122.

DWYER, J., et al. 1988. Unproven nutrition therapies for AIDS: What is the evidence? Nutr. Today 23, Mar./Apr., 25.

ENIG, M., MUNN, R., and KEENEY, M. 1978. Dietary fat and cancer trends: A critique. Federation Proc. 37, Jul., 2215.

FLEMING, C., and BERKNER, S. (Editors). 1987. Home Parenteral Nutrition. Philadelphia: J. B. Lippincott Co.

GRANT, J. 1980. Handbook of Total Parenteral Nutrition. Philadelphia: W. B. Saunders Co.

GRAY, R. 1983. Similarities between AIDS and protein-calorie malnutrition. Amer. J. Public Health 73, Nov., 1332.

GREENWALD, P., ERSHAW, A., and NOVELLI, W. (Editors). 1985. Cancer, Diet, and Nutrition: A Comprehensive Sourcebook. Chicago: Marquis Publications.

GRIMES, C., YOUNATHAN, M., and LEE, W. 1987. The effect of preoperative total parenteral nutrition on surgery outcomes. J. Am. Dietet. Assoc. 87, Sept., 1202.

HALPERN, S. (Editor). 1987. Quick Reference to Clinical Nutrition, 2nd Edition. Philadelphia: J. B. Lippincott Co.

HIU, Y. 1988. Handbook of Enteral and Parenteral Feedings. New York: John Wiley & Sons.

HOLLEB, A. 1986. The American Cancer Society Cancer Book. New York: Doubleday & Co.

HURLEY, R., and GALLAGER-ALLRED, C. 1980. Nutritional Care of Deteriorating Patients. Columbus: Ohio State University College of Medicine.

KERNER, J. (Editor). 1983. Manual of Pediatric Parenteral Nutrition. New York: John Wiley & Sons.

KÜBLER-ROSS, E. 1969. On Death and Dying. New York: Macmillan.

KÜBLER-ROSS, E. 1987. AIDS: The Ultimate Challenge. New York: Macmillan.

KURTZ, G., YARBOROUGH, M., and CURRERI, P. (Editors). 1981. Surgical Nutrition. New York: Churchill Livingstone.

LEBENTHAL, E. (Editor). 1986. Total Parenteral Nutrition: Indications, Utilization, Complications, and Pathophysiological Considerations. New York: Raven Press.

LIPKIN, E., et al. 1988. Mineral loss in the parenteral nutrition patient. Amer. J. Clin. Nutr. 47, Mar., 440.

LUNDHOLM, K., and DROTT, C. 1987. Optimal nutritional indexes in cancer patients. J. Parenteral/ Enteral Nutr. 11, Sept./Oct., 135-S.

MACKLIN, R. 1987. Mortal Choices: Ethical Dilemmas in Modern Medicine. Boston: Houghton Mifflin.

MARGIE, J., and BLOCH, A. 1983. Nutrition and the Cancer Patient. Radnor, PA: Chilton Book Co.

MCKUSICK, L. (Editor). 1986. What to Do About AIDS: Physicians and Mental Health Professionals Discuss the Issues. Berkeley: University of California Press.

MOORE, F. 1986. Current thoughts on malabsorption: Parenteral, enteral, and oral feeding. J. Am. Dietet. Assoc. 86, Sept., 1169.

NATIONAL CANCER INSTITUTE. 1985. Symposium on the Role of Nutrients in Carcinogenesis. New York: Plenum Press.

NATIONAL CANCER INSTITUTE. 1988. Eating Hints: Recipes and Tips for Better Nutrition During Cancer Therapy. Bethesda, MD: NCI.

NATIONAL DAIRY COUNCIL. 1985. Nutrition and the immune response. Dairy Counc. Dig. 56, Mar./Apr., 7.

NATIONAL DAIRY COUNCIL. 1986. Diet, nutrition, and cancer: New findings. Dairy Counc. Dig. 57, Mar./Apr., 7.

NEWELL, G., and ELLISON, N. (Editors). 1981. Nutrition and Cancer: Etiology and Treatment. New York: Raven Press.

OLSON, R. (Editor). 1988. Severe malnutrition in a young man with AIDS. Nutrition Rev. 46, Mar., 126.

O'SULLIVAN, P., LINKE, R., and DALTON, S. 1985. Evaluation of body weight and nutritional status among AIDS patients. J. Am. Dietet. Assoc. 85, Nov., 1483.

PALMER, S., and EKVALL, S. (Editors). 1978. Pediatric Nutrition in Developmental Disorders. Springfield, IL: Charles C. Thomas.

PEARSALL, P. 1987. Superimmunity. New York: Fawcett.

PESTANA, C. 1981. Fluids and Electrolytes in the Surgical Patient. Baltimore: Williams & Wilkins.

REDDY, B., and COHEN, L. (Editors). 1986. Diet, Nutrition, and Cancer: A Critical Evaluation. Boca Raton, FL: CRC Press.

RICKARD, K., et al. 1986. Advances in nutrition care of children with neoplastic diseases. J. Am. Dietet. Assoc. 86, Dec., 1666.

ROCKLAND COUNTY BOARD OF COOPERATIVE EDUCATION SERVICES. 1981. Doorway to Nutrition: A Nutrition Education Program for the Handicapped. West Nyack, NY: RCBCES.

ROKUSEK, C., and HEINRICHS, E. 1986. Nutrition and Feeding for the Developmentally Disabled. Pierre, SD: Child and Adult Nutrition Services.

ROMBEAU, J., and CALDWELL, M. 1986. Clinical Nutrition, Volume II: Total Parenteral Nutrition. Philadelphia: W. B. Saunders Co.

SCHREINER, J. 1988. Nutrition Handbook for AIDS. Available from author, PO Box 460112, Aurora, CO 80015.

SEAGRAN, J. 1981. The Joy of Eating (for cancer patients). Available from author, 5413 Avenida da Fiesta, La Jolla, CA 92037.

SELTZER, M. 1982. Specialized nutrition support: The standard of care. J. Parenteral/Enteral Nutr. *6,* May/Jun., 185.

SELTZER, M. 1984. Specialized nutrition support: Patterns of care. J. Parenteral/Enteral Nutr. *8,* Sept./Oct., 506.

SHAMBERGER, R. 1984. Nutrition and Cancer. New York: Plenum Press.

SHAW, J. 1988. Influence of stress, depletion, and/or malignant disease on the responsiveness of surgical patients to total parenteral nutrition. Amer. J. Clin. Nutr. *48,* Jul., 144.

SIMOPOULOS, A. 1987. Calories and energy expenditure in carcinogenesis: A conference report. J. Am. Dietet. Assoc. *87,* Jan., 92.

SPRINGER, N. 1982. Nutrition Casebook on Developmental Disabilities. Syracuse, NY: Syracuse University Press.

STEIN, T., and MERRITT, J. 1987. Specialized nutrition regimens for seriously ill patients. Nutrition Rev. *45,* Jun., 161.

TABER-PIKE, J., et al. 1987. Nutrition and AIDS. Campbell, CA: ARIS Project.

VETERANS ADMINISTRATION. 1988. VA cooperative trial of perioperative total parenteral nutrition in malnourished surgical patients. Amer. J. Clin. Nutr. *47,* Feb./Supp., 351.

WADE, J., and JAIN, R. 1984. Nutritional support: Enhancing the quality of life of the terminally ill patient with cancer. J. Am. Dietet. Assoc. *84,* Sept., 1044.

WINTERS, R., and HASSELMEYER, E. (Editors). 1975. Intravenous Feeding in the High Risk Infant. New York: John Wiley & Sons.

WODARSKI, L. 1985. Nutrition intervention in developmental disabilities: An interdisciplinary approach. J. Am. Dietet. Assoc. *85,* Feb., 218.

For journal subscriptions:

Journal of Nutrition, Growth, and Cancer. Food and Nutrition Press, 1 Trinity Square, Westport, CT 06880.

Journal of Parenteral and Enteral Nutrition. Williams & Wilkins, 428 East Preston Street, Baltimore, MD 21202.

Nutrition Support Services. 12849 Magnolia Boulevard, North Hollywood, CA 91607.

For audiovisual:

Your Cancer Diet. The Polished Apple, 3742 Seahorn Drive, Malibu, CA 90265.

For further information:

American Cancer Society, 261 Madison Avenue, New York, NY 10016.

ARIS Project, 595 Millich Drive, Suite 104, Campbell, CA 95008.

ASPEN, American Society for Parenteral and Enteral Nutrition, 8605 Cameron Street, Suite 500, Silver Spring, MD 20910.

Hospice Education Institute, Five Essex Square, Suite 3-B, PO Box 713, Essex, CT 06426.

Institute for the Advancement of Health, 16 East 53rd Street, New York, NY 10022.

National Cancer Institute, National Institutes of Health, Bethesda, MD 20892.

San Francisco AIDS Foundation, 333 Valencia Street, San Francisco, CA 94103.

Table 15.14   General Outline for Extended Illness Counseling

I.   Initial Session
   A.   General Guidelines
   B.   Patient Records
      1.   Medical History Form
      2.   Weight Chart
      3.   24-Hour Recall Form
   C.   Assignments
      1.   Food Intake Record
      2.   Diet History
   D.   Technician's Notes
II. Follow-up Session(s)
   A.   General Guidelines
   B.   Handouts
      1.   Personal Diet Plan
      2.   Cancer Guidelines
      3.   MRDD Guidelines
   C.   Technician's Notes

Counseling Guidelines—Extended Illness

Table 15.14 outlines the steps for diet counseling with patients with extended illnesses. The following material gives the details of each step.

I.   Initial Session

I.   A.   General Guidelines

1.   Use Medical History Form to assess patient's nutritional status.

2.   If possible, weigh patient and record on Weight Chart. The chart can be a helpful tool in visualization of weight status.

3.   If possible, assist patient in recording 24-hour recall of food intake using 24-Hour Recall Form. This will aid in keeping an accurate Food Intake Record.

4.   If possible, have patient keep daily Food Intake Record so that typical food intake patterns can be evaluated. Advise patient not to deviate from normal eating pattern. Stress the importance of recording food intake immediately after eating.

5. If possible, instruct patient to complete Diet History. (Use the Pre-test from Chapter 2.)
6. Record assessment and recommendation(s) using the SOAP method in Technician's Notes. This form can be kept in your files with a copy in the patient's medical records.

I. B. Patient Records

1. Medical History Form

Date _____ Referred by _____

Name _____ Date of birth _____

Address _____ Phone no. _____

Occupation _____ Hours per work week ____ Work phone no. _____

Educational background _____ Religious/ethnic background _____

Sex ____ Marital status _____

Household composition: Live alone _____ Spouse _____ Children/No. _____ Other: _____

General health status:

Physician _____ Address _____

Phone no. _____ Date of last visit _____

Ambulatory care required? _____ If so, describe: _____

Neuromuscular problems? _____ If so, how is eating affected? _____

Visual/auditory problems? _____ If so, describe: _____

Chewing difficulties? _____ If so, describe: _____

Appetite typically good? _____ fair? _____ poor? _____

Digestion/elimination difficulties? _____ If so, describe: _____

Food intolerances? _____ If so, describe: _____

Diabetes? _____ If so, describe: _____

Heart attack or stroke? _____ If so, describe: _____

Recent surgery, injury, or trauma? _____ If so, describe: _____

Cancer? _____ If so, describe: _____

Other: _____

Height _____ Weight _____ Frame _____

Triceps skinfold thickness _____ Mid-arm circumference _____

Mid-arm muscle circumference _____

Weight changes/problems? _____ If so, describe: _____

Clinical signs of nutritional status:

Skin _____ Mouth _____

Hair _____ Eyes _____

Teeth _____ Other: _____

Lab data:

Blood pressure _____

Cholesterol _____ Triglycerides _____ Lipoprotein profile _____

Fasting Blood Glucose _____

CBC _____

SUN _____ BUN _____ GFR _____

Serum: Urea _____ Uric acid _____ Creatinine _____ Ammonia _____

        Albumin _____ Electrolytes _____

Blood gases: _____ Fluid intake/output: _____

Bilirubin: Serum _____ Urine _____

SGOT _____ BSP _____ Alkaline phosphatase _____

Prothrombin time _____ Hematocrit _____ Hemoglobin _____

Other: _____

Medications taken regularly: _____

Prescribed by: _____ Date(s) prescribed: _____

Nutrition supplements taken regularly: _____

Prescribed by: _____ Date(s) prescribed: _____

Special diet prescription: _____

Prescribed by: _____ Date of prescription: _____

How closely is diet followed? Always adhered to __ Sometimes __ Rarely __ Never __

Type of housing: Room ____ Apartment ____ Home ____ Institution ____

Prepare own meals? _____ Dine out? Often (more than once a day) _____ Rarely _____

Food shopping done independently? _____ If not, describe required assistance: _____

_____

Eligible for food stamps? _____ If so, are they currently being used? _____

Cigarette smoker? _____ If so, how much: _____

Exercise regularly? _____ If so, describe: _____

    No. times per week _____ No. minutes per session _____

Comments: _____

2. Weight Chart

Starting weight _____   Reasonable weight _____

Date	No. weeks on diet	Weight	Comments

3. 24-Hour Recall Form

Date	Time	Food and amount

I. C. Assignments

1. Food Intake Record

Date and time	Duration of meal (min)	Food and amount	Where[a]	With whom	Associated activity[b]	Associated emotions[c]

[a]Such as hospital room, cafeteria, home kitchen.
[b]For example, watching television, reading, talking.
[c]Attitude: bored, anxious, frustrated, depressed, happy, angry, tense, etc.

2. Diet History

Use the Pre-test from Chapter 2 (p. 30) to provide a record of typical foods eaten.

I. D. Technician's Notes

Patient: _____   Date: _____

S (Subjective data—how patient feels):
O (Objective data—physical measurements including diet/nutritional status):
A (Assessment—acceptability of dietary progress/nutritional status):
P (Plan—diet prescription and instruction):
Comments:

II. Follow-up Session(s)

II. A. General Guidelines
1. If possible, weigh patient and record on Weight Chart.
2. Review assignments and discuss.
3. Individualize Personal Diet Plan and instruct patient in its use.
4. Instruct patient to self-evaluate adherence to Personal Diet Plan and to incorporate Cancer or MRDD Guidelines if pertinent.
5. Record evaluation and recommendation(s) using the SOAP method in Technician's Notes. This form can be kept in your files with a copy in the patient's medical records.

II. B. Handouts

1. Personal Diet Plan

Name _____

How to use diet plan:

1. *Oral intake:* Select a variety of foods from each of the Basic Food Groups. Include enough servings to provide sufficient calories and protein. Use nutrition supplements (and/or vitamin/mineral supplements) as prescribed. Divide food intake into several small feedings with supplementation as between-meal snacks.

2. *Enteral feedings:* Follow the specific directions provided by the physician/nutrition support team for the product(s) prescribed. Use only prescribed vitamin/mineral supplements and in the amounts required. Nutritional status needs to be continuously monitored. Undesirable side effects should be reported.

3. *Parenteral nutrition:* Follow the specific directions provided by the physician/nutrition support team for the product(s) prescribed. Use only prescribed vitamin/mineral supplements and in the amounts required. Nutritional status needs to be continuously monitored. Undesirable side effects should be reported. Hospital care is usually mandatory during treatment.

4. *Special requirements:* Use the Cancer Guidelines (Table 15.15), as well as the counseling advice of the dietitian/physician to individualize the diet to meet specific needs, desires, and requirements. Use the MRDD Guidelines (Table 15.16), as well as the counseling advice of the dietitian/physician, to individualize the diet to meet specific needs, desires, and requirements.

2. Cancer Guidelines

Table 15.15 lists some side effects specific to cancer and the appropriate diet-related guidelines.

3. MRDD Guidelines

Table 15.16 lists some common feeding problems and the suggested dietary guidelines.

II. C. Technician's Notes

Patient: _____   Date: _____

S (Subjective data—how patient feels):
O (Objective data—physical measurements including diet/nutritional status):
A (Assessment—acceptability of dietary progress/nutritional status):
P (Plan—diet prescription and instruction):
Comments:

Diet Counseling for Extended Illnesses Role Playing

Keeping in mind the preceding Suggested Readings and Counseling Guidelines, participate in the following role play situations. Select different partners for each situation, either classmates or co-workers, and elaborate on each role play situation to develop a patient/audience profile. You may want to use your product sheets from Steps 3, 4, and 5 or your handout from Step 6. Use the SOAP method to record in each patient's medical chart.

As a dietetic technician in nutrition care, do you consider yourself capable of conducting effective counseling sessions with patients suffering from trauma due to serious injury, surgery, or burns? Would you be able to counsel AIDS or cancer patients effectively? How about individuals with developmental disabilities and the associated feeding problems?

Role Play Situation 1. As a dietetic technician in a large metropolitan hospital, you are often asked to assist the clinical dietitians with postsurgical nutrition care plans. In discussing the case of an elderly female requiring enteral feedings, the dietitian asks you to explain the diet as you help to assess and counsel the patient. Follow the guidelines to complete the charts and provide the patient with an explanation of her individualized diet plan. Prepare a SOAP note that could be recorded in the patient's medical chart.

Role Play Situation 2. As a dietetic technician on the burn unit of a large private hospital, you are responsible for assisting pediatric patients in food selection, and for explaining the use of parenteral/enteral feedings. Counsel a severely burned teenaged male regarding the TPN plus Liposyn supplementation he is receiving during his recovery. Follow the guidelines to complete the charts and provide the patient with an individualized—and simplified—explanation of his diet plan. Prepare a SOAP note that could be inserted in the patient's medical chart.

Table 15.15   Cancer Guidelines[a]

Side effects	Guidelines	Additional suggestions
Decreased appetite	Encourage small, frequent meals and snacks—large amounts of food at one time may appear overpowering. Concentrate on nutritious foods that are high in calories and protein and vitamins, such as enriched milk (see opposite column), frappes, eggnog, cheese, eggs, custard, ice cream, pudding, peanut butter, yogurt, cream soups, fruits and vegetables, and juices. Encourage light to moderate exercise, when possible, to increase appetite. Experiment with ways to increase the flavor of foods such as seasonings and fruit juices. Keep favorite foods visible. Make mealtime fun and colorful. Encourage individual to help in actual food preparation (to arouse interest).	Recipe for enriched milk (high-calorie, high-protein): 1 quart whole milk $\frac{3}{4}$–1 cup nonfat dry milk powder Blend well. Serve cold as beverage, use in frappes and eggnog, use for cream soups and in cooking.
Nausea and vomiting	Immediately: Provide dry crackers or toast to reduce nausea. Try ice, cold carbonated beverages to settle stomach. Wipe face with cool water, loosen tight clothes, sit in cool, well-ventilated room. For prevention: Offer plain foods that are low in fats (avoid fried foods, gravy, margarine) and aroma (smell is often heightened). Provide liquids either 1 hour before or 1 hour after meals, rather than with meals (to decrease amount of food in stomach). Encourage individual to eat slowly, chew foods thoroughly, and relax. Since activity may slow digestion, the individual should rest or lie down after meals. Serve foods cold or warm; avoid hot foods. Offer frequent, small meals and snacks.	Observe the individual's intake for a couple of days and encourage the greatest intake when nausea occurs least often, for example, breakfast time.
Taste changes	Bitter and sweet tolerance changes. Serve food cold or at room temperature. Use seasonings (see opposite column) to flavor foods. Flavor milk and milk products. Try offering bland cheese. If meat products are not tolerated, select meat substitutes.	Seasonings Allow $\frac{1}{2}$ tsp dried herbs = $\frac{1}{2}$ tsp crushed herbs = 1 Tbsp chopped herbs. Allow $\frac{1}{4}$ tsp dried herbs for each 4 servings. Do not use too many kinds of seasonings in one recipe. Crush herbs in the palm of one hand with the fingertips of the other hand before adding to a dish. This permits faster flavor release. Add herbs to uncooked foods (salad dressing, fruits, juices) as long before serving as possible. Add herbs to soups and sauces toward the end of preparation and leave just long enough to lose their volatile oils (about 1 hour). Heat seasoned foods carefully as certain spices (cayenne, paprika, and curry blends) scorch easily and others (caraway) become bitter if overheated.

[a]From Howard and Herbold (1982).

(continued)

Table 15.15 *(Continued)*

Side effects	Guidelines	Additional suggestions
Constipation	Increase the amount of high fiber foods in the individual's diet—raw fruit and vegetables, nuts, popcorn, bran, whole grains, and bread. If individual refuses raw fruits, try adding them to gelatin. Encourage increased fluid intake, in the form of water and juices. Hot beverages, especially, may encourage bowel movements. Encourage light to moderate exercise, when possible.	Foods that are high in fiber may also be an irritant to sensitive intestinal tracts. Introduce these foods slowly, especially when advancing a diet from full liquid → to soft → to a regular diet with fiber included.
Low resistance to infection	Individuals with very low WBC counts may need a diet that avoids fresh fruits and vegetables (owing to their high bacteria count). Avoid food items that would be an excellent medium for hosting bacteria—i.e., raw seafoods or eggs. Use cooked and processed foods.	A *Reduced Bacteria Diet*[b] may be used for patients receiving bone marrow transplantation.
Sore or dry mouth and throat	Rinse mouth frequently. Offer mints or hard candy (like lemon drops) to stimulate saliva production. Use a straw or tilt head back to make swallowing more comfortable. Avoid foods that are extreme in temperature (either hot or cold). Avoid tart or acid foods such as citrus fruits, and highly seasoned or spicy foods. Offer soft and liquid foods, such as custard, ice cream, tuna salad, and scrambled eggs, or soften foods by dipping them in liquid. Moisten foods with margarine, gravy, cheese sauce, and cream.	The physician or dentist will have additional information regarding meticulous dental care.
Diarrhea	Begin by providing clear liquids (apple juice, gelatin, broth, popsicles) for 12 hours. Serve warm rather than hot foods (heat increases the natural movement of the GI tract). Limit fiber and gassy foods eaten (temporarily). These include dried cooked beans, cabbage, onions, raw fruits and vegetables, whole grains, nuts, popcorn, and carbonated beverages. Offer small, frequent meals and snacks, with beverages served between meals, rather than with them. Encourage rest after meals (to reduce peristalsis). Sometimes therapy may cause temporary "lactose intolerance"—diarrhea, bloating, and abdominal cramps due to inadequate digestion of milk or milk products. If diarrhea seems to be associated with milk or milk products, temporarily avoid these.	A low-lactose diet may be required. Many cheeses, because of the way they are made, contain no lactose. The following may be tolerated: Swiss, provolone, edam, blue, brick, muenster, colby, cheddar, pasteurized processed American, pasteurized processed Swiss, camembert, and mozzarella. Additionally, yogurt is usually well tolerated by most people who are lactose intolerant.
Weight loss	Encourage more between-meal snacks. Those which are low in fat provide fewer calories, but interfere less with the next meal (if this is a problem). Examples of good snacks include: *high-energy, high-protein*—milk, custard, pudding, beverages made with enriched milk, frappes, eggnog, cheese, eggs, peanut butter, yogurt, cream soups, small sandwiches. *low-fat*—jelly, honey, hard candy, fruit juices, sherbet, popsicles, gelatin, fruit, raw vegetables (low calorie).	Foods high in fat may contribute to nausea.

[b]Only cooked and processed foods and sterile water allowed. Avoid fresh fruits and vegetables. Disposable dishes and utensils should be used.

Table 15.16   MRDD Guidelines[a]

Feeding problem	Guidelines	Additional suggestions
Mechanical feeding problem ○ Asymmetrical tonic neck reflex ○ Moro ○ Tonic labyrinthine ○ Symmetrical tonic neck reflex	Feeding requires assistance to insure adequate dietary intake; consistency of foods needs to be modified to avoid choking, yet meals should be as tasty and appealing as possible.	Perform frequent diet analysis and nutritional assessment to assure optimal growth and health; use supplements if required.
Delayed feeding skills	Devise individualized diet based on nutritious, easy-to-eat foodstuffs; small, frequent meals may be more acceptable.	Monitor food intake and height/weight status; use of specially designed equipment and recipes can allot for self-preparation and self-feeding.
Behavior problem ○ Hyperactivity/misbehavior ○ Pica ○ Rumination ○ Anorexia nervosa	Provide varied diet with care to include acceptable, nutritious foods; monitor carefully to detect and correct any eating problems which can lead to nutritional deficiencies, and use supplements if necessary.	Monitor diet and height/weight status; behavioral management at mealtime may require psychological as well as nutritional support.
Overweight	Individualize diet to normalize weight in proportion to height; physical activity should be encouraged so that the diet need not be overly restrictive.	See Chapter 10.
Underweight	Individualize diet to normalize weight in proportion to height and to avoid malnutrition; use supplements if necessary.	See Chapter 10.
Anemia ○ Iron deficiency ○ Folic acid deficiency ○ Vitamin B_{12} deficiency	Individualize diet to include and emphasize foods appropriate for specific anemia; monitor physical and nutritional parameters carefully.	See Step 7 in this chapter.
Inborn error of metabolism ○ PKU ○ Galactosemia ○ MSUD ○ Others	Provide nutritionally adequate diet limited in specific nutrient which is improperly metabolized (i.e., phenylalanine, galactose, leucine, isoleucine, valine); monitor laboratory parameters carefully, and utilize special food products as available.	Adequate growth and development can be realized with *careful* dietary management.

[a]The nutrition care plan needs to be practical and usable, include the basic techniques for facilitation of eating with adaptive equipment, explain behavioral management and positioning techniques, and outline individualized diet/drug interactions (see Appendix IV). The Developmental Feeding Tool (Table 15.7) can provide additional guidance.

Role Play Situation 3.   As a dietetic technician in a hospice, your responsibilities include explaining to residents the need for optimal nutritional status. Prepare a brief outline and give a 15-minute talk on Supplements for Feeling Better. You may want to explain various parenteral/enteral preparations and their functions. Prepare a report on your talk for insertion in departmental files.

Role Play Situation 4.   As a dietetic technician employed by a state public health agency, you are asked to participate in a workshop on nutrition for the developmentally disabled to be conducted for the occupational/physical therapists in your agency. Prepare a brief outline and give a 15-minute talk on Feeding Problems and Diet Solutions in the Developmentally Disabled Adult. Prepare a report on your talk for insertion in departmental files.

STEP 9: POST-TEST ON OTHER CLINICAL CONDITIONS

In order to evaluate your understanding of the current diet therapies for recovery from anemia, trauma, and extended illnesses, complete the following Post-test. Answers are given in the Answer Key. Will your patients seeking to control nutritional anemias be able to use your nutrition guidelines successfully? Could those seeking to prevent anemia successfully use your guidelines as well? Do you now have a basic understanding of the role of diet therapy in the treatment of serious injury or burns, pre- and postsurgical conditions, cancer, AIDS, and developmental disabilities? Do you understand the functions of nutrition supplements, parenteral/enteral feedings, and the nutrition support team in clinical nutrition care?

Indicate whether you think the following statements are true (T) or false (F). Check your answers with the Answer Key.

_____ 1. Iron deficiency anemia is a common problem in this country, largely because of poor iron absorption and inadequate intakes of iron-rich foods.
_____ 2. Nonheme iron absorption can be increased with the simultaneous intake of foods rich in vitamin C.
_____ 3. Consumption of overcooked foods can contribute to a folic acid deficiency.
_____ 4. An excessive intake of folic acid can mask the presence of iron deficiency anemia.
_____ 5. Pernicious anemia is often due to dietary imbalance with an overemphasis on animal foods.
_____ 6. Pernicious anemia is usually treated with oral supplements of vitamin B_6.
_____ 7. Iron-binding capacity is increased with pernicious anemia.
_____ 8. Pica sometimes occurs in the iron-deficient individual, but may aggravate the problem.
_____ 9. Elemental diets are usually prescribed when the gastrointestinal tract is not functioning.
_____ 10. Tube feedings are usually started in amounts averaging 100–200 ml/hour.
_____ 11. Enteral feeding is safer than parenteral nutrition, and is less expensive.
_____ 12. Total parenteral nutrition is provided through a peripheral vein.
_____ 13. With long-term use of TPN, lipid emulsions should be provided several times a week.
_____ 14. Parenteral nutrition prevents the catabolic response of starvation plus stress.
_____ 15. Major surgery can cause body weight losses of up to 25% of preoperative weight.
_____ 16. Vitamin E supplementation is routinely prescribed after major surgery.
_____ 17. Patients with severe burns may require daily protein intakes of up to 4 g per kilogram of body weight.
_____ 18. Cancer treatments often lead to dietary problems and can cause specific nutritional deficiencies.
_____ 19. Granulocytopenia patients should increase fiber intake in the form of raw fruits and vegetables and salads.
_____ 20. Aggressive nutrition support is essential for all patients during all stages of AIDS.
_____ 21. Rumination usually leads to overweight.
_____ 22. Maple syrup urine disease (MSUD) requires a limited intake of maple syrup.
_____ 23. Self-motivation in dietary care should be discouraged for most MRDD individuals.

Select the answer that best completes the following statements and check your answers with the Answer Key.

_____ 24. A good source of dietary iron is
(a) oysters. (b) liver. (c) prune juice. (d) enriched bread. (e) baked potato. (f) a and b. (g) all of these.
_____ 25. EDTA can be found in
(a) oysters. (b) beer. (c) tuna fish salad. (d) root beer. (e) b, c, and d. (f) all of these.

_____ 26. Phytates and/or oxalates may be found in
(a) spinach salad. (b) devil's food cake. (c) rhubarb pie. (d) hot cocoa. (e) bran cereal. (f) oatmeal. (g) a and c. (h) all of these.

_____ 27. A good source of folic acid is
(a) bran. (b) liver. (c) spinach. (d) baked beans. (e) whole milk. (f) b, c, and d. (g) all of these.

_____ 28. An example of a nutrition supplement which might be used with patients requiring added calories is
(a) Polycose. (b) Sustacal. (c) Meritene. (d) b and c. (e) all of these.

_____ 29. An example of an elemental diet which might be used with patients requiring feedings low in residue is
(a) Vivonex-HN. (b) Precision-LR. (c) Flexical. (d) a and b. (e) all of these.

_____ 30. An example of an isotonic fat emulsion to provide essential fatty acids is
(a) Intralipid. (b) Liposyn. (c) Nutrament. (d) a and b. (e) all of these.

REFERENCES

DUDRICK, S. 1969. Can intravenous feeding as the sole means of nutrition support growth in the child and restore weight loss in an adult? An affirmative answer. Ann. Surgery *169,* Jun., 974.

HOWARD, R., and HERBOLD, N. 1982. Nutrition in Clinical Care, pp. 705–707. New York: McGraw-Hill.

SCHNEIDER, A., ANDERSON, C., and COURSIN, D. 1977. Nutritional Support of Medical Practice, pp. 85–86. New York: Harper & Row.

Recommended Dietary Allowances

Table AI.1 Recommended Daily Dietary Allowances[a]

Age (years)	Weight (kg)	Weight (lb)	Height (cm)	Height (in)	Protein (g)	Fat-soluble vitamins Vitamin A (μg RE)[b]	Vitamin D (μg)[c]	Vitamin E (mg α TE)[d]	Water-soluble vitamins Vitamin C (mg)	Thiamin (mg)	Riboflavin (mg)	Niacin (mg NE)[e]	Vitamin B_6 (mg)	Folacin (μg)[f]	Vitamin B_{12} (μg)	Minerals Calcium (mg)	Phosphorus (mg)	Magnesium (mg)	Iron (mg)	Zinc (mg)	Iodine (μg)
Infants																					
0.0–0.5	6	13	60	24	kg × 2.2	420	10	3	35	0.3	0.4	6	0.3	30	0.5[g]	360	240	50	10	3	40
0.5–1.0	9	20	71	28	kg × 2.0	400	10	4	35	0.5	0.6	8	0.6	45	1.5	540	360	70	15	5	50
Children																					
1–3	13	29	90	35	23	400	10	5	45	0.7	0.8	9	0.9	100	2.0	800	800	150	15	10	70
4–6	20	44	112	44	30	500	10	6	45	0.9	1.0	11	1.3	200	2.5	800	800	200	10	10	90
7–10	28	62	132	52	34	700	10	7	45	1.2	1.4	16	1.6	300	3.0	800	800	250	10	10	120
Males																					
11–14	45	99	157	62	45	1000	10	8	50	1.4	1.6	18	1.8	400	3.0	1200	1200	350	18	15	150
15–18	66	145	176	69	56	1000	10	10	60	1.4	1.7	18	2.0	400	3.0	1200	1200	400	18	15	150
19–22	70	154	177	70	56	1000	7.5	10	60	1.5	1.7	19	2.2	400	3.0	800	800	350	10	15	150
23–50	70	154	178	70	56	1000	5	10	60	1.4	1.6	18	2.2	400	3.0	800	800	350	10	15	150
51+	70	154	178	70	56	1000	5	10	60	1.2	1.4	16	2.2	400	3.0	800	800	350	10	15	150
Females																					
11–14	46	101	157	62	46	800	10	8	50	1.1	1.3	15	1.8	400	3.0	1200	1200	300	18	15	150
15–18	55	120	163	64	46	800	10	8	60	1.1	1.3	14	2.0	400	3.0	1200	1200	300	18	15	150
19–22	55	120	163	64	44	800	7.5	8	60	1.1	1.3	14	2.0	400	3.0	800	800	300	18	15	150
23–50	55	120	163	64	44	800	5	8	60	1.0	1.2	13	2.0	400	3.0	800	800	300	18	15	150
51+	55	120	163	64	44	800	5	8	60	1.0	1.2	13	2.0	400	3.0	800	800	300	10	15	150
Pregnant					+30	+200	+5	+2	+20	+0.4	+0.3	+2	+0.6	+400	+1.0	+400	+400	+150	[h]	+5	+25
Lactating					+20	+400	+5	+3	+40	+0.5	+0.5	+5	+0.5	+100	+1.0	+400	+400	+150	[h]	+10	+50

[a] National Research Council/Food and Nutrition Board. 1980. Designed for the maintenance of good nutrition of practically all healthy people in the United States. The allowances are intended to provide for individual variations among most normal persons as they live in the United States under usual environmental stresses. Diets should be based on a variety of common foods in order to provide other nutrients for which human requirements have been less well defined.

[b] Retinol equivalents. 1 retinol equivalent = 1 μg retinol or 6 μg β carotene.

[c] As cholecalciferol, 10 μg cholecalciferol = 400 I.U. of vitamin D.

[d] α-tocopherol equivalents. 1 mg d-α tocopherol = α T.E.

[e] 1 NE (niacin equivalent) is equal to 1 mg of niacin or 60 mg of dietary tryptophan.

[f] The folacin allowances refer to dietary sources as determined by Lactobacillus casei assay after treatment with enzymes (conjugases) to make polyglutamyl forms of the vitamin available to the test organism.

[g] The recommended dietary allowance for vitamin B_{12} in infants is based on average concentration of the vitamin in human milk. The allowances after weaning are based on energy intake (as recommended by the American Academy of Pediatrics) and consideration of other factors, such as intestinal absorption.

[h] The increased requirement during pregnancy cannot be met by the iron content of habitual American diets nor by the existing iron stores of many women; therefore the use of 30–60 mg of supplemental iron is recommended. Iron needs during lactation are not substantially different from those of nonpregnant women, but continued supplementation of the mother for 2–3 months after parturition is advisable in order to replenish stores depleted by pregnancy.

Table AI.2 Estimated Safe and Adequate Daily Dietary Intakes of Additional Selected Nutrients[a]

Age (years)	Vitamins Vitamin K (μg)	Biotin (μg)	Pantothenic acid (mg)	Trace elements Copper (mg)	Manganese (mg)	Fluoride (mg)	Chromium (mg)	Selenium (mg)	Molybdenum (mg)	Electrolytes Sodium (mg)	Potassium (mg)	Chloride (mg)
0–0.5	12	35	2	0.5–0.7	0.5–0.7	0.1–0.5	0.01–0.04	0.01–0.04	0.03–0.06	115–350	350–925	275–700
0.5–1	10–20	50	3	0.7–1.0	0.7–1.0	0.2–1.0	0.02–0.06	0.02–0.06	0.04–0.08	250–750	425–1275	400–1200
1–3	15–30	65	3	1.0–1.5	1.0–1.5	0.5–1.5	0.02–0.08	0.02–0.08	0.05–0.1	325–975	550–1650	500–1500
4–6	20–40	85	3–4	1.5–2.0	1.5–2.0	1.0–2.5	0.03–0.12	0.03–0.12	0.06–0.15	450–1350	775–2325	700–2100
7–10	30–60	120	4–5	2.0–2.5	2.0–3.0	1.5–2.5	0.05–0.2	0.05–0.2	0.1 –0.3	600–1800	1000–3000	925–2775
11+	50–100	100–200	4–7	2.0–3.0	2.5–5.0	1.5–2.5	0.05–0.2	0.05–0.2	0.15–0.5	900–2700	1525–4575	1400–4200
Adults	70–140	100–200	4–7	2.0–3.0	2.5–5.0	1.5–4.0	0.05–0.2	0.05–0.2	0.15–0.5	1100–3300	1875–5625	1700–5100

[a] Reprinted by permission from NUTRITION—CONCEPTS AND CONTROVERSIES by E. Hamilton and E. Whitney © 1982 by West Publishing Company. All rights reserved.

Table AI.3 Energy Allowances[a]

Age (years)	Weight (kg)	(lb)	Height (cm)	(in)	Energy needs[b] (cal)	Age (years)	Weight (kg)	(lb)	Height (cm)	(in)	Energy needs[b] (cal)
Infants						Females					
0.0–0.5	6	13	60	24	kg × 115 (95–145)	11–14	46	101	157	62	2200 (1500–3000)
0.5–1.0	9	20	71	28	kg × 105 (80–135)	15–18	55	120	163	64	2100 (1200–3000)
						19–22	55	120	163	64	2100 (1700–2500)
Children						23–50	55	120	163	64	2000 (1600–2400)
1–3	13	29	90	35	1300 (900–1800)	51–75	55	120	163	64	1800 (1400–2200)
4–6	20	44	112	44	1700 (1300–2300)	76+	55	120	163	64	1600 (1200–2000)
7–10	28	62	132	52	2400 (1650–3300)						
						Pregnant					+300
Males						Lactating					+500
11–14	45	99	157	62	2700 (2000–3700)						
15–18	66	145	176	69	2800 (2100–3900)						
19–22	70	154	177	70	2900 (2500–3300)						
23–50	70	154	178	70	2700 (2300–3100)						
51–75	70	154	178	70	2400 (2000–2800)						
76+	70	154	178	70	2050 (1650–2450)						

[a] Reprinted by permission from NUTRITION—CONCEPTS AND CONTROVERSIES by E. Hamilton and E. Whitney © 1982 by West Publishing Company. All rights reserved.

[b] The energy allowances for the young adults are for men and women doing light work. The allowances for the two older age groups represent mean energy needs over these age spans, allowing for a 2% decrease in basal (resting) metabolic rate per decade and a reduction in activity of 200 cal per day for men and women between 51 and 75 years, 500 cal for men over 75 years, and 400 cal for women over 75. The customary range of daily energy output, shown in parentheses, is based on a variation in energy needs of ±400 cal at any one age, emphasizing the wide range of energy intakes appropriate for any group of people. Energy allowances for children through age 18 are based on median energy intakes of children these ages followed in longitudinal growth studies. The values in parentheses are tenth and ninetieth percentiles of energy intake, to indicate the range of energy consumption among children of these ages.

Aids to Calculations:
Conversion Tables

Table AII.1   Weight Conversion

Ounces	Grams		Pounds	Grams	
$\frac{1}{16}$	1.772		1 (16 oz)	453.59	
$\frac{1}{8}$	3.544		2	907.18	
$\frac{1}{4}$	7.088		3	1360.78	(1.36 kg)
$\frac{1}{2}$	14.175		4	1814.37	(1.81 kg)
1	28.350		5	2267.96	(2.27 kg)
2	56.699		6	2721.55	(2.72 kg)
3	85.049		7	3175.15	(3.18 kg)
4	113.398		8	3628.74	(3.63 kg)
5	141.748		9	4082.33	(4.08 kg)
6	170.097		10	4535.92	(4.54 kg)
7	198.447				
8	226.796		1 g = 0.035274 oz		
9	255.146		1 kg = 2.2 lb		
10	283.495				
11	311.845				
12	340.194				
13	368.544				
14	396.893				
15	425.243				
16 (1 lb)	453.59				

Table AII.2   Liquid Measure Conversion

Fluid Ounces	Milliliters
1	29.57
2	59.15
3	88.72
4	118.29
5	147.87
6	177.44
7	207.01
8	236.58
9	266.16
10	295.73
11	325.30
12	354.88
13	384.45
14	414.02
15	443.59
16 (1 pt)	473.17
32 (1 qt)	946.33
128 (1 gal)	3785.32
1.01	30
1.35	40
1.69	50
16.91	500
33.815	1000 (1 L)

Table AII.3   Length and Volume Conversion

Length: 1 inch (in) = 2.54 centimeters (cm)
 1 foot (ft) = 30.48 centimeters (cm)
 3.3 feet (ft) = 1 meter (m)

Volume: 1.06 quarts = 1 liter (L)
 1 cup = 236 milliliters (ml)
 1 teaspoon (tsp) = 5 milliliters (ml)
 1 tablespoon (Tbsp) = 15 milliliters (ml)
 1 gallon = 3.8 liters (L)
 1 milliliter = 1 cubic centimeter (cc)

Table AII.4   Temperature, Energy, Etc. Conversion

Temperature: 212°F = 100°C (boiling point of water)
 98.6°F = 37°C (body temperature)
 32°F = 0°C (freezing point of water)

Temperature conversion equation: $°C = \frac{5}{9}(°F - 32)$
 $°F = \frac{9}{5}°C + 32$

Energy: 1 calorie = 4.2 joules (J)
 (calorie = the amount of heat energy necessary to raise 1 gram of water 1°C)
 1 kilocalorie (kcal) = 4.2 kilojoules (kJ)
 (kilocalorie = the amount of heat energy necessary to raise 1 kilogram of water 1°C)

Other: 1 retinol equivalent = 1 μ retinol
 6 μg β carotene
 12 μg other provitamin A
 3.33 I.U. vitamin activity from retinol
 10 I.U. vitamin A activity from β carotene

The Dietary Guidelines

Included below are several sets of nutrition guidelines developed by various sources. Changes will occur as scientific theory progresses, but these recommendations represent some temporary efforts made to simplify nutrition theory—as we now know it—into practical and healthful food habit guidelines for the general public. Pregnant women, children, and those with special health conditions need to seek individualized medical advice.

DIETARY GOALS FOR THE UNITED STATES[1]

1. To avoid overweight, consume only as much energy (calories) as is expended; if overweight, decrease energy intake and increase energy expenditure.
2. Increase the consumption of complex carbohydrates and "naturally occurring" sugars from about 28% of energy intake to about 48% of energy intake.
3. Reduce the consumption of refined and processed sugars by about 45% to account for about 10% of total energy intake.
4. Reduce overall fat consumption from approximately 40% to about 30% of energy intake.
5. Reduce saturated fat consumption to account for about 10% of total energy intake; balance that with polyunsaturated and monounsaturated fats, which should account for about 10% of energy intake each.
6. Reduce cholesterol consumption to about 300 mg a day.
7. Limit the intake of sodium by reducing the intake of salt to about 5 grams a day.

Meeting Dietary Goals

In order to meet the Dietary Goals, the following changes in food selection and preparation are suggested:

1. Increase consumption of fruits, vegetables, and whole grains.
2. Decrease the intake of sugars and foods containing large amounts of sugar (whether refined, corn sugar, syrups, molasses, or honey).
3. Decrease consumption of foods high in fat and replace some saturated fat with polyunsaturated fat.
4. Increase consumption of poultry and fish while decreasing consumption of meats relatively high in saturated fat.
5. Except for young children, substitute nonfat milk and low-fat milk products for whole milk and whole milk products.
6. Decrease consumption of butterfat, eggs, and other high-cholesterol sources. However, the egg is still recognized as a good source of protein for certain population groups.
7. Decrease consumption of salt and foods high in salt content.

[1]Senate Select Committee on Nutrition and Human Needs. Dec. 1977. Dietary Goals for the United States, 2nd edition. Washington, DC: Government Printing Office.

Total Energy Intake

Fat intake: 10% saturated + 10% polyunsaturated + 10% monounsaturated
                         = 30% of total energy intake

Protein intake: 12% protein = 12% of total energy intake

Carbohydrates: 48% complex carbohydrates and naturally occurring sugars
                              + 10% refined sugars
                                    = 58% of total energy intake

NUTRITION AND YOUR HEALTH: DIETARY GUIDELINES FOR AMERICANS[1]

1. *Eat a variety of foods.* Include selections of the following: fruits; vegetables; whole grain and enriched breads, cereals, and grain products; milk, cheese, and yogurt; meats, poultry, fish and eggs; and legumes (dried beans and peas).
2. *Maintain a reasonable weight.* To improve eating habits do the following: eat slowly, prepare smaller portions, and avoid "seconds." To lose weight do the following: increase physical activity, eat less fat and fatty foods, eat less sugar and sweets, and avoid too much alcohol.
3. *Avoid too much fat, saturated fat, and cholesterol.* Choose lean meat, fish, poultry, and dried beans and peas as your protein sources. Moderate your use of eggs and organ meats (such as liver). Limit your intake of butter, cream, hydrogenated margarines, shortenings, coconut oil, palm oil, and foods made from such products. Trim excess fat off meats. Broil, bake, or boil rather than fry. Read labels carefully to determine both amount and types of fat contained in food.
4. *Eat foods with adequate starch and fiber.* To eat more complex carbohydrates daily, substitute starches for fats and sugars and select foods which are good sources of fiber and starch, such as whole grain breads and cereals, fruits and vegetables, and dried beans and peas.
5. *Avoid too much sugar.* Use less of all sugars, including white sugar, brown sugar, raw sugar, honey, and syrups. Eat less of foods containing these sugars such as candy, soft drinks, ice cream, cakes, and cookies. Select fresh fruits or fruits canned without sugar or in light syrup rather than heavy syrup. Read food labels for clues on sugar content—if the names sucrose, glucose, maltose, dextrose, lactose, fructose, or syrups appear first, then there is a large amount of sugar. Remember, how often you eat sugar is as important as how much sugar you eat.
6. *Avoid too much sodium.* To avoid too much sodium, learn to enjoy the unsalted flavors of foods. Cook only with small amounts of added salt. Add little or no salt to food at the table. Limit your intake of salty foods such as potato chips, pretzels, salted nuts and popcorn, condiments (soy sauce, steak sauce, garlic salt), pickled foods, and cured meats. Read food labels carefully to determine the amounts of sodium in processed foods and snack items.
7. *If you drink alcohol, do so in moderation—and do not drive!*

TOWARD HEALTHFUL DIETS[2]

1. Select a nutritionally adequate diet from the foods available by consuming each day appropriate servings of dairy products, meats or legumes, vegetables and fruits, and cereals and breads.

[1]U.S. Department of Agriculture. Feb. 1980. Washington, DC: U.S. Department of Health and Human Services. Updated 1985.
[2]National Research Council/Food and Nutrition Board. 1980. Washington, DC: National Academy of Sciences.

2.   Select as wide a variety of foods in each of the major food groups as is practical in order to ensure a high probability of consuming adequate quantities of all essential nutrients.

3.   Adjust dietary energy intake and energy expenditure so as to maintain appropriate weight for height; if overweight, achieve appropriate weight reduction by decreasing total food and fat intake and by increasing physical activity.

4.   If the requirement for energy is low (that is, reducing diet), reduce consumption of foods such as alcohol, sugars, fats, and oils, which provide calories but few other essential nutrients.

5.   Use salt in moderation; adequate but safe intakes are considered to range between 3 and 8 grams of sodium chloride (salt) daily.

DIET AND CANCER: SIX RECOMMENDATIONS[1]

At this stage in the investigation of the relationship between diet and cancer, these recommendations seem eminently reasonable.

1.   Cut back on total fat to about 30% of total calories. (Remember that fat has more than twice as many calories per ounce as protein and carbohydrate.) For the sake of your heart, concentrate on reducing saturated fat, but because there is no evidence on the effects of very large habitual intakes of polyunsaturated fats, keep the proportion of these to no more than one-third of your total fat intake, with monounsaturates making up another third.

2.   Eat good amounts (the equivalent of two to four servings a day) of whole grain breads, whole grain, low-sugar cereals, and other grain products; citrus fruits and other good sources of vitamin C; and the dark green and deep yellow vegetables and fruits that are good sources of β carotene (vitamin A). Most of these are also good sources of all types of fiber.

3.   There is no indication that large supplements of any nutrients are useful—and they can be harmful. Increase your intake of vitamins C and A from foods, not pills. The same goes for selenium, an essential mineral which can be found in many foods. Some of the best sources are seafoods, meats (including lean meats), whole eggs, milk (including low-fat), and whole grains.

4.   For a number of reasons besides the possible carcinogenic effect, keep alcohol intake to no more than one or two drinks a day.

5.   Enjoy salt-pickled, salt-cured, and smoked foods occasionally and in moderation and minimize consumption of charcoal-broiled foods.

6.   Although the correlation between obesity and cancer seems to be more closely related to fat intake than to total calories in and of themselves, overweight has been implicated in certain types of carcinogenesis. Since overweight is also a risk factor for diabetes, hypertension and heart disease, it makes good sense to keep calories within the bounds necessary to control your weight.

[1]National Research Council Committee on Diet, Nutrition, and Cancer. July 1982. Report as interpreted by Jean Mayer, president of Tufts University and former chairman of the White House Conference on Food, Nutrition, and Health. © 1982, Washington Post Writers Group. Reprinted with permission.

Diet–Drug Interactions

A multitude of simple and complex interrelationships can develop—many as yet unrecognized—between an individual's food intake and nutritional status and the actions and side effects of over-the-counter and prescribed drugs. The following chart depicts some of the general interactions between food and medication. For the specifics in a handy pocketbook format, contact Food–Medication Interactions, PO Box 26464, Tempe, AZ 85282, or utilize the other pharmacology texts recommended in Appendix V.

Table AIV.1 Diet and Drug Interactions

Drug	Effects
Alcohol	Can cause malnutrition (see Table AIV.2).
Analgesics	Irritate gastrointestinal system; can cause anemia from blood loss.
Aspirin	Antagonizes vitamin K; 1–3 g causes 2 mg iron loss.
Antacids	Decrease nutrient absorption; cause deficiencies in iron, B vitamins.
Aluminum hydroxide gel	Inactivates thiamin; decreases absorption of vitamin A, phosphate; decreases calcium and vitamin D.
Mylanta	Inactivates thiamin; decreases absorption of vitamin A, phosphate.
Antibiotics	Alter taste of food; hamper nutrient absorption.
Neomycin	Decreases absorption of fat, carotene, lactose, potassium, calcium, iron, vitamins A, D, K, B_{12}, other nutrients.
Tetracycline	Impairs calcium metabolism; if taken during tooth formation permanent stains can occur.
Anticoagulant: Coumadin	Requires limited intakes of caffeine, foods high in vitamin K, proteolytic enzymes, papain, fried or boiled onions; cooking oil inhibits absorption.
Anti-convulsants	Impair nutrient metabolism and utilization.
Dilantin	Increases turnover vitamins D, K; decreases folic acid, vitamin B_{12}.
Antidepressants	Diminish salivary flow; increase appetite and may cause weight gain.
Monoamine oxidase inhibitors	Elevate blood pressure if taken with food sources of tyramine (see Table AIV.3).
Anti-fungal: Griseofulvin	High-fat meals enhance absorption.
Anti-gouts	Hamper nutrient absorption.
Allopurinol	Requires alkaline urine (see Table AIV.4).
Colchicine	Decreases absorption of fat, carotene, lactose, folic acid, vitamin B_{12}, potassium.
Probenecid	Requires alkaline urine (see Table AIV.4); decreases absorption of riboflavin.
Anti-hypertensives	Increase gastrointestinal motility.
Aldactone	Requires limited intake of high-potassium foods.
Reserpine	Causes carbohydrate intolerance; can cause weight gain.
Ser-Ap-Es	Has anti-B_6 effect; can cause anemia. (See Diuretics.)
Anti-infectives, urinary	Can irritate gastrointestinal tract, hamper nutrient absorption.
Furadantin	Requires adequate protein intake; decreases folic acid.
Trimethoprim	Decreases folic acid, B vitamins, vitamin K.

(continued)

Table AIV.1   *(Continued)*

Drug	Effects
Anti-inflammatories	Irritate gastrointestinal tract.
Motrin	May decrease appetite.
Antilipemics	Irritate gastrointestinal system, alter bile activity, hamper nutrient absorption.
Antineoplastics	Suppress appetite, hamper nutrient absorption, can cause nutrient deficiencies.
Antiparkinsonism: Levodopa	Requires limited intake of high-protein foods and foods high in B_6 (see Table AIV.5), and caffeine (see Table AIV.6); increases need for vitamins B_{12}, C.
Anti-spasmodics	Can irritate gastrointestinal tract, hamper nutrient absorption.
Azulfidine	Decreases absorption of iron and folic acid, and synthesis of vitamin K.
Anti-tubercular: INH	Can cause deficiencies of vitamins B_6, niacin.
Caffeine	Central nervous system stimulant; irritates gastrointestinal system (see Table AIV.6).
Corticosteroids	Increase potassium excretion; irritate gastrointestinal system.
Diuretics	Deplete potassium, cause electrolyte imbalance.
Aldomet	Increases need for dietary potassium, may increase need for folic acid, vitamin B_{12}.
Lasix	Increases need for dietary potassium.
Rauzide	Increases need for dietary potassium; can cause weight gain.
Triameterene	Conserves potassium so requires limited intake of high-potassium foods; decreases need for folic acid, vitamin B_{12}, calcium.
Laxatives	Cause electrolyte imbalance and nutrient deficiencies with prolonged use.
Mineral oil	Causes deficiencies in vitamins A, D, E, K.
Nutrients: Iron salts	Irritate gastrointestinal system, constipate.
Potassium chloride	Alters taste of foods; irritates gastrointestinal system.
Oral contraceptives	Increase appetite; alter absorption of folic acid, B_6.

Table AIV.2   Nutritional Effects of Chronic Alcohol Ingestion

Replaces food	→ Decreased nutrient intake
Contains 7 calories/g	→ No nutritional value
Decreased protein intake	→ Edema, muscle wasting
Thiamin deficiency	→ Neuropathy, psychosis
Folic acid deficiency	→ Anemia
Increased zinc excretion	→ Slowed wound healing
Increased potassium excretion	→ Muscle weakness
Increased magnesium excretion	→ Delirium tremens
Damages organs:	
Pancreas	→ Maldigestion of fat, protein
Liver	→ Blocked protein synthesis, increased triglyceride levels
Stomach	→ Anorexia, abdominal pain
Intestines	→ Impaired absorption of fat, thiamin, folic acid, vitamins B_6 and B_{12}
Alcohol abuse in pregnancy	→ Fetal alcohol syndrome

Table AIV.3   Food Sources of Tyramine

Yeast extracts
Cheese, aged
Sausage, bologna, salami
Fermented meats, aged beef
Cod, herring (dried, salted, pickled)
Chianti wines
Meat tenderizers, papaya products
Chicken livers
Pineapple, plums, raisins
Figs, avocados (overripe)
Broad beans (fava, Chinese pea pods)
Bananas
Licorice
Beer, ale, sherry
Yogurt, sour cream
Caffeine, chocolate, soy sauce (large amounts)

Table AIV.4   Urine Acidity/Alkalinity

Acidify urine	Alkalinize urine
Meat, poultry, fish	Milk, cream
Eggs	Nuts: Almonds, chestnuts
Cheese	Vegetables (all except*)
Lentils*	Fruits (all except*)
Peanut butter	
Nuts: Brazil, filberts, peanuts, walnuts	
Corn*	
Cranberries, plums, prunes*	
Breads, pasta, crackers	
Plain cakes, cookies	

**Table AIV.5
Foods High in Vitamin B$_6$**

Avocado	Peas, dried
Bananas	Tuna, salmon
Beans, dried	Vegetables, leafy green
Lean meats	Wheat germ
Milk	Yeast, brewer's

Table AIV.6   Caffeine Content

Food or beverage and amount	Caffeine content (approx. mg)
Coffee (6 oz)	
Automatic drip	180
Automatic perk	125
Instant	55
Decaffeinated	5
Soft drinks (12 oz)	
Mountain Dew	55
Mellow Yellow	50
Dr. Pepper	40
Pepsi Cola	40
Coca Cola	35
Tab	30
Tea (6 oz)	
Iced	70
Weak	20–45
Medium	50–60
Strong	70–100
Cocoa	
Chocolate candy (2 oz)	45
Baking chocolate (1 oz)	45
Milk chocolate (2 oz)	10
Cocoa powder (6 oz)	10

Appendix V

References

A. GENERAL REFERENCES

AMERICAN ACADEMY OF ALLERGY AND IMMUNOLOGY. 1984. Adverse Reactions to Foods, Publication No. NIH 84-2442. Washington, DC: Government Printing Office.

AMERICAN ACADEMY OF PEDIATRICS. 1985. Pediatric Nutrition Handbook. Elk Grove Village, IL: AAP.

AMERICAN CANCER SOCIETY/FLORIDA DIVISION. 1987. The Good Book of Nutrition. Lakeland, FL: ACS/Publix Supermarkets, Inc.

AMERICAN CANCER SOCIETY/OREGON DIVISION. 1986. Simply Nutritious! Recipes and Recommendations to Reduce the Risk of Cancer. Portland, OR: ACS.

AMERICAN DIETETIC ASSOCIATION. 1976. Professional Standards Review Manual. Chicago: ADA.

AMERICAN DIETETIC ASSOCIATION. 1978. Patient Care Audit: Quality Assurance Procedure Manual for Dietitians. Chicago: ADA.

AMERICAN DIETETIC ASSOCIATION. 1981. Handbook of Clinical Dietetics. New Haven, CT: Yale University Press.

AMERICAN DIETETIC ASSOCIATION. 1987. What You Should Know about Nutrition and Health. Chicago: ADA.

AMERICAN HEART ASSOCIATION. 1986. Dietary Guidelines for Healthy American Adults: A Statement for Physicians and Health Professionals. Dallas: AHA.

ANDERSON, J. 1984. Dr. Anderson's HCF Diet. Lexington, KY: HCF Diabetes Foundation.

ANDERSON, J. 1988. Nutrition Management of Metabolic Conditions: Professional Guide to HCF Diets. Lexington, KY: HCF Diabetes Foundation.

ARONSON, V. 1987. Thirty Days to Better Nutrition. Englewood Cliffs, NJ: Prentice-Hall.

ARONSON, V., FITZGERALD, B., and HEWES, L. 1990. Guidebook for Nutrition Counselors, 2nd Edition. Englewood Cliffs, NJ: Prentice-Hall.

BAKER, S., and HENRY, R. 1986. Parent's Guide to Nutrition: Healthy Eating from Birth through Adolescence. Reading, MA: Addison-Wesley.

BARKER, L. (Editor). 1982. The Psychology of Human Food Selection. Westport, CT: AVI Publishing Co.

BARNESS, M. (Editor). 1981. Nutrition and Medical Practice. Westport, CT: AVI Publishing Co.

BERNSTEIN, L. (Editor). 1985. Interviewing: A Guide for Health Professionals. Norwalk, CT: Appleton-Century-Crofts.

BOCK, A. 1982. Food Allergy: A Primer for People. Denver: AJ Publishing.

BRENEMAN, J. 1984. Basics of Food Allergy. Springfield, IL: Charles C. Thomas.

BRODY, J. 1981. Jane Brody's Nutrition Book. New York: W. W. Norton.

BRODY, J. 1985. Jane Brody's Good Food Book. New York: W. W. Norton.

BROSTOFF, J., and CHALLACOMBE, S. (Editors). 1987. Food Allergy and Intolerance. Philadelphia: W. B. Saunders Co.

BROWN, J. L. 1986. Physician Task Force on Hunger in America. Boston: Harvard University School of Public Health.

BROWNELL, K., and FOREYT, J. (Editors). 1986. Handbook of Eating Disorders. New York: Raven Press.

BURDMAN, G. 1986. Healthful Aging. Englewood Cliffs, NJ: Prentice-Hall.

CHICAGO'S WEST SUBURBAN DIETETIC ASSOCIATION. 1986. Nutritive Value of Convenience and Processed Foods. Chicago: American Dietetic Association.

COLORADO DEPARTMENT OF HEALTH. 1981. Colorado Self-Teaching Modules. Denver: Nutrition Services, Office of Health Care Services, CDH.

CONNOR, S., and CONNOR, W. 1986. The New American Diet. New York: Simon & Schuster.

COOPER, E. 1984. Stress, Immunity, and Aging. New York: M. Dekker.

CORNELL UNIVERSITY DEPARTMENT OF NUTRITION. 1982. Annotated Bibliography of Educational Materials. Ithaca, NY: Cornell University.

D'ANDREA, V., and SALOVEY, P. 1983. Peer Counseling: Skills and Perspectives. Palo Alto, CA: Science and Behavior Books.

DER MARDEROSIAN, A., and LIBERTI, L. 1987. A Clinical Guide to Natural Products in Medicine. Philadelphia: George F. Stickley Co.

DIKOVICS, A. 1987. Nutritional Assessment: Case Study Methods. Philadelphia: George F. Stickley Co.

DONG, F. 1984. All About Food Allergy. Philadelphia: George F. Stickley Co.

EISENBERG, A., EISENBERG, H., and EISENBERG, S. 1982. The Special Guest Cookbook. New York: Beaufort Books.

EGAN, G. 1982. The Skilled Helper. Monterey, CA: Brooks/Cole Publishing Co.

EGAN, J. 1987. Healthy High Fiber Cooking. Tucson, AZ: HP Books.

ELLENBOGEN, L. (Editor). 1981. Controversies in Nutrition, Volume 2: Contemporary Issues in Clinical Nutrition. New York: Churchill Livingstone.

ENDRES, J., and ROCKWELL, R. 1980. Food, Nutrition, and the Young Child. St. Louis: C. V. Mosby Co.

ENSIMINGER, A. 1983. Foods and Nutrition Encyclopedia. Clovis, CA: Pegasus Press.

ESCOTT-STUMP, S. 1988. Nutrition and Diagnosis-Related Care, 2nd Edition. Philadelphia: Lea & Febiger.

FELDMAN, E. (Editor). 1983. Nutrition in the Middle and Later Years. Littleton, MA: Wright·PSG.

FRANKLE, R., and YANG, M. 1988. Obesity and Weight Control. Rockville, MD: Aspen Publishers.

FRANZ, M. 1987. Fast Food Facts. Wayzata, MN: Diabetes Center, Inc.

FRANZ, M., HEDDING, B., and LEITCH, G. 1985. Opening the Door to Good Nutrition. Wayzata, MN: Diabetes Center, Inc.

FURIA, T. (Editor). 1980. CRC Handbook of Food Additives. Boca Raton, FL: CRC Press.

GILCHRIST, A. 1981. Foodborne Disease and Food Safety. Chicago: American Medical Association.

GOODHART, R., and SHILS, M. (Editors). 1980. Modern Nutrition in Health and Disease, 6th Edition. Philadelphia: Lea & Febiger.

GOOD HOUSEKEEPING INSTITUTE. 1984. Consumer Food and Nutrition Study. New York: GHI.

GOOD HOUSEKEEPING INSTITUTE. 1985. Food Attitude Study. New York: GHI.

GOODMAN, H., and MORSE, B. 1982. Just What the Doctor Ordered. New York: Henry Holt & Co.

GRAND, R., SUTPHEN, J., and DIETZ, W. 1987. Pediatric Nutrition: Theory and Practice. Stoneham, MA: Butterworth Publishers.

GREENWOOD, M. R. C. (Editor). 1983. Obesity. New York: Churchill Livingstone.

GUSSOW, J., and THOMAS, P. 1986. The Nutrition Debate: Sorting Out Some Answers. Palo Alto, CA: Bull Publishing Co.

GUTHRIE, H. 1986. Introductory Nutrition, 6th Edition. St. Louis: Times Mirror/Mosby.

HALPERN, S. (Editor). 1987. Quick Reference to Clinical Nutrition, 2nd Edition. Philadelphia: J. B. Lippincott Co.

HAMILTON, E., WHITNEY, E., and SIZER, F. 1988. Nutrition: Concepts and Controversies, 4th Edition. St. Paul: West Publishing Co.

HOLLI, B., and CALABRESE, J. 1986. Communication and Education Skills: The Dietitian's Guide. Philadelphia: Lea & Febiger.

HOPE, J., and BRIGHT-SEE, E. 1982. Everywoman's Book of Nutrition. Toronto, Canada: McGraw-Hill Ryerson.

HOWARD, R., and HERBOLD, N. 1982. Nutrition in Clinical Care. New York: McGraw-Hill.

HOWARD, R., and WINTER, H. (Editors). 1984. Nutrition and Feeding of Infants and Toddlers. Boston: Little, Brown & Co.

HURLEY, L. (Editor). 1987. Special Issues in Nutrition. Bethesda, MD: American Institute of Nutrition.

HUTCHINSON, M., and MONRO, H. 1986. Nutrition and Aging. Orlando, FL: Academic Press.

IOWA RESEARCH CLINIC. 1981. Intensive Workshop on Nutrition Counseling Manual. Iowa City: Iowa Research Clinic.

JASMUND, J. 1981. The Diet History: A Tool and a Process. East Lansing, MI: Michigan State University Press.

KANE, J. 1987. Exploring Careers in Dietetics and Nutrition. New York: Rosen Publishing Group.

KATCH, F., and MCARDLE, W. 1988. Nutrition, Weight Control, and Exercise, 2nd Edition. Philadelphia: Lea & Febiger.

KEYS, A., et al. 1950. The Biology of Human Starvation. Minneapolis: University of Minnesota Press.

KRAUSE, M., and MAHAN, L. 1984. Food, Nutrition, and Diet Therapy. Philadelphia: W. B. Saunders Co.

LANZ, S. 1983. Introduction to the Profession of Dietetics. Philadelphia: Lea & Febiger.

LINDSAY, A. 1988. The American Cancer Society Cookbook. New York: Hearst Books.

LONG, P. 1986. The Nutritional Ages of Women. New York: Macmillan.

LOWELL, J., KENNEY, J., and RASMUSSEN, A. 1987. Nutrition Assessment: Separating Fact, Fiction, and Fraud. Tucson, AZ: Nutrition Information Center.

MACKLIN, R. 1987. Mortal Choices: Ethical Dilemmas in Modern Medicine. Boston: Houghton Mifflin.

MAHAN, L., and REES, J. (Editors). 1984. Nutrition in Adolescence. St. Louis: Times Mirror/Mosby.

MARSHALL, C. 1983. Vitamins and Minerals: Help or Harm? Philadelphia: George F. Stickley Co.

MASON, M., WENBERG, B., and WELSCH, P. 1982. The Dynamics of Clinical Dietetics. New York: John Wiley & Sons.

MAYO CLINIC. 1988. Mayo Clinic Diet Manual: A Handbook of Dietary Practices, 6th Edition. Rochester, MN: Rochester Methodist Hospital.

MCDONALD, D., BUCKLE, R., and BERARDI, R. (Editors). 1983. Nutrition and Fitness Manual: A Summary of Research and Resources. Toronto, Canada: Ryerson Polytechnical Institute.

MCGEE, G. (Editor). 1987. Nutrition Misinformation and Mythology. Van Nuys, CA: PM, Inc.

METROPOLITAN LIFE INSURANCE CO. 1986. Eat Well, Be Well Cookbook. New York: Simon & Schuster.

MILLER, B., and KEANE, C. 1972. Encyclopedia of Medicine and Nursing. Philadelphia: W. B. Saunders Co.

MONK, A., and FRANZ, M. 1987. Convenience Food Facts. Wayzata, MN: Diabetes Center, Inc.

MORGAN, B. 1986. The Food and Drug Interaction Guide. New York: Simon & Schuster.

NATIONAL ACADEMY OF SCIENCES. 1980. Toward Healthful Diets. Washington, DC: NAS.

NATIONAL RESEARCH COUNCIL/FOOD AND NUTRITION BOARD. 1980. Recommended Dietary Allowances, 9th Edition. Washington, DC: National Academy of Sciences.

NATIONAL RESEARCH COUNCIL/FOOD AND NUTRITION BOARD. 1984. What is America Eating? Washington, DC: National Academy of Sciences.

NEUBERGER, A., and JUKES, T. (Editors). 1982. Human Nutrition: Current Issues and Controversies. Englewood, NJ: Jack K. Burgess, Inc.

NUTRITION FOUNDATION. 1988. Perspectives in Nutrition. Washington, DC: Nutrition Foundation, Inc.

OWEN, A., and FRANKLE, R. 1986. Nutrition in the Community: The Art of Delivering Services, 2nd Edition. St. Louis: Times Mirror/Mosby.

PEARSALL, P. 1987. Superimmunity. New York: Fawcett.

PENNINGTON, J., and CHURCH, H. 1985. Food Values of Portions Commonly Used, 14th Edition. Philadelphia: J. B. Lippincott Co.

PHYSICIANS DESK REFERENCE. 1989. Oradell, NJ: Medical Economics Co.

POWERS, D., and MOORE, A. 1986. Food-Medication Interactions. Phoenix, AZ: FMI, Inc.

PURTILO, R., and CASSEL, C. 1981. Ethical Dimensions in the Health Professions. Philadelphia: W. B. Saunders Co.

PYKE, M. 1981. Food Science and Technology. London, England: John Murray.

READER'S DIGEST. 1982. Eat Better, Live Better. Pleasantville, NY: Reader's Digest Assoc.

RECHEIGI, M. (Editor). 1982. CRC Handbook of Nutritive Value of Processed Foods. Boca Raton, FL: CRC Press.

REED, P. 1980. Nutrition: An Applied Science. St. Paul, MN: West Publishing Co.

RITCHEY, S., and TAPER, J. 1983. Maternal and Child Nutrition. New York: Harper & Row.

ROBERTS, H. (Editor). 1981. Food Safety. New York: John Wiley & Sons.

ROBERTSON, L., FINDERS, C., and RUPPENTHAL, B. 1986. Laurel's Kitchen: A Handbook for Vegetarian Cookery and Nutrition, 2nd Edition. Berkeley, CA: Ten Speed Press.

ROBINSON, C., and LAWLER, M. 1982. Nutrition and Therapeutic Nutrition, 16th Edition. New York: Macmillan.

ROBINSON, C., LAWLER, M., and GARWICK, A. 1982. Case Studies in Clinical Nutrition. New York: Macmillan.

ROE, D. 1985. Drug-induced Nutritional Deficiencies. Westport, CT: AVI Publishing Co.

ROE, D. 1987. Geriatric Nutrition. Englewood Cliffs, NJ: Prentice-Hall.

SAUBERLICH, H., SCALA, J., and DOWDY, R. 1974. Laboratory Tests for the Assessment of Nutritional Status. Boca Raton, FL: CRC Press.

SCARPA, I. (Editor). 1982. Sourcebook on Food and Nutrition. Chicago: Marquis Academic Media.

SCHEIDER, W. 1983. Nutrition: Basic Concepts and Applications. New York: McGraw-Hill.

SCHNEIDER, H., ANDERSON, C., and COURSIN, D. (Editors). 1983. Nutritional Support of Medical Practice, 2nd Edition. New York: Harper & Row.

SHILS, M., and YOUNG, V. 1988. Modern Nutrition in Health and Disease, 7th Edition. Philadelphia: Lea & Febiger.

SOCIETY FOR NUTRITION EDUCATION. 1980. Nutrition Information Resources for Professionals. Oakland, CA: SNE.

STARE, F., and ARONSON, V. 1982. Dear Dr. Stare: What Should I Eat? Philadelphia: George F. Stickley Co.

STARE, F., and ARONSON, V. 1983. Your Basic Guide to Nutrition. Philadelphia: George F. Stickley Co.

STARE, F., and ARONSON, V. 1985a. Food for Fitness After Fifty. Philadelphia: George F. Stickley Co.

STARE, F., and ARONSON, V. 1985b. Food for Today's Teens. Philadelphia: George F. Stickley Co.

STERN, B. 1987. The Good Book: The Complete Guide to the Most Popular Brand Name Foods in the U.S. New York: Dell.

STUNKARD, A., and STELLAR, E. (Editors). 1984. Eating and Its Disorders. New York: Raven Press.

SUCHER, K. 1989. Food and Culture in America: A Nutrition Handbook. New York: Van Nostrand Reinhold.

SZILARD, P. 1987. Food and Nutrition Information Guide. Littleton, CO: Libraries Unlimited, Inc.

TRUSWELL, A. (Editor). 1986. ABCs of Nutrition. London: British Medical Association.

TYLER, V. 1987. The New Honest Herbal. Philadelphia: George F. Stickley Co.

U.S. DEPARTMENT OF AGRICULTURE. 1977. Nutritive Value of American Foods in Common Units. Agriculture Handbook No. 456. Washington, DC: Government Printing Office.

U.S. DEPARTMENT OF AGRICULTURE. 1986. Dietary Guidelines and Your Diet. Washington, DC: Government Printing Office.

U.S. DEPARTMENT OF AGRICULTURE and U.S. DEPARTMENT OF HEALTH AND HUMAN SERVICES. 1985. Nutrition and Your Health: Dietary Guidelines for Americans, 2nd Edition. Washington, DC: Government Printing Office.

U.S. DEPARTMENT OF HEALTH AND HUMAN SERVICES. 1979. Healthy People: The Surgeon General's Report on Health Promotion and Disease Prevention, Publication No. 79-55071. Washington, DC: Government Printing Office.

U.S. SENATE SELECT COMMITTEE ON AGING, Subcommittee on Health and Long-term Care. 1984. Quackery: The $10 Billion Scandal, House Document No. 98-262. Washington, DC: Government Printing Office.

U.S. SENATE SELECT COMMITTEE ON NUTRITION AND HUMAN NEEDS. 1977. Dietary Goals for the U.S., 2nd Edition. Washington, DC: Government Printing Office.

U.S. SURGEON GENERAL. 1988. The Surgeon General's Report on Nutrition and Health. Washington, DC: Government Printing Office.

WALLACH, J. 1974. Interpretation of Diagnostic Tests. Boston: Little, Brown & Co.

WATKIN, D. 1983. Handbook of Nutrition, Health, and Aging. Park Ridge, NJ: Noyes Publications.

WICKHAM, S. 1982. Human Nutrition: A Self-Instructional Text. Bowie, MD: Robert J. Brady Co.

WILLIAMS, S. 1986. Essentials of Nutrition and Diet Therapy, 4th Edition. St. Louis: C. V. Mosby Co.

WILLIAMS, S., and WORTHINGTON-ROBERTS, B. 1988. Nutrition Throughout the Life Cycle. St. Louis: Times Mirror/Mosby.

WINICK, M. 1983. Nutrition and Drugs. New York: John Wiley & Sons.

WINICK, M. (Editor). 1986. Nutrition and Exercise. New York: John Wiley & Sons.

WORTHINGTON-ROBERTS, B., VERMEERSCH, J., and WILLIAMS, S. 1985. Nutrition in Pregnancy and Lactation, 2nd Edition. St. Louis: C. V. Mosby Co.

YETIV, J. 1986. Popular Nutritional Practices: A Scientific Appraisal. Toledo, OH: Popular Medicine Press.

ZEMAN, F., and NEY, D. 1988. Applications of Clinical Nutrition. Englewood Cliffs, NJ: Prentice-Hall.

B. JOURNAL AND NEWSLETTER SUBSCRIPTIONS

ADA Courier, American Dietetic Association, 216 West Jackson Boulevard, Chicago, IL 60606.

Annals of Internal Medicine, American College of Physicians, 4200 Pine Street, Philadelphia, PA 19104.

American Journal of Clinical Nutrition, 9650 Rockville Pike, Bethesda, MD 20014.

American Journal of Public Health, American Public Health Association, 1015 Fifteenth Street NW, Washington, DC 20005.

American Journal of Sports Medicine, Williams & Wilkins, 428 East Preston Street, Baltimore, MD 21202.

Bariatrician, American Society of Bariatric Physicians, 7430 East Caley Avenue, Suite 210, Englewood, CO 80111.

Behavioral Medicine Update, Society of Behavioral Medicine, Box 450, 600 North Wolfe Street, Baltimore, MD 21205.

Bulletin of the Pan American Health Organization, 525 23rd Street NW, Washington, DC 20037.

Cereal Foods World, 3340 Pilot Knob Road, St. Paul, MN 55121.

Consultant, Food Service Consultants Society International, 13227 8th Avenue NW, Seattle, WA 98177.

Cooking for Profit, P.O. Box 267, Fond du Lac, WI 54935.

Cornell Hotel and Restaurant Administration Quarterly, Cornell University, Ithaca, NY 14853.

Current Diet Review, P.O. Box 1914, Rialto, CA 92376.

Dairy Council Digest, National Dairy Council, 6300 North River Road, Rosemont, IL 60018.

Diabetes, American Diabetes Association, 1660 Duke Street, Alexandria, VA 22314.

Diabetes Care, American Diabetes Association, 1660 Duke Street, Alexandria, VA 22314.

Diabetes Forecast, American Diabetes Association, 1660 Duke Street, Alexandria, VA 22314.

Environmental Nutrition, 2112 Broadway, Suite 200, New York, NY 10023.

FDA Consumer, Food and Drug Administration, Superintendent of Documents, U.S. Government Printing Office, Washington, DC 20402.

Food and Nutrition Bulletin, United Nations Programme Office, Massachusetts Institute of Technology, Cambridge, MA 02139.

Food News for Consumers, Superintendent of Documents, U.S. Government Printing Office, Washington, DC 20402.

Food Service Marketing, 2132 Fordem Avenue, Madison, WI 53704.

Food Technology, 221 North La Salle Street, Suite 2120, Chicago, IL 60601.

Harvard Medical School Health Letter, Department of Continuing Education, 25 Shattuck Street, Boston, MA 02115.

Health and Social Work, 49 Sheridan Avenue, Albany, NY 12210.

Health Education Quarterly, John Wiley & Sons, 605 Third Avenue, New York, NY 10158.

Hospitals, 840 North Lake Shore Drive, Chicago, IL 60611.

International Journal of Eating Disorders, John Wiley & Sons, 605 Third Avenue, New York, NY 10158.

International Journal of Obesity, John Libbey & Co., 80–84 Bondway, London, England SW8 1SK.

International Obesity Newsletter, Route 1, Box 6A, Hettinger, ND 58639.

Journal of Allied Health, One Dupont Circle, Suite 300, Washington, DC 20036.

Journal of the American College of Nutrition, John Wiley & Sons, 605 Third Avenue, New York, NY 10158.

Journal of the American Dietetic Association, 216 West Jackson Boulevard, Chicago, IL 60606.

Journal of the American Medical Association, 535 North Dearborn Street, Chicago, IL 60610.

Journal of the Canadian Dietetic Association, 385 Yonge Street, Toronto, Canada M5B 1S1.

Journal of Food Protection, P.O. Box 701, Ames, IA 50010.

Journal of Food Science, 221 North La Salle Street, Suite 2120, Chicago, IL 60601.

Journal of Home Economics, 210 Massachusetts Avenue NW, Washington, DC 20036.

Journal of Nutrition, 9650 Rockville Pike, Bethesda, MD 20014.

Journal of Nutrition Education, Williams & Wilkins, 428 East Preston Street, Baltimore, MD 21202.

Journal of Nutrition for the Elderly, The Haworth Press, 75 Griswold Street, Binghamton, NY 13904.

Journal of Parenteral and Enteral Nutrition, Williams & Wilkins, 428 East Preston Street, Baltimore, MD 21202.

Lancet, 7 Adam Street, London, England WC2N 6AD.

Mayo Clinic Proceedings, 200 First Street Southwest, Plummer Building, Room 1035, Rochester, MN 55905.

Metabolism: Clinical and Experimental, Grune and Stratton, The Curtis Center, Independence Square West, Philadelphia, PA 19106.

New England Journal of Medicine, 10 Shattuck Street, Boston, MA 02115.

Nutrition Action Healthletter, Center for Science in the Public Interest, 1501 16th Street NW, Washington, DC 20036.

Nutrition and Health, Institute of Human Nutrition, Columbia University, 701 West 168th Street, New York, NY 10031.

Nutrition and the M.D., P.O. Box 2468, Van Nuys, CA 91404.

Nutrition Clinics, George F. Stickley Co., 210 West Washington Square, Philadelphia, PA 19106.

Nutrition News, National Dairy Council, 6300 North River Road, Rosemont, IL 60018.

Nutrition Research, Pergamon Journals, Inc., Fairview Park, Elmsford, NY 10523.

Nutrition Reviews, 1126 16th Street NW, Suite 111, Washington, DC 20036.

Nutrition Today, Williams & Wilkins, 428 East Preston Street, Baltimore, MD 21202.

Nutrition Week, Community Nutrition Institute, 2001 S Street NW, Washington, DC 20009.

Nutritional Support Services, 12849 Magnolia Boulevard, North Hollywood, CA 91607.

Pediatrics, American Academy of Pediatrics, P.O. Box 927, Elk Grove Village, IL 60009.

Primary Care, W. B. Saunders Co., 210 West Washington Square, Philadelphia, PA 19105.

Professional Nutritionist, Foremost Foods Company, 2226 Clay Street, San Francisco, CA 94115.

Restaurants and Institutions, 5 South Wabash Avenue, Chicago, IL 60603.

Running and FitNews, American Running and Fitness Association, 9310 Old Georgetown Road, Bethesda, MD 20814.

School Food Service Journal, 4101 East Iliff, Denver, CO 80222.

Science, 1515 Massachusetts Avenue NW, Washington, DC 20005.

Sports Medicine Digest, 14545 Friar Street, Suite 106, Van Nuys, CA 91411.

Sports-Nutrition News, P.O. Box 986, Evanston, IL 60204.

The Physician and Sportsmedicine, McGraw-Hill Publications, 4530 West 77th Street, Minneapolis, MN 55435.

Tufts University Diet and Nutrition Letter, P.O. Box 10948, Des Moines, IA 50940.
University of California, Berkeley Wellness Letter, P.O. Box 359162, Palm Coast, FL 32035.
Vegetarian Times, P.O. Box 570, Oak Park, IL 60303.

C. FOR FURTHER INFORMATION

American Academy of Allergy and Immunology, 611 East Wells Street, Milwaukee, WI 53202.
American Academy of Pediatrics, P.O. Box 1034, Evanston, IL 60204.
American Alliance for Health, Physical Education, Recreation, and Dance, 1900 Association Drive, Reston, VA 22091.
American Anorexia Nervosa Association, 133 Cedar Lane, Teaneck, NJ 07666.
American Association of Retired Persons, 1225 Connecticut Avenue NW, Washington, DC 20036.
American Celiac Society, 45 Gifford Avenue, Jersey City, NJ 07304.
American College of Sports Medicine, P.O. Box 1440, Indianapolis, IN 46206.
American Dental Association, 211 East Chicago Avenue, Chicago, IL 60611.
American Diabetes Association, 1660 Duke Street, Alexandria, VA 22314.
American Dietetic Association, 216 West Jackson Boulevard, Chicago, IL 60606.
American Heart Association, 7320 Greenville Avenue, Dallas, TX 75231.
American Home Economics Association, 2010 Massachusetts Avenue NW, Washington, DC 20036.
American Institute of Nutrition, 9650 Rockville Pike, Bethesda, MD 20014.
American Medical Association, 535 North Dearborn Street, Chicago, IL 60610.
American Public Health Association, 1015 15th Street NW, Washington, DC 20005.
American Red Cross, 430 17th Street NW, Washington, DC 20006.
American Society for Clinical Nutrition, Inc., 9650 Rockville Pike, Bethesda, MD 20014.
American Society for Parenteral and Enteral Nutrition, 428 East Preston Street, Baltimore, MD 21202.
Anorexia Nervosa and Association Disorders, P.O. Box 271, Highland Park, IL 60035.
Canadian Diabetes Association, 1491 Yonge Street, Toronto, Ontario, Canada M5G 1EZ.
Chicago Nutrition Association, 8158 South Kedzie Avenue, Chicago, IL 60652.
Community Nutrition Institute, 2001 S Street NW, Washington, DC 20009.
Consumer and Food Economics Research Division, Federal Center Building, Hyattsville, MD 20782.
Consumer Information Center, The Consumer Information Catalog, Health Services Administration, Rockville, MD 20857.
Diabetes Center, Inc., P.O. Box 739, Wayzata, MN 55391.
Food and Agriculture Organization (FAO), Via delle Terme di Caracalla, 0100 Rome, Italy.
Food and Agriculture Organization of the United Nations (FAO), North American Regional Office, 1325 C Street SW, Washington, DC 20025.
Food and Drug Administration (FDA), 5600 Fishers Lane, Rockville, MD 20852.
Food and Nutrition Information Education Resources Center (FNIERC), National Agricultural Library, 10301 Baltimore Boulevard, Room 304, Beltsville, MD 20705.
Gluten Intolerance Group, P.O. Box 23053, Seattle, WA 98102.
Human Nutrition Research Division, Agricultural Research Center, Beltsville, MD 20705.
Institute of Food Technologists, 221 North La Salle Street, Chicago, IL 60601.
La Leche League International, Inc., P.O. Box 1209, Franklin Park, IL 60131.
Los Angeles District California Dietetic Association, P.O. Box 3506, Santa Monica, CA 90403.
March of Dimes Foundation, 1274 Mamoroneck Avenue, White Plains, NY 10605.
Meals for Millions/Freedom from Hunger Foundation, 1800 Olympic Boulevard, P.O. Drawer 680, Santa Monica, CA 90406.
National Academy of Sciences/National Research Council, 2101 Constitution Avenue NW, Washington, DC 20418.
National Anorexic Aid Society, P.O. Box 29461, Columbus, OH 43229.
National Diabetes Information Clearinghouse, P.O. Box NDIC, Bethesda, MD 20892.
National Heart, Lung, and Blood Institute, National Institutes of Health, Bethesda, MD 20892.
National High Blood Pressure Education Program, National Heart, Lung, and Blood Institute, 120/80 National Institutes of Health, Bethesda, MD 20892.
National Institute of Allergy and Infectious Disease, National Institutes of Health, Bethesda, MD 20892.
National Restaurant Association, 5 South Wabash Avenue, Chicago, IL 60603.
Nutrition and Health Associates, P.O. Box 11102, Tallahassee, FL 32303.
Office of Child Development, Office of Education, Public Health Service, Washington, DC 20204.
President's Council on Physical Fitness and Sports, 450 5th Street NW, Suite 7103, Washington, DC 20001.
Society for Nutrition Education, 1700 Broadway, Suite 300, Oakland, CA 94612.

United Fresh Fruit and Vegetable Association, 1019 19th Street NW, Washington, DC 20036.
U.S. Government Printing Office, The Superintendent of Documents, Washington, DC 20402.
Worldwatch Institute, 1776 Massachusetts Avenue NW, Washington, DC 20036.

D.   IF YOU STILL NEED MORE

State health departments, local health agencies, accredited colleges, hospitals, medical and dental schools with nutritionists can be excellent sources of reliable information. Sports medicine centers with nutritionists and RDs in private practice can also serve as reliable nutrition information resources. For computer software reviews, send for:

Computer Software for Nutrition and Food Education, Pennsylvania State University, University Park, PA 16802.
Journal of Dietetic Software (annual review), P.O. Box 2565, Norman, OK 73070.

Answer Key

CHAPTER 1

Page 7

(1)b. (2)c. (3)a. (4)a. (5)b. (6)c. (7)d. (8)c. (9)d. (10)a. (11)d. (12)a.

Pages 15–16

Section A. (1)d. (2)i. (3)a. (4)g. (5)h. (6)j. (7)e. (8)b. (9)f. (10)l. (11)c. (12)k.

Pages 26–27

(1)d. (2)a. (3)d. (4)a. (5)d. (6)d. (7)c. (8)b. (9)a. (10)d. (11)b. (12)c. (13)d. (14)b. (15)c. The facts about sensible dieting and professional weight loss counseling are discussed in following chapters.

CHAPTER 2

Page 45

(1) A degree in nutrition is usually indicative of the higher level of nutrition knowledge (but see Chapter 6 for discussion of pseudonutritionists). (2) The more "often" checks, the better; it is important to discern where patients are obtaining their nutrition information or misinformation. (3)d. (4)b. (5)b; accuracy requires recording food intake immediately after eating. (6)c. (7)d.

CHAPTER 3

Pages 68–70

(1)c. (2)d. (3)d. (4)b. (5)c. (6)f. (7)c. (8)a. (9)b. (10)c. (11)a. (12)b. (13)d. (14)c. (15)b. (16)b. (17)b. (18)c. (19)A—e. D—a. E—k. K—h. Thiamin—b. Riboflavin—j. Niacin—g. Pyridoxine—f. Folic acid— i. B_{12}—d. C—c. (20) Calcium—j. Phosphorus—n. Sodium—a. Chloride—e. Potassium—b. Magnesium—i. Sulfur—m. Iron—k. Manganese—l. Copper—f. Iodine—h. Zinc—c. Cobalt—g. Chromium— d.

CHAPTER 4

Page 82

(1)F. (2)F. (3)F. (4)T. (5)F. (6)T. (7)F.

Page 85

(1)F. (2)F. (3)T. (4)T. (5)T. (6)F. (7)T. (8)F.

Pages 101–104

(1)F. (2)T. (3)F. (4)T. (5)T. (6)T. (7)F. (8)F. (9)T. (10)F. (11)F. (12)T. (13)d. (14)b.

CHAPTER 5

Page 119

Section I.   (1)F. (2)T. (3)F. (4)T. (5)F. (6)F. (7)F. (8)T. (9)T. (10)F. (11)T. (12)f. (13)g. (14)d. (15)i.
Section II.   (1)T. (2)T. (3)T. (4)F. (5)F. (6)T. (7)e. (8)e. (9)d. (10)f.

CHAPTER 6

Page 132

(1)F. (2)T. (3)F. (4)F. (5)F. (6)T. (7)F. (8)T. (9)e. (10)d.

CHAPTER 7

Page 153

Section I.   (1)F. (2)F. (3)F. (4)F. (5)T. (6)F. (7)F. (8)F. (9)F. (10)T.
Section II.   (1)T. (2)T. (3)F. (4)T. (5)F. (6)T. (7)F. (8)T. (9)F. (10)F. (11)T. (12)F. (13)e. (14)c. (15)e.

CHAPTER 8

Page 188

Section I.   (1)F. (2)F. (3)F. (4)F. (5)T. (6)F. (7)F. (8)F. (9)F. (10)F. (11)F. (12)F. (13)T.
Section II.   (1)T. (2)T. (3)F. (4)F. (5)F. (6)F. (7)F. (8)F. (9)T. (10)F. (11)T. (12)F. (13)F. (14)T. (15)F. (16)T. (17)F. (18)T. (19)F. (20)F. (21)f. (22)b. (23)d. (24)a.

CHAPTER 9

Pages 212–213

Section I.   (1)T. (2)F. (3)T. (4)F. (5)T. (6)F. (7)F. (8)F. (9)F. (10)F. (11)F. (12)T.
Section II.   (1)T. (2)F. (3)F. (4)T. (5)F. (6)F. (7)T. (8)F. (9)T. (10)F. (11)F. (12)T. (13)a. (14)e. (15)e. (16)b.

CHAPTER 10

Pages 249–250

Section I.   (1)F. (2)F. (3)F. (4)F. (5)F. (6)F. (7)T. (8)F. (9)T. (10)F. (11)F. (12)F. (13)F. (14)F. (15)F. (16)F. (17)F. (18)T. (19)T. (20)F.
Section II.   (1)F. (2)F. (3)T. (4)F. (5)T. (6)T. (7)F. (8)T. (9)F. (10)F. (11)F. (12)F. (13)T. (14)T. (15)d. (16)e.

CHAPTER 11

Pages 281–282

Section I.   (1)T. (2)T. (3)F. (4)F. (5)F. (6)T. (7)T. (8)F. (9)F. (10)T. (11)T. (12)T. (13)F. (14)T. (15)F. (16)T. (17)T. (18)g. (19)f.

Section II.   (1)F. (2)T. (3)F. (4)T. (5)F. (6)F. (7)F. (8)T. (9)F. (10)F. (11)F. (12)T. (13)F. (14)F. (15)T. (16)T. (17)T. (18)F. (19)F. (20)F. (21)c. (22)f. (23)e. (24)g. (25)c. (26)e.

CHAPTER 12

Pages 306–307

Section I.   (1)T. (2)T. (3)F. (4)T. (5)F. (6)T. (7)T. (8)T. (9)F. (10)f. (11)e. (12)e.

Section II.   (1)T. (2)T. (3)F. (4)F. (5)T. (6)T. (7)T. (8)F. (9)T. (10)T. (11)F. (12)F. (13)T. (14)T. (15)T. (16)T. (17)T. (18)F.

Section III.   (1)T. (2)T. (3)T. (4)F. (5)T. (6)T. (7)T. (8)F. (9)F. (10)F. (11)F. (12)T. (13)F. (14)F. (15)F. (16)T. (17)f. (18)g.

CHAPTER 13

Pages 333–334

Section I.   (1)F. (2)F. (3)F. (4)T. (5)T. (6)T. (7)e. (8)d.

Section II.   (1)T. (2)T. (3)F. (4)T. (5)F. (6)T. (7)T. (8)T. (9)T. (10)T.

Section III.   (1)T. (2)F. (3)F. (4)F. (5)F. (6)T. (7)T. (8)F. (9)T. (10)F. (11)F. (12)F. (13)f. (14)g. (15)f.

CHAPTER 14

Pages 367–369

(1)F. (2)T. (3)T. (4)T. (5)F. (6)T. (7)F. (8)F. (9)T. (10)F. (11)F. (12)F. (13)F. (14)F. (15)F. (16)T. (17)T. (18)T. (19)T. (20)F. (21)T. (22)T. (23)T. (24)T. (25)T. (26)g. (27)g. (28)g. (29)f. (30)f.

CHAPTER 15

Pages 412–413

(1)T. (2)T. (3)T. (4)F. (5)F. (6)F. (7)F. (8)T. (9)F. (10)F. (11)T. (12)F. (13)T. (14)F. (15)T. (16)F. (17)T. (18)T. (19)F. (20)F. (21)F. (22)F. (23)F. (24)g. (25)e. (26)h. (27)f. (28)e. (29)e. (30)d.

Index of Terms

This Index includes only those terms defined in the margins throughout the text. Topical listings can be found in the Table of Contents.

Psychosis, 98
Public hospital, 17
Pulmonary, 313
Purines, 197
Purpura, 344
Pyuria, 344

Q

Quackery, 71

R

Reanastamosis, 224
Reasonable weight, 37
Reflexology, 125
Registered Dietitian (R.D.), 5
Renal, 343
Renal threshold, 268
Retina, 256
Retinopathy, 344
Rheumatic heart disease, 286
RNA (riboneucleic acid), 76
Role play, 10
Rotation diet, 143
Rumination, 390

S

Salmonella, 77
Saturated fat, 63
Scapula, 221
Scoliosis, 391
Senility, 197
Septic, 343
Seventh Day Adventist, 39
Spastic colon, 32
Specialty hospital, 17
Stabilizers, 92
Steatorrhea, 224
Steatosis, 338
Sterol, 290
Stomatitis, 386
Stool, 31
Supplemental feeding, 9
Sweeteners, 92
Systemic lupus erythematosus, 343

T

Tachycardia, 263
Taco, 110
Tahini, 107
Tetracycline, 374
Texturizers, 92
Thickeners, 92
Thyroid, 32
Thyroxine, 139
Tibia, 241
Tofu, 57
Tortilla, 110
Toxemia (eclamptogenic), 139
Toxicology, 89
TPN (total parenteral nutrition), 23
Triglycerides, 32
Tryptophan, 194
Tube feeding, 9
Tuberculosis, 85
TVP (textured vegetable-protein), 107
24-hour recall, 11

U

Ulcer, 32
Ulcerative colitis (spastic colon), 32
Unsaturated fat, 63
Urea, 337
Uremia, 344

V

Vegetarian, 39
Villi, 196
Viscosity, 315
"Vitamins"
  B_{15}, 123
  B_{17}, 123
Voluntary health agency, 24

W

Wernicke-Korsakoff syndrome, 339
WIC (Women, Infants, Children), 24
Wilson's disease, 343

Z

Zen macrobiotics, 107